Biological Effects and Dosimetry of Nonionizing Radiation

Radiofrequency and Microwave Energies

NATO ADVANCED STUDY INSTITUTES SERIES

A series of edited volumes comprising multifaceted studies of contemporary scientific issues by some of the best scientific minds in the world, assembled in cooperation with NATO Scientific Affairs Division.

Series A: Life Sciences

Recent Volumes in this Series

Volume 43—Advanced Topics in Radiosensitizers of Hypoxic Cells
edited by A. Breccia, C. Rimondi, and G. E. Adams

Volume 44—Cell Regulation by Intracellular Signals
edited by Stéphane Swillens and Jacques E. Dumond

Volume 45—Structural Molecular Biology:
edited by David B. Davies, Wolfram Saenger, and Steven S. Danyluk

Volume 46—Post-Harvest Physiology and Crop Preservation
edited by Morris Lieberman

Volume 47—Targeting of Drugs
edited by Gregory Gregoriadis, Judith Senior, and André Trouet

Volume 48—Neurotransmitter Interaction and Compartmentation
edited by H. F. Bradford

Volume 49—Biological Effects and Dosimetry of Nonionizing Radiation
edited by Martino Grandolfo, Sol M. Michaelson, and Alessandro Rindi

Volume 50—Somatic Cell Genetics
edited by C. Thomas Caskey and D. Christopher Robbins

Volume 51—Factors in Formation and Regression of the Atherosclerotic Plaque
edited by Gustav R. V. Born, Alberico L. Catapano, and Rodolfo Paoletti

Volume 52—Chemical Carcinogenesis
edited by Claudio Nicolini

This series is published by an international board of publishers in conjunction with NATO Scientific Affairs Division

A Life Sciences B Physics	Plenum Publishing Corporation London and New York
C Mathematical and Physical Sciences	D. Reidel Publishing Company Dordrecht, The Netherlands and Hingham, Massachusetts, USA
D Behavioral and Social Sciences E Applied Sciences	Martinus Nijhoff Publishers The Hague, The Netherlands

Biological Effects and Dosimetry of Nonionizing Radiation

Radiofrequency and Microwave Energies

Edited by

Martino Grandolfo

Superior Institute of Health
Rome, Italy

Sol M. Michaelson

University of Rochester Medical Center
Rochester, New York

and

Alessandro Rindi

National Institute of Nuclear Physics
Frascati, Italy

PLENUM PRESS • NEW YORK AND LONDON

Published in cooperation with NATO Scientific Affairs Division

Library of Congress Cataloging in Publication Data

NATO Advanced Study Institute on Advances in Biological Effects and Dosimetry of Low Energy Electromagnetic Fields (1981: Erice, Italy)
Biological effects and dosimetry of nonionizing radiation.

(NATO advanced study institutes series. Series A, Life sciences; v. 49)
"Proceedings of a NATO Advanced Study Institute on Advances in Biological Effects and Dosimetry of Low Energy Electromagnetic Fields which was also the fourth course of the International School of Radiation Damage and Protection of the Ettore Majorana Center for Scientific Culture, held March 28–April 8, 1981, in Erice, Italy"—T.p. verso.
Includes bibliographical references and index.
1. Microwaves—Physiological effect—Congresses. 2. Radio waves—Physiological effect—Congresses. I. Grandolfo, Martino. II. Michaelson, Sol M. III. Rindi, Alessandro. IV. North Atlantic Treaty Organization. Division of Scientific Affairs. V. International School of Radiation Damage and Protection (4th: 1981: Erice, Italy). VI. Title. VII. Series. [DNLM: 1. Radiation, Non-ionizing—Congresses. 2. Radiation dosage—Congresses. QT 162.U4 N279b 1981]
QP82.2.M5N37 1981 574.19′151 82-7598
ISBN 0-306-41017-6 AACR2

Proceedings of a NATO Advanced Study Institute on Advances in Biological Effects and Dosimetry of Low Energy Electromagnetic Fields which was also the Fourth Course of the International School of Radiation Damage and Protection of the Ettore Majorana Center for Scientific Culture, held March 28–April 8, 1981, in Erice, Italy.

Printed in the United States of America

PREFACE

During the last 35 years, there has been considerable development and increase in the number of devices that emit nonionizing radiant energies. These energies such as radiofrequency including microwaves are used in all sectors of our society for military, industrial, telecommunications, medical, and consumer applications. This increase in sources of nonionizing radiant energies has resulted in growing interest on the part of government regulatory agencies, industrial and military physicians, research workers, clinicians, and environmentalists. Although there is information on biologic effects and potential hazards to man from exposure to microwave/radiofrequency energies, considerable confusion and misinformation has permeated not only the public press but also some scientific and technical publications.

Because of the complexity of the interactions of nonionizing radiation in biological systems, an inter-disciplinary approach is necessary to assess and elucidate the problems that evolve as this field advances and as the use of these energies expands. It is important to maintain a proper perspective and assess realistically the biomedical effects of these radiant energies so that the worker or general public will not be unduly exposed nor will research, development and beneficial utilization of these energies be hampered or restricted by an undue concern for effects which may be nonexistent or minimal in comparison to other environmental hazards.

To address these problems, the International School of Radiation Damage and Protection of the"ETTORE MAJORANA" Centre for Scientific Culture in Erice, Italy has planned four courses on Nonionizing Radiation Protection to cover the most important of these energies. The first course which this book represents was devoted to consideration of microwave/radiofrequency energies.

This book is addressed to persons working in universities, research institutes, government and industrial laboratories. After a detailed review of the fundamentals of the physics and biology connected with the interaction of low-energy electromagnetic radiation with living matter, the lectures provide an updating of the techniques developed for the dosimetry of these energies and a critical analysis of the biological effects of radiofrequency and microwave radiation in relation to the establishment of safety standards.

Martino Grandolfo
Sol M. Michaelson
Alessandro Rindi

ACKNOWLEDGEMENTS

This Fourth Course of the International School of Radiation Damage and Protection of the "Ettore Majorana" Centre for Scientific Culture directed by Professor A. Zichichi has been held as a NATO Advanced Study Institute.

We are indebted to the Associazione Italiana Protezione Radioazioni, the Italian Ministery of Public Education, the Italian Ministry of Scientific and Technological Research, the Istituto Superiore di Sanita, the RAI-Radiotelevisione Italiana, and the Sicilian Regional Government for sponsoring the Course.

We acknowledge with appreciation the cooperation and contributions of: Mrs. Franca Grisanti, Mr. Giacomo Monteleone and Basilia Scolaro Toscano of the Istituto Superiore di Sanita, Rome, Italy and Mrs. Nancy Scott and the staff of the University of Rochester Radiation Biology and Biophysics Word Processing Center.

One of us (M.G.) especially wishes to personally thank Dr. Simonetta Battisti and Dr. Paolo Vecchia for helpful and simulating discussions pertaining to our objectives.

Martino Grandolfo
Sol M. Michaelson
Alessandro Rindi

CONTENTS

HISTORY OF THE GENESIS AND DEVELOPMENT OF THE STUDY OF EFFECTS OF LOW ENERGY ELECTROMAGNETIC FIELDS

Herman P. Schwan

Department of Bioengineering *
University of Pennsylvania
Philadelphia, PA 19104
and
Institut für Biophysik der Universität des Saarlandes
(Boris Rajewsky-Institut)
Homburg/Saar, West-Germany

Any review of this topic should include consideration of the development of the field of nonionizing radiation biohazard research in the broader context of the development of the biophysical interdisciplinary sciences. Hence I shall structure my lecture in three parts:

1. The development of Biomedical Engineering and Biophysics.

2. History of the nonionizing radiation field before World War 2.

3. History after World War 2.

I shall furthermore distinguish between three different approaches:

The biophysical approach, largely concerned with molecular and cellular considerations.
The bioengineering approach, primarily concerned with more macroscopic considerations such as absorption phenomena and the distribution of absorbed energy in man and animals.
And finally,
Experimental work of a biological or medical nature.

---

* Permanent address

1. DEVELOPMENT OF BIOMEDICAL ENGINEERING AND BIOPHYSICS

Biomedical engineering, medical physics and Biophysics developed at about the same time. Beginnings date about 40 to 50 years back and took place in a number of different institutions and laboratories. At that time no real difference could be conceived between these fields. I myself became associated with these interdisciplinary activities in 1937. At that time I became a technician at the Institute for Physical Foundations in Medicine, established about 1922 in Frankfurt, Germany, and now the Max Planck Institute for Biophysics. Another laboratory was headed by Otto Glasser at the Cleveland Clinic and a biophysics laboratory existed at Cold Spring Harbor with Hugo Fricke and Howard Curtis. No doubt more such interdisciplinary laboratories were in existence. After the second world war an increasing number of such interdisciplinary laboratories emerged. Departments of biomedical engineering and biophysics developed as formal training programs were established beginning in 1961. This was largely due to a far reaching decision by NIH to support these developments and the formation of biophysical and biomedical engineering societies in the USA and abroad.

During these early developments engineers and physicists joined with medical doctors, attracted by the possibility to apply the analytical power of the physical sciences and its instrumental capabilities to problems in medicine and biology. There are several distinct features of all these early and most present efforts in biophysics and bioengineering.

1. We note that no particular laboratory was primarily basic or applied in orientation. As a matter of fact both basic and applied work developed hand in hand.
2. The more basic oriented work was in many cases conceived as necessary to solve some practical problems. We may term it purpose oriented basic research.

Earlier efforts concentrated on the effects of ionizing radiation. Other topics included certain other therapeutic and diagnostic approaches and more basically oriented work of a biophysical nature. In particular the work concerned with electrical and acoustic properties of cells and tissues and biopolymers deserves special mentioning at this occasion. After the second world war various organizational patterns emerged. The Annual Conferences of Engineering in Medicine and Biology in the USA took place since 1947. They were originally primarily concerned with ionizing radiation and failed to attract large numbers of engineers in attendance as they turned to more biomedically engineering oriented topics since 1958. The Biophysical Society in the USA formed at about the same time and decided to concentrate its interests on purely basic problems, related to molecular biology and to membrane physiology. The ionizing radiation fields became the primary interest of the

Radiation Research Society in the USA and other national societies. The international Medical Physics Organization provided for effective international cooperation. The interest of these medical physics organizations in nonionizing radiations was small. Biological and medical ultrasound went its own way by forming the Medical Ultrasonic Institute and organizing meetings under the auspices of the Acoustical Society. The now thriving community of nonionizing radiation scientists recently formed the Bioelectromagnetic Society.

The various organizations interested in more basic aspects of biophysics cooperate rather well. So do apparently national and international organizations in medical physics. But the bioengineering community appears to be badly split, with at least six thriving societies operating independently in the USA alone; largely unaware of each other's activities. The International Federation of Medical and Biological Engineering was conceived to provide an international roof organization and to establish coordination and needed exchange of ideas and cross fertilization. But it has not been able so far to correct this situation. As a matter of fact its activities and announcements of meetings are not longer communicated to a large fraction of all biomedical engineers in the USA. But all biophysicists know about the meetings of the International Union of Pure and Applied Biophysics, the roof organization of all biophysical societies.

These developments therefore could not fail to affect the distribution of more basic and applied interests. The biophysical societies and the International Union of Pure and Applied Biophysics continue to concentrate on basic interests, primarily molecular biology and membrane biophysics. Certainly nonionizing radiation bioeffect are so far of no interest to them. The International Organization of Medical Physics and its national member organizations continue to represent a good mixture of applied and basic interests, primarily in the field of ionizing radiation and related technology. Finally in the large number of existing biomedical engineering societies interest in basic as well as applied work exists, with a much more diverse mixture of independent subdisciplines. The tremedous scope of these subdisciplines is readily appreciated by anyone who cares to examine the programs of many meetings which take place in the total field of biological and medical engineering every year.

Something else becomes apparent if one compares recent programs of Federation meetings and Annual Conferences on Medical and Biological Engineering with those from the early sixties. Earlier the spectrum of specialities included many areas with a rather strong basic orientation, while in more recent years these meetings have become more practically oriented. Many outstanding bioengineers therefore no longer attend these meetings and join meetings of other organizations where they now feel more at home. This has had far reaching consequences.

This development is regretable since interaction with other interdisciplinary societies active in the biophysical and bioengineering fields can only be fruitful. For example, the interaction of electrical fields with biomolecules and cells is of vital interest to all those who are concerned with the possibility of more subtle "nonthermal" effects of RF- and MW-fields. But little awareness exist in our ranks about the extended knowledge available. Closer interaction with physical chemists and biophysicists studying cellular and molecular responses would be most productive, I suspect. Only one meeting was recently held, which attempted to bridge the gap. It took place 1980 in Houston at the occasion of the annual meeting of the Chemical Society.

2. HISTORY BEFORE WORLD WAR II

Let me now summarize the earlier developments of the field of electromagnetic nonionizing radiation, including RF and microwaves. The bioengineering approach has been eminently productive. It continues through the total history of the field with major contributions in recent times to a point where it will be possible to achieve a refined understanding of tolerable thermal loads and to propose more detailed standards of safe exposure than in the 1960's.

Very early interest in the biological effects of high frequency fields dates back to the turn of the century and such names as Tesla and d'Arsonval. But it was at first in the late twenties and thirties that a rather substantial research effort was undertaken. One motivation for this effort was the invention of ultrashortwave diathermy by Shereshewsky in the USA and Schliephake and Esau abroad. Another motivation was the interest in the electrical properties of tissues for its own sake. For the first time the technology had arrived to generate hundreds of Watts of power with frequencies up to 100 MHz and more. The relevant technology was almost immediately applied with the intent to provide penetrating heat for therapeutic purposes. This effort and related research resulted in hundred of scientific papers emerging primarily from Germany, Austria, the United States and Russia.

The total Work may be conveniently divided into three parts:

a. Biophysical studies at the cellular and molecular level;
b. Bioengineering studies concerned with macroscopic aspects such as the spatial distribution of field strength and energy absorption;
c. Biomedical experimentation, primarily concerned with actual experimental work with animals, nerve preparation, etc.

a. Biophysical studies

Biophysical studies were primarily conducted in Germany and the United States. Dielectric properties of cell suspensions and eventually single cells were undertaken and theoretical insight was gained how alternating currents penetrate into cells and what mechanism account for the dielectric properties of cells. Beginning with the late thirties, dielectric properties of biopolymers, primarily proteins, were determined and interpreted in terms of appropriate physical models.

The Biophysical studies proved singularly successful. They assessed correctly many features of the electrical characteristics of cellular and molecular biological structures and permitted an understanding of the response of such microscopic and submicroscopic bio-systems to alternating electrical fields. The models proposed have never been successfully challenged to my knowledge and additional work after the second world war proved supportive of the concepts developed.

Interest in the electrical properties of cells and tissues began almost immediately with the introduction of techniques to measure such properties near the turn of the century. Already in 1910 Höber performed a decisive experiment. He measured the electrical resistivity with a simple but ingenious technique at very high frequencies, then only available in form of damped oscillation. Comparison of this value with the low frequency resistivity demonstrated a strong frequency dependance of the resistivity. Höber postulated that this dispersive behaviour could be best explained by the existence of a cell membrane which would be penetrated only by currents of a sufficiently high frequency. He was the first to postulate the existence of biological membranes on the basis of electrical measurements. His concepts were of course debated for some time. But they eventually prevailed. Höber's work could only increase the interest in such measurements. It appeared possible to deduce from such measurements some insight into the structure of biological media and to learn thereby more about the phenomena of excitability and other aspects of bioelectricity. With the invention of undampened waves during World War I techniques of measurement improved. A rather large number of measurements were taken by electrophysiologists and biophysicists. Perhaps the first ones to introduce the concept of equivalent electrical circuits and to suggest mechanism responsible for the frequency dependencies observed were Lullies and Gildemeister. But the range of frequencies covered was still too small, and electrode polarization, not yet recognized as a major trouble maker, made many reported results erroneous. The first major attempt to systematically measure the resistivity of tissues over a broad frequency spectrum was undertaken by Rajewsky and his collegues at the Institute for Physical Foundations of Medicine in Frankfurt. It extended from a few KHz to 100 MHz. Strongly dispersive behavior was noted and it became clear that the applicability of low frequency data to evaluate the merits of high frequency diathermy techniques was in question. Dänzer at the Frankfurt Institute measured the resistivity of blood and successfully applied quantitative field theory to explain this behavior. At another laboratory, headed by Pätzold at Siemens-Reiniger in Erlangen, good data of both resistivity and dielectric constant were obtained at 25, 50 and 100 MHz. These data and those of the Rajewsky group are still used and entirely adequate as recent measurements with modern instrumentation in our laboratory demonstrated.

At the same time a major effort developed in the USA. Fricke, Cole and Curtis introduced advanced instrumentation and theory and applied them to cellular suspensions with great success. Their work and the work of Dänzer resulted in an understanding of the dispersive behavior of these systems. The RF-dispersion was found to be a Maxwell-Wagner relaxation effect due to inhomogeneous structure caused by the existence of membranes separating the cell interior from the external phase. But the additional relaxation effects at ELF and MW had to await the development of further advances after World War II.

During this period between the two world wars interest in dielectric properties was by no means restricted to biological media. A large effort on dielectric properties was undertaken resulting in substantial advances in the understanding of such properties. Debye developed his concept of polar molecules and received the Nobel Prize for this singular achievement. During these years dielectric theory was perfected. In the late 30's the concept of polar molecules was applied to biological molecules. First Arrhenius and shortly thereafter Oncley studied protein properties. Particularly Oncley and his collegues measured properties with precision over most of the RF-range. They then applied the Debye theory, modifying itt by incorporating the rotational diffusion constants calculated before by the wellknown French physicist Perrin for ellipoids. The results explained the dispersive behavior of proteins. In summary then, two important theories of dielectric dispersive behavior had been successfully applied to biological materials by the beginning of the 1940's: The theory of inhomogeneous media, i.e. the Maxwell Wagner effect, accounted for cellular behavior in the RF-range and appropriately considered the existence of biological membranes. The Debye's theory of polar molecules, in modified form explained protein data at RF-frequencies.

Why do I dwell to some extent on these early developments? First of all, they provided the fundaments for developments in the biophysical field for advances after World War II. And second, they provided insight into the mode of interaction of electrical fields with biological matter. One might ask, what have properties to do with the interaction of fields? When one measures dielectric properties of cells, electric signals must be applied to the cells. The measured response characterizes the response of the cells to the electrical fields. The results obtained already clearly demonstrated for many cellular systems that the ability of high frequency or microwave fields to polarize cell membranes is many orders of magnitude weaker than the corresponding ability of low frequency fields. Clearly, cell membranes must have truly amazing abilities to compensate for this tremendeous disadvantage of high frequency fields if they can respond to such fields in a biologically significant manner. The results of Oncley permit us to make a similar statement about proteins: From the dipol moment obtained and applying the Langevin equation, it is apparent that very large field strength values of many KV/cm must be applied before a significant orientation effect of the protein to an applied field can be expected. Obviously, mechanism of interaction which determine measurable properties can be evaluated from such properties. This, of course, does not exclude the possibility that other interactions which do not reflect upon the parameters investigated may exist.

b. Bioengineering studies

Bioengineering studies might also be considered biophysical on a macroscopic level. The work before 1940 attempted to assess the penetration of ultrashortwave frequency electrical and magnetic fields into tissues and to develop improved technology in order to achieve the goal of penetrating heat. Theoretical understanding had to be based on a knowledge of the dielectric properties of tissues and hence, it is not surprising that such properties were determined up to 100 MHz by 1938.

This more macroscopically oriented bioengineering work before World War II led to improvements in the technology of diathermy treatments and the realization that increase in frequency should be beneficial to UHF therapeutic applications. This work was in good part conducted at the Max Planck Institute of Biophysics under Rajewsky and in the research laboratories of Siemens at Erlangen, headed by Paetzold. This work, as that of a more biophysical orientation, moved along systematically, building on past knowledge.

Particularly at the Siemens laboratory advances were made in the perfection of various techniques to provide deeper penetration and phantom techniques introduced to measure heat deposition patterns. With other words, experimental arrangements with appropriate layers of subcutenous fat and muscle tissues were utilized for the stated purpose. The concept of frequency specific treatments was introduced as follows: Different dielectric properties of various tissues were assumed and a layer arrangement such as skin on top of fat on top of muscle. Then it could be readily shown that for a constant high frequency current those tissues heat optimally whose parameters match the frequency properly. Hence, it was thought, one had to merely tune in the appropriate wavelength in order to achieve a tissue selective heating effect. The theory was correct in principle. However the eventual application of actual tissue data showed that the theory had in practice no utility except for one result: The higher the frequency, the better is the penetration to deeper tissues. This result substantially supported the drive for higher frequencies for diathermy purposes and thereby suggested the introduction of microwave frequencies for diathermy purposes.

c. Biomedical observations

This work includes results reporting the response of patients to partial body irradiations and a number of exposures of biological systems such as bacterial colonies, etc.

The medically oriented experimental work before the second world war led almost immediately to a split between two different schools of thought. One had it that whatever therapeutic or other effect was observed was caused by a noticeable temperature increase and that, therefore, the results observed were due to heat and not caused by electrical fields per se. The other school of thought believed that aside from obvious thermal effects direct field interactions termed specific nonthermal or athermal are important. This controversy, so similar to the one taking place today, led to many publications of variable quality. The debate was never settled and these papers are largely forgotten. But for those interested in this subject matter the books by Schliephake and by Liebesny should be rewarding while Rajewsky's monograph on the biophysics of ultrashortwaves provides broader insight and hundreds of relevant references.

However several models were discussed which might explain more subtle and direct field interactions. For example the concept of specific heat was debated for some time. It had been proposed that it is not the general volume heating which explains the beneficial therapeutic effects of shortwave treatment. Instead it was suggested that heat is generated selectively at specific sites of microscopic dimensions which might be responsible for biological effects. A number of papers were published by Dora Kulka, Liebesny, N.N. Malov and others in Austria, Germany and Russia. It took some time before it became evident that at cellular dimensions selective temperature elevations must be very small. Another phenomena which had been observed was that of cells in suspension forming chains under the influence of high frequency fields. Muth reported it first in 1937 and Krasny-Ergen attempted its theoretical treatment. It is of some interest to consider some relevant speculations by Krasny-Ergen. He considers the balance between Brownian movement and the forces which act on dispersed particles near a surface. He also states that this balance is affected by electrical fields, and cites experiments by Schliephake and Compère who measured surface tension and observed that it is affected by high frequency fields. Krasny-Ergen also suggested that cellular boundary potentials may well be altered. Agglutination should thereby also be affected and the formation of membrane systems. Wilkins, much later, observed in Heller's laboratory that the electrophoretic movement of charged colloidal particles appears changed by RF-fields. This report may well relate to these early suggestions of Krasny-Ergen. Krasny-Ergen also suggested that the viscosity of biological solutions may be affected by high frequency fields since micelles are formed. He furthermore demonstrated the existence of rotating fields near cell surfaces caused by alternating fields and implicitly suggested that such fields might be biologically significant. Only two of these ideas were followed up. That of specific heat and, after the second world war, that of pearl chain formation. All other suggestions, originally of a purely qualitative nature, were forgotten. A systematic persusal of the literature before the last world war might well reveal a large number of additional ideas worthy of checking out.

What remains from all these efforts before the second world war? Obviously a great deal had been done to understand the RF-properties of cell suspensions and tissues. Most of the collected data are still valid and quoted in the literature. Also a good start had been made on dielectric properties of proteins. The more macroscopically oriented bioengineering approach led to improved diathermy techniques and the realization that higher frequencies are more advantageous. The more medically and biologically oriented experimental work introduced the controversy of thermal vs nonthermal effects. Almost all of this work has been forgotten even though several interesting speculations about nonthermal mechanism were advanced.

3. DEVELOPMENT AFTER WORLD WAR II

Most of the activities summarized above came to an abrupt end with the beginning of World War 2. But almost immediately thereafter work resumed and benefitted from a number of technical advances made during the war. Reliable magnestrons had been invented and the frequency range extended from a few hundred MHz to many thousands. Waveguides had been introduced and techniques developed to measure dielectric properties well into the microwave range. Modern instrumentation permitted vastly increased accuracy. It was needed to separate significant but weak capacitive currents from the strong conductive ones prevelant at low frequencies in cell suspensions and tissues. Advanced amplifier techniques contributed materially to the fields of axonology and electrobiology.

After the second world war the scene shifted largely to the United States. Powerful and reliable magnetrons were now available operating at 2.450 MHz and an extensive medical effort began at the Mayo Clinic, undertaken by Krusen and his colleagues and at a number of other institutions. It was at the Mayo Clinic where microwave hazards first became the topic of an open scientific meeting. The Office of Naval Research had started a small but effective program almost immediately after the war which continues to this day. During the late fifties and early sixties the Tri-service meetings took place. Much excellent research was conducted during this time.

When the Tri-Service meetings came to an end a comparatively quiet period started which lasted to the late sixties and early seventies. However during this time the American National Standards Institute had formed a committee concerned with the development of guide numbers of microwave radiation safety. It adopted after lengthy deliberations a standard of 10 mW/cm^2 for exposures longer than 0.1 hr. This value had been set already much earlier by the Navy, following a meeting which it organized in 1953. The ANSI committee also set a standard for short time exposure which was based on physical considerations and then available results.

During this time reports were received to an increasing extent from Russia about experiments which indicated all sorts of subtle sensitivities. They motivated Russia and other eastern countries to adopt a standard 1000 times smaller than the one in use in the western world. These reports, several Congressional inquiries and increasing concern by various government agencies led to renewed interest in the field and to the comparatively large activity which ensued during the seventies.

a. Biophysical Studies

Dielectric measurements on blood and tissues up to nearly 1 GHz were conducted in the USA and Germany. A significant effort developed in England. A number of investigators including Cook, Buchanan and then Grant applied pertinent microwave dielectric measuring techniques to water, electrolytes, protein solutions, blood and some tissues with increasing accuracy. This extended effort continues to this day.

The cellular work, primarily done by Cole and by Fricke and Curtis before World War II was eventually extended to the non-linear level. It culminated in the extensive effort which was undertaken on the giant squid axon and the Hodgkin-Huxley equations. This work is recognized as one of the outstanding contributions of modern science.

After the second world war modern techniques enabled us to considerably extend the range of observation from a few Hz to GHz and to classify entirely different relaxation effects characteristic of the dielectric properties of cells and tissues. Three major dielectric relaxation effects were noted occurring at ELF, RF and GHz frequencies. Major efforts in these fields developed in my laboratory and then in the laboratories of Carstensen at Rochester, Grant in London and Hanai in Japan. Contributions included:

Investigation of a large number of systems including blood, bacteria, subcellular organelles and vesicle systems as well as artificial membranes. This included the development of a large number of closed form solutions which characterize the Maxwell-Wagner RF-dispersion range and are useful to extract cellular parameters.

Extension of the range of observation to the difficult range of low frequencies and discovery of entirely new relaxation effects. Identification of the mechanism responsible for these low frequency relaxation processes included the discovery that counter ion movement is frequently responsible for substantial induced dipol moments and associated relaxation effects.

Extension of the range of observation to microwave frequencies and observation of an additional relaxation effect in the GHz-range which could be used to state that tissue water and normal water appear to be identical from a dielectric point of view.

Observation of a relaxation effect of biopolymers in the UHF range which is in part due to protein bound water and, perhaps, partially due to rotation of polar subgroups.

The macromolecular work after World War II was an extension of the concepts which Peter Debye, Kirkwood and Lars Onsager had developed. These efforts provided refined insight based on elaboration of the principles developed before the war. They added to the Debye-Oncley model of polar biopolymers consideration of counter ion cloud relaxation effects and protein bound water in our laboratory and that of Grant. Some work established dielectric saturation of some biopolymers at about 50 KV/cm in agreement with the prediction of Langevin equation.

It has been sometimes stated that during the Tri-Service period no effort was undertaken which dealt with the possibility of nonthermal field effects and that it was taken for granted that only thermal effects prevailed. This is incorrect. Herrick and her colleagues had already confirmed earlier observation on pearl chain formation of erythrocytes during the early fifties. Much effort was undertaken in our laboratory to understand these field induced forces or "induction forces" as Krasny-Ergen had called them. For example, Heller's observation of the preferential movement of microorganism in alternating fields explained by the rotational effects of the field. The threshold field strength values needed to cause all sorts of effects induced by alternating fields acting on cells were estimated theoretically in agreement with the experiment. It was also found that the time constant needed to cause the effect changes inversely with the square of the field strength and that, therefore, pulsed fields can be no more effective than continuous fields of the same average power. This sort of work and related efforts to affect cells by applying alternating electrical fields has become in very recent times again of interest. For example, efforts are underway to break cells dielectrically and to fuse them using the pearl chain principle into larger vesicles. Other work concerns the question, how and if electrical fields cause conformational changes in membranes.

The implications of all these results to the nonionizing radiation fields are not yet entirely clear. The previously noted difficulty to apply with microwaves noticeable potentials across membranes was again confirmed. The unliklihood to cause by nonthermal intensities of microwaves noticeable orientation effects of biopolymers was also further confirmed. The question what fields are necessary to cause noticeable displacements of the counter ion atmosphere is so far unanswered. One of the present difficulties is that the theoretical formulation of the counter ion relaxation effect by Schwarz is apparently not applicable to biological cells. Another, that much more experimental material is needed to clearly separate the relative contributions of various relaxation effects to low frequency admittance problems.

The dielectric data collected sofar do not suggest any subtle mechanism for field interactions of ELF, RF and microwave fields with biological matter at nonthermal intensities. This of course, as previously noted, simply means that subtle direct field interactions do not reveal themselves in the substantial changes of biological structure needed to be detectable by dielectric spectroscopy. Nevertheless, whatever polarization mechanism has been considered sofar is too slow to be evoked by microwaves. And the responses noted sofar dielectrically are entirely linear at field strength levels of a few V/cm in situ. This suggests that the considered disturbances caused by the field are of small magnitude compared with those caused by thermal motion.

The dielectric spectroscopy data do not suggest any direct nonthermal field interaction mechanism. But the work with field induced forces ("induction" forces) is not necessarily so clear to evaluate. At first glance it appears from the few quantitative experimental data sofar available and from theoretical equations that these forces can be neglected at nonthermal levels of RF- or MW-fields, i.e. below about 1 V/cm in situ. However, the experimental material is still limited. In addition the theoretical approach has been only partially successful since it is based on the assumption that threshold field values may be defined by equating the potential energy due to field application and thermal energy. But the definition of potential energy for lossy media remains obscure to this day. We also note that for typical cell size sofar predicted threshold intensities for significant field effects are by no means much larger than the limit of thermal effects of about 1 V/cm. Clearly, more work in this area should be undertaken before definite statements are appropriate.

b. Bioengineering efforts

Bioengineering efforts continued after the second world war primarily in the USA, first at my laboratory at the University of Pennsylvania and somewhat later that of Lehmann and Guy at the University of Washington in Seattle. Then Johnson and his colleagues Durney and Gandhi at the University of Utah in Salt Lake City entered this field and eventually at many other places bioengineering efforts started. This consequent effort, carried through with ever increasing sophistication has yielded today a rather detailed insight into the patterns of heat deposition caused by microwave and RF exposure. This work is also yielding now actual temperature elevations and thereby provides, hopefully, in the near future a refined insight in thermally tolerable microwave exposure levels.

The work during the fifties and early sixties concentrated first on the determination of absorption coefficients and evaluation of reflectance phenomena at tissue interfaces, their effect on absorbed energy and spatial distributions of the specific absorption rate (SAR) in layered tissue arrangements of practical interest. This work was of particular interest for therapeutic purposes and led to suggestion that such therapy is best conducted at low microwave frequencies, i.e. at 915 MHz. As the interest in radiation health hazards increased early spherical models of man were introduced and relative absorption cross section (average SAR values) already calculated and experimentally determined about twenty years ago. These early data demonstrated a resonance effect at lower microwave frequencies for man. But it was not very pronounced with the spherical model and, hence, did not enter into the health standard discussions taking place shortly after.

The bioengineering effort during the 1970's profited very much from further advances in the computer field and numerical analytical techniques. Further, the development of phantom techniques and the application of infraredsensing devices permitted evaluation of complex heating patterns in complex body shapes. This effort provided rather detailed data of the average specific absorption rate (SAR) and its spatial distribution. Good agreement between theory, numerical calculation and experiment was achieved. The physical processes responsible for the observed results, including various resonance phenomena and energy exchange between various body compartments could be understood.

In addition work was undertaken to determine under what circumstances "hot spots" can be generated. Several studies have been published which translate patterns of SAR-values into actual temperature elevations. Some of these utilize highly advanced models of the thermoregulatory system of man. I shall assume that details of these productive approaches will be summarized by Dr.Guy and others at this meeting.

c. Biomedical Experiments

A large number of experimental data have been collected during the past two decades. No systematic effort has been undertaken to my knowledge to sort out these data. For example what data clearly establish thermal responses, what data appear to be of a nonthermal origin, what data are due to pulsed fields, what data can be explained by the RF-hearing phenomena? Several lectures at this meeting will deal with this body of results. I shall therefore not attempt to summarize this work except for some results which have been particularly interesting.

Studies were conducted at ELF, RF- and MW-fields indicating that the noted subthermal responses were sensitive to modulation characteristics and apparently to a lesser extent to the carrier frequency. This work, primarily conducted by Adey and his colleagues has been partially confirmed by others. The results appear to be exceedingly dependant on all sorts of experimental parameters not yet defined. On the other hand, Fröhlich suggested theoretically the existence of high frequency selective sensitivities at high MW-frequencies. Experimental data by Berteaud, Grundler and Keilman appear to confirm this prediction. But again experimental details are sofar not yet transparent and need to be modified. It is too early to evaluate the biological significance of these carrier or modulation frequency sensitive results. In both cases nonlinear mechanism are strongly indicated. These topics will be dealt with in several lectures at this meeting.

SUMMARY

What can be learned from all the distant and more recent history? First of all the interaction between the three fields indicated, namely medical research, bioengineering and biophysics has been regretably poor for most of the time. Most deplorable is the almost entire neglect of appreciation for the work of the biophysicists and the significance of their work. But also the interaction between the biomedical field and the bioengineering field has been poor even though it is now rapidly improving and appropriate microwave field exposure techniques are appreciated to an increasing extent by the biomedical experimenter. The main contribution of the bioengineering field, i.e. the study of the mode of propagation of microwaves into man and animals, yielded significant results in spite of the complexity of the problem. But it cannot go beyond the establishment of detailed dose rate maps and, hopefully, resultant temperature elevations. The understanding of other than thermal effects, if there are any, has to come from the biophysicists primarily.

The following conclusions summarize the historical development of the microwave hazard field:

1. The bioengineering area has been moving through its historical development step by step in a logical fashion. It has brought us to a threshold of reasonable founded thermal standards of safety provided that some more detailed work is done on thermoregulatory aspects. Local heat generation either due to partial irradiation or spatially selective body absorptions must be also considered.
2. The biophysical area is fairly well advanced. It is not presently suggestive of subtle mechanisms. Some call it therefore irrelevant or outdated. Good science is never outdated. The biophysical knowledge cannot be neglected because its present implications are unacceptable to some. At that, it

may well become some day extended to more complex situations than dealt with presently. Present and future biophysics are our only hope to achieve an understanding of nonthermal subtle effects, if there are any.

3. The biomedical experimental evidence is supportive of significant thermal effects appearing somewhere above 10 mW/cm^2 for man and probably in the range of 1 to 10 mW/cm^2 for smaller animals. It does not suggest so far any scientific principles which may aid us in formulating nonthermal standards of exposure. This situation has prevailed for more than four decades and is not likely to change soon.

ACKNOWLEDGEMENT

Support by the Alexander von Humboldt-Stiftung, Germany, and by the Office of Naval Research, USA, is gratefully acknowledged.

SOURCES AND APPLICATIONS OF RADIOFREQUENCY (RF) AND MICROWAVE ENERGY

Michael H. Repacholi

Radiation Protection Bureau
Health and Welfare Canada
Ottawa, Ontario K1A 0L2

INTRODUCTION

Advances in the development of sources of microwave and radiofrequency energy, especially in the production of solid state devices, together with the accompanying reduction in costs, have allowed the application of this technology to diversify and proliferate into industry, medicine, commerce, research, and the home. It is not uncommon to find microwave or RF systems in individual houses, in automobiles, in private aircraft and on boats.

The International Telecommunication Union[1] has mediated rational use of the electromagnetic spectrum by subdividing the part of the spectrum commonly used for telecommunications (radio spectrum) into nine frequency bands, seven of which are in the radiofrequency and microwave range (Table 1). The whole radio spectrum refers to radiofrequency radiation, but microwaves are normally defined as a subsection within this spectrum. Unfortunately, the frequency range for microwaves has not been rigidly defined by any universal convention. Recently, the World Health Organization[2] defined radiofrequency as 100 kHz - 300 MHz, and microwaves as 300 MHz to 300 GHz. For purposes of this presentation, sources and applications of electromagnetic energy in the frequency range 100 kHz to 300 GHz will be included. Specific allocations of frequencies or frequency bands are then given to particular applications, some of which are shown in Table 1.

SOURCES

<u>Natural Background</u>. Microwave and radiofrequency electro-

Table 1. Nomenclature of frequency band designations used in radiocommunications and some typical applications.

BAND NO.	DESIGN-ATION	FREQUENCY RANGE*	WAVELENGTH	METRIC SUBDIVISION	TYPICAL APPLICATIONS
5	LF	30 - 300 kHz	10 - 1 km	kilometric waves	power line carrier, marine and aeronautical mobile, radionavigation, radiolocation
6	MF	300 - 3000 kHz	1 - 0.1 km	hectometric waves	communications, radionavigation, marine, radiophone, amateur, industrial RF heating equipment, AM broadcast
7	HF	3 - 30 MHz	100 - 10 m	decametric waves	citizens band, amateur, medical diathermy, AM broadcast, international communications, industrial RF equipment
8	VHF	30 - 300 MHz	10 - 1 m	metric waves	police, fire, amateur, FM, VHF-TV industrial RF equipment, FM broadcast
9	UHF	300 - 3000 MHz	1 - 0.1 m	decimetric waves	short range broadcast, communications, amateur radio, taxi, police, fire, radar, citizens band, radionavigation, UHF-TV, microwave ovens, medical diathermy, industrial heating.
10	SHF	3 - 30 GHz	10 - 1 cm	centimetric waves	satellite communications, radar, amateur radio, microwave relay, airborne weather radar
11	EHF	30 - 300 GHz	10 - 1 mm	millimetric waves	terrain avoidance, radar, microwave relay

NOTE 1. Band number "N" extends from 0.3×10^N to 3×10^N Hz.

NOTE 2. Hz = hertz, k = kilo (10^3), M = mega (10^6), G = giga (10^9).

* lower limit exclusive, upper limit inclusive

magnetic radiations occur naturally in the environment from the sun and galaxies, and from earth. The earth's electromagnetic biosphere is determined predominantly by its electric and magnetic fields and atmospheric discharges (lightning). Radiofrequency emission from the sun is composed of a quiet permanent part coming from the entire surface (measured from a quiet sun) and a superimposed variable part emitted from centres of activity (measured during sunspot activity) as shown[3] in Figure 1. The quiet sun component corresponds to emissions during minimum sunspot activity, whereas the slowly varying component corresponds to emissions during maximum sunspot activity. The spectra of bursts (lasting a few seconds to a few minutes) and storms (lasting for hours) correspond to their maximum values and are plotted in terms of flux density per unit bandwidth.

Extraterrestrial. Background microwave and radiofrequency radiation from the sun and other extraterrestrial sources has been estimated by Osepchuk.[4] Using the data of Kundu,[3] the solar spectral noise emission is found to have an integrated flux for frequencies below 30 GHz of approximately:

2×10^{-7} μW/cm^2 for quiet sun

10^{-5} μW/cm^2 for bursts (lasting for minutes).

For frequencies up to 300 GHz, one can approximate the microwave flux by adding the value derived from Allen,[3] who reports a flux of 8×10^{-6} μW/cm^2 for microwaves below 100 GHz, to that of Sinton[5,6] who reports a microwave flux of 6×10^{-6} μW/cm^2 between

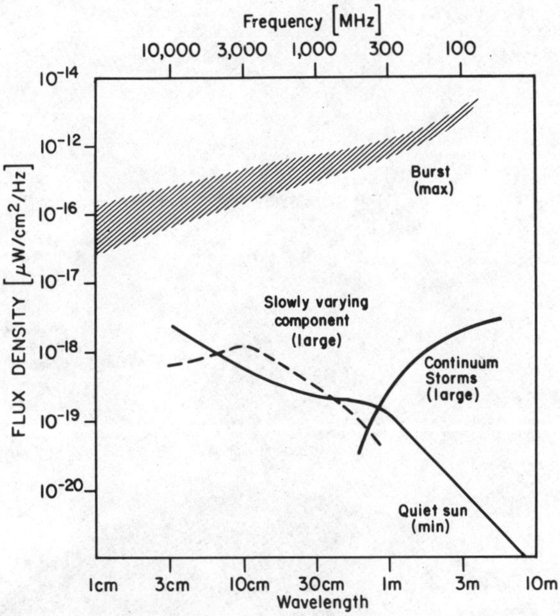

Figure 1. The spectra of various components of radiofrequency and microwave emissions from the sun.[3]

100 - 300 GHz. An integrated flux of 1.4×10^{-5} μW/cm^2 for a quiet sun is obtained. Bursts and high sunspot activity could increase this value to about 10^{-3} μW/cm^2.

Earth. All media with an absolute temperature greater than 0°K emit electromagnetic radiation. This thermal emission is a result of the accelerations experienced by individual charges in the course of their thermal motion. The thermal emission from the earth or any hot body can be determined using the black body equation. The emitted flux S is approximately

$$\frac{dS}{dt} = \frac{10^{-36}}{9} f^2 T \quad \mu W/cm^2/Hz$$

or

$$S = 0.3\left(\frac{f}{300}\right)^3 T/300 \ \mu W/cm^2$$

where f is the frequency in GHz and the body temperature T is in $^\circ$K. In this equation an emissivity of 1 is assumed, which is a reasonable approximation (normally within 10%). Using this equation the thermal noise from the earth (surface temperature at approximately 20°C) has been calculated[4] to be 0.3 μW/cm^2 when integrated up to 300 GHz or 0.0003 μW/cm^2 when integrated up to 30 GHz.

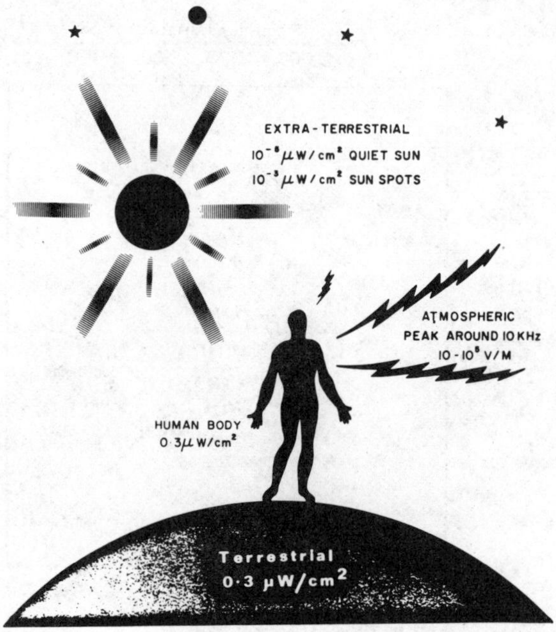

Figure 2. Natural sources of microwave and radiofrequency radiation integrated flux for frequencies up to 300 GHz.

Further details of the distribution of intensities of natural sources of radio emission are provided by Minin.[7] Increased electric field intensities occur during thunderstorms. The intensity of thunderstorm activity is always a minimum in the morning hours and increases toward night. During winter, maximum activity occurs in the middle of the night, and during summer in the mid afternoon. Electromagnetic fields with a wide frequency range (atmospheric noise) are created during thunderstorms. Their maximum intensity occurs at about 10 kHz and decreases at higher frequencies. Electric field strengths during local storms can vary[8] up to about 10^5 V/m.

Human Emission. The human body emits thermal energy in the frequency range 10 kHz to 300 GHz. The same black body equation as given above can be applied to human emission. Here radiant emittance integrated up to 300 GHz is calculated[4] to be approximately 0.3 μW/cm^2.

A summary of the various natural sources of microwaves and radiofrequency radiation is given in Figure 2.

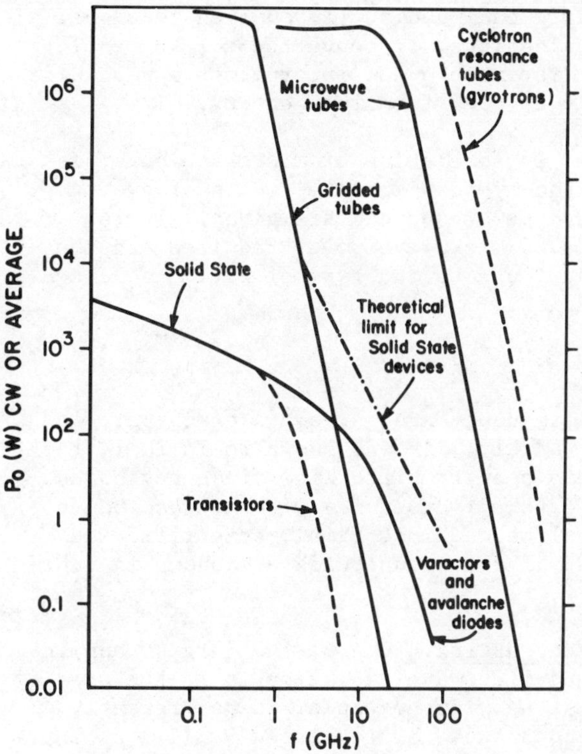

Figure 3.
Typical maximum limits of average power from various microwave power sources (adapted from[8]).

Man-Made Sources. There are four basic types of man-made devices for generating radiofrequency and microwave energy: power-grid tubes; linear beam tubes such as klystrons; cross-field devices such as magnetrons and amplitrons; and solid state devices.

Linear-beam tubes and crossed-field devices are used in most industrial microwave applications. Some industrial and consumer microwave applications use tubes with power outputs up to 100 kW. Solid-state microwave devices have been developed in the past 15-20 years and include transistors for applications below 1 GHz and avalanche diodes for applications above 1 GHz.

Once microwave energy is generated, it can be transmitted to an applicator or antenna through a waveguide or coaxial transmission line. Waveguides can be rectangular or circular in shape, and are normally constructed of a conducting metal, such as aluminum, brass or copper, or a non-conducting substance with a thin conducting coat on its inner surface. The waveguide is normally at ground potential and allows the transmission of high power microwaves over distances of up to about 100 meters.

Radiating antennas such as parabolic reflectors are used to transit microwave energy through free space or through a dielectric material. Transmitted energy can be directly applied to a specialized devise, used in communications, or converted to another form of energy, such as heat. Microwave ovens incorporate a waveguide to deliver microwave energy to cook food in a cavity.

The "state of the art" in generation of microwave power is shown[8] in Figure 3. Here the typical maximum limits of average power from various microwave power sources are given. It is apparent that the magnitude of microwave power required and the frequency of operation contribute to the type of device selected for any particular application.

APPLICATIONS

Applications of radiofrequency and microwave energy are now widespread and increasing rapidly. As was shown in Table 1, the ITU had subdivided the radio spectrum into nine frequency bands for telecommunications. Certain frequencies within these bands have been designated for unlicenced industrial, scientific and medical (ISM) applications. These frequencies are shown in Table 2.

Communications and Broadcasting. One of the largest applications of radiofrequency and microwave radiation is in the area of communications and broadcasting. For example, it was recently reported[9] that in the United States there existed 9 million broadcasting transmitters, hundreds of thousands of microwave communi-

Table 2. Frequencies designated for unlicenced use world-wide in industrial, scientific and medical applications (World Administrative Radio Conference, Geneva, 1979).

ISM Band Frequencies
*6.78 MHz ± 1.5 kHz
13.56 MHz ± 6.78 kHz
27.12 MHz ± 160 kHz
40.68 MHz ± 20 kHz
*†433.92 MHz ± 0.87 MHz
915 MHz ± 13 MHz
2.45 GHz ± 50 MHz
5.80 GHz ± 75 MHz
24.125 GHz ± 125 MHz
*61.0 GHz ± 250 MHz
*122.5 GHz ± 0.5 GHz
*245 GHz ± 1 GHz

* Special authorization required for use.

† Authorized for use in certain countries only.

Table 3. Frequencies assigned for commercial radio and television transmission with typical characteristic parameters[10]

Frequency Band (MHz)	Application	Tower Height (m)	Maximum ERP (kW)	Field Intensity (mV/m)	Power Density ($\mu W/cm^2$)
0.535-1.605	AM Radio				
54-88	VHF TV ch.2-6	305	100	807	1.73
88-108	FM Radio	152	100	1023	2.78
174-216	VHF TV ch.7-13	305	316	191	0.1
470-890	UHF TV	305	5000	380	0.38

cations towers, tens of thousands of radar antennas and almost 30 million citizen band (CB) radios.

Broadcasting and communications has been regulated to operate within assigned frequency bands. For commercial radio and television transmission, these have been assigned as shown in Table 3. For broadcasting, actual powers of tens of kilowatts and effective radiated powers (ERP) up to megawatts are radiated and directed toward homes in a radius of up to 50 miles from the antenna. The actual maximum allowable ERP, and the electric field intensity (with equivalent plane wave power density) at ground level one mile from broadcast transmitters are also shown in Table 3.[10] Broadcast - antenna installations are normally located on high towers, and comprise radiating antennas for VHF and UHF TV stations, as well as some for FM radio stations. Efficient broadcasting is achieved by directing omnidirection radiation towards the horizon from antennas hundreds of meters above the ground. The power densities measured in the vicinity of transmitting towers and in areas accessible to the general public are small,[11] below 0.1 $\mu W/cm^2$.

Exposure of the United States population to the "general radiofrequency environment" is dominated by radio and television broadcast transmission. From measurements made in 15 major United States cities, the median population exposure to radiations in the frequency range 54 - 900 MHz was found[11,12] to be 0.005 $\mu W/cm^2$. Although these estimates do not include the contribution from AM broadcast, it is known that if this contribution was added, the 0.005 $\mu W/cm^2$ value would not increase by more than a factor of two. From the same survey it was estimated that 99% of the United States population is exposed to less than 1 $\mu W/cm^2$ (54 - 900 MHz). Sources operating at frequencies outside the broadcast bands do not contribute significantly to general population exposure.[13]

Power density levels measured[14] inside buildings close to

broadcast antennas varied from less than 1 μW/cm^2 to 97 μW/cm^2. At an unshielded location on the roof of one building, a value of 230 μW/cm^2 was recorded.

Broadcast transmitters may constitute a radiation hazard for the maintenance crews servicing the towers while the transmitters are operating. In this case the exposure conditions cannot be evaluated theoretically, but some measurements were performed[15] for a single FM station located on Mt. Wilson, California. The station operates at an ERP of 105 kW from a tower 36 m high and the antenna located 24 m above the ground. A power density of 180 mW/cm^2 was measured in several locations on the tower structure. Similar exposure levels may occur on towers close to the antennas for many FM stations. TV towers may also have high intensity fields close to the antennas.

Microwave Relay Towers. Microwave relay towers[12] are located across the country-side and employ antennas radiating highly directional beams of up to 12 watts each at frequencies of 4 or 6 GHz. Radiation levels on the ground emitted from towers[8] some 15-25 m high are less than 1 μW/cm^2.

Mobile Communications Devices. Personal communication devices, such as citizen band (CB) radios mounted on cars, or hand-held such as walkie-talkies have become very popular over the past few years. Portable and mobile transmitters[16] can operate at frequencies in the VHF band from 30 - 54 MHz and 132 - 174 MHz and in the UHF band 403 - 512 MHz with a maximum permitted power of 100 W. The electric field intensity from the antenna of these transmitters mounted on a vehicle depends on the type of antenna (usually a base loaded whip), the distance from the antenna and the location of the antenna on the vehicle, transmitter operating frequency and power, shape of the vehicle, and geometry of nearby objects.[17] With a large number of variables influencing the electric field, it is not possible to estimate theoretically the field intensity at a given location.

Janes[12] has compiled the available data on electric field strengths in and around radio-equipped vehicles. Substantial fields (up to 1350 V/m) occur near the antenna, but that these fields fall off rapidly as the distance from the antenna increases. It is difficult to interpret these data in terms of human exposure because most measurements are conducted in the near-field where the fields are quite complex, so that the absorption in the human body may be quite different[18,19]. Operation of these devices is intermittent which also complicates this assessment of partial, non-uniform human exposure.

Even less data has been compiled on the electric fields surrounding walkie-talkie devices. These devices can operate at certain frequencies in the range 30 - 512 MHz and have an output power typically up to about 6 W. Electric field intensities[16] at the eye of operators can be from 134 to 212 V/m. Lambdin[20] also found electric fields up to 212 V/m at 7.5 cm from the antenna of a 164 MHz device operating at 1.8 W. This field reduced to about 20 V/m at just over 10 cm from the antenna. At 12 cm from the antenna of a 2.5 W hand-held device, a maximum electric field of 205 V/m and maximum magnetic field of 0.9 A/m were recorded.[21] As with CB radios, it is difficult to determine the patterns of radiation absorption in tissue since exposure occurs in the near field and a number of variables complicate the assessment.

Telemetry transmitters operating in the frequency range 10 - 1000 MHz are used to give continuous, omnidirectional data transmission from small body mounted antennas. These can be used by athletes and patients to allow continuous recording of parameters such as pulse rate. Following a study[22] of these body mounted devices, it was suggested that for safety reasons the transmitter power should not exceed 100 mW, and for practical reasons should operate in the frequency range 75 - 160 MHz. It appears that the 100 mW value is rather conservative.

Satellite Communications. Satellite communications earth terminals are continuous wave sources that operate[23] at frequencies around 2 - 8 GHz and effective radiated powers in excess of 1 MW. The antennas are circular cross-section paraboloids. Hankin et al[23] have compiled the anticipated characteristics of some satellite communication systems, and these are shown in Table 4. In this table, f is the transmitting frequency, P is the power delivered to the antenna (transmitter power), D is the antenna diameter, R is the distance of the near field (= $D^2/5.66\lambda$) from the antenna, λ is the wavelength of the radiation, W_{MAX} is the maximum near-field power density along the beam axis (= $16\eta P/\pi D^2$) and η is the aperture efficiency (normally 0.5 to 0.75). The table also indicates the distance from the antenna that one would expect power density levels of 10 and 1 mW/cm^2.

Satellite communications systems may produce high power densities, but because they are normally located in sparsely populated areas, and the beams are well collimated - the off-axis levels decrease to 1% of on-axis levels for angles greater than 5° from the central beam axis[23], the probability of being exposed is quite small.

Radars. Radars can be divided into high power (acquisition and tracking for civilian and military use) and medium to low power (on-board aircraft and marine craft, and speed-control). High power radars used in conjunction with satellite systems have average effective radiated powers (ERP) up to 31.6 GW, while experimental systems[24] can have an average ERP up to 3 TW (TW = 10^{12} W).

Table 4. Characteristics of several communications systems.[23]

System	f (GHz)	P (kW)	D (m)	Rn (km)	W_{max} (mW/cm²)	Distance (km) from antenna for power density of 10 mW/cm²	1 mW/cm²
LET	8.1	2.5	4.6	0.1	30.4	0.25	0.8
AN/TSC-54	8.1	8	5.5	0.14	50.8	0.46	1.45
AN/FSC-9	8.1	20	18.3	1.6	7.6	6.2	19.7
Intelsat	6.25	5	29.6	3.2	0.73	-	-
Goldstone Venus	2.38	450	25.9	0.94	97.3	4.2	13.2
Goldstone Mars	2.38	450	64.0	5.8	16.8	9.7	33.4

Acquisition and tracking radars typically operate[23] at 1 - 9 GHz, have transmitter powers up to 150 kW. Acquisition, radars normally have rotating antennas which reduce the radiation level at a given location. Tracking radars on the other hand, because they have non-rotational antennas and are capable of producing significant radiation levels over large areas are normally located in remote regions. Near airports or military bases persons may be exposed to sidelobe or secondary radiation from radars with stationary or rotating antennas. Average power density levels can be as high as between 10 and 100 μW/cm² at distances up to 0.8 km from these systems.[25]

Low-medium power weather radars in aircraft are usually located in the nose under a microwave-transparent radome (housing). They typically operate at 5.4 or 9.375 GHz with peak powers of 20 - 100 kW and normally use a horn-fed parabolic dish antenna. Approximate power densities[26] of 13.5 mW/cm² occur at the radome surface to less than 3 mW/cm² at a distance 1 m.

In another survey of weather radars in aircraft, no intensity exceeding 10 mW/cm² was found at distances beyond 6 m, and for distances greater than 2 - 3 m from the antenna the power density decreased proportionally to the inverse square of the distance.[27] The largest "leakage" field observed in the cockpit (which was just above the antenna) was a pulse-peak E-field of 800 V/m (170 mW/cm²), but an average E-field of 19 V/m (0.1 mW/cm²). In aircraft cockpits radiation levels were not found[28] to exceed 0.2 mW/cm², however if the radars were inadvertently left operating while on the ground passengers in waiting rooms could be exposed to levels around 1 mW/cm².

Measurements around three air traffic control radars yielded a wide range of field intensities.[27] These operated at frequencies in the 2.7 to 2.9 GHz band at peak and average powers of 425 - 550 kW and 375 - 475 W, respectively. An airport surveillance radar produced a power density of 10 mW/cm^2 at a point near head height and 60 cm in front of the reflector. Two higher power devices (peak power 2.5 and 4 MW) produced more intense fields: 10 and 0.1 mW/cm^2 at distances from the source of 36 and 397 m, respectively, and 15 and 1.2 mW/cm^2 at 9.5 and 83 m, respectively.

The characteristics of three typical low power radars used on naval ships have been studies by Stuchly and Mann.[29] These radars operated at 1.3 - 9.4 GHz with average powers of 7.5 to 600 W. While their antennas were rotating the maximum power density to occupied areas was small, however, if the antennas stopped, considerable power levels existed close to the antennas. For smaller marine craft the average power density of radars at the antenna's turning circle radius was found[30] to be between 50 - 250 $\mu W/cm^2$.

Traffic speed measuring radars can be either hand-held or mounted on a vehicle, and operate via a conical horn antenna at a frequency of 10.525 GHz and have a transmitter power of approximately 0.1 W. These continuous wave devices measure the speed of a vehicle from the Doppler frequency shift of the returning signal. The maximum power density at the antenna surface was found[31] to vary from 170 - 400 $\mu W/cm^2$, but falls off to 24 $\mu W/cm^2$ at 3 m and 0.2 $\mu W/cm^2$ at 30 m. Using the formula for determining the average power density in the far field zone ($= PG/4\pi R^2$) at a distance R from an antenna having a gain G and an average power P fed to the antenna, Stuchly[17] estimates the maximum power density at 9 cm from the antenna to be 3.6 mW/cm^2.

Radiation from most radars is pulsed with pulse widths and pulse repetition frequencies that produce an average transmitter power at least two orders of magnitude less than the peak power. In addition many radar antennas rotate through 360° or oscillate in a sector scan so that the average power density at a given location will be much less than values obtained for a stationary antenna. The contribution of radars to the general environment is less than 0.005 $\mu W/cm^2$.

Heating. Microwave and radiofrequency energy for heat production have found application in industry, commerce and the home. Probably the most popular application is in heating or cooking food. Most microwave heating involves devices operating at ISM band frequencies of 915 or 2450 MHz.

Microwave Ovens. Rapid advances in microwave technology, resulting in lower magnetron and hence microwave oven prices, have lead to significant sales of these devices in North America. Over 2.5 million microwave ovens are expected[32] to be sold in the United States in 1981.

Microwave ovens can be considered as low power devices - typically domestic ovens have average powers of around 600 W and industrial ovens 1.5 kW or more. With large numbers of microwave ovens being sold in homes, virtually an uncontrolled environment, concerns were expressed that leakage-radiation could pose potential health hazards. Earlier surveys in Canada indicated that a real problem existed in restaurants, fast food outlets and other commerical establishments using microwave ovens designed for domestic use.[33] The introduction of regulations in Canada under the Radiation Emitting Devices Act in 1974 and their subsequent amendment in 1979 to prevent commercial establishments using domestic ovens has alleviated concerns about leakage radiation from domestic and commercial microwave ovens.

Regulations concerning leakage radiation from microwave ovens are similar throughout the World. A maximum leakage of 1 mW/cm^2 at 5 cm from the outer surface is specified for new ovens, rising to 5 mW/cm^2 at 5 cm for ovens in use. A load of 275 ml water is normally placed inside the domestic and commercial oven during leakage measurements. Specifications for industrial microwave ovens are also included in the Canadian regulations but not in the United States regulations. Personal exposure from microwave ovens is small due to a rapid decrease of the power density with increasing distances from the oven.[34] For an oven leaking 5 mW/cm^2 at 5 cm, the power density at 0.3 m is less than 0.15 mW/cm^2 and at 1 m is about 10 μW/cm^2.

Surveys of 15 different conveyorized industrial microwave heating systems operating at 915 or 2450 MHz with output powers of 2 - 60 kW indicated that maximum leakage (mostly up to 25 mW/cm^2, some to 70 mW/cm^2) occurred[35] at the conveyor slot. However exposures at eye level of the operator did not exceed 4 mW/cm^2. In another survey[36] of industrial microwave power devices operating at the standard magnetron frequencies of 915 and 2450 MHz and output powers of 2 - 120 kW, and used for filament and film drying, food processing, doughnut proofing, and precooking, maximum leakage levels reached 190 mW/cm^2. However the maximum potential exposure for all operators under normal working conditions was found to be approximately 1 mW/cm^2.

<u>Dielectric (RF) Heaters</u>. Dielectric heaters utilize radiofrequency energy for heat processing of dielectric materials. Typically RF heaters generate heat by means of an RF generator that produces oscillating fields of electromagnetic energy and comprises a power supply and control circuitry, a hydraulic press, a parallel plate applicator (die) and a system for supporting and moving processed material. These devices have been in use for more than 30 years and although no documented numbers of these

Table 5. Exposures (corrected for average duty cycle) to operators of various dielectric (RF) heaters.[38]

Heater Type	Number of Units	Above 1 mW/cm^2		Above 10 mW/cm^2	
		-	%	-	%
Sewing Machine	33	19	58	13	39
Shuttle Tray	16	10	63	1	6
Turntable	4	2	50	0	0
Pressure Sealed Applicator	21	0	0	0	0
Edge-Glue Dryer	7	0	0	0	0
All	81	31	38	14	17

units is available, it is estimated that approximately 20,000 exist in the United States.[37] RF heaters are used to heat, melt or cure materials such as plastic, glue or rubber.

RF heaters operate within the frequency range 3 - 70 MHz with a few (used for molding plastics) operating at 300-400 MHz. Most heaters used for sealing operate between 13 - 40 MHz with a few wood glueing devices operating at frequencies as low as 3 - 6 MHz. Heaters that are poorly designed or shielded can emit stray RF electromagnetic energy that could be hazardous to health. In a recent survey of dielectric heaters in Canada,[38] the intensities of the electric and magnetic fields in the vicinity of 82 devices were measured. The devices operated at frequencies between 4 - 51 MHz and their output power ranged from 0.5 - 90 kW. Heaters normally operated at frequencies allocated for ISM uses, namely 13.56, 27.12 and 40.68 MHz, with most operating at 27.12 MHz. The survey indicated that many types of RF heaters existed, but that these could be grouped into 5 categories: sewing machine, shuttle tray, turntable, pressure sealed applicators and edge glue dryers. A summary of the operator exposures received from the various types of RF heater is given in Table 5. These exposures were corrected for duty cycle (fraction of on-time to total time during normal operation), giving values of equivalent plane wave power density above 10 mW/cm^2 in many cases for both the sewing machine and shuttle tray type heaters. Similarly high RF fields have been recorded by Conover et al[39] in the United States and Hansson Mild[40] in Sweden.

Clearly RF heaters represent a major concern with respect to operator exposure. Values of electric and magnetic field strengths, even when corrected for duty cycle, still exceed acceptable limits. Of particular concern is that RF heaters operate at frequencies in or near the region of human resonant absorption[41] (60 - 100 MHz).

Hence workers near RF heaters can absorb considerable amounts of stray energy. Contact (electrical) of the worker with a ground plane can shift the frequency at which maximum absorption rate occurs to well within the frequency band of most RF heaters. The problems of stray fields from the RF heaters can be relatively easily solved by proper design and appropriate location of shields for the RF fields.

<u>Welding</u>. High frequency radiation welding can be used to produce such products as longitudinal butt seams in pipes or tubes. This occurs either by the induction or contact method. Induction coils can be used to generate heat via high frequency currents in the workpiece without touching it. In the contact method small metal shoes slide along the workpiece to convey the current and thus heating, directly into the metal. Phenomena peculiar to HF current such as the "skin" and "proximity" effect are common to both the contact and induction method, and have an effect on the efficiency of heating. The "skin effect" is the tendency of HF current to flow at shallow depths in the metal. The "proximity effect" is the tendency of HF currents to concentrate at that point where the feed and return conductors are at closest proximity. The combination of the skin and proximity effects result in a concentration of heat at the surfaces to be joined. A typical HF welder is shown schemmatically in Figure 4, where a pipe seam is being welded at the point where the two sides (conductors) are squeezed together. The pipe is made seamless by a bite-tip which shaves the weld smooth. The impeder is a ferrite core inside an insulat-

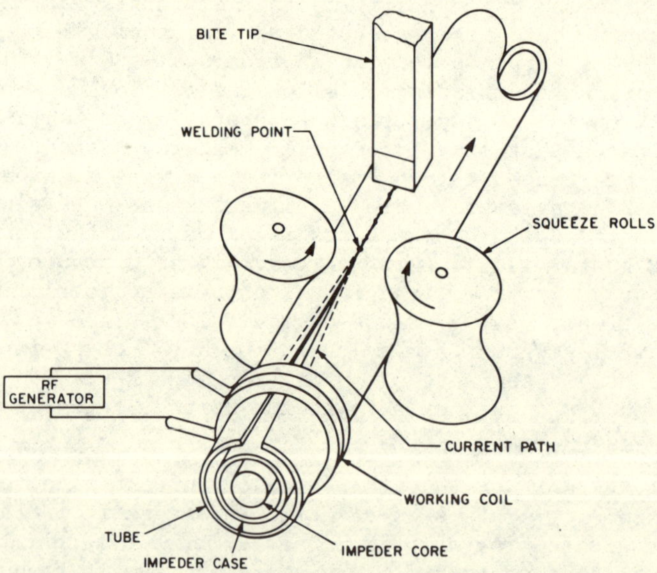

Figure 4. Radiofrequency welder used to produce seamless pipes or tubes.

ing case - this combination produces a high resistance to currents induced by both the electric and magnetic fields and causes a greater flow of current in the pipe while reducing the current flow needed in the coil.

Industrial welders operate at a frequency of about 400 kHz and have an output power around 400 kW. A survey conducted on a smaller welder[42] operating at a nominal frequency of 2.2 MHz gave radiated emissions at frequencies up to 100 MHz and above. The unit was pulsed with a pulse width of approximately 20 μs with off-times of 200 μs (duty cycle 1:10). The strengths of electric and magnetic fields were such that no one in the working area would be exposed to an equivalent plane wave power density of more than 1 mW/cm^2. Much more information is needed before any kind of an assessment can be made of human exposure to these devices.

Medical Applications

Diagnostic Techniques. Non-ionizing electromagnetic radiation techniques used or having potential application in medical diagnosis have recently been reviewed by Iskander and Durney.[43] In brief, techniques have been developed to measure changes in fluid accummulation in the lungs using low frequency (20 - 100 kHz) to detect current flow (higher air volumes) and hence less fluid in the lungs cause higher resistance to current flow), or using 915 MHz microwaves to detect changes in dielectric properties. Electromagnetic imaging using microwaves, especially to visualize lung tissue, is still being researched. Microwave radiometry to detect "hot spots", such as those produced by malignant lumps in the breast, may have an advantage over infrared thermography because microwaves emitted from greater depths can travel with lower attenuation to the surface. Efforts are presently being focused on developing an electromagnetic flow meter to non-invasively monitor to flow of blood in humans. Stuchly et al[44] have recently described a technique for monitoring the movements of arterial walls using a low-power, 10.525 GHz Doppler radar.

Hyperthermia. All the techniques described above use low power radiation. However high power non-ionizing electromagnetic radiation has been used for hyperthermia in the treatment of cancer. This has recently been reviewed by Johnson et al[45] and Short and Turner.[46] Cancer therapy using hyperthermia makes use of the fact that most malignant cells are more sensitive to heat (41 - 45°C) than normal cells. In addition, many tumours above 1 cm diameter have a poorer blood supply than surrounding normal tissue, so that heat dissipation of the tumour is less than that of the surrounding normal tissue. Non-ionizing, electromagnetic radiation hyperthermia modalities include capacitative, inductive and UHF-microwave techniques. Applications of radiofrequency heating involve the use of 13.56 and 27.12 MHz fields while microwave heating is conducted with 2450, 915 and 434 MHz (the latter only outside North America). Most radiofrequency- and microwave-induced hyperthermia treatments are conducted as a part of research programs.

Diathermy. Diathermy is the application of radiofrequency or microwave energy to generate heat in body tissues. Therapeutic diathermy is used in the treatment of such conditions as pain, arthritis, muscle spasm, by producing deep heating without excessive temperature elevation of the skin surface or subcutaneous fatty tissue. Short-wave diathermy devices operate at frequencies from 10 to 100 MHz (predominantly at 27.12 MHz) while microwave diathermy equipment operates from 300 - 100,000 MHz (normally at 2450 MHz, but used experimentaly at 915 MHz). Therapeutic diathermy involves the use of one or two applicators, or conducting cables to applying energy to the treatment area for a specified period of time.

Leakage radiation from the applicators of both microwave and shortwave diathermy devices have been the subject of recent studies [47,48,49]. Measurements made[47] at 5 cm from the interface between a tissue - equivalent phantom and a microwave diathermy appplicator indicated leakage levels from 10.4 to 44 mW/cm^2. Exposures to the operators (standing at the control console) during microwave diathermy treatment were reported[48] to be up to 1.3 mW/cm^2. From a questionnaire survey of medical microwave and short-wave devices in Canada[50] it was found that about ten times more short-wave than microwave diathermy devices are used in therapy. As a result of this and the fact that only a few manufacturers for microwave diathermy devices exist, Health and Welfare Canada[51] issued a set of safety guidelines in lieu of mandatory regulations to induce manufacturers to reduce leakage radiation levels.

Leakage radiation levels from short-wave diathermy devices represent a greater problem. Operators of these devices can be exposed[48] from applicators or RF cables to field strengths up to 0.47 A/m and 250 V/m (equivalent to free space power densities of 8.3 and 16.6 mW/cm^2 respectively). Similar results have been reported by Stuchly et al.[49] In the latter study, Stuchly et al also found that high exposures occurred in untreated areas of patients during all treatment protocols. Exposures were found to be as high as 710 V/m or 1.35 A/m to the eyes, 2650 V/m or 1.6 A/m to the gonadal area during certain treatments. As a result of these surveys it is evident that greater protection can be afforded by shielding the RF cables (between the RF generator and the applicators) and educating the operator with regard to where and where not to stand during treatments. Patient exposure to untreated areas could be reduced by better design of the applicators.

Electrosurgical Devices. Electrosurgical devices are used

for cutting and cauterizing tissue and are found in virtually every operating room and many doctors' offices and clinics in the United States.[21] They operate at frequencies from 0.5 to 2.4 MHz, but may emit a spectrum of frequencies up to 100 MHz. Continuous wave (cw) operation is used for cutting and an amplitude modulation (10's of kHz) of the cw is used when coagulation is desired. Measurements of the electric and magnetic field strengths at 16 cm from the probe lead of a solid state and a spark-gap type electrosurgical unit, gave values of 1000 V/m and 0.71 A/m when the power was at maximum. Fields of up to 690 V/m and 0.58 A/m were measured at power levels normally used. These fields translate to equivalent plane-wave power densities of up to 265 mW/cm^2 at maximum power, and about 100 mW/cm^2 under normal operating conditions. Such fields could present potential health hazards to the operators and possibly produce electromagnetic interference to the other electromedical devices such as patient monitoring and life support systems.[21]

Microwave Blood Warmers. Microwave blood warmers operate at 2450 MHz and are a special type of microwave heating device similar to a microwave oven, but designed to heat blood to physiological temperatures prior to transfusion. Earlier models of these devices were found to haemolyze blood either by overheating or by producing an excessive rate of heating. This was partly due to the design of the device and partly as a result of untrained operators incorrectly placing the bags of blood into the oven cavity. Subsequent to this, guidelines for these devices were introduced in Canada.[52]

Other Sources

Satellite Solar Power. The United States Department of Energy is presently considering the use of geosynchronous satellites in space to collect solar energy, convert it to microwave energy and transmit it to large, earth-based receiving/rectifying antennas (rectenna). The microwave energy generated at each satellite would be transmitted to earth in the form of a narrow beam of continuous wave radiation having a frequency of 2.45 GHz. The power density at the centre of the rectenna would be 23 mW/cm^2, at the edge of the rectenna 1 mW/cm^2, at the rectenna site exclusion boundary 0.1 mW/cm^2, at the first sidelobe (approximately 9 km from centre of rectenna) 0.08 mW/cm^2, and at the grating (subsequent) sidelobes (spacings 400 km) would be less than 0.01 mW/cm^2. Non-occupational exposure would normally be less than 0.1 mW/cm^2. Workers at the rectenna site could be exposed to 23 mW/cm^2 or higher (if reflections are considered). Workers in space could be exposed to power densities of the order of W/cm^2. Humans in aeroplanes flying through the main beam would be exposed to much less than 23 mW/cm^2 because of shielding by the metal shell of the plane. Although special precautions may be necessary for workers within the rectenna boundry, the exposure of less than 0.1 mW/cm^2

to the general public living near the rectenna sites, should not cause any particular concerns.

Video Display Units (VDU). VDU's have been much maligned in the past few years, being suggested (in the press) as responsible for the production of cataracts and miscarriages. They have been erroneously implicated as sources of hazardous microwave and radiofrequency emissions. Surveys conducted by NIOSH[54] have indicated that there are no microwave emissions, except for an extremely small component due to heat emitted from the electronics. Besides visible radiation, radiofrequency fields (15 - 21 kHz) having electric field strengths up to 1000 V/m and magnetic field strengths up to 0.65 A/m have been measured at the back of some VDU's where the "flyback" transformer was located close to the outer casing and no shielding was provided by the outer cover (unpublished surveys - Radiation Protection Bureau (1981), P.S. Ruggera - personal communication (1981)). However, at the normal operator position these fields are very low (less than 10 V/m). Because of the very low absorption of energy by the human body at these frequencies, no adverse health effects would be expected.

Coronas. During inclement weather, water droplets or icicles on high voltage transmission lines (345 - 765 kV) provide sources of corona discharges having a radiofrequency component that can interfere with low-level AM radio signals. Similar spurious signals may be heard on radios during lightning discharges or from arcing across high voltage insulators. This noise produces insignificantly small levels of radiofrequency radiation into the environment.[12]

CONCLUSIONS

The general ambient environment is dominated by radiofrequency and microwave emissions from radio and television transmission, especially in the broadcast band 54 - 900 MHz. Over 99% of the population is continuously exposed to power densities of less than 1 $\mu W/cm^2$. Contributions to the ambient environment from microwave relay transmitters, mobile communications systems and low-power radars can be considered negligible.

In certain cases, occupational exposure levels can exceed 1 mW/cm^2 or more. Examples of these situations include maintenance crews on broadcast towers and around high power radars, workers using dielectric RF heaters, operators of electrosurgical units, microwave and short-wave diathermy devices, and personnel working near antennas of mobile communications equipment. As a result of government regulations and improved designs there does not appear to be any health hazard from domestic and industrial microwave ovens.

Some devices are difficult to assess in terms of potential

adverse health effects because they radiate non-uniform fields. For example highly localized, partial body exposure occurs near the antenna of a walkie-talkie or CB radio, or close to an electro-surgical unit. The strength of these fields decrease rapidly with distance from the device. Investigations of power absorption under near-field illumination conditions needs to be investigated before an adequate assessment can be made on health effects from human exposure.

ACKNOWLEDGEMENTS

I would like to extend my sincere appreciation to Dr. John M. Osepchuk for his assistance and helpful advice in the preparation of this manuscript. My thanks to Dr. Maria Stuchly and Dr. Peter Waight for their reviews. Finally my thanks to Mrs. Judy Smith for typing the text and Mr. David Lecuyer for preparing many of the drawings.

REFERENCES

1. "Radio regulations", Published by the General Secretariat of the International Telecommunication Union Pub. No. ISBN 92-61-00181-5, 1976 Edition revised (1979).
2. "Environmental health criteria for radiofrequency and micro-waves", World Health Organization, Geneva (1980).
3. M.R. Kundu, "Solar Radio Astronomy", Interscience Publishers, New York (1965).
4. J.M. Osepchuk, Review of environmental electromagnetic fields, Personal communication (1980).
5. W.M. Sinton, Detection of millimetre wave solar radiation, Phys. Rev. 86:424 (1952).
6. W.M. Sinton, Observations of solar and lunar radiation at 1.5 millimetres, J. Opt. Soc. Amer. 45:975 (1955).
7. B.A. Minin, "Microwaves and human safety. Part I." Published from Russian - available from U.S. Dept. of Commerce, National Technical Information Service (JPRS 65506-1) August (1975).
8. J.M. Osepchuk, Sources and basic characteristics of microwave/RF radiation, Bull. N.Y. Acad. Med. 55(11), 976-998 (1979).
9. P. Gwynne, S. Begley and M. Hager, The flap over the zap, Newsweek 92(3), 87-88 (1978).
10. R.A. Tell, Broadcast radiation: How safe is safe, IEEE Spectrum, August, pp. 43-51 (1972).
11. R.A. Tell and E.D. Mantiply, Population exposure to VHF and UHF broadcast radiation in the United States, Proc. IEEE 68(1), 6-12 (1980).
12. D.E. Janes, Radiation surveys - measurement of leakage emis-sions and potential exposure fields, Bull. N.Y. Acad. 55(11), 1021-1041 (1979).

13. D.E. Janes, R.A. Tell, T.W. Athey and N.N. Hankin, Radiofrequency radiation levels in urban areas, Radio Science (Suppl.), 12:49-56 (1977).

14. R.A. Tell and N.N. Hankin, "Measurement of radiofrequency field intensity in buildings with close proximity to broadcast stations", U.S. Environmental Protection Agency Techn. Note ORP/EAD 78-3, Las Vegas, Nevada (1978).

15. R.A. Tell, "A measurement of RF field intensities in the immediate vicinity of an FM broadcast station antenna", Techn. Note ORP/EDA-76-2, U.S. Environmental Protection Agency (1976).

16. J. Adams, M. Kanda, J. Shafter and Y. Wu, "Near-field electric field strength levels of EM environments applicable to automotive systems, National Bureau of Standards Report, Boulder, Colorado (1977).

17. M.A. Stuchly, Potentially hazardous microwave radiation sources - a review, J. Microwave Power, 12(4): 369-381 (1977).

18. Q. Balzano, O. Garay and R. Steel, Energy deposition in biological tissue near portable radio transmitters at VHF and UHF, IEEE Pub. 77Ch1176-7VT, 25-39 (1977).

19. Q. Balzano, O. Garay and R. Steel, Energy deposition in simulated human operators of 800 MHz portable transmitters, IEEE Trans. Vehic. Techn. VT-27, 174-181 (1978).

20. D. Lambdin, "An investigation of energy densities in the vicinity of vehicles with mobile communications equipment and near hand-held walkie-talkies, Tech. Note ORP/EAD 79-2, Las Vegas, Nevada, U.S. Environmental Protection Agency (1979).

21. P.S. Ruggera, Near-field measurements of RF fields, in Symposium on biological effects and measurements of radio frequency/microwaves. U.S. Dept. of Health, Education and Welfare Pub. No. (FDA) 77-8026, pp. 104-113 (1977).

22. P.A. Neukomm, Biotelemetry antennas: the problem of small body-mounted antennas. Proc. Biosigma 78, Paris (1978).

23. N.N. Hankin, R.A. Tell, T.W. Athey and D.E. Janes, High power radiofrequency and microwave radiation sources. A study of relative environmental significance. Proceedings of 9th Midyear Topical Symposium of the Health Physics Society, Boulder, Colorado, editors: P.L. Carson, W.R. Hendee and D.C. Hunt (1976).

24. N.N. Hankin, An evaluation of selected satellite communication systems as sources of environmental microwave radiation, Environmental Protection Agency Report EPA-520/2-74-008, Silver Springs, Maryland, pp. 56 (1974).

25. N.N. Hankin, Exposure levels and potential biologic effects of the PAVE PAWS radar system, Panel on the extent of radiation from the PAVE PAWS radar system. Washington, D.C., Nat. Aca. Sci., p. 40 (1979).

26. R.A. Tell, N.N. Hankin and D.E. Janes, Aircraft radar measure-

ments in the near field, in Proc. 9th Midyear Topical Symp., P.C. Carson, W.R. Hendee and D.C. Hunt, ed., Health Physics Society, Boulder, Colorado (1976).

27. E.B. Larsen and J.F. Shafer, "Surveys of electromagnetic field intensities near representative high-power RAA transmitting antennas", U.S. Dept. of Transport, Federal Aviation Administration Publication FAA-RD-77-179 (1977).
28. Z.R. Glazer and G.M. Heimer, Determination and elimination of hazardous microwave fields aboard naval ships, IEEE Trans. Microwave Theory and Technique. MTT-19, 232-238 (1971).
29. M.A. Stuchly and R. Mann, "Survey of naval radars", Internal Report, Radiation Protection Bureau, Health and Welfare Canada (1977).
30. D. Peak, D. Conover, W. Herman and R. Shuping, "Measurement of power density from marine radar", U.S. Dept. of Health, Education and Welfare Pub. (FDA) 76-8004, Rockville, Maryland (1975).
31. N.N. Hankin, "Radiation characteristics of traffic radar systems", U.S. Environmental Protection Agency Techn. Note ORP/EAD 76-1, Silver Springs, Maryland (1976).
32. J.M. Osepchuk, Life begins at forty: microwave tubes, Invited paper: International Electronic Devices Meeting, IEEE Washington, D.C., December 28, 1977. Also as Technical Memorandum T-1030, Raytheon Co. Research Division (1977).
33. M.A. Stuchly, M.H. Repacholi and D. Lecuyer, The impact of regulations on microwave ovens in Canada, Health Physics 37:137-144 (1979).
34. Safety from microwave hazards in using microwave power equipment - an IMPI policy statement, J. Microwave Power 10:333-341 (1975).
35. J.A. Eure, J.W. Nicolls and R.L. Elder, Radiation exposure from industrial microwave applications, Am. J. Public Health 62:1573-1577 (1972).
36. R.L. Elder, J.A. Eure and J.W. Nicolls, Radiation leakage control of industrial microwave power devices, J. Microwave Power, 9:51-61 (1974).
37. "Radiofrequency (RF) sealers and heaters: potential health hazards and their prevention", Joint NIOSH/OSHA Current Intelligence Bulletin 33, United States Dept. of Health, Education and Welfare (National Institute for Occupational Safety and Health) - United States Dept. of Labour (Occupational Safety and Health Administration), December 4 (1979).
38. M.A. Stuchly, M.H. Repacholi, D. Lecuyer and R. Mann, Radiofrequency survey of dielectric (RF) heaters in Canada, J. Microwave Power 15(2):113-121 (1980).
39. D.L. Conover, W.E. Murray, E.D. Foley, J.M. Lary and W.H. Parr, Measurement of electric- and magnetic-field strengths from industrial radio-frequency (6-38 MHz) plastic sealers, Proc. IEEE 68(1):17-20 (1980).

40. K.H. Hansson Mild, Occupational exposure to radiofrequency electromagnetic fields, Proc. IEEE 68(1):12-17 (1980).
41. C.H. Durney, M.F. Iskander, H. Massoudi, S.J. Allen and J.C. Mitchell, "Radiofrequency Radiation Dosimetry Handbook, 3rd edition, Report SAM-TR-80-32, U.S.A.F. School of Aerospace Medicine, Brooks Air Force Base, Texas 78235, pp. 136 (1980).
42. R.A. Facey, "Radiofrequency Hazards from Tungsten Inert Gas (TIG) Welding Units", Ontario Hydro Information Report SSD-IR-80-11, Safety Services Department, Ontario Hydro, Canada (1980).
43. M.F. Iskander and C.H. Durney, Electromagnetic techniques for medical diagnosis: a review, Proc. IEEE, 68(1):126-132 (1980).
44. S.S. Stuchly, M. Goldberg, A. Thansandote and B. Carraro, Monitoring of arterial wall movement by microwave Doppler radar, Symp. Electromagnetic Fields in Biological Systems, Ottawa, June 27-30 (1978).
45. R.J.R. Johnson, J.R. Subjeck, D.Z. Moreau, H. Kowal and D. Yakar, Radiation and hyperthermia, Bull. N.Y. Acad. Med. 55(11):1193-1204 (1979).
46. J.G. Short and P.F. Turner, Physical hyperthermia and cancer therapy, Proc. IEEE, 68(1):133-142 (1980).
47. H. Bassen, G. Kantor, P. Ruggera and D. Witters, "Leakage in the proximity of microwave diathermy applicators used on human and animal models," U.S. Dept. Health, Education and Welfare Pub. (FDA) 79-8073, Rockville, Maryland (1978).
48. P.S. Ruggera, "Measurements of emission levels during microwave and shortwave diathermy treatments", U.S. Dept. Health and Human Services Pub. (FDA) 80-8119, Rockville, Maryland, (1980).
49. M.A. Stuchly, M.H. Repacholi, D.W. Lecuyer and R.D. Mann, Exposure to the operator and patient during short-wave diathermy treatment, Health Physics (in press) (1981).
50. Health and Welfare Canada, "Canada-wide survey of non-ionizing radiation emitting medical devices. Part I: Short-wave and microwave devices", Environmental Health Directorate Pub. 80-EHD-52 (1980).
51. "Guidelines for microwave diathermy devices", Health and Welfare Canada, Health Protection Branch Pub. I.L. No. 585, September 19 (1980).
52. "Guidelines for microwave blood warmers", Health and Welfare Canada, Health Protection Branch Pub. I.L. No. 539, October 12 (1978).
53. J.S. Krebs, L.N. Heynick and P. Polson, "An assessment of the potential impact of microwave radiation from a solar power satellite", Special Report SRI International, Proj. #LSU8141. Prepared for Environmental Protection Agency, Research Triangle Park, North Carolina (1980).

54. C.E. Moss, W.E. Murray, W.H. Parr, J. Messite and G.J. Karches, "A report on electromagnetic radiation surveys of video display terminals," U.S. Dept. of Health, Education and Welfare (NIOSH) Pub. No. 78-129, Cincinatti, Ohio (1977).

FUNDAMENTALS OF THE CLASSICAL THEORY OF ELECTROMAGNETIC FIELDS

Martino Grandolfo

Radiation Laboratory, Istituto Superiore di Sanità

00161 Rome, Italy

INTRODUCTION

Charge is one of the fundamental physical quantities in terms of which all other physical quantities can be ultimately defined. The charge associated with an object is a measure of its electrical content. In nature charge is found in two forms, positive and negative charges. Objects possessing similar charges repel one another, whereas objects possessing dissimilar charges attract one another. Matter is made up of atoms that are composed of a positively charge nucleus surrounded by a "cloud" of electrons. In its ground state an atom has no net charge, being the positive and negative charges perfectly balanced.

Two very strange phenomena were known to the greeks: that if a piece of amber was rubbed it could lift up little pieces of papyrus, and that there was a strange rock from the island of Magnesia which attracted iron. The reason why these were the only phenomena in which the effects of electricity and magnetism were apparent is due to the fantastic precision of the balancing of charges existing in nature. After the greeks, scientists discovered new phenomena that were really only different aspects of the old amber and lodestone effects, but today is clearly realized that most of chemistry, physics and biology is concerned with the electromagnetic interaction.

During the latter half of eighteenth century Coulomb investigated the forces between electrically charged objects. He found that the force between two such objects acted along the line joning them, that it was proportional to the product of their charges, and that it was inversely proportional to the square of their separation, showing a striking similarity to the law of gravitation. The discovery of the magnetic effects associated with electric currents (current is the term introduced to describe the movement of charges) came early in the nineteenth century. Oersted observed that a current flowing in a loop of wire exerted magnetic forces on permanent magnets. Subsequently, Ampère showed that the magnetic force resulting from the flow of current in a circuit can be considered as a sum of contributions from infinitesimal segments of the circuit. The force due to each segment falls off inversely as the square of the distance. Scientists thought of the electric and magnetic forces primarly in terms of the "action-at-a-distance" concept. The beginning of the change toward a "field theory" view of the interactions came in the first half of the nineteenth century.

Faraday introduced lines of force which, at an arbitrary point in space, point in the direction of the force that would be exerted on a test charge located at that point. The number of lines of force per unit area was made proportional to the magnitude of the force. His fundamental idea was that charged objects establish a field in the region of space around them and that the interaction between objects occurs via this field. Faraday's discovery of electromagnetic induction, in which a time-varying magnetic field through a circuit induces voltage in the circuit, established the importance of the concept of magnetic field. Gauss, contemporary of Faraday, was able to relate the number of lines of force out of a region to the total charge within the region. This was the first mathematical formulation of classical field theory.

Maxwell accepted the idea that the electric and magnetic fields were the fundamental quantities and was able to devise a set of partial differential equations obeyed by these fields. He immediately noted that the equations predicted that an electromagnetic disturbance originating at one charged object would travel out as a wave with a speed that could be deduced from electrical and magnetic measurements. The predicted speed, within the relatively small experimental error of measurement, agreed with the speed of light. Maxwell had provided convincing evidence of the superiority of a field theory to an action-at-a-distance theory and also established the link between electromagnetism and optics. Neither quantum mechanics nor the special theory of relativity has in any way reduced the significance of the electromagnetic field equations Maxwell proposed over one hundred years ago. Scientists of the nineteenth century tried to understand a wave model of light in terms of the transverse vibrations of a hypothetical elastic medium which they named the ether, whose properties soon resulted very unrealistic. In terms of the Maxwell's equations the electric and magnetic fields are the fundamental entities concerned with optics and electromagnetism and there is no need to introduce the ether at all. A few years later Hertz produced electromagnetic waves of several centimeters wavelength in the laboratory. From this time Maxwell's equations have received universal acceptance, and optics has been treated as a branch of electromagnetism.

Early in the twentieth century Max Planck introduced the quantum concept and shortly afterward Einstein predicted the existence of the photon and used Planck's quantum hypothesis to deduce the law of the photoelectric effect. Whereas a wave theory predicts a continuous distribution of energy in a wave, the existence of photons requires that the energy in an electromagnetic wave be quantized in discrete packets as for a corpuscular theory. For some time this apparent contradiction provided a serious impediment to the development of quantum theory. It is now recognized that both the corpuscular and wave points of view simultaneously have their merits; the wave picture correctly describes the average behaviour of the photons but the energy is carried by the photons in discrete amounts. For long wavelength radiation, such as radio-frequency and microwaves (non ionizing radiation) the photon energy is very small and ordinary sources provide such enormous numbers of photons that their discreteness is not of practical importance. The incorporation of wave-particle duality into a single theory of electromagnetism falls into the realm of quantum electrodynamics.

The above brief account provides some insight into the historical development of the classical theory of fields and, by no means, constitutes a complete history of events, making only reference to some of the more important contributions.

THE ALGEBRA AND CALCULUS OF VECTORS

In Physics we encounter some quantities, such as velocity, force, electric field, to which we attribute both a magnitude and a direction. Such physical quantities are called vector quantities; a quantity possessing only a magnitude is termed a scalar quantity (mass, volume, charge, etc.). In specifying the direction of a vector we need a system of reference axes. We shall start with cartesian coordinates, for which the axes x, y, and z are mutually perpendicular. We may now specify a vector $\vec{P}$ by stating the components P_x, P_y, and P_z. If $\vec{i}$, $\vec{j}$, and $\vec{k}$ are vectors of unit magnitude in the directions of the axes x, y, and z, respectively, we can write

$$\vec{P} = P_x\vec{i} + P_y\vec{j} + P_z\vec{k} \tag{1}$$

Two different methods of multiplying two vectors $\vec{P}$ and $\vec{Q}$ are defined. They are designated symbolically by $\vec{P} \cdot \vec{Q}$ and $\vec{P} \times \vec{Q}$.

The scalar product $\vec{P} \cdot \vec{Q}$ is defined as a scalar whose magnitude is equal to

$$\vec{P} \cdot \vec{Q} = P\,Q\cos\vartheta \tag{2}$$

being P and Q the magnitudes of vectors and ϑ the angle between them. In terms of their components we find

$$\vec{P} \cdot \vec{Q} = P_xQ_x + P_yQ_y + P_zQ_z \tag{3}$$

The vector product $\vec{P} \times \vec{Q}$ is defined as a vector whose direction is that of advance of a right-handed screw rotating from $\vec{P}$ to $\vec{Q}$, and whose magnitude is

$$|\vec{P} \times \vec{Q}| = P\,Q \sin\vartheta \tag{4}$$

In terms of components a useful rule may be derived, such as

$$\vec{P} \times \vec{Q} = \begin{vmatrix} \vec{i} & \vec{j} & \vec{k} \\ P_x & P_y & P_z \\ Q_x & Q_y & Q_z \end{vmatrix} \tag{5}$$

Theorems which follow from the above are:

$$\vec{P} \cdot \vec{P} = P^2 \;; \quad \vec{P} \cdot \vec{Q} = \vec{Q} \cdot \vec{P} \;; \quad \vec{P} \times \vec{P} = 0 \;; \quad \vec{P} \times \vec{Q} = -\vec{Q} \times \vec{P}$$

Let $\varphi(x,y,z)$ represent a scalar field of the coordinates and, possibly, the time. Examples of such a function are temperature, pressure, the electrostatic potential. Let $\vec{A}(x,y,z)$ represent a vector field of coordinates and, possibly, the time. The most frequent example of such a function will be the velocity of a fluid, or the electric and magnetic fields. We now introduce a differential operator (called nabla, or del) which is also a vector (has components), namely,

$$\nabla = \vec{i}\,\frac{\partial}{\partial x} + \vec{j}\,\frac{\partial}{\partial y} + \vec{k}\,\frac{\partial}{\partial z} \tag{6}$$

The gradient of a scalar field φ is by definition the same as $\nabla\varphi$. From Eq.6, we have

$$\text{grad}\,\varphi = \nabla\varphi = \vec{i}\,\frac{\partial\varphi}{\partial x} + \vec{j}\,\frac{\partial\varphi}{\partial y} + \vec{k}\,\frac{\partial\varphi}{\partial z} \tag{7}$$

which is a vector function of the coordinates. The physical meaning is best understood by imagining that, as in Fig.1, we draw surfaces (or lines in two dimensions) along which φ has successive constant values, such as 0,10,20,....... It would be possible to prove that the vector $\nabla\varphi$, at any point, (i) is in the direction at right angles to the surfaces we have drawn,(ii) is in the direction in which φ increases most rapidly, and (iii) has for its magnitude the rate of change of φ with respect to distance in that direction, or $(d\varphi/ds)_{max}$, where ds is an element of distance. In electrostatics, equipotential surfaces (V = constant) and lines of force are mutually perpendicular, the electric field $\vec{E}$ being

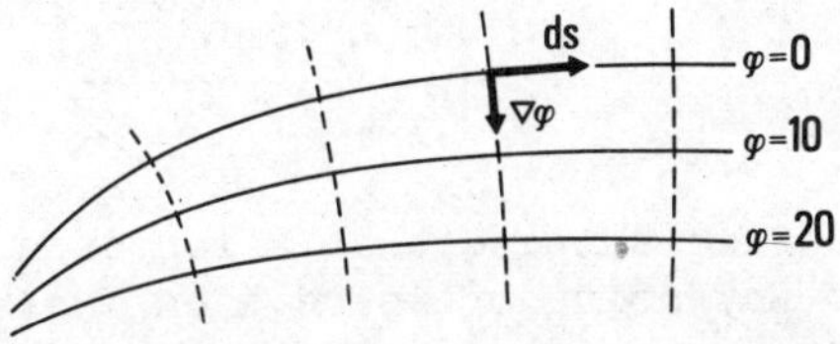

Fig.1 - Relation between the vector $\nabla\varphi$ (the gradient) and the surfaces along which φ has constant values.

$$\vec{E} = - \text{grad } V = - \nabla V \tag{8}$$

The divergence of a vector field $\vec{A}$ is by definition the same as $\nabla\cdot\vec{A}$. From Eqs.3 and 6, we see that the divergence of $\vec{A}$ is

$$\nabla\cdot\vec{A} = \frac{\partial A_x}{\partial x} + \frac{\partial A_y}{\partial y} + \frac{\partial A_z}{\partial z} \tag{9}$$

where A_x, A_y, and A_z are the components of $\vec{A}$ and may themselves be functions of the coördinates. The divergence of a vector is a scalar. Its physical meaning is best seen in connection with the flow of a fluid; if $\vec{A}$ represents the quantity of fluid flowing per unit time and per unit area through an area perpendicular to $\vec{A}$, then A_x, A_y, and A_z will be the quantities passing per unit time through unit area at right angles to the x-, y-, and z-axis, respectively. We see that $\nabla\cdot\vec{A}$ is the net rate of volume flow out per unit time. In a region where $\nabla\cdot\vec{A}$ is positive, the net flow from a small region is outward, or "diverging". If such a region does not contain a source of fluid, we must conclude that the fluid is draining away and the density decreasing. Mathematical formulation of this statement leads to what we will term the equation of continuity.

The curl of a vector field $\vec{A}$, sometimes called the rotation of $\vec{A}$ (rot $\vec{A}$), by definition is

$$\text{curl } \vec{A} = \text{rot } \vec{A} = \nabla \times \vec{A} \tag{10}$$

From Eqs.5 and 6, we see that curl $\vec{A}$ is

$$\nabla \times \vec{A} = \begin{vmatrix} \vec{i} & \vec{j} & \vec{k} \\ \partial/\partial x & \partial/\partial y & \partial/\partial z \\ A_x & A_y & A_z \end{vmatrix} \tag{11}$$

which is a vector. If we suppose that $\vec{A}$ represents the linear velocity $\vec{v}$ of a fluid at any point of space, then $\nabla \times \vec{A}$ is proportional to the angular velocity of the fluid at the point considered. Among possible successive applications of ∇, the following double applications are important: (i) The divergence of the gradient, $\nabla \cdot \nabla = \nabla^2$, is called the Laplacian. It may operate on either a scalar or a vector function. If we recall that $\vec{p} \cdot \vec{p} = p^2 = p_x^2 + p_y^2 + p_z^2$, we have

$$\nabla^2 \varphi = \nabla \cdot \nabla \varphi = \frac{\partial^2 \varphi}{\partial x^2} + \frac{\partial^2 \varphi}{\partial y^2} + \frac{\partial^2 \varphi}{\partial z^2} \tag{12}$$

and

$$\nabla^2 \vec{A} = \nabla \cdot \nabla \vec{A} = \frac{\partial^2 A_x}{\partial x^2} + \frac{\partial^2 A_y}{\partial y^2} = \frac{\partial^2 A_z}{\partial z^2} \tag{13}$$

(ii) The curl of the curl, for which the following expansion will be prove useful:

$$\nabla \times \nabla \times \vec{A} = \nabla (\nabla \cdot \vec{A}) - \nabla \cdot \nabla \vec{A} \tag{14}$$

(iii) The curl of the gradient, for which it is possible to show that

$$\nabla \times \nabla \varphi = 0 \tag{15}$$

Since a vector whose curl is everywhere zero is called irrotational, we see that the gradient of a scalar function is always irrotational. Similarly, for the divergence of the curl is

$$\nabla \cdot \nabla \times \vec{A} = 0 \tag{16}$$

for any vector $\vec{A}$. A vector, such as the curl of any vector function, whose divergence is everywhere zero is called solenoidal. In advanced vector analysis it is proved that any vector function may be written as the sum of two parts,one of which is irrotational and the other solenoidal.

In order to analyse elementary line and surface integrals, consider first a curve with a given positive direction (Fig.2a). If ds is a curve or arc length element, a vector $\vec{ds}$ of the same length pointing in the positive tangent direction is called the vectorial curve element. If $\vec{A}$ is an arbitrary vector field, we have

$$\vec{A} \cdot \vec{ds} = A_s ds \tag{17}$$

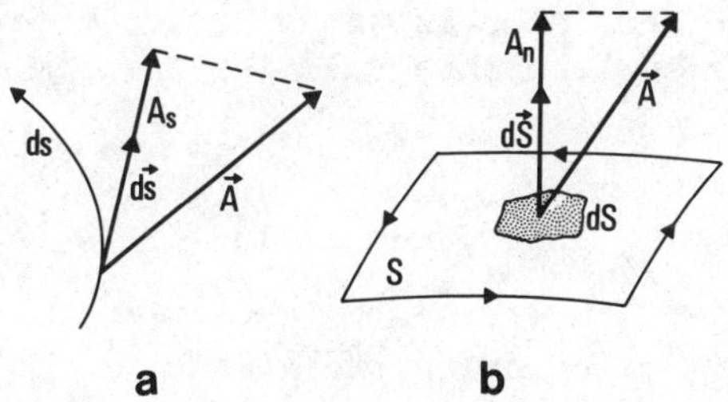

Fig.2 - (a) Vectorial line element $\vec{ds}$, (b) Vectorial surface element $d\vec{S}$.

A_s being the tangential component of $\vec{A}$. This expression, if integrated between two points of the curve, is called a line integral

$$\int_a^b \vec{A} \cdot \vec{ds} = \int_a^b A_s ds \tag{18}$$

For closed curves we usually write $\oint \vec{A}\cdot d\vec{s}$ for a line integral.

In Fig.2b we have a surface S bounded by an oriented closed curve. A scalar surface element dS may be used for definition of a corresponding vectorial element

$$d\vec{S} = dS\,\vec{n} \tag{19}$$

$\vec{n}$ being the positive normal vector of the surface element as defined in accordance with the positive direction of the peripheral curve. For an arbitrary vector field $\vec{A}$ we now have

$$\vec{A}\cdot d\vec{S} = A_n\, dS \tag{20}$$

and a surface integral for a bound region as in Fig.2b is defined as

$$\int_S \vec{A}\cdot d\vec{S} = \int_S A_n\, dS \tag{21}$$

The divergence theorem, also known as Gauss' theorem, enables to go from a volume to a surface integral. The theorem states that

$$\int_V \nabla\cdot \vec{A}\, dV = \int_S \vec{A}\cdot d\vec{S} \tag{22}$$

where S is the surface bounding the volume V. The volume integral of the divergence of a vector function is then equal to the surface integral of the vector over the surface of that volume. The physical meaning of this theorem is best seen in the case where $\vec{A}$ stands for the velocity at any point in a fluid. In this case $\int_V \nabla\cdot\vec{A}\, dV$ represents the rate at which fluid is diverging from V and $\int_S \vec{A}\cdot d\vec{S}$ gives the net rate of flow out across the S surface surrounding V. The two should be equal, as the divergence theorem tells us.

A second fundamental theorem of vector calculus is the Stokes' theorem, which enables to go from a surface integral to a line integral. The theorem states that

$$\int_S (\nabla \times \vec{A}) \cdot d\vec{S} = \oint \vec{A}\cdot d\vec{s} \tag{23}$$

where the line integral is taken around the periphery of the surface S. The surface integral of the curl of a vector function is then equal to the line integral of the function around the surface. If S is a closed surface there is no periphery and the line integral is zero. As stated above, by definition $\vec{A}$ is irrotational if $\nabla \times \vec{A} = 0$ everywhere. Then

$$\oint \vec{A}\cdot d\vec{s} = \int_S (\nabla \times \vec{A}) \cdot d\vec{S} = 0 \qquad (24)$$

for any closed path, and hence may be put equal to an exact differential. An irrotational vector has, then, the following properties:

i) its curl is everywhere zero (by definition);

ii) its integral around any closed path is zero;

iii) it is the gradient of a scalar function V.

If $\vec{A}$ represents a vector field, V will represent the potential associated with the field.

Similarly, by definition, if $\vec{A}$ is solenoidal, $\nabla \cdot \vec{A} = 0$ everywhere. Then, by Eq.22,

$$\int_S \vec{A} \cdot d\vec{S} = \int_V \nabla \cdot \vec{A}\, dV = 0$$

for any closed surface S. A solenoidal vector $\vec{A}$ can be, then, expressed as the curl of another vector $\vec{B}$ (a vector potential function), that is,

$$\vec{A} = \nabla \times \vec{B} \qquad (25)$$

Sometimes in order to specify the position of a point P in space, instead of using a Cartesian coordinate system it is better to choose spherical coordinates, which are the distance r from the origin, the latitude ϑ measured from a chosen pole, and the longitude φ measured around the polar axis, as shown in Fig.6. Let $\vec{e}_r$, $\vec{e}_\vartheta$, and $\vec{e}_\varphi$ be unit vectors in the directions of increasing r, ϑ, and φ, respectively. It would be possible to prove that in spherical coordinates the operator ∇ is

$$\nabla = \vec{e}_r \frac{\partial}{\partial r} + \vec{e}_\vartheta \frac{1}{r}\frac{\partial}{\partial \vartheta} + \vec{e}_\varphi \frac{1}{r \sin\vartheta} \frac{\partial}{\partial \varphi} \qquad (26)$$

This expression will be of great future value.

THE MAXWELL'S EQUATIONS

Maxwell pulled together various bits of knowledge concerning electromagnetism into a coherent, unified theory. He was the first to realize that Gauss, Ampère, and Faraday laws, when written in a suitably more general mathematical form and with a necessary modification to Ampère's law to take account of the possibility of time varying electric fields, yield a set of four equations from which all electric and magnetic phenomena can be derived. Maxwell's equations, expressing the relationship between the fields and the sources (charges and currents), as well as the interconnection between time-varying electric and magnetic fields, and Lorentz equation , expressing the force acting on a charge moving under the action of the same fields, summarize all the basic knowledge of electricity and magnetism that has been accumulated during centuries. The further development of the classical theory of electromagnetism consists, not of the introduction of new fundamental laws, but rather of the examination of the consequences of Maxwell's equations, usually after making some appropriate approximations. Therefore, though most of the basic ideas, except for Maxwell's displacement current, were previously known, the field laws of electricity and magnetism are now generally referred to as Maxwell's equations. Below we enumerate the laws, mathematically and verbally, and mention a significant physical consequence of each.

Gauss' law for the general case of a continuous charge distribution is written as

$$\Phi_S(\vec{E}) = \int_S \vec{E} \cdot d\vec{S} = \frac{1}{\varepsilon_0} \int_V \rho dV = \frac{Q}{\varepsilon_0} \tag{27}$$

where $\Phi_S(\vec{E}) = \int_S \vec{E} \cdot d\vec{S}$ is the net electric flux emerging from a closed surface S, ε_0 is the vacuum permittivity, and ρ is the charge density. According to Gauss' law, $\Phi_S(\vec{E})$ is proportional to the total charge Q contained within the surface. A physical consequence: the electric field associated with a stationary point charge is a central inverse-square field. This in turn is related to Coulomb's law of electric force. According to the divergence theorem, it is always possible to transform the surface integral in Gauss'law into a volume integral as follows:

$$\int_S \vec{E} \cdot d\vec{S} = \int_V \nabla \cdot \vec{E} \, dV \tag{28}$$

where the integration is throughout that volume contained by the surface. The volume integral in Gauss'law is also taken throughout the volume enclosed by the surface so that we can write

$$\int_V \nabla \cdot \vec{E} \, dV = \frac{1}{\varepsilon_0} \int_V \rho \, dV \tag{29}$$

The equality of these two integrals for an arbitrary volume V implies that the integrands are identical; that is,

$$\nabla \cdot \vec{E} = \frac{\rho}{\varepsilon_0} \tag{30}$$

This is Maxwell's first equation in its differential form.

Due to the fact that isolated free magnetic poles do not seem to exist, magnetic lines are always closed lines, neither beginning nor ending on magnetic "charges". It is thus not possible to construct a closed surface through which more magnetic lines emerge than enter, or vice-versa, as was the case of electric lines. This means that the surface integral of the magnetic field over any closed surface is zero, and Gauss'law for magnetism is

$$\int_S \vec{H} \cdot d\vec{S} = 0 \tag{31}$$

The same reasoning applied above, implies that

$$\nabla \cdot \vec{H} = 0 \tag{32}$$

This is Maxwell's fourth equation.

The consideration of the magnetic field around a long, straight current led Ampère to establish one of the basic equations of electromagnetism holding for all current arrangements and for all closed paths, which can be stated as follows: the line integral of the magnetic field around any closed path C is equal to the current I threading C namely,

$$\oint \vec{H} \cdot d\vec{s} = I \tag{33}$$

This equation, however, is inconsistent with the law of conservation of charge when there are time-varying fields. In Ampère's law the current I is the total current passing through any surface S bounded by the closed curve C. If we let the closed path C shrink to a single point, as shown in Fig.3, the surface S bounded by C becomes a closed surface, and Ampère's law reduces to

$$0 = I \tag{34}$$

for an arbitrary closed surface S. However, since the net current outward through a closed surface is the rate at which electric charge Q is transported across this surface out of the region inside S, the law of conservation of electric charge implies that

$$I = -\frac{dQ}{dt} \tag{35}$$

where Q is the net charge inside S. Therefore Ampère's law and the law of conservation of charge are consistent only if $dQ/dt = 0$, namely if the net charge within every closed surface remains unchanged as time elapses. Maxwell published a proposed generalization of Ampère's law that could be valid under all circumstances. Maxwell's theory uses Gauss'law (27) for electric field

$$\int_S \vec{E} \cdot d\vec{S} = \frac{Q}{\varepsilon_o} \tag{36}$$

from which dQ/dt can be evaluated:

$$\varepsilon_o \int_S \frac{d\vec{E}}{dt} \cdot d\vec{S} = \frac{dQ}{dt} \tag{37}$$

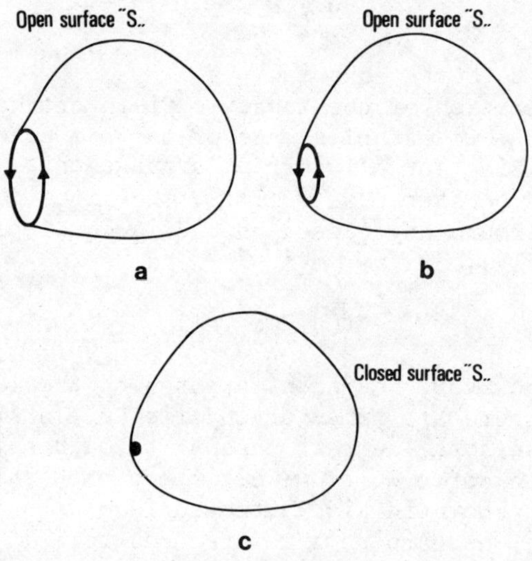

Fig.3 - (a) S is an open surface bounded by the closed path C. (b) When the path C starts to shrink to a point. (c) C is shrunk to a point and the surface S becomes closed.

A quantity I' is defined by

$$I' = I + \int_S \varepsilon_o \frac{d\vec{E}}{dt} \cdot d\vec{S} \tag{38}$$

where I is the current through the surface S; although the term

$$\int_S \varepsilon_o \frac{d\vec{E}}{dt} \cdot d\vec{S}$$

does not represent a flow of electric charge, it does have the dimensions of a current, and it is traditionally called the displacement current. If S is a closed surface, Eqs.35 and 37 imply that

$$I' = -\frac{dQ}{dt} + \frac{dQ}{dt} = 0 \tag{39}$$

The replacement of I in Ampère's law by I' gives the generalization called the Maxwell-Ampère's law,

$$\oint \vec{H} \cdot d\vec{s} = I + \int_S \varepsilon_o \frac{d\vec{E}}{dt} \cdot d\vec{S} \tag{40}$$

When the curve C shrinks to a point and S consequently becomes a closed surface, the Maxwell-Ampère's law gives I' = 0 , which is consistent with Eq.39. And for the steady-state, since $d\vec{E}/dt$ is then zero, the Maxwell-Ampère's law reduces to Ampère's law. Eq.40 may be written in an alternative form in terms of current density (that is the current per unit area). By definition, the total current through the surface S is

$$I = \int_S \vec{j} \cdot d\vec{S}$$

and the alternative form for Maxwell-Ampère's law become

$$\oint \vec{H} \cdot d\vec{s} = \int_S (\vec{j} + \varepsilon_o \frac{\partial \vec{E}}{\partial t}) \cdot d\vec{S} \tag{41}$$

which has general validity. The partial derivative is used since $\vec{E}$ may be a function of position as well of time.

The interpretation of the displacement current is difficult since there is no physical movement of charge associated with it. However, there are magnetic effects associated with the displacement current, which are the same as would arise from a real current equal to the displacement current. This is true in general: whenever an electric field varies with time or charges are moving a magnetic field is produced. Using Stokes' theorem stated above, the line integral of Eq.41 can be transformed into a surface integral, leading to the equation

$$\oint \vec{H} \cdot d\vec{s} = \int_S (\nabla \times \vec{H}) \cdot d\vec{S} \qquad (42)$$

Therefore, Maxwell-Ampère's law may be written as

$$\int_S (\nabla \times \vec{H}) \cdot d\vec{S} = \int_S (\vec{j} + \varepsilon_o \frac{\partial \vec{E}}{\partial t}) \cdot d\vec{S} \qquad (43)$$

which implies

$$\nabla \times \vec{H} = \vec{j} + \varepsilon_o \frac{\partial \vec{E}}{\partial t} \qquad (44)$$

This is the Maxwell's second equation.

In a region where a magnetic field is changing, there is an electric field which is related to the time rate of change of the magnetic field. A physical consequence is that a moving magnet or a changing magnetic flux can induce a current in a coil. The fundamental relationship between the electric field $\vec{E}$ and the time rate of change $\partial\vec{H}/\partial t$ of the magnetic field which is inferred from the results of a tremendous variety of experiments is Faraday's law

$$\oint \vec{E} \cdot d\vec{s} = - \mu_o \int_S \frac{\partial \vec{H}}{\partial t} \cdot d\vec{S} \qquad (45)$$

where S is any open surface bounded by an arbitrary closed curve C, and μ_o is the vacuum permeability. By definition of magnetic flux $\Phi_S(\vec{H})$

$$\Phi_S(\vec{H}) = \int_S \vec{H} \cdot d\vec{S} \qquad (46)$$

so that Eq.45 may be written as

$$\oint \vec{E} \cdot d\vec{s} = -\mu_o \frac{d\Phi_S(\vec{H})}{dt} \qquad (47)$$

Applying Stokes' theorem to the line integral in Eq.45 yields

$$\oint \vec{E} \cdot d\vec{s} = \int_S (\nabla \times \vec{E}) \cdot d\vec{S} \qquad (48)$$

so that

$$\int_S (\nabla \times \vec{E}) \cdot d\vec{S} = - \int_S \mu_o \frac{\partial \vec{H}}{\partial t} \cdot d\vec{S} \qquad (49)$$

which implies

$$\nabla \times \vec{E} = -\mu_o \frac{\partial \vec{H}}{\partial t} \tag{50}$$

This is Maxwell's third equation.

In Table 1 we summarize the four Maxwell's equations, written in both their integral and differential form.

Table 1 - Integral and differential form of Maxwell's equations

Equation	Integral form	Differential form
1	$\int_S \vec{E} \cdot d\vec{S} = \frac{Q}{\varepsilon_o}$	$\nabla \cdot \vec{E} = \frac{\rho}{\varepsilon_o}$
2	$\oint \vec{H} \cdot d\vec{s} = \int_S (\vec{j} + \varepsilon_o \frac{\partial \vec{E}}{\partial t}) \cdot d\vec{S}$	$\nabla \times \vec{H} = \vec{j} + \varepsilon_o \frac{\partial \vec{E}}{\partial t}$
3	$\oint \vec{E} \cdot d\vec{s} = -\mu_o \frac{d\,\Phi(H)}{dt}$	$\nabla \times \vec{E} = -\mu_o \frac{\partial \vec{H}}{\partial t}$
4	$\int_S \vec{H} \cdot d\vec{S} = 0$	$\nabla \cdot \vec{H} = 0$

The four Maxwell's equations express the relationship that exist between electric and magnetic field vectors $\vec{E}$ and $\vec{H}$. They have been developed in vacuum, where $\varepsilon = \varepsilon_o$ and $\mu = \mu_o$. To take account of the electrical and magnetic properties of matter, as they will be treated in later lectures, we will introduce the new field vectors

$D = \varepsilon\vec{E}$, and $\vec{B} = \mu\vec{H}$.

A term-by-term correspondence of differential form of Maxwell's equations to their integral form is evident. Differential equations relate derivatives of $\vec{E}$ and $\vec{H}$, both time and space derivatives, to charge and current densities. They are local equations. The fields in the neighborhood of a point, both the spatial and temporal neighborhood, are related to the charge and current at that point. Thus the idea of action-at-a-distance is completely missing from these equations. Nevertheless, it is in the nature of a differential equation that although the equation itself spans only an infinitesimal neighborhood, the solution of the equation spans a finite, or possibly even an infinite, range of space and time. It is possible to notice an interesting thing about the set of equations shown in Table 1, when the case is treated in which nothing depends on the time, called the static case. In the static case all charges are permanently fixed in space, or if they do move, they move as a steady flow in a circuit, so ρ and $\vec{j}$ are constant in time. In these circumstances, all of the terms in the Maxwell equations which are time derivatives of the field are zero. In this case, the Maxwell's equations become:

$$\begin{cases} \nabla \cdot \vec{E} = \rho/\varepsilon_o \\ \nabla \times \vec{H} = \vec{j} \\ \nabla \times \vec{E} = 0 \\ \nabla \cdot \vec{H} = 0 \end{cases} \tag{51}$$

and the electric and magnetic fields are not interconnected. This means that electricity and magnetism are distinct phenomena as long as charges and currents are static. The interdependence of $\vec{E}$ and $\vec{H}$ does not appear until there are changes in charges or currents, as when a condenser is charged, or a magnet moved. Only when there are sufficiently rapid changes, so that the time derivatives in Maxwell equations become significant, will $\vec{E}$ and $\vec{H}$ depend on each other. Later we shall show how Maxwell's equations for free space directly point to the existence of electromagnetic waves and deduce some of the properties of the waves.

SOLVING MAXWELL'S EQUATIONS

Now we would like to solve Maxwell's equations. We begin with the simplest of the equations, namely,

$$\nabla \cdot \vec{H} = 0 \tag{52}$$

which implies that $\vec{H}$ is everywhere solenoidal. As stated before a solenoidal vector can be always expressed as the curl of another vector. So, if we write

$$\vec{H} = \frac{1}{\mu_o} \nabla \times \vec{A} \tag{53}$$

where $\vec{H}$ is written for free space, we have already solved one of Maxwell's equations. The vector field $\vec{A}$, called magnetic vector potential, is of great interest and simplifies many computations, as we illustrate later. If we take into account Eq.53 and differentiate with respect to t the third Maxwell's equation, we may write

$$\nabla \times \vec{E} = - \frac{\partial}{\partial t} (\nabla \times \vec{A}) \tag{54}$$

Since we can differentiate either with respect to time or to space first, we can also write Eq.54 as

$$\nabla \times \vec{E} + \frac{\partial}{\partial t} (\nabla \times \vec{A}) = \nabla \times (\vec{E} + \frac{\partial \vec{A}}{\partial t}) = 0 \tag{55}$$

Since $\vec{E} + \partial\vec{A}/\partial t$ is an irrotational vector, it is the gradient of some scalar function V. For technical convenience, we take it to be the gradient of $-V$, and we set

$$\vec{E} + \frac{\partial \vec{A}}{\partial t} = - \nabla V \tag{56}$$

From Eq.56 we deduce that

$$\vec{E} = - \frac{\partial \vec{A}}{\partial t} - \nabla V \tag{57}$$

We have solved two of Maxwell's equations already, and we have found that to describe the electromagnetic fields $\vec{E}$ and $\vec{H}$, we need four potential functions: a scalar potential V and a vector potential $\vec{A}$, which corresponds, of course, to the three components A_x, A_y, and A_z.

Previously we focused our attention on the Maxwell's equations which did not involve any currents or charges. Now we return to the two remaining equations which will give us the relations between the potentials and the sources ρ and $\vec{j}$. Once we can determine $\vec{A}$ and V from the currents and charges, we can always get $\vec{E}$ and $\vec{H}$ from Eqs.53 and 57. Substituting Eq.57 in the first Maxwell's equation, we get

$$\nabla \cdot (- \nabla V - \frac{\partial \vec{A}}{\partial t}) = \rho / \varepsilon_o \tag{58}$$

which we can write also as

$$- \nabla^2 V - \frac{\partial}{\partial t} \nabla \cdot \vec{A} = \frac{\rho}{\varepsilon_o} \tag{59}$$

This is our first equation relating V and $\vec{A}$ to the sources. The final equation will result the most complicated. We write the second Maxwell's equations as

$$\nabla \times \vec{H} - \varepsilon_o \frac{\partial \vec{E}}{\partial t} = \vec{j} \qquad (60)$$

and then substitute for $\vec{H}$ and $\vec{E}$ in terms of the potential:

$$\nabla \times \left(\frac{1}{\mu_o} \nabla \times \vec{A}\right) - \varepsilon_o \frac{\partial}{\partial t}\left(- \nabla V - \frac{\partial \vec{A}}{\partial t}\right) = \vec{j} \qquad (61)$$

Taking into account the algebraic identity $\nabla \times (\nabla \times \vec{A}) = \nabla(\nabla \cdot \vec{A}) - \nabla^2 \vec{A}$ and the relation $\varepsilon_o \mu_o = 1/c^2$ we get

$$- c^2 \nabla^2 \vec{A} + c^2 \nabla (\nabla \cdot \vec{A}) + \frac{\partial}{\partial t} \nabla V + \frac{\partial^2 \vec{A}}{\partial t^2} = \frac{1}{\varepsilon_o} \vec{j} \qquad (62)$$

To simplify Eq.62 we can now make use of the freedom to choose arbitrarily the divergence of $\vec{A}$. This freedom arises from the fact that if $\vec{H}$ is given, the equation $1/\mu_o \text{ rot } \vec{A} = 1/\mu_o \nabla \times \vec{A} = \vec{H}$ does not determine $\vec{A}$ completely. A theorem of vector analysis states that to determine $\vec{A}$ in full detail we must be given not only its curl, namely $\mu_o \vec{H}$, but also its divergence. If only its curl is given, then, with due regard for the proper boundary conditions, we are at liberty to specify the divergence of $\vec{A}$ as we please. Choosing the $\nabla \cdot \vec{A}$ is called "choosing a gauge". What we are going to do now is to use our choice to fix things so that the equations for $\vec{A}$ and for V are separated but have the same form. We can do this by taking

$$\nabla \cdot \vec{A} = - \frac{1}{c^2} \frac{\partial V}{\partial t} \qquad (63)$$

which is called the Lorentz gauge.

When we do that, the two middle terms in $\vec{A}$ and V in Eq.62 cancel, and that equation becomes much simpler:

$$\nabla^2 \vec{A} - \frac{1}{c^2} \frac{\partial^2 \vec{A}}{\partial t^2} = - \frac{\vec{j}}{\varepsilon_o c^2} \qquad (64)$$

wheras our equation for V (Eq.59), takes on the same form

$$\nabla^2 V - \frac{1}{c^2} \frac{\partial^2 V}{\partial t^2} = - \frac{\rho}{\varepsilon_o} \qquad (65)$$

Maxwell's equations have led us to a new kind of equation for the potentials V and $\vec{A}$ but to the same mathematical form for all four functions V, A_x, A_y, and A_z. Moreover, Eqs.64 and 65 are nicely separated, going V and $\vec{A}$ with the charge and current densities, respectively. Once we learn how to solve these equations, we can get H and $\vec{E}$ from $1/\mu_o \nabla x \vec{A}$ (Eq.53) and $- \partial\vec{A}/\partial t - \nabla V$ (Eq.57). We have another form of the electromagnetic laws exactly equivalent to Maxwell's equations, but much simpler to handle in many situations.

In free space, where $\rho = 0$ and $\vec{j} = 0$, Eqs.64 and 65 take on the simpler form

$$\nabla^2 V - \frac{1}{c^2} \frac{\partial^2 V}{\partial t^2} = 0 \tag{66}$$

$$\nabla^2 \vec{A} - \frac{1}{c^2} \frac{\partial^2 \vec{A}}{\partial t^2} = 0 \tag{67}$$

Thus in free space the scalar potential V and the vector potential $\vec{A}$ satisfy the same mathematical equation describing in physics the propagation of mechanical waves, namely sound waves, or waves on a stretched string, moving out at the speed c.

It is possible to show that if we let Ψ stand for any of the four quantities V, $\vec{A}$, $\vec{H}$, and $\vec{E}$, the same general three-dimensional wave equation

$$\nabla^2 \Psi - \frac{1}{c^2} \frac{\partial^2 \Psi}{\partial t^2} = 0 \tag{68}$$

is always satisfied.

RADIATION FROM A SHORT ANTENNA

As an important example of the implications of Maxwell's four equations taken together, we will consider the radiation emitted by an idealized short antenna, the limiting case of an antenna whose length tends to zero.

As a first step we evaluate the magnitude of the static dipole field at the point P. The potential at the point P due to the charges +q and -q, shown in Fig.4, is

$$V = \frac{1}{4\pi\varepsilon_o} \left(\frac{q}{r_1} - \frac{q}{r_2}\right) = \frac{q}{4\pi\varepsilon_o} \cdot \frac{r_2 - r_1}{r_1 r_2}$$

For $\ell \ll r$, we can set

$$r_1 r_2 \simeq r^2 \quad \text{and} \quad r_2 - r_1 \simeq \ell \cos\vartheta$$

Therefore

$$V = \frac{q\ell\cos\vartheta}{4\pi\varepsilon_o r^2} = \frac{p_e\cdot\cos\vartheta}{4\pi\varepsilon_o r^2} \tag{69}$$

being $p_e = q\cdot\ell$ the electrical dipole moment associated with the electrical dipole.

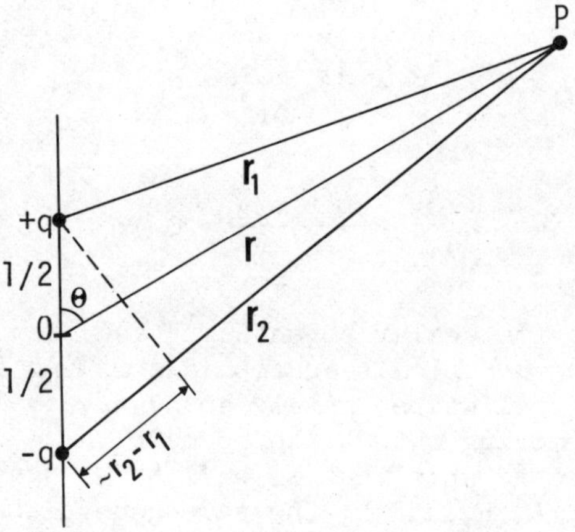

Fig.4 - The static dipole field at the point P.

Let us take the point O at the center of the dipole as the origin of a spherical polar coordinate system.

If V is the potential and $\vec{E} = \vec{e}_r E_r + \vec{e}_\vartheta E_\vartheta + \vec{e}_\varphi E_\varphi$ ($\vec{e}_r$, $\vec{e}_\vartheta$ and $\vec{e}_\varphi$ clearly are unit vectors in the direction of increasing r, and φ, respectively) is the static dipole field at the point P(r, ϑ, φ), for spherical coordinates we obtain

$$\vec{E} = -\nabla V = \left(\frac{\partial V}{\partial r}\right)\vec{e}_r + \frac{1}{r}\left(\frac{\partial V}{\partial\vartheta}\right)\vec{e}_\vartheta + \frac{1}{r\sin\vartheta}\left(\frac{\partial V}{\partial\varphi}\right)\vec{e}_\varphi$$

Consequently, the spherical components of $\vec{E}$ at P are

$$E_r = -\frac{\partial V}{\partial r} = \frac{2p_e\cos\vartheta}{4\pi\varepsilon_o r^3} \tag{70}$$

$$E_\vartheta = -\frac{1}{r}\frac{\partial V}{\partial \vartheta} = \frac{p_e \sin\vartheta}{4\pi\varepsilon_o r^3} \tag{71}$$

and, since V is independent of φ,

$$E_\varphi = -\frac{1}{r\sin\vartheta}\frac{\partial V}{\partial\varphi} = 0 \tag{72}$$

In order to evaluate the components of $\vec{H}$ at P (r, ϑ, φ), we recall that if we consider a portion of length $d\vec{l}$ of a thin wire carrying a steady current i, its contribution to $\vec{H}$ at P (Biot-Savart Law, Fig.5) is

$$d\vec{H} = \frac{i\,d\ell}{4\pi}\frac{\sin\vartheta}{r^2}\vec{e}_\varphi \tag{73}$$

Since $\ell \ll r$, we can take $d\ell \simeq \ell$ and $d\vec{H} \simeq \vec{H}$.

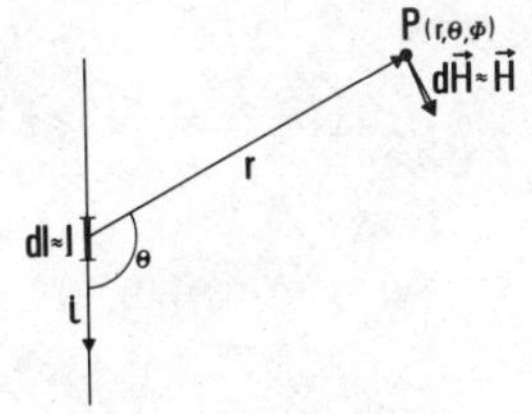

Fig.5 - Contribution to $\vec{H}$ at P caused by a portion of length dl of a thin wire carrying a steady current i (Biot-Savart Law).

Consequently, the spherical components of $\vec{H}$ at P are

$$H_r = 0$$

$$H_\vartheta = 0 \qquad (74)$$

$$H_\varphi = \frac{i d\ell}{4\pi} \cdot \frac{\sin\vartheta}{r^2}$$

We are now ready to evaluate the radiation pattern of an oscillating dipole.

The antenna we are interested in, far removed from the ground and other objects, consists of two straight wires with an a.c. generator connected between them, as in Fig.6, and metal spheres at their free ends. Owing to the presence of the generator, electrons are sent up and down the wires and charges on the spheres are periodically reversed so that the antenna has an alternating electric moment, given by

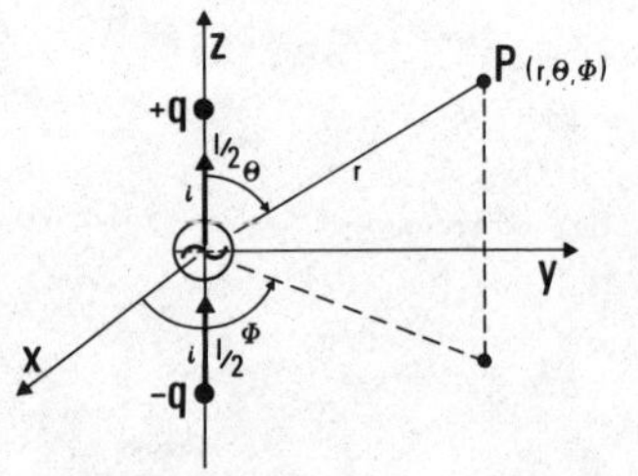

Fig.6 - Evaluating the field of the oscillating Hertzian dipole at a point $P(r,\vartheta,\varphi)$.

$$p_e = q \cdot \ell \qquad (75)$$

where q is the charge at the metal spheres and ℓ is the length of the antenna ($\ell \to 0$).

It is assumed that, at any instant, the current i in the antenna has the same value at every cross section of the wire, and is given by

$$i = I \cos \omega t \tag{76}$$

where ω is the angular frequency.

The problem is to find at any instant the field of the oscillating dipole at point $P(r,\vartheta,\varphi)$, as shown in Fig.6. Since

$$i = \frac{dq}{dt} \tag{77}$$

the charge at one end of the antenna as a function of t is given by

$$q = \int_0^t i\, dt' = \int_0^t I \cos \omega t' dt' = \frac{I}{\omega} \sin \omega t \tag{78}$$

and the dipole electric moment has magnitude

$$p_e = q\ell = \frac{I\cdot \ell}{\omega} \sin \omega t \tag{79}$$

We assume that the antenna is so short that $\ell \ll r$, and the distance from the point P to any part of the dipole is practically equal to r. Since electromagnetic effects travel with the speed c in vacuum or air, the time required for an electromagnetic interaction to travel from the antenna to P is then r/c. Consequently, the electric field at P at an instant t will be determined by the electric moment of the antenna at an earlier instant, say τ, given by the formula

$$\tau = t - \frac{r}{c} \tag{80}$$

and called the retarded time. Thus, the effects felt at P at an instant t are caused not by the current and electric moment expressed by Eqs.75 and 76, but by their earlier values, namely,

$$i = I \cos \omega t \tag{81}$$

and

$$p_e = \frac{I\ell}{\omega} \sin \omega t \tag{82}$$

As usual in all perturbative methods, we write $\vec{E}_o$ and $\vec{H}_o$ for the first approximation to the complete fields $\vec{E}$ and $\vec{H}$.

To get our first approximation to $\vec{E}$ and $\vec{H}$ at P we substitute the time-dependent expression for p_e (Eqs.81 and 82) into the static components stated above, and find that

$$\begin{cases} E_{or} = \dfrac{2\, I\ell \cos\vartheta}{4\pi\varepsilon_o \omega r^3} \sin\omega\tau \\ \\ E_{o\vartheta} = \dfrac{I\ell \sin\vartheta}{4\pi\varepsilon_o\omega r^3} \sin\omega\tau \\ \\ E_{o\varphi} = 0 \end{cases} \tag{83}$$

and

$$\begin{cases} H_{or} = 0 \\ \\ H_{o\vartheta} = 0 \\ \\ H_{o\varphi} = \dfrac{I\ell \sin\vartheta}{4\pi r^2} \cos\omega\tau \end{cases} \tag{84}$$

At least roughly, one can say that the fields $\vec{E}_o$ and $\vec{H}_o$ are produced directly by the charges on the ends of the antenna and by the current flowing in the antenna, respectively.

These fields are, of course, only an approximation to the correct field because, as indicated by Maxwell's second and third equations, a changing electric field produces a changing magnetic field and a changing magnetic field produces a changing electric field. Both of these extra fields will in turn generate time varying fields, and so on, and only the resultants of all these fields will satisfy Maxwell's equations. However, we would expect that the exact fields reduce, close enough to the antenna, to those expressed by Eqs.83 and 84. From this point of view, the combination of the fields $\vec{E}_o$ and $\vec{H}_o$ is called the local field of the antenna, and the region where this field is a sufficiently good approximation is called the near zone, or reactive zone or Fresnel region. Note that

$$\omega\tau = \omega\left(t - \frac{r}{c}\right) = \omega t - \frac{\omega r}{c} = \omega t - Kr \tag{85}$$

where $K = 2\pi/\lambda = \omega/c$ is the wave propagation constant; when $r \to 0$, as in the near zone, $\tau \to t$.

As stated above the fields $\vec{E}_o$ and $\vec{H}_o$ do not satisfy Maxwell's free-space equations exactly, but it is possible to proceed to use in a self-consistent manner the simplest components to uncover discrepancies which in turn will guide in searching successive corrections. It is possible to show that this method converges, and when these extra contributions are added to the time-varying dipole field we get the complete electromagnetic field

$$\begin{cases} E_r = \dfrac{2\, I\ell \cos\vartheta}{4\pi\varepsilon_0 \omega r^3} \sin\omega\tau + \dfrac{2\, I\ell\cos\vartheta}{4\pi\varepsilon_0 c r^2}\cos\omega\tau \\ E_\vartheta = \dfrac{I\ell\sin\vartheta}{4\pi\varepsilon_0\omega r^3}\sin\omega\tau + \dfrac{I\ell\sin\vartheta}{4\pi\varepsilon_0 c r^2}\cos\omega\tau - \dfrac{I\ell\omega\sin\vartheta}{4\pi\varepsilon_0 c^2 r}\sin\omega\tau \\ E_\varphi = 0 \end{cases} \tag{86}$$

and

$$\begin{cases} H_r = 0 \\ H_\vartheta = 0 \\ H_\varphi = \dfrac{I\ell\sin\vartheta}{4\pi r^2}\cos\omega\tau - \dfrac{\omega I\ell\sin\vartheta}{4\pi c r}\sin\omega\tau \end{cases} \tag{87}$$

The same general results can be obtained using directly Maxwell's equations and the procedures previously described. The electric field about the dipole no longer is the same as the static field. In fact, the time-dependent field even includes closed lines, as shown in Fig.7, that are detached from the dipole. For r small enough, however, the exact field reduces to the local fields $\vec{E}_0$ and $\vec{H}_0$. If we consider the opposite extreme and let r grow large, the dominant terms in the complete field are the terms in r^{-1}, and these fields reduce to

$$\vec{E} = -\frac{\omega I\ell\sin\vartheta}{4\pi\varepsilon_0 c^2 r}\sin\omega\tau\cdot\vec{e}_\vartheta = \frac{\omega I\ell\sin\vartheta}{4\pi\varepsilon_0 c^2 r}\sin(Kr-\omega t)\cdot\vec{e}_\vartheta \tag{88}$$

and

$$\vec{H} = -\frac{\omega I\ell\sin\vartheta}{4\pi c r}\sin\omega\tau\cdot\vec{e}_\varphi = \frac{\omega I\ell\sin\vartheta}{4\pi c r}\sin(Kr-\omega t)\,\vec{e}_\varphi \tag{89}$$

The region where this approximation is applicable is called the far zone of the antenna, or the radiative zone, or Fraunhofer region.

In this region the fields $\vec{E}$ and $\vec{H}$ are mutually perpendicular

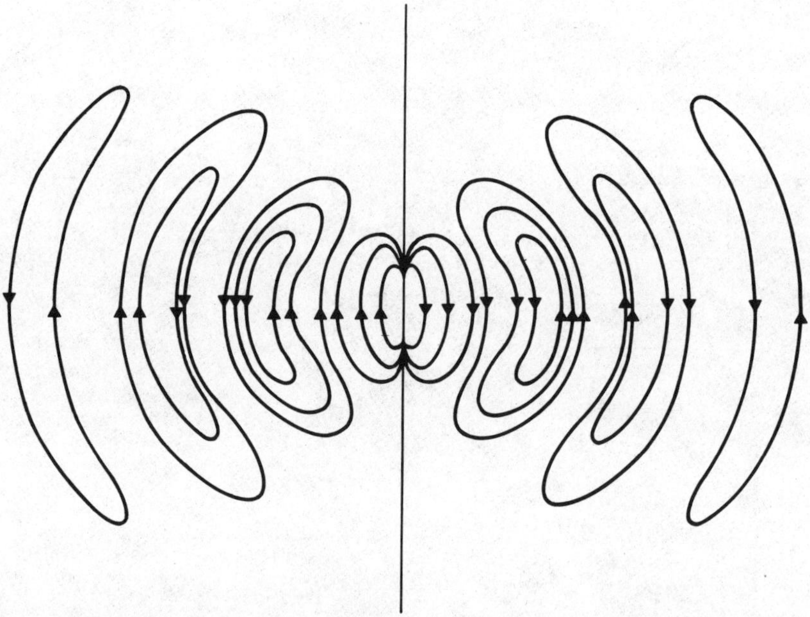

Fig.7 - The time-dependent electric field about the Hertzian dipole.

and, in contrast to the near zone (where $\vec{H}$ is $\pi/2$ radiant out of phase with $\vec{E}$), they are in phase with each other. These features are illustrated in Fig.8.

If we consider, as shown in Fig.9, a point P in the far zone of the antenna so close to the y axis that

$$|x| \ll y \quad ; \quad |z| \ll y$$

the following approximations then hold at P:

$$r \simeq y \ , \ \sin\vartheta \simeq \sin\frac{\pi}{2} \simeq 1$$

and

$$\vec{e}_r \simeq \vec{j} \ , \ \vec{e}_\vartheta \simeq -\vec{k} \ , \ \vec{e}_\varphi \simeq -\vec{i}$$

where $\vec{i}$, $\vec{j}$ and $\vec{k}$ are unit vectors in the direction of increasing x, y, and z respectively.

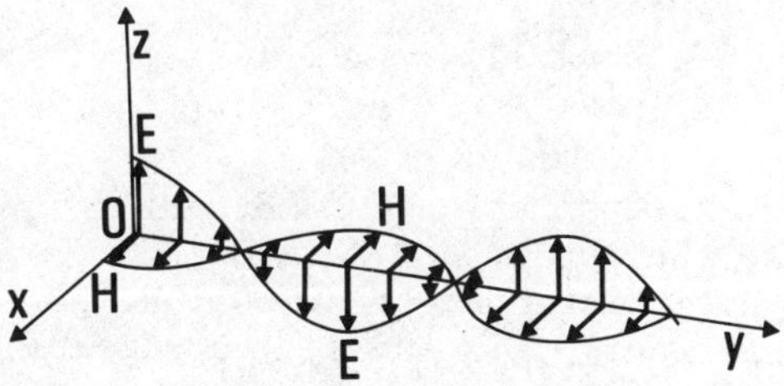

Fig.8 - A wave moving in the y direction, described at a fixed value of t by the vectors $\vec{E}$ and $\vec{H}$.

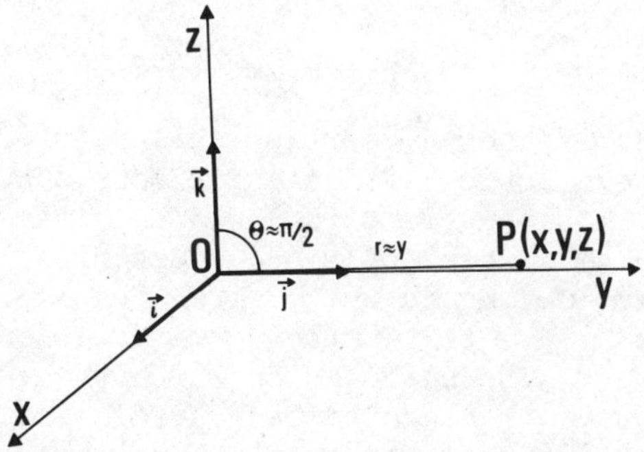

Fig.9 - A point P in the far zone of the antenna very close to the y axis.

When we make these approximations in (88) and (89), and change the signs of fields to simplify equations, we get the approximate formulas

$$\vec{E} = \frac{\omega I \ell}{4\pi\varepsilon_o c^2 y} \sin (Ky - \omega t)\, \vec{k} \tag{90}$$

$$\vec{H} = \frac{\omega I \ell}{4\pi\, cy} \sin (Ky - \omega t)\, \vec{i} \tag{91}$$

Eqs.90 and 91 are exact solutions of Maxwell's equations, called plane waves. Since the function $\frac{1}{y}$ does not change considerably if y is large enough, as it is in our assumptions, the coefficients of the sine factors in Eqs.70, 71 and 73, representing peak values of the fields, can be regarded as constants and denoted by E_p and H_p respectively. In terms of the new symbols, a plane wave moving in the +y direction, is described by

$$\vec{E} = E_p \sin (Ky - \omega t)\, \vec{k} \tag{92}$$

and

$$\vec{H} = H_p \sin (Ky - \omega t)\, \vec{i} \tag{93}$$

where, recalling that $c = 1/\sqrt{\varepsilon_o \mu_o}$, the constant peak values E_p and H_p satisfy the equation

$$E_p = Z_o H_p \tag{94}$$

The parameter $Z_o = \sqrt{\mu_o/\varepsilon_o}$ is called the intrinsic impedance of free space.

Note that Eqs.92 and 93, derived making further approximations in the approximate solutions for the far zone prove to be an exact solution of Maxwell's equations, and not only far from the origin, but for any value of y. Maps of $\vec{E}$ and $\vec{H}$ describing, at a fixed value of t , a plane wave moving in the y direction are shown in Fig.10.

The quantity $Ky - \omega t \pm \varphi_o$ (being φ_o a constant) is called the phase of $\vec{E}$ and $\vec{H}$. The surfaces on which the phase is constant at a fixed instant of time are called surfaces of constant phase pertaining to that instant. The vector $\vec{K}$ pointing in the direction of propagation of a plane wave and having magnitude equal to the propagation constant K is the wave propagation vector. At any point P, the vector $\vec{E}$ in Eq.92 is perpendicular to the propagation vector $\vec{K}$, and the field is called a transverse electric wave (a TE wave). Similarly, $\vec{H}$ in Eq.93 is perpendicular to $\vec{K}$, and therefore is called a transverse magnetic wave (a TM wave). Since both $\vec{E}$ and $\vec{H}$ are per-

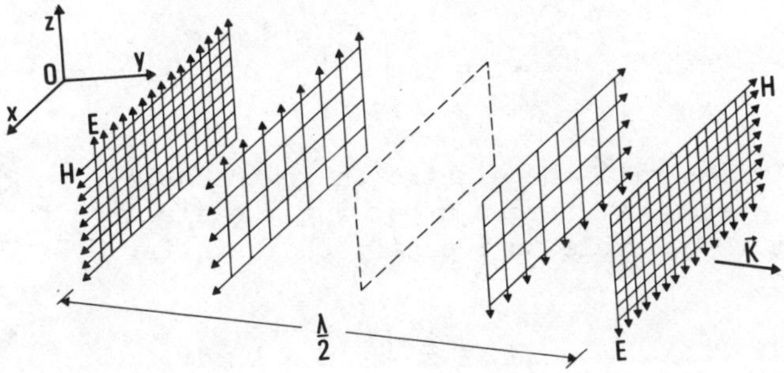

Fig.10 - Maps of $\vec{E}$ and $\vec{H}$ describing, at a fixed value of t, a plane wave moving in the y direction.

pendicular to $\vec{K}$, this wave is a transverse electromagnetic wave (a TEM wave). In plane waves vectors $\vec{E}$ and $\vec{H}$ at any point are parallel to a fixed line (in this case, the z and x axis, respectively), and for this reason they are said to be linearly polarized. The frequency of plane waves, namely $\nu = \omega/2\pi$, is a constant and, therefore, they are called monochromatic. From Eqs. 92 and 93 formulas for linearly polarized plane monochromatic TEM waves moving in any direction can be constructed and written as

$$\vec{E} = \vec{E}_p \cos(\vec{K} \cdot \vec{r} - \omega t + \varphi_o) \tag{95}$$

$$\vec{H} = \vec{H}_p \cos(\vec{K} \cdot \vec{r} - \omega t + \varphi_o) \tag{96}$$

where $\vec{H}_p = 1/\mu_o\omega(\vec{K} \times \vec{E}_p)$, $\vec{E}_p$ being a constant vector normal to $\vec{K}$. Eqs.95 and 96 are, of course, solutions of the wave equation 68.

The theory of the Hertzian dipole serves as a starting point to the study of actual antennas. Note, however, that even in the case of the simplest actual antennas, the current usually does not have the same value at every cross section of the wire, and the proximity of the ground may cause the image of the antenna in the ground to play an essential role.

ENERGY FLOW IN THE ELECTROMAGNETIC FIELD

By computing the work done in establishing a static electric field it is possible to show that the quantity

$$W_E = \frac{1}{2}\int_V \vec{E}\cdot\vec{D}\;dV \qquad (97)$$

can be identified with the electrostatic potential energy in the volume of the system of charges producing the electric field. In a similar way it is possible to identify the quantity

$$W_M = \frac{1}{2}\int_V \vec{H}\cdot\vec{B}\;dV \qquad (98)$$

with the energy stored in the magnetic field. This section is devoted to analyse the applicability of these expressions to nonstatic situations. If the scalar product of the second Maxwell's equation with $\vec{E}$ is taken, and the resulting equation is substracted from the scalar product of the third Maxwell's equation with $\vec{H}$, the resulting equation is

$$\vec{H}\cdot\nabla\times\vec{E} - \vec{E}\cdot\nabla\times\vec{H} = \mu_o\,\vec{H}\cdot\frac{\partial\vec{H}}{\partial t} - \varepsilon_o\,\vec{E}\cdot\frac{\partial\vec{E}}{\partial t} - \vec{E}\cdot\vec{j} \quad (99)$$

The left side of this expression can be converted into a divergence by using the identity

$$\nabla\cdot(\vec{A}\times\vec{B}) = \vec{B}\cdot\nabla\times\vec{A} - \vec{A}\cdot\nabla\times\vec{B} \qquad (100)$$

to obtain

$$\nabla\cdot(\vec{E}\times\vec{H}) = -\vec{H}\cdot\frac{\partial\vec{B}}{\partial t} - \vec{E}\cdot\frac{\partial\vec{D}}{\partial t} - \vec{E}\cdot\vec{j} \qquad (101)$$

where $\vec{B}=\mu_o\vec{H}$ and $\vec{D}=\varepsilon_o\vec{E}$ in vacuum. Being in free space μ_o and ε_o constants independent of the field variable and time, the time derivatives on the right of (101) can be written as

$$\vec{H}\cdot\frac{\partial\vec{B}}{\partial t} = \vec{H}\cdot\frac{\partial}{\partial t}(\mu_o\,\vec{H}) = \frac{1}{2}\mu_o\frac{\partial\vec{H}^2}{\partial t} = \frac{\partial}{\partial t}\left(\frac{1}{2}\vec{H}\cdot\vec{B}\right) \quad (102)$$

and

$$\vec{E} \cdot \frac{\partial \vec{D}}{\partial t} = \vec{E} \cdot \frac{\partial}{\partial t} (\varepsilon_o \vec{E}) = \frac{1}{2} \varepsilon_o \frac{\partial \vec{E}^2}{\partial t} = \frac{\partial}{\partial t} (\frac{1}{2} \vec{E} \cdot \vec{D}) \tag{103}$$

Using these relationships, Eq.101 takes the form

$$\nabla \cdot (\vec{E} \times \vec{H}) = - \frac{\partial}{\partial t} \left[\frac{1}{2} (\vec{E} \cdot \vec{D} + \vec{B} \cdot \vec{H}) \right] - \vec{j} \cdot \vec{E} \tag{104}$$

The first term on the right is the time derivative of the sum of the electric and magnetic energy densities; the second term is, in many cases, just the negative of the Joule heating rate per unit volume. Integrating over a fixed volume V bounded by the surface S gives

$$\int_V \nabla \cdot (\vec{E} \times \vec{H}) \, dV = - \frac{\partial}{\partial t} \int_V \frac{1}{2} (\vec{E} \cdot \vec{D} + \vec{B} \cdot \vec{H}) \, dV - \int_V \vec{j} \cdot \vec{E} \, dV \tag{105}$$

Applying the divergence theorem to the left side, we obtain

$$\int_S (\vec{E} \times \vec{H}) \cdot d\vec{S} = - \frac{\partial}{\partial t} \int_V \frac{1}{2} (\vec{E} \cdot \vec{D} + \vec{B} \cdot \vec{H}) \, dV - \int_V \vec{j} \cdot \vec{E} \, dV \tag{106}$$

Rewriting this equation:

$$- \int_V \vec{j} \cdot \vec{E} \, dV = \frac{\partial}{\partial t} \int_V \frac{1}{2} (\vec{E} \cdot \vec{D} + \vec{B} \cdot \vec{H}) \, dV + \int_S (\vec{E} \times \vec{H}) \cdot d\vec{S} \tag{107}$$

makes it clear that the $\vec{j} \cdot \vec{E}$ term is comprised of two parts: the rate of change of electromagnetic energy stored in V, and a surface integral. The left side of Eq.107 is the power transferred into the electromagnetic field through the motion of free charge in volume V. Since the surface integral in Eq.107 involves only the electric and magnetic fields, it is feasible to interpret this term as the rate of energy flow across the surface. It is tempting to interpret $\vec{E} \times \vec{H}$ itself as the energy flow per unit time per unit area. The latter interpretation, however, leads to certain inconsistencies, and a complete analysis involves the concepts of electromagnetic momentum and angular momentum. The only interpretation which survives careful scruting is that

$$\int_S (\vec{E} \times \vec{H}) \, d\vec{S}$$

represents the rate at which electromagnetic energy crosses the closed surface S. The vector $\vec{E} \times \vec{H}$ is known as the Poynting vector, and is usually represented by the symbol $\vec{S}$. Equation 107 thus expresses the conservation of energy in a fixed volume V. Since the vector $\vec{E} \times \vec{H}$ points in the direction in which the electromagnetic wave is travelling, an electromagnetic wave transports energy in the direction in which is travelling.

REFERENCES

1. R. P. Feynman, R. B. Leighton and M. Sands, "Lectures on Physics," Addison Wesley, Reading (1964).
2. C. H. Durney and C. C. Johnson, "Introduction to modern electromagnetics," McGraw-Hill Company, New York (1969).
3. V. Rojansky, "Electromagnetic Fields and Waves," Prentice Hall Inc., London (1971).
4. L. D. Landau and E. M. Lifshitz, "The classical theory of fields," Pergamon Press, Oxford (1962).
5. R. L. Armstrong and J. D. King, "The electromagnetic interaction," Prentice Hall Inc., London (1973).

FUNDAMENTALS OF THE INTERACTIONS OF RADIO-FREQUENCY AND MICROWAVE ENERGIES WITH MATTER

Maria A. Stuchly

Radiation Protection Bureau, Health and Welfare Canada
Ottawa, Ontario K1A 0L2, and

Department of Electrical Engineering, University of Ottawa, Ottawa, Ontario

INTRODUCTION

A relatively large segment of the electromagnetic spectrum is occupied by radio-frequencies (RF) and microwaves (MW). The lower part between a few tens of kilohertz (kHz) and 300 megahertz (MHz) is called radio-frequencies, while the upper part between 300 MHz and 300 gigahertz (GHz) is named microwaves. The corresponding wavelengths extend from a few tens of kilometres (km) to 1 metre (m) for radio-frequencies and from 1 m to 1 millimetre (mm) for microwaves. The quantum energies at these frequencies are very small and not capable of altering the intramolecular structure nor breaking any intermolecular bonds. The maximum quantum energy (at 300 GHz) is 1.2×10^{-3} electronvolt (eV), while a disruption of the weekest hydrogen bond requires 0.08 eV, for comparison, the thermal motion energy at 30°C is 2.6×10^{-2} eV.

The interaction of RF and MW radiation with matter is described by Maxwell's equations reflecting the wave-like rather than the particulate nature of the interaction. The wavelengths of the radiation are much greater than the dimensions of atomic or molecular structures. However, the wavelengths are comparable to dimensions of many objects, including biological bodies, and electrical circuit components. This contributes to a complexity of physical interactions and subsequently their mathematical representation.

Physical aspects of the interactions of RF and microwave radiation with matter, including biological systems, can be described in two separate but interrelated ways. Macroscopic interactions are expressed in terms of classical electrodynamics (i.e., Faraday's induction law, Maxwell's equations). The interactions are determined by the electric permittivity and magnetic permeability of the medium. The solutions are sought in terms of the distribution of the electric and magnetic fields inside and outside of a given object. In case of lossy objects, the absorbed power i.e. the rate of energy absorption is of interest.

Microscopic interactions are expressed in terms of occurences on atomic, molecular or cellular levels caused by the applied RF or microwave fields. A specific mechanism of interaction may be due to an electric field or magnetic field or both. Types of microscopic interactions depend on the structure of a given medium and vary with the frequency of the applied field.

The electric permittivity and magnetic permeability are macroscopic expressions of microscopic interactions. Both are complex numbers, the permittivity describes the interactions in response to the electric field, the permeability represents the interactions with the magnetic field. Most frequently, relative values normalized to (in reference to) those of the vacuum are used.

In the field of biological effects and interactions of non-ionizing electromagnetic radiations with living matter, it is customary to refer to a description of macroscopic interactions as dosimetry, and to describe microscopic interactions and their macroscopic representation as biophysics or interaction mechanisms.

The objective of this contribution is to present fundamental principles of the interactions of RF and microwaves with matter with special reference to biological substances and systems. To meet this objective the propagation of waves in lossless and lossy dielectrics is described including relationships between wavelength, attenuation and phase constant as well as the intrinsic properties of the medium, (i.e. the permittivity and the permeability), and the radiation frequency. A description of wave propagation in presence of metals and dielectric interfaces follows. Macroscopic and molecular properties of dielectrics are discussed in general terms and examples of the properties of biological media are given. The electromagnetic energy flow and its conversion into heat are also briefly outlined. It is concluded that the interactions of RF and MW with living matter are complex functions of radiation characteristics (frequency, intensity, polarization), object parameters (size, shape, internal structure, permittivity distribution) and the surroundings (radiation source - object configuration, presence of scattering objects nearby).

Macroscopic Representation of Fields and Matter

Matter may be considered as an aggregate of particles some of which possess electric charges, and some of which act as magnetic dipoles. Because of the presence of charged particles and magnetic dipoles, the electromagnetic field within matter is extremely complex. However, in dealing with electromagnetic fields, they can be considered on the "macroscopic" scale. In this case, the "smoothened" fields are obtained by averaging the fields over volumes large compared with the molecular dimensions, but very small compared with the dimensions of the object.

In the macroscopic theory of electromagnetic fields the field in matter is fully described by two vectors, the electric field vector, E, and the magnetic field vector, H, analogously to these two vectors being necessary and sufficient to define the electromagnetic field in free space. The macroscopic properties of matter defining the interactions with the electromagnetic field are expressed by the complex permittivity, and complex permeability.

The permittivity describes the interaction of matter with the electric field vector, and can be expressed as[1]

$$\hat{\varepsilon} = \varepsilon' - j\varepsilon'' \tag{1}$$

where ε' is the dielectric constance and ε'' is the loss factor. The permittivity, in general is a tensor. For an isotropic, linear and time invariant material $\hat{\varepsilon}$ is a scalar. Only anisotropic materials have a tensor permittivity, in which case the permittivity depends on the direction of the applied electric field. The dielectric constant, ε', is a measure of the ability to store electric field energy. The loss factor, ε'', describes the fraction of the energy dissipated in the material. Frequently, the relative permittivity is used, i.e. the permittivity normalized to that of free space (vacuum)

$$\hat{\varepsilon}_r = \varepsilon'_r - j\varepsilon''_r = \frac{\hat{\varepsilon}}{\varepsilon_o} = \frac{\varepsilon'}{\varepsilon_o} - j\,\frac{\varepsilon''}{\varepsilon_o} \tag{2}$$

where ε_o is the permittivity of the free space, $\varepsilon_o \simeq 8.85 \times 10^{-12}$F/m. The loss factor, ε'', is related to the conductivity of the material, σ, in the following way

$$\varepsilon''_r = \frac{\sigma}{\omega\varepsilon_o}\,, \tag{3}$$

where $\omega = 2\pi f$, f is the frequency. The unit of conductivity is siemens per metre (S/m). The conductivity σ consists of two terms, the static conductivity and conductivity due to the polar rotation as it is explained in the section on molecular interactions.

Frequently a parameter called the loss tangent, $\tan\delta$ is used. It is defined as:

$$\tan\delta = \frac{\varepsilon''}{\varepsilon'} = \frac{\sigma}{\omega\varepsilon'_r\varepsilon_o} \qquad (4)$$

The permeability describes the interaction of matter with the magnetic field[1], and can be expressed as:

$$\hat{\mu} = \mu' - j\mu'' \qquad (5)$$

Similarly like the permittivity, the permeability in general is a tensor, unless the material is isotropic, linear and time-invariant, in which case $\hat{\mu}$ is a scalar. The real part of the permeability, μ', is a measure of the ability to store the magnetic field energy, while the imaginary part, μ'', defines the fraction of the energy dissipated in the material. The relative permeability indicates that the values are normalized to the permeability of the free space (vacuum).

$$\hat{\mu}_r = \mu'_r - j\mu''_r = \frac{\hat{\mu}}{\mu_o} = \frac{\mu'}{\mu_o} - j\,\frac{\mu''}{\mu_o} \qquad (6)$$

where μ_o is the permeability of the free space, $\mu_o \simeq 1.26 \times 10^{-6}$H/m.

Depending on their parameters, namely σ, ε' and $\hat{\mu}$, materials can be divided into groups. Only a relatively small group of materials has the permeability, $\hat{\mu}$, different from that of the free space μ_o. The most common magnetic materials are ferrites. Biological materials are non-magnetic, and their permeability is equal to that of the free-space, μ_o.

Furthermore, depending on the values of the conductivity, σ, and the dielectric constant, materials are divided into conductors and dielectrics. A perfect conductor has infinitely large conductivity, $\sigma = \infty$. Practical conductors, so called good conductors satisfy the condition, $\sigma \gg \omega\varepsilon$ i.e., the conduction current density is large compared with the displacement current density. Values of the static conductivity for a few materials are given in Table 1.

Similarly, a perfect dielectric has $\sigma = 0$ and therefore is lossless, the propagation of electromagnetic waves through it occurs without attenuation. Free space is a perfect dielectric. Materials such as teflon, polyethylene, some plastics and glass are good approximations of a perfect dielectric at radio and microwave frequencies. Imperfect dielectrics satisfy the condition $\sigma \ll \omega\varepsilon$. The electromagnetic wave propagating through an imperfect dielectric is attenuated at a rate dependent on $\hat{\varepsilon}$ (i.e. both σ and ε'). These dielectrics are frequency referred to as lossy

Table 1. Static Conductivities (f=0) of a Few Materials

Material	Conductivity (S/m)	Material	Conductivity (S/m)
Silver	6.1×10^7	Sea Water	4
Copper	5.8×10^7	Fresh Water	10^{-3}
Gold	4.1×10^7	Distilled Water	2×10^{-4}
Aluminum	3.5×10^7	Dry Soil	10^{-5}
Brass	1.5×10^7	Glass	10^{-10}-10^{-14}
Lead	4.8×10^6	Mica	10^{-11}-10^{-15}

dielectrics. Biological substances and tissues belong to this group.

Wave Propagation in Matter

Maxwell's equations for an homogeneous, linear and source free (containing no free charges) medium, when an harmoic variation of the fields with time is assumed ($e^{j\omega t}$), are[2]:

$$\nabla \times \vec{E} = -j\omega\hat{\mu}\vec{H} \tag{7}$$

$$\nabla \times \vec{H} = j\omega\hat{\varepsilon}\vec{E} \tag{8}$$

$$\nabla\vec{E} = 0 \tag{9}$$

$$\nabla\vec{H} = 0 \tag{10}$$

where $\vec{E}$ is the electric field vector and $\vec{H}$ is the magnetic field vector.

Differentiating eq. (7) and (8) with respect to time, substituting one equation into the other and using the vector identity $\nabla \times \nabla \times \vec{E} = \nabla(\nabla\vec{E}) - \nabla^2\vec{E}$, the wave equations are obtained[2]

$$\nabla^2 E - \hat{\gamma}^2\vec{E}^2 = 0 \tag{11}$$

$$\nabla^2\vec{H} - \hat{\gamma}^2\vec{H}^2 = 0 \tag{12}$$

where

$$\hat{\gamma} = j\omega\sqrt{\hat{\varepsilon}\hat{\mu}} = \alpha + j\beta \tag{13}$$

$\hat{\gamma}$ is the complex propagation constant, α is the attenuation constant and β is the phase constant.

Let us assume that the medium having the permittivity $\hat{\varepsilon}$ and the permeability $\hat{\mu}$, not only does not contain free charges

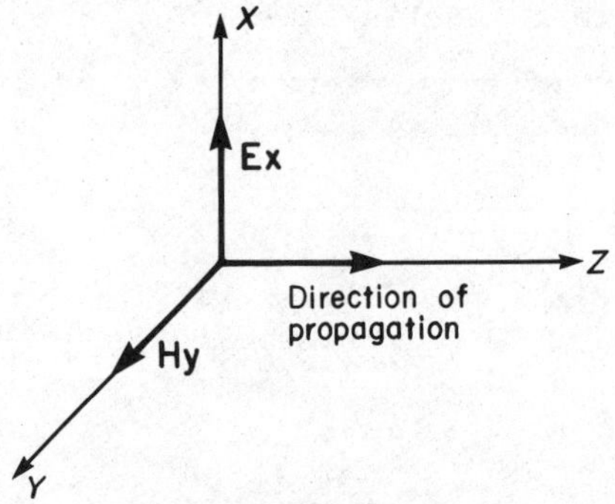

Figure 1. A plane wave representation.

(assumed earlier), but is also infinite, then one of the solutions of the wave equations can be then obtained assuming that the field vectors $\vec{E}$ and $\vec{H}$ depend only on z (in Cartesian coordinates) and time, t. The solution of the wave equations is then a plane wave

$$\vec{E} = \vec{E}_0 e^{j\omega t - \hat{\gamma} z} = \vec{E}_0 e^{-\alpha z} e^{-j(\omega t - \beta z)} \tag{14}$$

$$\vec{H} = \vec{H}_0 e^{j\omega t - \hat{\gamma} z} = \vec{H}_0 e^{-\alpha z} e^{-j(\omega t - \beta z)} \tag{15}$$

propagating in the z direction and having a complex propagation factor $\hat{\gamma}$, as shown in Fig. 1. It is apparent, that for a medium having a complex propagation constant, $\hat{\gamma}$, as the wave progresses through the medium (in z directions), its amplitude decreases exponentially at a rate determined by α, while its phase changes are described by β. These two parameters are dependent on the intrinsic properties of the matter. For non-magnetic materials, i.e. $\hat{\mu} = \mu_0$

$$\alpha = \frac{\omega}{c} \sqrt{\frac{\varepsilon'_r}{2}} \left[\sqrt{1 + \left(\frac{\varepsilon''_r}{\varepsilon'_r}\right)^2} - 1\right]^{1/2} \tag{16}$$

$$\beta = \frac{\omega}{c} \sqrt{\frac{\varepsilon'_r}{2}} \left[\sqrt{1 + \left(\frac{\varepsilon''_r}{\varepsilon'_r}\right)^2} + 1\right]^{1/2} \tag{17}$$

where $\omega = 2\pi f$, and $c = 1 \sqrt{\varepsilon_o \hat{\mu}_o}$ is the velocity of light.

The wavelength in the medium is

$$\lambda = \frac{\lambda_0}{\sqrt{\frac{\varepsilon_r'}{2}\left[\sqrt{1 + \left(\frac{\varepsilon_r''}{\varepsilon_r'}\right)^2} + 1\right]^{1/2}}} \qquad (18)$$

where λ_0 is the wavelength in free space for the same frequency. For a given frequency, the wavelength in the medium is always shorter than in the free space.

The phase velocity of the wave along the direction of propagation is given by

$$v_p = \frac{\omega}{\beta} = \frac{c}{\sqrt{\frac{\varepsilon_r'}{2}\left[\sqrt{1 + \left(\frac{\varepsilon_r''}{\varepsilon_r'}\right)^2} + 1\right]^{1/2}}} \qquad (19)$$

and is less than the phase velocity in the free space.

For a perfect dielectric the following relationships apply

$$\alpha = 0$$

$$\beta = \frac{\omega}{c}\sqrt{\varepsilon_r'}$$

$$\lambda_\varepsilon = \lambda_o / \sqrt{\varepsilon_r} \qquad (20)$$

$$v_p = c/\sqrt{\varepsilon_r'}$$

Another useful parameter for characterizing a medium is the intrinsic impedance. It is defined as the ratio of the electric field to the magnetic field.

$$\hat{Z} = \frac{E}{H} = \sqrt{\frac{\hat{\mu}}{\hat{\varepsilon}}} \qquad (21)$$

The intrinsic impedance is a complex quantity, which can be represented in the polar form. For $\hat{\mu} = \mu_o$

$$\hat{Z} = |Z|\, e^{j\xi}$$

$$|Z| = \sqrt{\frac{\mu_o}{\varepsilon_o}}\,[\varepsilon_r'^2 + \varepsilon_r''^2]^{-1/4} \qquad (23)$$

$$\tan 2\xi = \varepsilon''/\varepsilon' = \tan\delta$$

$$\xi = \delta/2 \tag{22}$$

In the free space the intrinsic impedance is $Z_o = \sqrt{\dfrac{\mu_o}{\varepsilon_o}}\ 120\pi \simeq 377\Omega$.

In the free space or a perfect dielectric occupying unbound space the electric and magnetic field vectors of an electromagnetic wave are in phase. However, in a lossy medium the electric field vector is advanced or retarded in phase with respect to the magnetic field vector, depending whether the magnetic loss factor, μ'', or the dielectric loss factor, ε'', is greater. If $\mu'' = 0$, the electric field vector is advanced. A plane wave propagating in a lossy dielectric is illustrated in Fig. 2. Table 2 lists the propagation parameters for three imperfect dielectrics at a frequency, f_d (for each), at which $\sigma = \omega\varepsilon'$ (see a condition for imperfect dielectric).

The rate of energy flow out through a given enclosed surface is[2]

$$W = \oint_S \vec{P}.\vec{n}\ ds \tag{23}$$

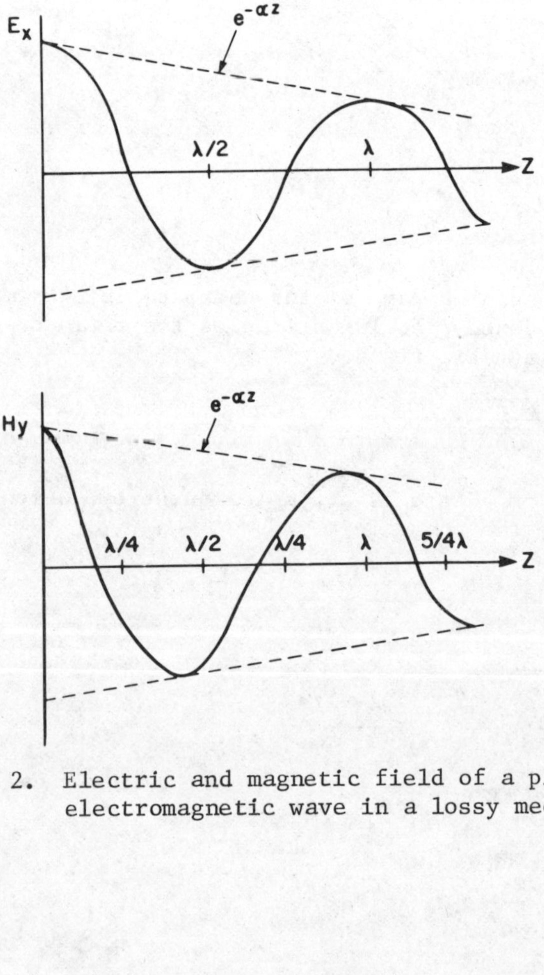

Figure 2. Electric and magnetic field of a plane electromagnetic wave in a lossy medium.

Table 2. Propagation parameters.

Material	σ (S/m)	ε'_r	f_d	α (Np/m)	β/β_o	v_p/c	$\lambda\varepsilon/\lambda$	$\lvert z\rvert$ (Ω)
Mica	10^{-11}	6	0.03 Hz	$77\text{x}10^{-4}$	2.45	0.41	0.41	154
Dry Soil	10^{-5}	5	36 kHz	$84\text{x}10^{-5}$	2.24	0.45	0.45	169
Sea Water	4	80	0.9 GHz	84.3	8.94	0.11	0.11	42

where

$$\vec{P} = \vec{E} \times \vec{H} \tag{24}$$

and $\vec{P}$ is called the Poynting vector, $\vec{n}$ is a unit vector normal to the surface element ds. For an imperfect dielectric with $\hat{\mu} = \mu_o$

$$\int_S \vec{P}.\vec{n}\, ds = -\frac{1}{2}\int_V \sigma\vec{E}\,\vec{E}^*\, dv + j\frac{\omega}{2}\int_V(\mu_o\vec{H}\vec{H}^* - \varepsilon'\vec{E}\vec{E}^*)\, dv \tag{25}$$

where the asterics denotes the complex conjugale, and V is the volume enclosed within the surface S. In eq. (25) Re § $\vec{P} . \vec{n}$ ds represents the total power dissipated within the volume V enclosed by the surface S, or if a unit volume is chosen, it represents the power dissipation density.

$$\text{Re} \int \vec{P}.\vec{n}\, ds = -\frac{1}{2}\int_V \sigma|E|^2\, dv \tag{26}$$

is the power dissipated within volume V, and

$$P_d = \frac{1}{2}\sigma|\vec{E}|^2 = \frac{1}{2}\omega\varepsilon_o\varepsilon''_r\,|\vec{E}|^2 \tag{27}$$

is the power dissipated in a unit volume, assuming that the electric field intensity within that volume is constant.

The imaginary power of W (eq. (23)) represents the difference in the mean values of the energy stored in the magnetic and electric field. When a unit volume is considered the stored energy densities associated with the electric and magnetic fields in the medium are (nonmagnetic medium)

$$W_e = \frac{1}{2}\varepsilon'\,|\vec{E}|^2 = \frac{1}{2}\varepsilon'_r\,\varepsilon_o|\vec{E}|^2 \tag{28}$$

$$W_m = \frac{1}{2}\mu_o\,|\vec{H}|^2 \tag{29}$$

Let us consider now plane waves in an imperfect conductor. The approximate propagation parameters can be obtained from eq. (16) to (19) and (21), by taking into account the condition $\sigma/\omega\varepsilon' >> 1$.

$$\alpha_c \simeq \sqrt{\pi f \mu_o \sigma} \tag{30}$$

$$\beta_c \simeq \sqrt{\pi f \mu_o \sigma} \tag{31}$$

$$\lambda_c \simeq \sqrt{\frac{4\pi}{f \mu_o \sigma}} \tag{32}$$

$$v_{pc} = \sqrt{\frac{4\pi f}{\mu_o \sigma}} \tag{33}$$

$$Z_c = \sqrt{\frac{j\omega\mu_o}{\sigma}} \tag{34}$$

The wavelength in copper for a few frequencies is given in Table 3. ($\lambda_c = 0.415/\sqrt{f}$).

Comparing the attenuation per wavelength with the wavelength in conductors, it is apparent that the waves are very rapidly attenuated with distance.

A parameter called the skin depth or the penetration depth δ, is defined as a distance at which the field is attenuated by a factor e^{-1} or 0.368. From this definition and eq (30) it follows that

$$\delta = \frac{1}{\sqrt{\pi f \mu_o \sigma}} \tag{35}$$

The penetration depth (see Table 3) is only a fraction of the wavelength in the conductor and a minute fraction of the wavelength in free space.

Table 3. Wavelength in copper.

Frequency	10 MHz	100 MHz	1 GHz	10 GHz
Wavelength (mm)	0.13	0.041	0.013	0.004
Skin Depth (mm)	0.021	0.0066	2.1×10^{-3}	0.66×10^{-3}

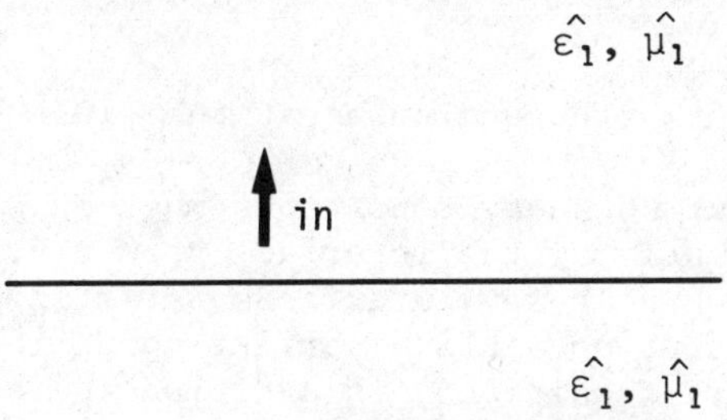

Figure 3. Boundary between two media.

Wave Reflection and Transmission at Boundaries

In practice, an electromagnetic wave on its way of propagation encounters objects having different intrinsic properties. Most physical structures and certainly biological systems are non-uniform in terms of their electromagnetic properties. Maxwell's equations have to be satisfied at any medium, as well as at the boundaries between the media.

At any boundary between two media the following conditions have to be satisfied[2], Fig. 3,

$$i_n \times (\vec{E}_1 - \vec{E}_2) = 0 \tag{36}$$

$$i_n \times (\vec{H}_1 - \vec{H}_2) = \vec{J} \tag{37}$$

$$i_n \cdot (\vec{D}_1 - \vec{D}_2) = \rho \tag{38}$$

$$i_n \cdot (\vec{B}_1 - \vec{B}_2) = 0 \tag{39}$$

where i_n is a unit vector normal to the boundary.

In case of a boundary between two dielectrics, when there are no surface currents nor changes, the boundary conditions[2] state that

$$E_{t1} = E_{t2} \tag{40}$$

$$H_{t1} = H_{t2} \tag{41}$$

the tangential electric and magnetic fields on both sides of the boundary are equal, and

$$\varepsilon_1 E_{n1} = \varepsilon_2 E_{n2} \tag{42}$$

$$\mu_1 H_{n1} = \mu_2 H_{n2} \tag{43}$$

the normal components are continuous at the dielectric interface.

The set of four boundary conditions must be satisfied at any interface independently of the interface geometry. Let us consider the wave propagation at a few interfaces, starting with a plane wave normally incident on a plane perfect conductor, Fig. 4. To satisfy the boundary conditions, in addition to the incident wave, there is the reflected wave. The two waves are of equal amplitude and together form a standing wave in such a way, that the resultant electric and magnetic fields satisfy the boundary conditions, i.e. the electric field (tangential) is zero at the interface, while the magnetic field is maximum.

If a uniform plane wave is normally incident on a dielectric boundary as shown in Fig. 5, there is a reflected wave normal to the interface and the transmitted wave which travels in the direction normal to the interface. The reflection coefficient is equal to

$$\hat{\Gamma} = \frac{E_1^r}{E_1^i} = \frac{\hat{Z}_2 - \hat{Z}_1}{\hat{Z}_2 + \hat{Z}_1} \tag{44}$$

where $\hat{Z}$ is the medium intrinsic impedance. For a medium having $\hat{\mu}_1 = \hat{\mu}_2 = \mu_0$

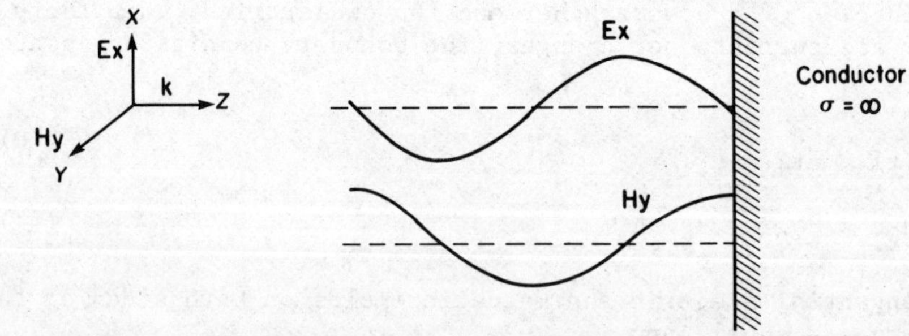

Figure 4. Reflection of a uniform plane wave from a perfect conductor

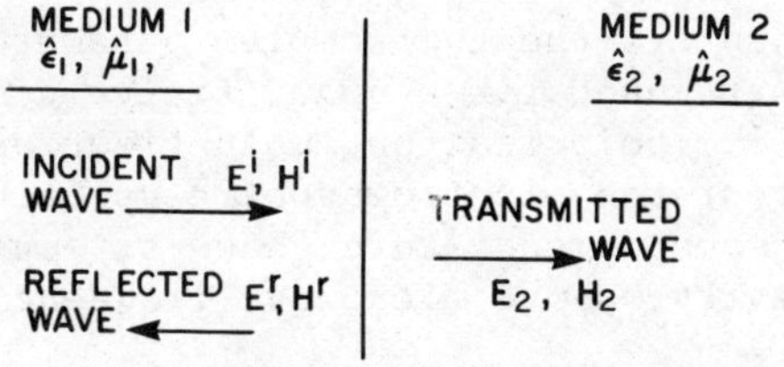

Figure 5. Reflection and transmission at a plane boundary between two media.

$$\hat{\Gamma} = \frac{\sqrt{\hat{\varepsilon}_1} - \sqrt{\hat{\varepsilon}_2}}{\sqrt{\hat{\varepsilon}_1} + \sqrt{\hat{\varepsilon}_2}} \tag{45}$$

For the wave incident on a dielectric interface at an oblique angle (Fig. 6) the direction of the transmitted wave is described by the Snell's law of refraction

$$\frac{\sin \Theta_t}{\sin \Theta_i} = \frac{\beta_1}{\beta_2} \tag{46}$$

where β_1 and β_2 are the phase constants of medium 1 and 2.

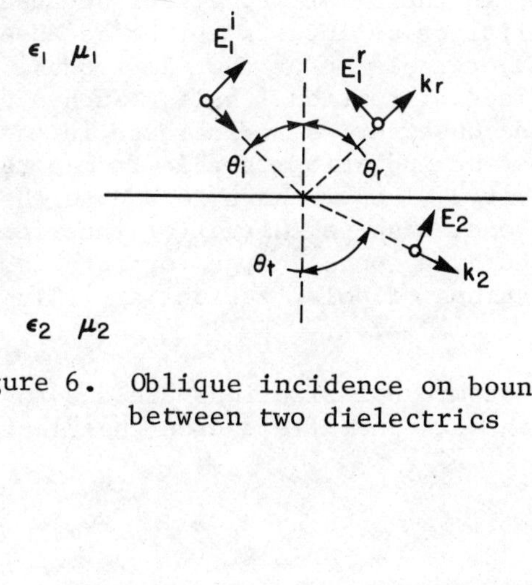

Figure 6. Oblique incidence on boundary between two dielectrics

Molecular Properties of Dielectrics

In previous chapters the two complex parameters, permittivity and permeability, were used for a quantitative description of matter. They describe polarization, magnetization and conduction throughout the part of the electromagnetic spectrum extending from DC to X-rays (with some nomenclature changes, e.g. refraction index instead of permittivity, above microwave frequencies).

On a microscopic level matter can be simplistically considered to consist of positive atomic nuclei surrounded by negative electrons. The application of an external electric field results in a slight displacement of the electrons in respect to the nuclei; induced dipole moments result and cause the so-called electronic polarization of materials. When atoms of different types form molecules, they normally do not share their electrons symmetrically, as the electron clouds are displaced eccentrically toward the stronger binding atoms. Thus atoms acquire charges of opposite polarity, and an external field acting on these net charges tends to change the equilibrium positions of the atoms themselves. By this displacement of charged atoms or groups of atoms with respect to each other, a second type of induced dipole moment is created; it represents the atomic polarization of the dielectric. The asymmetric charge distribution between the unlike partners of a molecule gives rise to permanent dipole moments which exist also in the absence of an external field. Such moments experience a torque in an applied field that tends to orient them in the field direction. Consequently, an orientation (or dipole) polarization can arise.

These three mechanisms of polarization[1], characterized by an electronic polarizability, an atomic polarizability and an orientation or dipole polarizability are due to charges that are locally bound in atoms, in molecules, or in the structures of solids and liquids. In addition, charge carriers usually exist that can migrate for some distance through the dielectric. When such carriers are impeded in their motion, either because they become trapped in the material or on interfaces, or because they cannot be freely discharged or replaced at the electrodes, space charges and a macroscopic field distortion result. Such a distortion appears to an outside observer as an increase in the capacitance of the sample and may be indistinguishable from a real rise of the dielectric permittivity. Thus we have to add to the polarization mechanisms a fourth one, a space charge (or interfacial) polarization, characterized by a space-charge (or interfacial) polarizability. The mechanisms of polarization[1] are illustrated in Fig. 7.

Electronic and atomic polarizations are due to the displacing force exercised by the external field upon the electrons and atoms,

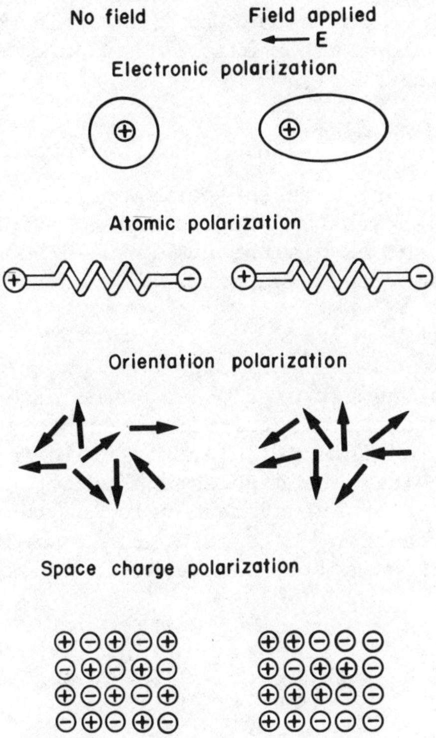

Figure 7. Mechanisms of polarization.

and measure the induced moments thus created. The orientation polarization, on the contrary, arises from the torgue action of the field on the existing permanent moments of the molecules.

Since the field-induced rotation of polar molecules[3,4] is one of the basic mechanisms underlying interactions of electromagnetic fields with matter at radio and microwave frequencies let us examine this process closer. Polar molecules e.g. water, proteins, when subjected to an electric field, attempt to align themselves with the field. Orientation is hindered by the thermal (Brownian) motion of the molecules. Frictional forces, that are dependent upon the rate of orientation (the frequency of the applied field) and the relaxation time, determine the degree of orientation. The relaxation time depends on the viscosity of the solvent, the size and shape of the dipoles, temperature and the nature of the solute-solvent bonds. Only partial orientation takes place when moderate values of the electric field are applied. The degree of orientation is proportional to the strength of the directing field until the saturation occurs. The number of dipoles oriented along a specific direction Θ and $\Theta + \Delta\Theta$ in respect to the z axis when the electric field direction is along the z axis is (assuming uniform field of a relatively low frequency)

$$\Delta N = A \exp(\mu E_r \cos\Theta/kT)\Delta N_o \tag{47}$$

where: A is a constant, μ is the permanent dipole moment, E_r is the directing field, k is the Boltzmann's constant, T is the temperature in ^oK, and ΔN_o is the number of dipoles oriented in the direction $\Theta + \Delta\Theta$ without an external electric field.

$$\Delta N_o = 1/2\ N \sin \Theta\Delta\Theta \tag{48}$$

where N is the total number of dipoles. The directing field is smaller than the internal electric field due to the reaction field of the dipole, and the internal electric field is never greater than the applied field. The dipoles are directed by the field to the extent determined by the average value of the function cos Θ (for a random distribution it is zero, for a perfect alignment it is one). This function called the Langevin function is equal to:

$$L(\mu E_r/kT) = \sqrt{\cos \Theta} = \text{cotanh}\ (\mu E_r/kT) - kT/\mu E_r. \tag{49}$$

For small values of $\mu E_r/kT(\mu E_r/kT < 1)$ the Langevin function is linear and equal to

$$L(\mu E_r/kT) = \mu E_r/3kT \tag{50}$$

Let us calculate the effect of a directing field of 2 V/cm (an equivalent plane wave power density in air 10 mW/cm^2) on protein molecules having the dipole moments of 420 Debye units (Haemoglobin) at room temperature ($T = 300^oK$).

$$L = \mu E_r/3kT = \frac{420 \times 10^{-18} \times (2/300)}{3 \times 1.38 \times 10^{-16} \times 300} = 2.3 \times 10^{-5}.$$

(1 Debye unit, which is roughly equal to the dipole moment of a system consisting of a positive and a negative electron charge separated by a distance of 2 nm, is equal to 10^{-18} esu. 1 esu of electric field strength is equal to 300 V/cm). It can be, therefore, seen that the percentage of the dipoles oriented by the field of 2 V/cm in a unit volume is negligibly small. The field intensities required for saturation are a few to a few hundred of kV/cm depending on the molecule dipolar moment.

The degree of orientation of the dipoles in the directing field decreases with the frequency of the field above a certain frequency owing to the phase lag between the motion of the dipoles and the oscillations of the field. At these frequencies the combined effects of the viscosity, molecular size and shape, and solute-solvent bonding prevent the molecular motion from being in phase with the applied field. As the frequency is further increased a stage is reached where none of the dipoles is able to keep up with the field and the system then behaves like a non-polar material i.e., the value of ε' will lie between 2-5 and ε'' will diminish to zero. Within the range at which dielectric dispersion occurs lies the relaxation frequency f_r at which ε'' (the absorption of energy per cycle of applied field) reaches a maximum. Note, however, that transfer of energy from the field to the medium per unit volume of medium increases with frequency and later level off.

Electrical Properties of Biological Materials

Biological materials, from the point of view of the interactions with electromagnetic fields, are lossy dielectrics[5,6]. Their permeability, $\hat{\mu}$, is equal to that of free space, μ_o. Their permittivity is complex, at frequencies above a few tens of kHz scalar, and varies depending on the materials composition, temperature and field frequency. The dielectric properties are greatly influenced by water, which constitutes from 30 to 80 percent of biological materials and tissues.

Water appears in two forms as free water and bound water. The relaxation of free water takes place at a frequency of approximately 25 GHz at 37°C, and the relaxation frequency is a function of temperature. An increase in the temperature causes an increase in the relaxation frequency. Bound water has many definitions according to the experimental techniques being employed to investigate it. A suitable general designation would be to refer to bound water as molecules held in nonrandom orientations at or near the surface of a macromolecule. Considerable differences of opinion exist as to how much water in the vicinity of the macromolecule may be considered to be different from free water. The relaxation frequency of bound water depending on the molecule the water is attached to and the solvent viscosity occurs between 100 and 1000 MHz. Protein molecules are highly charged with the number of positive and negative charges nearly equal and the charge distribution on the surface highly uniform. Due to large dimensions of the molecules a relatively small asymmetry in the charge distribution results in a large dipole moment. The relaxation frequencies are between 100 kHz and 50 MHz. For many proteins more than one relaxation time have been observed and attributed to nonspherical shape of the molecules. The relaxation frequencies for amino acids and peptides are typically between 0.5 and 3 GHz.

Average values of the permittivity for high-water-content and low water content tissues are given in Table 4.

Table 4. Relative Dielectric Constant and Conductivity of Biological Media at Microwave Frequencies.

Frequency (MHz)	Wavelength (cm)	High Water Content Media		Low Water Content Media	
		ε'	σ(S/m)	ε'	σ(mS/m)
10	3 000	160	0.625	-	-
100	300	72	0.889	7.5	19.1-75.9
300	100	54	1.37	5.7	31.6-107
915	33	51	1.60	5.6	55.6-147
2 450	12	47	2.21	5.5	96.4-213
3 000	10	46	2.26	5.5	110 -234
5 000	6	44	3.92	5.5	162 -309
10 000	3	40	10.3	4.5	324 -549

Summary

The interaction of the electromagnetic waves at radio and microwave frequencies with matter can be described in terms of the complex permittivity and complex permeability, which are a macroscopic reflection of molecular interactions. These parameters are employed in Maxwell's equations, and theoretically it is possible to quantify the fields outside and inside of any object. In practice, in many cases, the difficulties in solving Maxwell's equations for complex geometries and highly non-uniform properties of the object, are unsurmountable.

Biological materials can be identified, in general, as lossy isotropic dielectrics. Their permeability is equal to that of free space, while their permittivity is a complex scalar. The basic molecular interaction mechanism involves relaxation phenomena due to the rotation of polar molecules such as water, amino acids, protein, lipids, etc., and the space-charge polarization. The energy of the electromagnetic field is converted into the kinetic energy of molecules or charges in these relaxation processes, and subsequently it is converted into heat. Other molecular interactions involving unique properties of biological matter e.g. non-equilibrium systems and cooperative phenomena are not discussed here. Also, the non-linear phenomena which many occur at very high intensities of the field are not dealt with.

The interaction of RF and MW radiation depends on the characteristics of the radiation, such as the frequency, polarization and intensity, the biological object characteristics, namely the geometry (size and shape), internal structure and permittivity distribution, and finally the surroundings i.e. the source-object interactions (near-field of a radiator), presence of other objects nearby.

REFERENCES

1. A.R. von Hippel, "Dielectrics and Waves", John Wiley & Sons, Inc., London (1954).
2. N.N. Rao, "Elements of Engineering Electromagnetics", Prentice-Hall, Inc., Englewood Cliffs, N.J. (1977).
3. C.J.F. Bottcher and P. Bordwijk, "Theory of Electric Polarization", Vol. II, Elsevier Publ. Co., Amsterdam (1978).
4. M.A. Stuchly, "Interaction of Radiofrequency and Microwave Radiation with Living Systems - A Review of Mechanisms", Radiat. Environ. Biophysics, Vol. 16, pp. 1-4 (1979).
5. E.H. Grant, R.J. Sheppard and G.P. South, "Dielectric Behaviour of Biological Molecules in Solutions", Clarendon Press, Oxford,(1978).
6. H.P. Schwan and K.R. Foster, "RF-Field Interactions with Biological Systems: Electrical Properties and Biophysical Mechanisms", Proc. IEEE, Vol. 68, pp. 104-113 (1980).

INSTRUMENTATION FOR MEASUREMENT OF ELECTROMAGNETIC FIELDS: EQUIPMENT, CALIBRATIONS AND SELECTED APPLICATIONS PART I - RADIOFREQUENCY FIELDS

Richard A. Tell

US Environmental Protection Agency
Office of Radiation Programs
Nonionizing Radiation Surveillance Branch
P.O. Box 18416
Las Vegas, Nevada 89114

THE NEED TO MEASURE ELECTROMAGNETIC FIELDS

Determination of radiofrequency electromagnetic field exposure is necessary in both biological effects research work concerned with electromagnetic field effects and the assessment of possible hazards to exposed individuals. The situations include laboratory exposure of animals and human exposures in both the work place and non-occupational settings for determining compliance with applicable safety standards. Because of the common complications introduced by the environment such as multipath reflections and absorption caused by intervening attenuative media, resort is often made to a direct measurement of the ambient fields in lieu of the often impossible task of accurate mathematical computation.

THE VARIETY OF FACTORS SURROUNDING MEASUREMENTS

Measurements of electromagnetic fields from a hazard point of view are subject to a number of factors which can influence measurement accuracy and impose special requirements on instrumentation performance.

Reactive and Radiated Fields Close to Antennas

Figure 1, taken from Swicord (1971), depicts the electric and magnetic fields very near to a dipole element due to charge motion along the element.

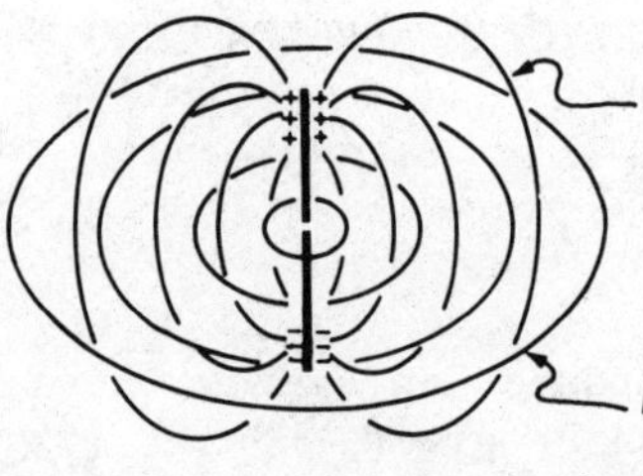

Figure 1. Electric and magnetic fields very near to a dipole element due to charge motion along the element [taken from Swicord (1971)].

The electric E and magnetic H fields produce in turn induced magnetic and electric fields, respectively. These fields are given mathematically as

$$E_r = 2A\ Z_o \cos\theta \left[\frac{1}{2\pi}\left(\frac{\lambda}{r}\right)^2 - \frac{j}{(2\pi)^2}\left(\frac{\lambda}{r}\right)^3\right] \tag{1}$$

$$E_\theta = A\ Z_o \sin\theta \left[j\left(\frac{\lambda}{r}\right) + \frac{1}{2\pi}\left(\frac{\lambda}{r}\right)^2 - \frac{j}{(2\pi)^2}\left(\frac{\lambda}{r}\right)^3\right] \tag{2}$$

$$H_\phi = A \sin\theta \left[j\left(\frac{\lambda}{r}\right) + \frac{1}{2\pi}\left(\frac{\lambda}{r}\right)^2\right] \tag{3}$$

where

$$A = I_o L\ e^{j\omega(t-r/c)}$$

$Z_o = \frac{1}{\varepsilon_o c}$ = impedance of free space

L = length of dipole
I_o = current in antenna
ω = angular frequency = $2\pi f$
f = frequency
λ = wavelength
r = distance from dipole
θ = angle between direction of dipole and direction of vector r
c = speed of light = 3×10^8 m/S

When r is very much smaller than λ, the λ/r^3 term dominates and this region is commonly referred to as the reactive zone or near field. As λ/r approaches 1, the λ/r^2 and λ/r terms become more pronounced and this region is referred to as the intermediate field or the radiating near-field zone. When r becomes large with respect to λ, the only significant term becomes λ/r. In this, the so-called far-field case, the first equation may be neglected and

$$E_\theta = A\, Z_o \sin\theta \left[j\left(\frac{\lambda}{r}\right) \right] \tag{4}$$

$$H_\phi = A \sin\theta \left[j\left(\frac{\lambda}{R}\right) \right] \tag{5}$$

In the far field E and H are related by a constant, Z_o, the impedance of free space and E and H are mutually orthogonal.

Most electromagnetic fields of hazard concern are in the close proximity to radiating structures such as antennas; in these regions the electromagnetic field structure may be highly inhomogenous and there may typically be substantial variations in the wave impedance from as small as a few ohms to thousands of ohms. Thus the electric E and magnetic H fields do not in general have the same and constant relationship as exists in the far field of a radiation source; i.e., in some regions there may exist almost pure E fields and in other regions almost pure H fields. In regions somewhat removed from the immediate vicinity of the antenna or the reactive zone but still within the radiative near-field region, there can be strong spatial oscillation caused by the distribution of current on the radiating structure. This property is particularly evident with highly directive (high gain) antennas. It is important to note that an instrument that responds to the E field will indicate not only the radiated field, but will measure the resultant of the vector addition of all field components given by equations (1) and (2). In the near-field although the reactive components do not contribute to the net flow of radiated energy, they can couple into material and thus affect energy absorption.

Frequency Ranges-Multiple Frequencies

The radiofrequency spectrum of practical interest extends from nominally 10 kHz to 100 GHz and frequently there may exist simultaneous emissions on several frequencies due to a multiplicity of radiating sources.

Polarization

Electromagnetic fields of concern may exhibit various polarizations ranging from linear to elliptical. In a general sense, from a hazard survey point of view, the polarization(s) may not be known prior to measurements.

Modulation Properties

Fields in general will have imposed on them some form of modulation depending upon the nature of the source. These modulations may consist of amplitude and frequency modulation of voice and video information in the case of broadcast stations, pulse modulation in the case of radars, and simple 60 or 50 Hz amplitude modulation related to the ac power supply for high power continuous wave generators commonly used in biological effects research work.

Intermittent Emissions

The on-off nature of many emitters such as land-mobile and portable communications equipment, and certain industrial operations such as radiofrequency heat sealers, can introduce complications in accurate measurement of exposure fields.

Radiofrequency Interference (RFI)

Instrumentation used to measure field intensity must be capable of accurate measurement without error introduced by interference from strong radiofrequency fields.

Safety Considerations

Equipment must be compatible for use in a variety of situations without introducing significant, additional hazards due to the measurement itself; e.g., small, lightweight, portable instruments are desired for electromagnetic radiation surveys on broadcast towers.

Environmental Conditions

Instrumentation will frequently be subjected to a wide range of temperature and humidity, particularly in outdoor measurements.

SPECIFICATION OF THE FIELDS

Electromagnetic fields are made up of electric field E components measured in units of volts/meter (V/m) and magnetic field H components measured in units of amperes/meters (A/m). The ratio of these two components is called the electromagnetic wave impedance Z. In terms of the magnitudes of these vectors,

$$Z = \frac{E}{H} \tag{6}$$

In free space at distances of many wavelengths (far field) from a source of radiation, this ratio is a constant (does not vary with distance from the source) and is equal to Z_o, the intrinsic impedance of free space where $Z_o = 377$ ohms. In the far-field the incident power density magnitude S of the electromagnetic wave is often found from

$$S = EH = \frac{E^2}{Z_o} = H^2 Z_o \quad \text{where} \tag{7}$$

S is visualized as the <u>net</u> power per unit area emerging through a location in space. S is the unit which has most commonly been used in measurements of electromagnetic field intensity even though it is rarely if ever the field parameter actually measured. More commonly, field sensors actually are sensitive to E^2 or H^2 but are calibrated to read in terms of the plane wave equivalent power density. Use of the concept of power density, although useful in many situations for envisioning the rate of energy absorption by a target, can lead to a misconception of the actual situation.

Bowman (1970) has discussed the selection of a suitable field parameter; a suitable field parameter for quantifying hazardous electromagnetic fields is dependent on the relevancy of the parameter to the potential hazard and on the ease of measuring the parameter. Bowman points out that except for very simple fields, power density is least suitable because (a) the power density of some very strong fields can be small, and (b) power density is a relatively difficult parameter to measure. Power density is a vector quantity given by the time average of $|\underline{E} \times \underline{H}|$. In complicated fields, it is much easier to measure the scaler magnitudes E and H (see for example Moore School Report No. 63-23, "Feasibility Studies of Poynting Vector Measurements", University of Pennsylvania, Moore School of Electrical Engineering, July 31, 1963). This can be illustrated via two examples. Imagine an incident wave impinging upon a reflective surface. At some point in front of this surface the wave has some incident power density. If the surface is a good reflector, the reflected wave power density may be equal to the incident wave density such that there exists a net zero power flow through the unit of space. Even though the net power density at this point may be zero, the resultant electric field strength may be double the incident value and thus there exists a major discrepancy between power density and the potential hazard associated with exposure to this field.

Fortunately, most so-called power density monitors, because they actually sense the square of the electric field, indicate the equivalent power density which would be associated with the resultant electric field strength sensed at the point, but they are not sensing the actual power density which is zero.

Another area of ambiguity in using instruments with such calibrations is in near-field situations wherein the electric and magnetic fields, do not necessarily have the same relationship as they do in the far field where $\frac{E}{H} = 377$ ohms. When the wave impedance is other than the far-field value of 377 ohms, the monitor will still indicate the apparent far-field equivalent power density. This means that one can still arrive at what the electric or magnetic field amplitude value is by solving backward for either E or H from

$$S = \frac{E^2}{377} = 377\ H^2$$

However, since the actual wave impedance may be other than 377 ohms, no knowledge can be gained of the other field parameter without measurement with a device sensitive to the other field component.

Bowman (1970) has proposed the use of energy density units for specifying the intensity of electromagnetic fields. The energy density of a wave is given as

$$U = U_E + U_H = \frac{1}{2}(\varepsilon_o E^2 + \mu_o H^2) \quad \text{where} \tag{8}$$

U_E and U_H are the electric and magnetic field energy densities respectively in units of energy per unit volume or joules per cubic meter (J/m^3), ε_o is the permittivity of free space = 8.854×10^{-12} Farad/m, μ_o is the permeability of free space = 1.257×10^{-6} Henry/m, and E and H are the electric and magnetic field strength magnitudes in units of V/m and A/m. In the far field $U_E = U_H$.

There is a certain attractiveness in specifying exposure fields in this fashion. This derives from two considerations: (a) except for non-thermal biological effects thermal heating is proportional to U, U_E, and U_H; (b) it is convenient to use the same units for stating the intensities of the total field, the electric field, and the magnetic field. The latter consideration would seem to perhaps lead to clearer visualization of the relative impact of electric and magnetic field coupling with biological systems in the near-field.

Despite these propositions it has become common practice to specify fields in terms of their electric and magnetic field strength magnitudes or the plane wave equivalent power density.

TYPES OF MEASUREMENTS

Measurements of electromagnetic fields can be classified as broadband or narrowband. Broadband measurements are accomplished with instruments which possess a frequency independent sensitivity and indicate the intensity of the field without providing information on the frequency of the field. Such devices are commonly used for both radiofrequency hazard surveys and determining the exposure levels of animals used in biological effects research.

Narrowband measurements are accomplished with instruments which possess frequency selectivity and tuneability in their design. Instruments commonly used with these characteristics are field strength meters and spectrum analyzers and are used when measurements of emissions on specific frequencies are required. This can become important when multiple sources on different frequencies are illuminiating a given area and it is required to determine the contribution to exposure from each individual source.

Finally, the approaches used in electromagnetic field measurements may vary according to the nature of the exposure situation; i.e., whether the measurements are being made in a laboratory environment where the conditions are under good control or in typical non-laboratory situations where the field configuration may be more complicated because of reflections and near-field properties of antennas, the climatic conditions may be adverse and where there may be severe constraints imposed by difficult measurement locations.

BROADBAND INSTRUMENTATION

Desirable Characteristics of Broadband Instruments

There are a number of characteristics for broadband measurement instruments which are desirable. These include:

Portability. Because in general broadband instrumentation is used for assessing the electromagnetic fields in various awkward environments, it is important that the instrument be completely portable; i.e., it should be as reasonably small and lightweight as possible, and be battery powered to permit operation in locations where access to the commercial AC mains is not possible.

Readability. The instrument's readout should preferably be of the analog type and be capable of being read at arms length.

Responsiveness to one field parameter. Instruments designed to sense either the electric or magnetic field should exhibit negligible response to the other field parameters. Aslan (1976) has discussed a transmission line technique for evaluating the electric field response of magnetic field sensors.

Spatial resolvability of the field. It is important that broadband survey instruments represent a small cross section to the ambient fields. In general this means that the sensitive probe element be less than a wavelength long at the highest intended frequency so that oscillations in this field due to standing wave formations can be resolved.

Non-perturbation of the field. The probe should possess the property of not perturbing the fields which are to be measured by introducing significant scattering and reflections. This is important because one would like to know the value of the field in the absence of the probe. This quality is most often achieved by making the probe elements very small and using some form of high impedance connecting cable between the probe and the electronics package. Such techniques are elaborated on by Rudge and Knox (1970) and Swicord (1971).

Isotropicity. It is desirable that the orientation of the sensing probe not affect the instrument reading since there may be multiple emissions to monitor at a given point in space. Since these fields may be arriving from different directions and the resultant field magnitude is wanted, the probe must be non-directional, preferably in all three planes of possible polarization.

Interference. An important consideration in modern instruments is possible interference with proper operation. This can arise from direct case penetration of the electronic package by the electromagnetic field being measured or pickup of the field on the leads connecting the probe to the electronics package and conduction of these unwanted signals into the readout circuitry. Kucia (1972) examined the effects of capacitive coupling of the probe to the source of radiation and the effects of improperly balanced probe circuits becoming sensitive to electric field potentials. This particular phenomenon may be particularily apparent at low frequencies where the cables connecting the probe to the electronics become more conductive. Langlet (1978) investigated the detrimental effects of common-mode pickup of low frequency fields of magnetron modulators by the sensing probe of several commercial survey meters. Because of the very high input impedance of the instrumentation circuitry typically used, it is common to see cable flexure effects exhibited as momentary deflections on the meter readout. Depending on the severity of this charge sensitivity, the length of time that the erroneous deflection persists can vary from a virtual instantaneous transient to a long-lived perturbation of meter response of a second or greater. Operators of such instruments must be careful not to report erroneous readings of field intensity when measuring near to high voltage sources such as video display devices and television receivers.

Frequency response. Ideally, the frequency response of a broadband instrument should be flat within the desired frequency range and steeply fall both below and above this range. Thus, out of band responses should be kept to an absolute minimum to avoid the problem of signals which fall outside the range of applicability for the instrument causing erroneously high indicated values of field intensity leading to erroneous assessment of the potential hazard. Unless special precautions are taken both loop and dipole configured probes may exhibit undesirable positive errors in the region of the resonance frequency for the probe. The frequency response of commercial instruments is typically specified as within $\pm$ 2 dB over their intended range of operation. Since manufacturer's specifications are frequently based on measurements at a limited number of frequencies, considerable effort is required to fully evaluate an instrument's frequency response.

Average and peak detection. Instruments employed for broadband measurements normally respond to the root-mean-square (rms) value of the field amplitude. This is consistent with the usual specification of maximum permissible intensities in rms units in safety standards except in the case of pulsed fields where in some standards the absolute instantaneous peak intensity is specified.

Multiple signal addition. It is useful for broadband instruments, particularly ones to be employed in hazard surveys, to properly add together the field intensities from signals on different frequencies within its passband. For example, in cases where there are several signals of concern the instrument should indicate the summation of the total with minimum error. For sensors operated as square law devices such errors do not exist or are negligible.

Response time. Response time is the time required for an instrument to respond to changes in the applied field intensity and indicate the proper value on its indicating device. This property is an important one from two practical points of view: (a) fields which are rapidly changing in time such as scanning radar beams and signals associated with certain types of frequently intermittent transmissions such as public service communications equipment. In a practical sense the response times of most available survey instruments are such that accurate measurements of scanning radar fields are not possible and the antennas must be stopped to ensure a proper measurement; (b) the rapid surveying of large regions wherein standing waves exist with consequent significant variations in field amplitudes over small distances. In this case, if the meter response is quite slow, the operator must be more careful in traversing the area to look for peaks in field intensity. This means that typically more time is required to evaluate the exposure situation.

Maximum hold feature. It is sometimes convenient for an instrument to possess the ability to remember the maximum field intensity sensed during some period of time. This feature has been implemented in different ways including analog and digital techniques.

Stability. Aside from absolute accuracy, frequency response, and isotropicity, stability is one of the most important aspects of broadband survey type instruments. This derives from the practical problem of assessing possibly hazardous exposures in typical conditions. Thus if the meter zero set-point drifts, the problem of conducting the survey is greatly increased meaning in some cases that the operator must remove himself from the field and/or that shielding material must be placed about the probe before rezeroing the instrument. Both of these situations are awkward and can lead to introduction of some uncertainty in the survey results. It is important for instruments employed in outdoor measurements to possess particularly good thermal stability since they will often be subjected to large temperature cycles.

Absolute accuracy. It is desirable for broadband instruments to possess an absolute measurement accuracy of at least ± 1 dB or better. Absolute accuracy refers to the response accuracy of the instrument when employed at a frequency for which a known calibration exists. This uncertainty relates to the manufacturer's or user's ability to know the absolute intensity of the calibrating field. In practice, because there is always some variation in isotropic response, i.e., no probe is perfectly isotropic, it is conventional to calibrate an instrument with the probe oriented to the midpoint of its isotropic response. This is typically accomplished by finding the maximum and minimum response of the probe by rotating it in the calibration field and comparing the mean value of response to the known field intensity.

Dynamic range. Wide dynamic range in broadband survey instruments is desirable. This permits a better definition of the actual range of electromagnetic field exposure levels in a given circumstance. For hazard determinations, a response capability from at least 3-10 dB above the applicable safety limit to 10 dB below the limit is desirable. Depending upon the safety limit used, which varies widely according to country of origin and exposure frequency, this implies that a universally useful instrument would have a fairly large dynamic range, namely on the order of 50-60 dB. There are some practical constraints on the maximum sensitivity useful with broadband instruments, at least for those employed in environmental situations. Because of the nature of man's electromagnetic environmment it is common to find a multiplicity of radiofrequency signals, with intensities of 100 nW/cm^2 or less in urban areas (Tell and Mantiply, 1980). Thus in developed countries it is common to have man-made electromagnetic radiation backgrounds in this range. In a practical sense, instruments designed for broadband detection of signals much less than 100 nW/cm^2 (this corresponds to 0.6 V/m) will exhibit significant variations in response due to the continually changing fields with time, making their usefulness somewhat questionable.

Recorder output. It is useful to have available a recorder output connection which provides a voltage proportional to the analog meter reading. This output is useful in laboratory applications where it may be used for long-term recording or more accurate digital voltmeter reading of intensity than can be derived from a visual observation of the meter.

THERMOMETRIC BASED INSTRUMENTATION

The term thermometric is used here to describe that class of broadband instruments which relies on the interaction of an electromagnetic field with some sensory mechanism that ultimately results in an increase in temperature within the sensor. It is this increase in temperature which is in turn quantitatively related to the field intensity. A discussion of thermometric based instrumentation is partitioned according to bolometric devices, thermally sensitive chemicals, and thermocouple devices.

Bolometric Devices

Bolometric devices such as thermistors and barretters operate on the principle that a resistance change with temperature in the device is measurable by means of a sensitive bridge circuit. The disadvantages of thermally sensitive devices are that they respond to any form of heating, are subject to burnout if overloaded, and have relatively slow response time. Meter reading variations due to ambient temperature fluctuations can be reduced by using more than one detector in a differential configuration where one of the sensors is used to sense the ambient temperature.

There have been a number of devices developed in the past which employed thermistors for the detection of electromagnetic fields. Perhaps the most notable was the Ramcore models 1200 and 1270 manufactured by Ramcore, Inc., USA. Descriptions of evaluative tests of these devices are given by Crapuchettes (1970) and Moore et al. (1970). The Ramcore, no longer manufactured, made use of a series of small antennas including pyramidal horns and flat, pancake configured spirals with a thermistor detector. Moore et al. (1970) discuss the polarization sensitivity of this instrument pointing out the need to hold the probe parallel to a linearily polarized electric field or to make two readings 90 degrees apart to arrive at the actual field intensity. They also claim that the instrument exhibited a rather unstable zero adjustment, presumably due to thermal instability in the circuitry.

A bolometric device is one which exhibits a heating effect due to interaction with or absorption of electromagnetic energy. Certain forms of resistive films may be placed in this category. Several approaches, making use of thermally sensitive films, have been tried in the development of radiofrequency sensors. One of the more interesting was the development of a form of Golay cell described by Fletcher and Woods (1969). A summary of the principles of operation of this device has been given by Bowman (1974). The sensor consists of two thin-walled air-filled spheres connected by tubes to a sensitive differential pressure transducer.

One sphere is coated with a resistive film that is heated by the electromagnetic field to produce a pressure differential between the spheres. The non-coated sphere provides compensation for changes in ambient temperature or pressure. Aside from the scattering effects of the other parts of the instrument, the symmetry of the energy absorbing sphere produces an isotropic response to fields of arbitrary complexity. Bowman (1974) states that "for wavelengths much longer than the diameter of the sphere and if the surface resistivity of the sphere is large enough, the response of the sensor will be determined to a good approximation solely by the value of E^2 at the position of the sensor regardless of the configuration of the field. For long wavelengths the unperturbed electric field will be essentially uniform over the sphere for any field configuration. The currents in the coating when the sphere is introduced into the field will be due to the final tangential field over the sphere; and, for a large surface resistivity, the final tangential field will not differ significantly from the unperturbed field. Thus, the response of the sensor, to a good approximation, will not be affected by the magnetic field and the sensor will have the same response coefficient for E^2 in a reactive near-field or standing-wave field as it would for a simple plane-wave field." A device patterned after this description was marketed for a while by the Wayne-Kerr Com-pany Limited, New Malden, Surrey, England.

A combination of resistive films with liquid crystal coatings have been used for laboratory measurement of electromagnetic fields. Bendix Corporation Research Laboratories (1970) developed a prototype liquid crystal microwave power density meter. The device consists of a Mylar membrane with resistive and liquid crystal coatings which serves as a large area sensing element and uses direct current electrical power for bias and calibration of the membrane. One side of the Mylar is metalized with a thin layer of nichrome to a resistivity of approximately 377 ohms per square. A thin layer of liquid crystals is also applied to the Mylar. When a microwave field is incident on the structure, microwave energy is converted into heat by the metalized layer. The colors scattered by the liquid crystals are a function of the temperature distribution over the membrane.

The nichrome layer is very thin compared with skin depth at microwave frequencies. The resistivity is, therefore, the same for both direct currents and currents oscillating at microwave frequencies. This equivalence serves as the simple and fundamental method of calibration. Direct currents are passed through the membrane, and the resultant temperature increase serves both as a biasing means to obtain the liquid crystal color threshold and a means of calibration by substitution. Tests on the prototype device showed a maximum sensitivity of about 5 mW/cm^2. Problems such as uniformity of the nichrome coating deposition, baffling from infrared radiation, and selection of a low-heat-capacity binding material for a faster response must be solved before this instrument can be manufactured.

Recently a similar but simple device manufactured under the name of Micro-Check and distributed by Micro-Check Industries Ltd., Alberta, Canada, was introduced, designed for the microwave oven survey market. This device consists of a plastic substrate with strips of resistive coating to absorb microwave leakage fields and a layer of liquid crystals to detect changes in the temperature of the resistive strips caused by microwave absorption. The manufacturer claims that the Micro-Check will indicate the presence of microwave oven leakage fields of 5 mW/cm^2 or greater when used in accordance with instructions.

Thermally Sensitive Chemicals

Levine and Moore (1970) describe the use of sponges soaked in 0.3 molar cobaltous chloride ($CoCl_2.6H_2O$) to study the effects of load positions within a microwave oven cavity on leakage levels. Cobaltous chloride is a reddish-pink color when dissolved in water but becomes deep blue when partially or completely dehydrated. Sponges measuring 16.0 cm x 9.0 cm x 0.7 cm were first impregnated with about 50 ml of the solution and placed in a nonabsorptive holder, placed in the oven and allowed to partially dehydrate by operation of the oven. By observing the disappearance of the pink coloration of the sponges, they were able to quantitatively assess standing wave patterns within the oven cavity. Although the technique is inexpensive, it provides no quantitative measures of the incident microwave field intensity.

Conover (1971) investigated the use of lithium fluoride (LiF) thermoluminescent dosimetry (TLD) material as a dosimeter for microwave radiation. Teflon discs impregnated with LiF were subjected to saturation exposures (approximately 10^5 R) of gamma radiation and these irradiated dosimeters were then exposed to microwave radiation at 2450 MHz. Analysis of the relative light output data for the treatment groups and the control group (which received no microwave radiation) showed that there were no significant differences between groups indicating that this technique was not useful. Additional research on selecting an absorptive medium for the TLD discs to be placed within during microwave irradiation might prove effective but has not been investigated.

Thermocouple Devices

In terms of thermometric based devices, thermocouples have proved to be most effective in electromagnetic field instrumentation. The thermocouple produces a dc voltage as a result of the rise in temperature caused by the absorption of electromagnetic energy and has the advantage of requiring only a millivoltmeter to determine the exposure field intensity. The circuitry of the millivoltmeter is much simpler than the complex bridge circuitry required with bolometers. There are numerous papers in the literature describing and evaluating various instrumentation techniques using thermocouples. Swicord (1971) presents information on the Narda model 8100 instrument which is designed to operate at 915 MHz and 2450 MHz. Figure 2 illustrates the two axis electric field sensitive probe used in the Narda model 8100. Note that in this case two mutually perpendicular dipolar elements are used which have thermocouples across their junctions. Although the probe actually senses E^2 the associated readout is calibrated in units of plane-wave equivalent power density (mW/cm^2). Measurements are independent of x, y polarization of incident radiation propagating in the z direction. The components of the E vector will be properly added regardless of the polarization, provided the squares of the E field components are added. The simple addition of the magnitude of the vector components of E would create an eliptically polarized receiving probe. The probe uses a novel configuration of thin-film vacuum-evaporated thermocouple elements

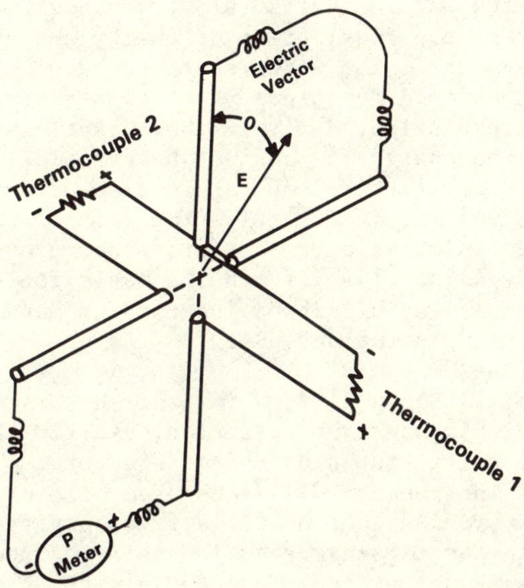

Figure 2. Pictorial diagram of two-axis electric field sensitive probe used in the Narda Microwave Corporation model 8100 survey instrument. [Compliments of the Narda Microwave Corporation, New York, USA].

which function as both antenna and detector. The manufacturer claims temperature insensitivity due to the close proximity of the hot and cold junctions. These elements will respond to infrared radiation and the possibility of detecting infrared rather than microwave frequencies is eliminated by the use of a styrofoam spacer sphere which functions as an infrared shield as well as a distance guide for survey measurements.

Hopfer (1972) has described a broadband thermocouple based instrument which uses a resistive mesh sensor. The mesh is constructed from strips consisting of alternating segments of bismuth and nichrone films, suitably heat sinked at alternate junction points. This configuration is sensitive to incident radiation in two polarizations and thus is also not purely isotropic.

Aslan (1972) describes a probe using thin-film thermocouple techniques to construct an array of extremely lossy dipoles making possible an electromagnetic radiation monitor having a 3-dB bandwidth of 300 MHz to 18 GHz, and an isotropic response which is independent of polarization. Figure 3 illustrates the relationship of the three mutually orthogonal probe elements which are contained within a 5-cm sphere. Each antenna probe element consists of a series of distributed thermocouple film elements. The probe elements are composed of thin films of overlapping antimony and bismuth deposited upon a thin plastic substrate, creating alternate cold and hot junctions. The hot junctions are formed at the center of the narrow strips having relatively high resistance, thereby allowing for the dissipation of energy and the resultant increase in temperature. The wider sections have a low resistance and thus function as cold junctions, the low resistance allowing little energy to be dissipated within these sections. The broad areas distribute the energy and conduct heat rapidly into the substrate so that very little temperature rise occurs. The resultant dc output voltage is directly proportional to the energy dissipated in the resistive portion of the thermocouple. The design outlined by Aslan (1972) forms the basis for several electric field sensitive, broadband instruments manufactured by the Narda Microwave Corporation, USA.

Thermocouples, although limited in their ultimate sensitivity as detectors of electromagnetic radiation, exhibit the desirable characteristic of being true square-law detectors. This means that thermocouple instruments will accurately indicate the resultant intensity of simultaneous multiple frequency fields and will correctly indicate the time-averaged intensity of modulated fields. Instruments using diode detector elements must be operated only within their square-law region to insure accurate indications when used in simultaneous, multiple frequency fields or modulated fields.

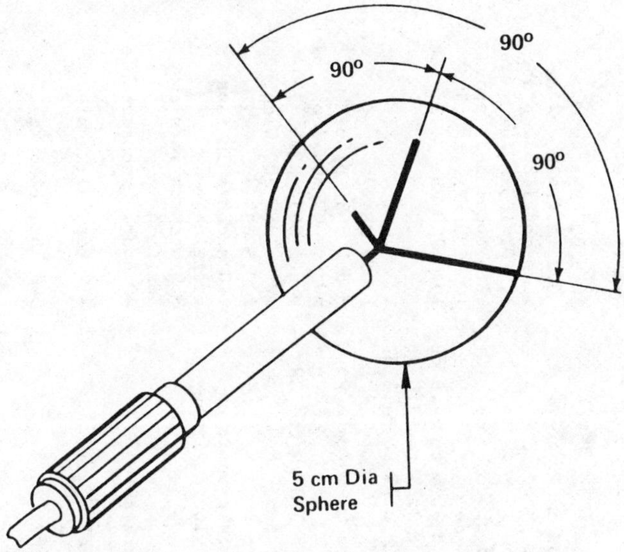

Figure 3. Illustration of geometric relationship of three mutually orthogonal detection elements contained within a 5-cm sphere [taken from Aslan (1972)].

Table 1 provides information on several of the more popular thermocouple, broadband instruments manufactured in the US useful for practical measurements of electromagnetic fields. The magnetic field instruments manufactured by Narda employ a design described by Aslan (1976) that incorporates three mutually orthogonal two-turn coils which are terminated in thin film thermocouple elements. Specifications provided for instruments in Table 1 are taken from manufacturer's literature. Methods for evaluation of instrument performance characteristics may be found in technical reports of the Bureau of Radiological Health (BRH, 1970; Herman and Witters, 1980).

In addition to commercially available instruments many practical measurements may be accomplished by use of calibrated receiving antennas in combination with radiofrequency power meters. It is required that a calibration factor for the antenna be known so that the received power indicated on the power meter can be related to the intensity of the incident field illuminating the antenna. A description of antenna factors is given in the treatment of narrowband instrumentation. This measurement method is subject to the polarization sensitivity of the antenna. Although the method can produce very accurate measures of the electromag-

Table 1. Summary of Specifications of Three Commercially Available Thermocouple Based Broadband Electromagnetic Field Survey Instruments[1]

	General Microwave RAHAM Model 2	Narda Model 8606	Narda Model 8607
Field parameter which instrument senses	Electric field	Electric field	Magnetic field
Frequency Range	0.3 - 18.0 GHz	0.3 - 26.0 GHz	10 - 300 MHz
Indicated full scale measuring ranges	2 mW/cm^2 20 mW/cm^2 200 mW/cm^2	0.2, 2.0, 20, mW/cm^2 with model 8621 probe 1, 10, 100 mW/cm^2 with model 8623 probe	0.2, 2.0. 20, mW/cm^2 with model 8631 probe 1, 10, 100 mW/cm^2 with model 8633 probe
Frequency response	± 1.0 dB	1-12 GHz ± 0.75 dB 0.85 - 16 GHz, + 0.75 to -1.0 dB 0.30 - 18 GHz, + 0.75 to -3.0 dB 0.30 - 26 GHz, + 0.75 to -4.5 dB	10 -200 mHz, ± 0.5 dB 10 - 300 mHz, ± 2.0 dB
Calibration accuracy	± 0.5 dB at 2.45 GHz	± 0.5 dB[3]	± 0.5 dB[3]
Overload level	0.5 W/cm^2 average	Model 8621 probe 60 mW/cm^2 CW 60 W/cm^2 peak Model 8623 probe 300 mW/cm^2 CW 300 W/cm^2 peak	Model 8631 probe 60 mW/cm^2 CW 60 W/cm^2 peak Model 8633 probe 300 mW/cm^2 CW 300 W/cm^2 peak
Isotropicity	± 0.5 dB[2]	0.5 dB[2]	± 0.5 dB[2]
Response time	1.5 seconds	1.0 seconds in fast position 3.0 seconds in slow position	1.0 seconds in fast position 3.0 seconds in slow position
Operating time	500 hours (non-rechargeable)	40 hours (rechargeable)	40 hours (rechargeable)
Recorder output	0.124 V for full scale	3 V for full scale	3 V for full scale
Weight	3.25 lbs. (1.46 kg)	5.8 lbs. (2.6 kg)	5.8 lbs. (2.6 kg)

(1) Specifications provided in this table are taken from published manufacturer's descriptive literature.
(2) Maximum deviation from energy incident from any direction except from/through handle.
(3) At each of several specific calibration frequencies.

netic field intensity, it is important that the user know a priori the frequency of emission since in general the antenna calibration factor will be frequency dependent. Often, if several frequencies are simultaneously present, the use of separate tuneable or fixed bandpass filters as well as inherent frequency selectivity in the antenna can effectively insure accurate measurement of the emission of interest.

DIODE BASED INSTRUMENTS

The nonlinear characteristics of semiconductor diodes can be used to detect radiofrequency energy. The nonlinearity is used to convert the radiofrequency signal to a dc signal for detection. Suitable filtering of the radiofrequency signal must be provided to prevent coupling into the dc circuitry.

Diode detectors have a region of linear detection and a region of square-law detection. The linear region occurs for input signals of about 3-4 mW and larger while the square-law region occurs for input signals of about 0.1 mW and less. Rudge and Knox (1970) discuss the use of diodes as direct electromagnetic sensors.

An advantage of diode detection is that it is not a thermal process and ambient temperature changes do not significantly influence the voltage output. Although temperature variations can influence the current-voltage characteristic of a diode and consequently the detector sensitivity this is usually a second-order effect and will be negligible for normal ambient temperature changes. Several other advantages of diode detectors for use in broadband, electromagnetic field instrumentation include (a) low cost and small size, (b) high burnout levels, (c) simplicity of associated circuitry for reading the field intensity and (d) high sensitivity.

Bowman (1974) described a broadband, isotropic field sensor based on a design using diode detectors. Three small dipolar elements with diodes at the dipole center gaps are placed about the periphery of an equilateral triangular cross section tube for support. The dipoles are arranged in such a manner that they are each orthogonal to the others. The small separation of the dipole centers is provided to minimize the induction of differential mode radiofrequency currents on the connecting lines from the diodes to the associated electronics circuitry. High resistance leads are used to convey the detected, dc voltage from the diodes. These high resistance lines tend to introduce very little perturbation of the field being measured and also provide filtering so that only the dc value of the rectified signal at the diode is conducted to the electronics.

For low-level signals the diodes operate within their square-law region and the outputs from each of the three detector channels are simply summed in a summing amplifier. For higher intensity fields, a non-linear characteristic in the summing amplifier is used to compensate for the diode detectors' departure from square-law response.

A disadvantage associated with diode detection with high-level fields is the non-square law region response which can lead to improper indication of the intensity of multiple frequency emissions. Bowman (1974) indicates that this error will be positive (i.e., the instrument will tend to read high) and can be as high as 3 dB if two fields of identical strength are present. This same phenomenon can influence measurements of the time-average intensity of modulated signals and must be evaluated to assess the actual uncertainty in measurements.

Several instruments have been developed making use of diode detectors. The National Bureau of Standards has extended the original design of Bowman, Larsen, and Belscher (1970) to create several models suitable for different applications (Belscher, 1975).

An instrument using a diode detector with a short monopole sensing antenna has been developed by Instruments for Industry, Inc., and is their model EFS-1. This device is sensitive, of course, to only one polarization but another model, the RHM-2 consists of basically three EFS-1 units combined into a single unit. This unit is described by Ruggera (1976). Both units possess a dynamic range of 1-300 V/m and a flat frequency response from 10 kHz to 220 MHz. Ruggera (1977) and Hurt and Allen (1979) provide information on the use of the EFS-1 and an evaluation of its accuracy.

A diode based instrument manufactured by the General Microwave Corporation, model RAHAM-4, is an isotropic survey instrument designed for coverage of the 10 MHz to 26 GHz frequency range. Hopfer and Adler (1980) describe a new version of the model 4 which reportedly possesses broadband frequency coverage down to 200 kHz.

A new broadband instrument based on the NBS design (Bowman, 1974) has recently been introduced by Holaday Industries, Inc., which employs diode detection principles in combination with several unique instrumentation approaches. Figure 4 is a block diagram of the Holaday model 3001 instrument. The two major innovations in the 3001 are (a) the incorporation of digital circuitry to correct for the diodes' response over a very large field strength range, extending the instruments useable dynamic range to approximately 60 dB, and (b) the use of a full-time automatic zero adjustment circuit freeing the operator from ever having to check the zero setting and virtually eliminating instrument drift.

The first feature is accomplished by using a digital read-only-memory (ROM) which stores the response curves for the detection probe diodes. The detector output voltage is used to determine the actual field strength via a look-up table technique; i.e., the ROM has stored in it the value of voltage that would be associated with a true square law response from the diode. This proper value obtained from the ROM is used in the determination of the field level. The automatic zero feature is implemented by a multiplexing technique. A multiplexer switching circuit sequentially samples the output voltage conducted from each of the three diode detectors via high resistivity lines and in addition, reads a value from a fourth reference lead which is terminated at the sensitive probe but is not connected to a detector element. By referencing each of the three detector outputs to this reference lead output at a rate of approximately 7000 times per second, the instrument continually compensates for variations in amplifier circuitry gain variations. This particular feature is extremely useful since the operator need not concern himself with checking the zero set while in precarious situations where it might be difficult or impossible to properly shield the detector.

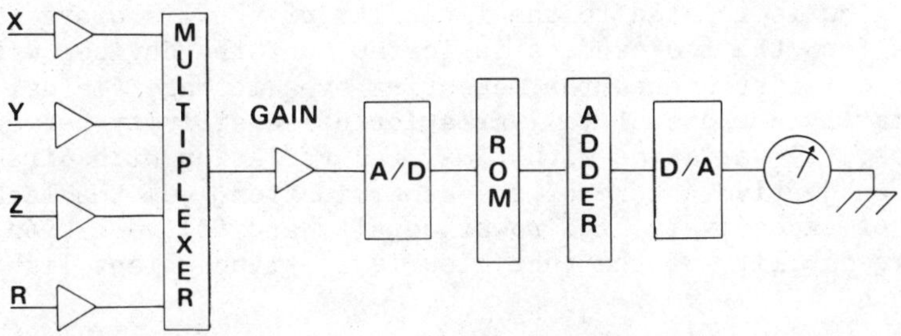

Figure 4. Simplified block diagram of the Holaday Industries, Inc., model 3001 instrument. A reference channel, R, is used to provide automatic zero-set and a read-only-memory (ROM) is implemented for correcting the diode detector response for non-square law operation.

The design of measurement probes based on the principle of diode detection has been extended to very small probes suitable for implantation in biological tissue. Bassen (1977) described a miniature electric field probe consisting of three, mutually orthogonal dipoles each 2.5 mm long mounted in an I-beam configuration. A fiber optically-linked telemetry system is used to read the voltage from the diode detector which provides radiofrequency interference immunity and enhances accuracy by eliminating cable scatter. This probe is useable over the frequency range of 0.2 to 12 GHz and exhibits a sensitivity permitting the detection of an 8.7 V/m field at 2.5 GHz with a 10 dB signal to noise ratio in a 1 Hz bandwidth or a 27.5 V/m field in a 2 kHz bandwidth. Cheung et al. (1976) discuss applications of small probes to the measurement of internal fields in biological media and methods for their calibration. Although these very small probes are only practically useful in the laboratory, they permit extremely high spatial resolution of electromagnetic fields and find particular application in exploring the field structure inside of small devices such as animal holders used in biological effects research work.

Table 2 provides a summary of the performance characteristics of several commercially available, broadband, diode based instruments for measuring electromagnetic fields. These specifications are taken from the manufacturers' literature.

Preignited Neon-Mercury Tubes

Moore et al. (1970) and Klein et al. (1970) report on the evaluation of a preignited neon-mercury glow tube type detector which was designed to detect microwave oven leakage. The degree of tube glow is related to the intensity of the microwave field. Findings from the two studies indicated that the devices were not satisfactory instruments for measuring oven leakage fields. This was primarily because of (a) variation of sensitivity between instruments, (b) variation with time, (c) variation with direction, (d) the subjective nature of the determination, (e) the lack of warning of excessively high power density and (f) variation of visual readability of the tube glow level with ambient lighting conditions.

PERSONNEL DOSIMETERS

Since the beginning of concerns over hazardous exposure of personnel to high intensity electromagnetic fields, there have been attempts to devise a practical dosimeter that could be worn on the person. In 1958 Ely (1958) provided a description of a field trial of what was known as the Richardson microwave dosimeter. This small, pocket sized unit consisted of a small gelatin capsule which contained a thermistor for detecting increases in the gelatin temperature. The thermistor was followed by a one or two stage dc transistor amplifier circuit and an indicating meter.

Table 2. Summary of Specifications for Two Commercially Available Diode Based Broadband Electromagnetic Field Survey Instruments (1)

	General Microwave RAHAM Model 4	Holaday Model 3002	
Field parameter which instrument senses	Electric field	Electric field	Magnetic field
Frequency range	10 MHz - 26 GHz	0.5 MHz -6 GHz	5 MHz - 300 MHz
Indicated full scale measuring ranges	0.02, 0.2, 2, 20 mW/cm^2	10^4, 10^5, 10^6, 10^7 V^2/m^2	0.1, 1, 10, 100 A^2/m^2(2)
Frequency response	± 2 dB	0.5 - 6 GHz ±2 dB 1 MHz - 1 GHz ±1 dB 3 MHz - 500 MHz ±0.5 dB	5 MHz - 300 MHz ±2 dB 10 MHz - 200 MHz ±1
Calibration accuracy	± 0.5 dB at 2.45 GHz	±0.5 dB at selected calibration frequencies	
Overload level	0.5 W/cm^2 average 150 W- S/cm 30 W/cm^2 peak	8 x full scale	
Isotropicity	± 0.5 dB (3)	±0.5 dB (3)	
Response time	1.5 seconds	<1 second Peak hold 5 mS (4)	
Operating time	900 hours (non-rechargeable)	28 hours (non-rechargeable)	
Recorder output	0.124 V for full scale	1.0 V for full scale	
Weight	3.25 lbs. (1.46 kg)	6.5 lbs. (2.9 kg)	

(1) Specifications provided in this table are taken from published manufacturer's descriptive literature.
(2) Meter indications are in field strength units squared.
(3) Maximum deviation from energy incident from any direction except from/through handle.
(4) A maximum hold circuit retains maximum field strength value.
(5) This instrument has a low level probe and a high level probe. Overload specification is for each one.

The gelatin mass was intended to simulate an avascular body structure which, principally because of its water content, would be heated by an electromagnetic field. The impression provided in Ely's account is that this instrument was not a calibrated device and due to significant variation in instrument readings due to changes in ambient temperature was not useful for indicating exposure to even intense microwave fields. Ely also commented on the fact that there existed an immediate response to the heating effect due to pickup of radiofrequency energy directly on the thermistor leads and subsequently a response due to actual heating of the gelatin mass.

Crapuchettes (1970) briefly mentioned a small pocket sized radiofrequency dosimeter designated as the model C-1 produced by Scientific Protection Devices, Inc. Apparently this device was manufactured for only a short time and there is no technical description of its operation.

Minin (1974) describes several Soviet versions of small radiofrequency dosimeters. These units have all made use of some form of small antenna probe, usually a small loop, a diode detector unit, and some form of accumulative readout mechanism. The use of both mechanical and electro-chemical (such as the hydrogen coulometer) forms of memory are described. Thus the intent is to retain information on the product of exposure level and time. Minin discusses the use of both orthogonally arranged loop sensors and mechanically driven, by small motor, loops to improve their isotropicity response. It is pointed out that chemical integrators are not desirable because of their susceptibility to jolting from movement of the individual. Nonlinearity in integration due to the nonlinear detector diode characteristic is also mentioned as a shortcoming of these designs. A single turn loop type of dosimeter is described by Minin which used a mercury capillary coulometer to measure exposure. This device is claimed to have a response sensitivity of 0.01 mm of electrolyte travel/μW hour/cm^2, a memory volume of 4000 μW-hour/cm^2 or 14.4 J/cm^2 and an upper frequency limit of 1 GHz. It is not clear what the isotropic response or frequency response is.

Iskander, Durney, and Jaggard (1980) describe initial development activities toward realizing a microwave personnel dosimeter using three printed circuit orthogonal dipoles using diode detectors and high resistance leads to a microcoulometer for integration over a period of time. A major problem associated with any personnel dosimeter is the interaction of the body with the instrument leading to erroneously indicated values of exposure.

Kornberg et al. (1980) described the development of a small personnel dosimeter designed for use in 60 Hz fields associated with work around electrical power systems. In this design, microelectronics are used to sort the field amplitudes into ranges so that after a period of time, the dosimeter can be read to determine not only the range of exposure levels but the length of time that the dosimeter was exposed at each range of field intensity. This type of active processing of exposure data is needed to meaningfully assess personnel exposure to radiofrequency fields when continual observation and logging of exposure level data is not practical. The problem of body proximity to the detector becomes more critical at radiofrequencies and severe constraints on frequency response appear to be inescapable.

NARROWBAND, SELECTIVELY TUNED INSTRUMENTATION

Narrowband measurement systems may be characterized as more sophisticated than broadband field meters. This is so because of the more complicated task of being able to measure the amplitude of frequency specific signals. These systems are typically bulky, not necessarily portable, and most often require external antennas for sensing of the electric or magnetic field. The narrowband measurement techniques coupled with antennas, usually a sizeable fraction of a wavelength in size, yield very high field intensity measurement sensitivities.

Spectrum Analyzers

A spectrum analyzer is an instrument which graphically displays voltage or power as a function of frequency on a cathode ray tube (CRT). It is thus a form of a swept radiofrequency receiver which can be used to analyze signals in the frequency domain. Although there are numerous advantages to spectrum analyzers for certain forms of signal analysis, the principle feature useful for making electromagnetic field measurements is its ability to present a display of individual signal components over a very wide range of frequencies in a very short observation period. Thus the spectrum analyzer permits quick determination of signals of interest when conducting an environmental electromagnetic field evaluation which would take a much longer time to accomplish with a tuned receiver.

The type of spectrum analyzer most used in the radiofrequency or microwave region is the swept-tuned analyzer. Swept-tuned analyzers are tuned by electronically sweeping them over their frequency range. Therefore, the frequency components of a spectrum are sampled sequentially in time. The block diagram of a swept superheterodyne spectrum analyzer is shown in Figure 5. Hewlett-Packard (1974) describes the analyzer as basically a narrow-band receiver which is electronically tuned in frequency by applying a saw-tooth voltage to the frequency control element of a voltage tuned local oscillator (VTO). This same saw-tooth voltage is simultaneously applied to the horizontal deflection plates of the CRT. The output from the receiver is synchronously applied to the vertical deflection plates of the CRT and a plot of amplitude versus frequency is displayed.

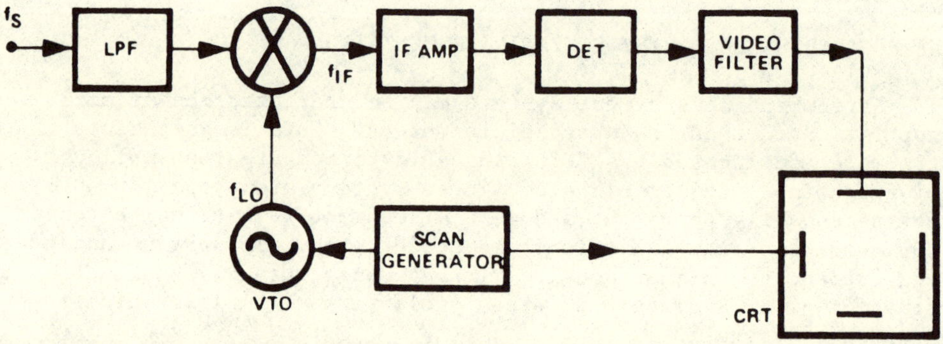

Figure 5. Block diagram of a swept superheterodyne spectrum analyzer.

The analyzer is tuned through its frequency range by varying the voltage on the local oscillator (LO). The LO frequency is mixed with the input signal to produce an intermediate frequency (IF). When the frequency difference between the input signal and the LO frequency is equal to the IF frequency, then there is a response on the analyzer.

The advantages of the superheterodyne technique are considerable. It obtains high sensitivity through the use of IF amplifiers, and many decades in frequency can be tuned. Also, the resolution can be varied by changing the bandwidth of the IF filters. Some spectrum analyzers employ electronically controlled frequency tracking filters on the front-end to enhance overall selectivity and minimize spurious responses. In some designs there exist external control lines which are interfaced to a controlling computer.

There are two aspects of spectrum analyzers which must be considered when applying them to the measurement of radiofrequency signals. When used to detect pulsed signals, such as from a radar, care must be taken to insure that the bandwidth of the IF filter (this is the filter which determines frequency resolution in the analyzer) is sufficient to permit response to the peak of an incident pulse; i.e., for response to pulsed signals the proper IF bandwidth is determined by the width of the pulse, being wider for narrower pulses. An IF, or resolution bandwidth, of approximately 3 MHz is usually sufficient to permit accurate response to the amplitude of pulses from most radar systems. However, if too narrow of an IF bandwidth is used, there can occur what is called pulse desensitization. This is a phenomenon wherein the filter bandwidth, which has an associated time constant, is so narrow that a narrow pulse which has high frequency content can not produce full output from the filter. In this case, the analyzer is desensitized and erroneously low values of peak signal strength will be indicated. Pulse desensitization can be corrected for by a special determination of the impulse bandwidth of the IF filter.

Another feature of the spectrum analyzer is that it is a peak detector; i.e., it responds, or attempts to respond, to the instantaneous amplitude of the input signal. If the time-average or rms value of signals are desired (these signals could be simple unmodulated signals which are varying slowly in time due to fade or operational characteristics or they could consist of complex, modulated radiofrequency carriers) then some form of data processing is required. Such processing may consist of simple photographic techniques using variable persistence phosphor CRTs or more complicated digital processing in a controlling computer.

The spectrum analyzer display is most commonly calibrated in units of radiofrequency power delivered to the input terminal in units of milliwatts or dBm where 0dBm = 1 mW. The dBm units are preferred since spectrum analyzers normally possess a logarithmic display format such that a rather large dynamic range of signal levels may be viewed.

Field Strength Meters

A field strength meter can be thought of as a tuneable, narrowband radiofrequency voltmeter. The field strength meter, or receiver as it is commonly referred to, is similar to a radio receiver in that it contains manually tuneable circuitry, usually using superheterodyne techniques, manually tuned front-end filtering, and an indicating meter movement calibrated in terms of the radiofrequency voltage applied to the input terminal of the receiver. In a literal sense a calibrated radio receiver (one which has a calibrated radiofrequency voltage meter) becomes a field strength meter only when it has associated with it some form of calibrated antenna. In practice one must know the calibration factor (antenna factor) of the antenna to be able to interpret the receiver's indicated voltage in terms of the actual intensity or strength of the electromagnetic field illuminating the sense antenna.

A field strength meter may consist of a receiver and loop antenna combined into an integral system. Such a unit, although only sensitive to the magnetic field component of an electromagnetic wave, may be calibrated in terms of the equivalent electric field strength which would occur in a plane-wave environment. This derives from the fact that measurements of the magnetic field are less subject to proximity effects of near-by obstacles such as the operator and conventionally, broadcast engineers are mostly interested in the electric field intensity from a broadcast point of view. This points out the need to be aware of the principle of operation of the device used for making field intensity measurements if one wishes to properly interpret results, especially in near-field situations. Since the relationship of E/H = 377 ohms is used in such an instrument's calibration the actual magnetic field strength can always be properly obtained by calculation. But only in the far field of a source will the indicated electric field strength be correct.

The nominal input impedance of most radiofrequency measurement equipment is 50 ohms. Thus when using either a spectrum analyzer or field strength receiver for field strength measurements the operator must insure that the impedance of the calibrated antenna is also 50 ohms or that its calibration was established when used with a 50 ohm detection system. In practice this is usually not a problem in that most antenna systems developed for such measurements are designed and calibrated for use with 50 ohm receivers or spectrum analyzers.

Field strength meters or receivers, in contrast to spectrum analyzers, often contain specialized detector functions. For example, such receivers may feature three basic detector types; (a) an average responding detector, (b) an instantaneous peak detector, and (c) a so-called quasi-peak detector. The quasi-peak detector function possesses a rapid attack time, as in the peak detector, and a relatively fast decay time. This permits convenient determination of the peak value of rapidly changing pulsed signals.

Calibrated Receiving Antennas

Antennas used for making measurements of electromagnetic field intensity can be characterized in several ways. Passive antennas simply contain no electronically active devices such as transistors or integrated circuits. Passive antennas are most common for use in electromagnetic field strength measurements. Active antennas contain some form of active device which is typically used to transform impedance, introduce gain, or shape the frequency response of the antenna. There are tuned antennas which exhibit specific resonant frequencies at which the efficiency of the antenna increases and broadband antennas which possess relatively small variations in their calibration factor with frequency. Most antennas possess specific polarizations which means that they must be properly aligned with the field vector of choice; alternatively, if the antenna is linearily polarized, three separate and mutually orthogonal measurements of the field vector can be made from which the resultant field may be determined. Equation 9 is the mathematical expression of this definition of electric field strength.

$$E = \sqrt{E_x^2 + E_y^2 + E_z^2} \tag{9}$$

Antennas may also be classified according to their directivity, i.e., their beam-width.

The choice of an antenna for a specific measurement task is best determined by the nature of both the source of radiation and the measurement environment. For example if the field intensity of a rapidly moving beam of radiation is to be measured, wherein the received signal level is continually changing thereby making the proper orientation of the antenna difficult, it is advisable to use a relatively low directivity or broad beamed receiving antenna. Such a choice permits more accurate alignment of the main axis of the reception antenna with the incident field, often by purely visual means. Thus uncertainty in the measured field strength due to misalignment of the reception antenna is reduced.

The received signal voltage obtained from a receiving antenna may be related to the strength of the illuminating field by knowledge of the antenna factor. The antenna factor is defined as the multiplicative factor by which the receiver voltage is multiplied to obtain the field strength, or

$$E = V(AF) \tag{10}$$

where

E = incident electric field strength (V/m)
V = antenna voltage at receiver input terminal (V)
AF = antenna factor (m^{-1})

In logarithmic units

$$E(dB\mu V/m) = V(dB\mu V) + AF(dBm^{-1}) \tag{11}$$

Figure 6 is an example of the antenna factor for a calibrated dipole antenna. At each frequency the dipole must be readjusted for resonance, typically by shortening or lengthening telescopic elements. It should be noted that the higher the gain of an antenna, i.e., the higher its efficiency, the lower the antenna factor will be. Appendix A provides a derivation of equation 11.

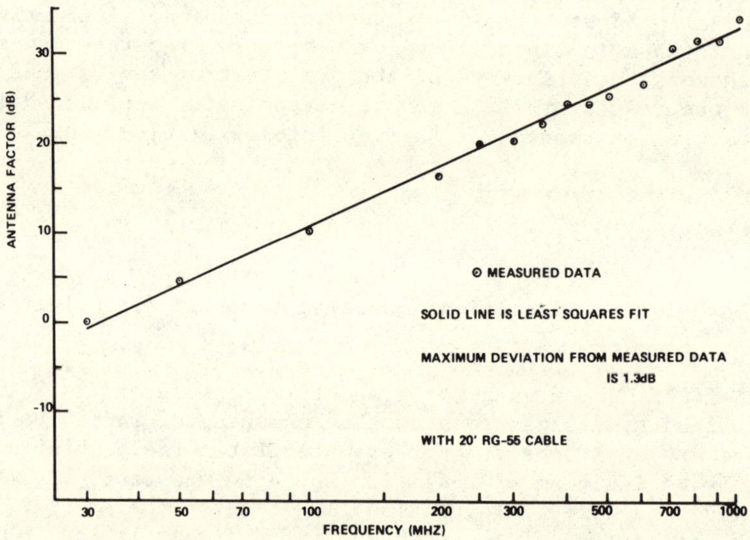

Figure 6. The measured antenna factor for three separate, adjustable dipole receiving antennas as a function of frequency. Straight line is the least square fit of the measured data. Note that at each frequency the dipole must be readjusted for resonance.

For instrumentation which possesses an impedance of 50 ohms, a signal power measured in dBm units may be converted to equivalent voltage in dBμV by the correction factor of 107 dB, i.e.,

$$V(dB\mu V) = P(dBm) + 107 \text{ dB}.$$

Appendix B provides a derivation of the 107 dB correction factor.

To completely determine the strength of an arbitrary electromagnetic field it is convenient to use specialized antennas consisting of assemblies of dipole elements to create an approximation to an isotropic receiver. Figure 7 illustrates an example of such an assembly installed on a measurement van. In practice separate coaxial cables are brought down to the detection equipment from each dipole element. The received field strength is read sequentially from each dipole and processed in a small computer to obtain the value given by equation 9.

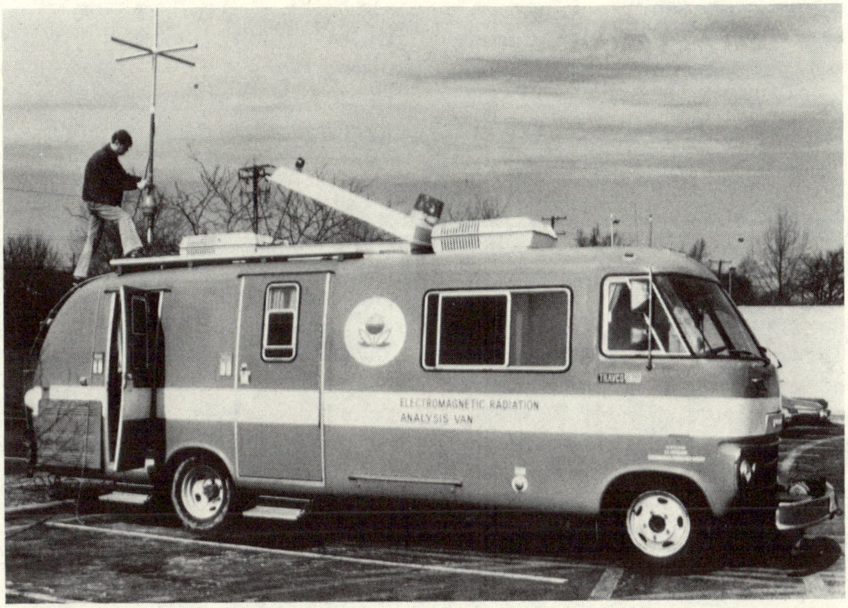

Figure 7. A large mobile electromagnetic field measurement van illustrating an orthogonal, calibrated measurement antenna system for absolute field strength measurements in the VHF frequency range.

Since in general the antenna factor is a function of frequency, making large numbers of field strength measurements can become tedious due to separate antenna corrections required at each frequency. For this reason it is desirable to have broadband antennas for which the antenna factor is a constant, eliminating the use of different antenna factors across the spectrum of interest.

A unique antenna system developed at the National Bureau of Standards and referred to by its developers as a broadband, isotropic, real-time, electric-field sensor (Kanda, Ries, and Belsher, 1980) consists of three resistively loaded dipoles mounted orthogonally to each other. An electronics amplification package is used to increase the induced signal levels of the antenna resulting in a sensitivity of about 20 μV/m. Below 200 MHz the cable signal pick-up begins to compete with the antenna elements themselves and the overall system sensitivity becomes greater which is revealed by decreasing antenna factor values. This antenna system has been used in several measurement problems inside of building structures where larger antennas would not have been feasible or would not necessarily resolve the complex field patterns caused by multiple reflections. A switch on the electronics package permits two ranges of sensitivity thereby making measurements possible in either moderately weak or relatively intense signal environments.

Automated Measurement Systems

An automated measurement system is an assembly of equipment which permits collection of radiofrequency field strength data with some form of digital control of the various elements of the system. Several approaches to automated measurements have been developed. Most automated systems have been applied to the measurement of band occupancy; i.e., the determination of the presence of radio signals on given frequencies (Hagn, et al. 1971; McMahon, 1973; Matheson, 1977). Such studies are primarily designed to aid in efficient spectrum management techniques. Tell (1976) has described an automated system which is used for collecting environmental field intensity data through the use of a computer automated spectrum analyzer with associated antenna systems.

Figure 8 is a block diagram of a typical automated measurement system. Any such system consists of a remotely, digitally controlled receiver or spectrum analyzer, appropriately calibrated receiving antennas, antenna switching hardware, and a digital computer to effect the actual control. Usually, some form of mass storage device is used, such as a magnetic tape drive or rotating disc memory system, to store applications software and data resulting from the measurement process. Figure 8 depicts the use of an orthogonal antenna system, individual elements of which are automatically selected for connection to the input of the spectrum analyzer.

Several special features possible when using automated field strength measurement systems are worthy of discussion. Since antenna systems composed of several individual elements, as in the case of three mutually orthogonal dipoles, may be used in routine measurements, any one element will only provide field strength data associated with the element's particular polarization plane. In general it is necessary to perform the vector addition of these field components; such addition is readily accomplished in the computing controller used by the system. The resultant electric field strength, as given in equation 9 is formed by squaring each of the individual field strength components, summing, and extraction of the square root of this sum. Note that in the case of a spectrum analyzer the output signal is normally given directly in power units and since power is proportional to the square of the input voltage from the antenna and thus the square of the field strength, it is not necessary to square each value of data obtained from the analyzer by the computer. This can result in a reduction in processing time.

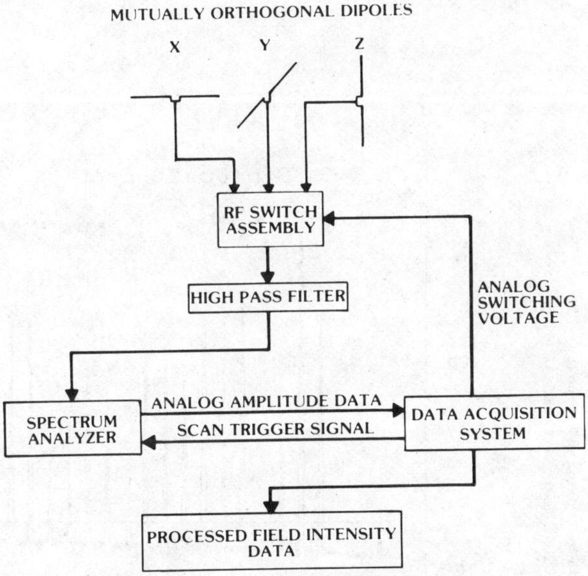

Figure 8. Block diagram of a typical automated radiofrequency measurement system consisting of calibrated receiving antennas and a computer controlled spectrum analyzer.

Another valuable feature of computer based systems is the ability to perform signal averaging. Thus in the case of signals whose amplitudes vary in time, it is straight forward to perform continual computations on the incoming signal values to obtain the time-average of the amplitude. In a similar fashion the computer may be programmed to check each signal value to determine if it is greater or lesser than the previous sample value. Consequently peak retention software routines may be implemented which permit the maximum value of signals at each frequency to be retained in memory and used for further analysis after some suitable observation period.

Spectral integration of measured amplitude spectra is often of interest to find the resultant exposure intensity of a complete band of individual signals. Figure 9 illustrates a typical measured spectrum of signals obtained in New York City with an automated measurement system as plotted on the internal thermal printer contained within the computer. Note that the ordinate is labeled in units of electric field strength in dBμV/m. These values of resultant electric field strength are the time averaged amplitudes of the signals obtained over a sample period of several minutes. Although the strengths of the individual FM radio stations

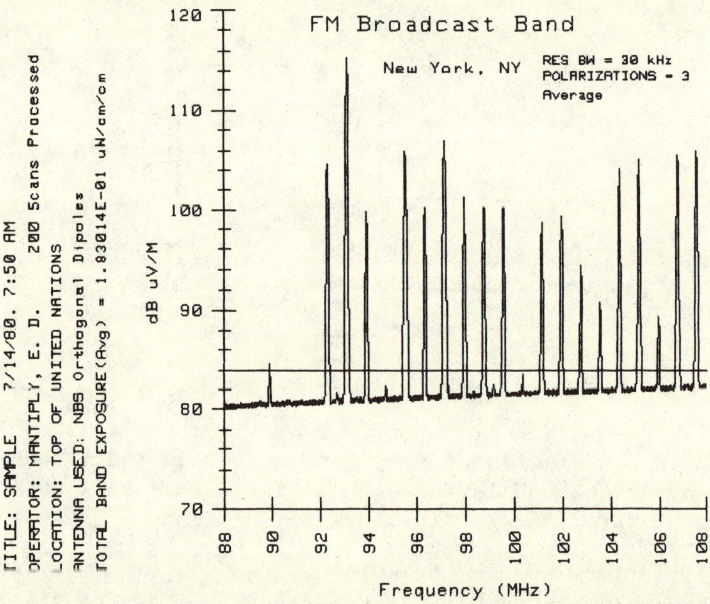

Figure 9. Graphical output of measured spectrum of FM broadcast signals obtained with an automated measurement system in New York City. The vertical axis represents the resultant electric field strength in units of dBμV/m. These values of field strength are averaged over a short observation period by the computer. The horizontal line represents a threshold value for integrating the power density equivalents of all of the signals; signals above the threshold are included in the summation process, the result of which is printed at the side of the graph.

are directly given, an integration of this spectrum by the computer in effect converts each measured field strength value to the equivalent plane wave power density using the relation of equation 7, sums up the power densities of all signals, and prints out the value of band power density in units of $\mu W/cm^2$ at the side of the graph.

Probably the single most powerful advantage of automated radiofrequency measurement systems is the ability to store in the computer's memory the antenna factor data which allows automatic correction of the incoming data from the spectrum analyzer to directly obtain field strength. In reality it is useful to store the antenna correction data in a mathematical form as a function of frequency. This allows computation of appropriate antenna factors over any selected part of the spectrum for which the system is employed. In fact expressions for many different antennas may be stored and accessed by appropriate input from the operator.

Upon completion of a spectral measurement the processed data is typically written into a tape or flexible disc file for subsequent computerized access and/or re-evaluation. It is apparent that automated systems permit a rapid and accurate indication of the field intensities of large numbers of signals when conducting environmental evaluations.

Figure 10 is a picture of an automated system installed in a four-wheel drive utility vehicle designed for environmental measurement and analysis over a large frequency range. This photo shows a steerable dish antenna mounted on top of the vehicle for measurements in the 1-12 GHz band which features selection of individual horizontal and vertical polarization components. A small gasoline powered generator is used to provide ac power for the instrumentation.

Signal Processing

There are several types of signal processing which are of particular value in the measurement of radar signals. Radars represent a considerable problem in environmental measurements; this problem is principally related to (a) the moving beam of radiation which typically illuminates a given measurement area for only a fraction of a second and (b) the task of determining the average field intensity of the pulsed emission. Since the spectrum analyzer, when used with a sufficiently wide IF bandwidth, will properly respond to the instantaneous peak signal level of the radar, the average signal level must usually be

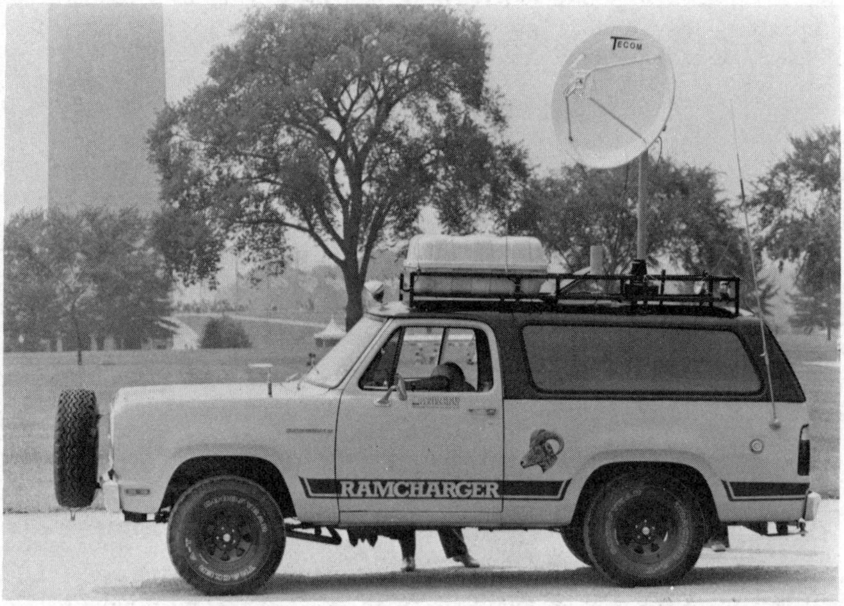

Figure 10. An automated radiofrequency measurement system installed in a four-wheel drive utility vehicle designed for environmental measurement and analysis over a large frequency range. The photograph shows a steerable parabolic dish antenna which features selection of individual horizontal and vertical polarization components.

determined by measuring the duty cycle of the radar emission. Duty cycle is given by

$$D = t(PRF) \tag{12}$$

where

D = duty cycle
t = pulse width (s)

PRF = pulse repetion frequency (Hz)

From a knowledge of the duty cycle and the peak incident power density, the average power density is given by

$$S_{av} = D \cdot S_{pk} \tag{13}$$

This means that the PRF and pulse width must be measured through some technique. Commonly this is accomplished by observing the radar signal in the time domain; Tell (1975) has reported on measurements of both PRF and pulse width of air traffic control radars using a manually operated spectrum analyzer. Computer enhanced spectrum analysis techniques permit more rapid and accurate assessments of these parameters and consequently the duty cycle by which the peak field intensity may be corrected to obtain the average value.

One area deserving special mention is the long-term time averaged field intensity of a rotating radar due to the movement of the radar's beam of radiation over the area of interest. Thus it is desirable to measure the apparent rotational duty cycle of the radar antenna and this is a relatively convenient matter for an automated measurement system. In essence, the technique consists of monitoring in time the variation in peak field intensity over one or more complete rotations of the antenna. The computer is then used to find the mathematical average of the field intensity values and relate this average value to that measured as the main beam of the radar passes by the measurement site. This antenna rotational duty cycle may then be used to correct the measured field strengths and arrive at a true average value, averaged not only over the transmitter duty cycle but also the time rate of change of the beam direction. An example measurement of the peak signal arriving from a rotating radar is illustrated in Figure 11. Here one complete antenna rotation is apparent from the presence of two main beam peaks of signal observed on the left and the right of the display. The distance between the two peaks corresponds to 360 degrees of antenna rotation.

The ultimate accuracy of any field strength measurement system is dependent on the accuracy of the antenna factors used in the measurement process. When employing antennas mounted on vehicles it is preferable to calibrate the receiving antennas in place as they will be used and to fully characterize any influence of the vehicle on the antenna patterns. Tell et al. (1976) describe a technique for measuring the radiation pattern of several antennas, including orthogonal dipolar arrays, for the measurement van shown in Figure 7. For this case, the entire van system was rotated on a large turntable and pattern varitions were measured using the equipment in the vehicle. From an analy-

Operator: Michael R. Molony 03/23/81. 2:51 PM
Location: LAB, EPA ROOM 521, BLDG C

Sweep Time = 20 sec Res BW = 3 MHz

Reference Level = 0 dBm
Scale Div = 10 dB/

Antenna Rotational Duty Cycle Center freq = 1.3311 GHz

Peaks measured at:
Location 1: 220 -16.60dBm Location 2: 827 -16.90dBm

Radar Rotation Rate:
Seconds/Rotation: 12.14 R P M 4.942

Main Beam Reference: -16.747 dBm

Antenna duty cycle: -20.581 dBm

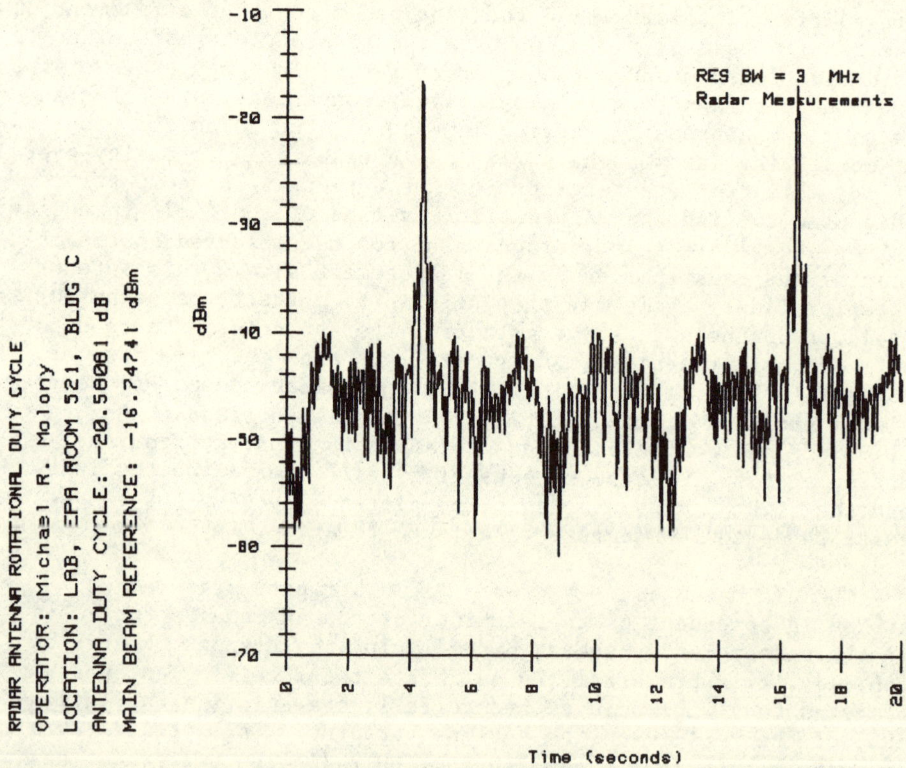

Figure 11. An example measurement of the antenna rotational duty cycle of a common air traffic control radar using an automated measurement system. The two tall peaks represent main beam alignment with the receiving location from one full rotation.

sis of these data it was concluded that a worst case error of ±2.5 dB was associated with the measurement system. This uncertainty figure is primarily related to the absolute accuracy of the antenna factors and pattern variations of individual antenna elements.

Electro-Optical Crystals

Bassen and Peterson (1976) have described a unique narrow-band electric field probe based on the property of an electro-optical crystal to modulate a laser beam. A small (1 mm x 1 mm x 20 mm) lithium niobate crystal is imbedded in either a dipole or loop antenna. A laser beam, passing through the crystal is modulated by the action of the crystal. Because of the electro-optical crystal's very fast response time, the instantaneous voltage applied to the crystal is converted without degradation to laser beam amplitude modulation. Thus this system is able to measure the waveform of the field being measured whether it is a sinusoidal signal or a complex waveform (short pulsed radiofrequency, multi-frequency radiofrequency, or transient electromagnetic pulse, EMP). The laser beam after transmission through the crystal is detected with a semiconductor PIN (positive-intrinsic-negative) photodiode detector whose output is delivered to a radiofrequency spectrum analyzer which permits recovery of both the frequency and amplitude of the field illuminating the crystal detector system. Bassen and Peterson (1976) found a maximum sensitivity of 1 V/m when using a 30 cm long dipole antenna with a 30 Hz bandwidth on the spectrum analyzer. They surmise that with the use of an integrated optical modulator, the dipole length could be reduced to 3 cm with the same overall sensitivity.

Calibration of Instrumentation

The calibration of instrumentation is complicated by a number of problems including (a) the size of the instrument, (b) the intensity range over which it is desired to calibrate the equipment and (c) the frequency range over which calibrations are to be performed. For example, if relatively large receiving antennas are to be calibrated, a volume of space sufficiently large to uniformly illuminate the antenna is required. This also places more difficult constraints on insuring a reflection free area for the calibration process. If very high field intensities are to be used this usually requires relatively high power generating equipment.

Calibration methods pertinent to field strength measuring equipment include (a) free space standard field methods, (b) guided wave methods and (c) transfer probe methods.

Free Space Radiated Field Techniques. This technique consists of creating a standard or known field intensity at some point in space. The broadband probe or antenna is placed in this standard field and the instrument response is noted. In any technique requiring the radiation of a field, reflections can introduce uncertainties in the calibrating field. This arises because, in general, the field is calculated from known properties of the transmitting antenna and it is virtually impossible to account theoretically for the reflections which may introduce multipath fields into the region of interest causing the actual field strength to be different from the calculated value. More severe reflections cause greater uncertainties.

Standard gain transmitting horn antennas are commonly used to establish highly accurate electromagnetic field intensities, primarily in the microwave range above 1 GHz. Commonly, microwave calibrations are conducted within anechoic chambers; an anechoic chamber is a room which is lined with microwave anechoic or nonreflective material. The purpose of the anechoic chamber is to create a reflectionless environment in the vicinity of the antenna or broadband probe which is being calibrated. Such chambers are extremely expensive and often require considerable floor space. Aslan (1979) described the use of standard gain horn antennas and a so-called anechoic sled apparatus for averaging out multipath interference. Two parallel panels, surfaced with anechoic material face one another. By varying the distance between the probe being calibrated and the back panel, it is possible to chose a position which minimizes the influence of reflections.

The field in front of the transmitting horn is calculated based on the physical dimensions of the horn. To achieve higher field intensities with limited transmitter power, illumination of the probe is accomplished within the near-field of the horn. Swicord et al. (1976) describe radiated field techniques with emphasis on determination of the uncertainty in the calibration. Larsen (1979) outlines a method for computing the on-axis gain of the horn. Following Larsen's procedure several parameters are developed for the horn according to Figure 12 taken from his work. Each physical dimension is divided by the free-space wavelength to obtain wavelength normalized values where A and B are the wavelength normalized width and height of the horn aperature, L_E and L_H are the wavelength normalized values of the slant distances to the central axis of the horn and D is the wavelength normalized value of the distance from the front surface of the horn. Accordingly

$$\alpha = A^2\left[\frac{1}{L_H} + \frac{1}{D}\right] \quad \text{and} \quad \beta = B^2\left[\frac{1}{L_E} + \frac{1}{D}\right] \tag{14}$$

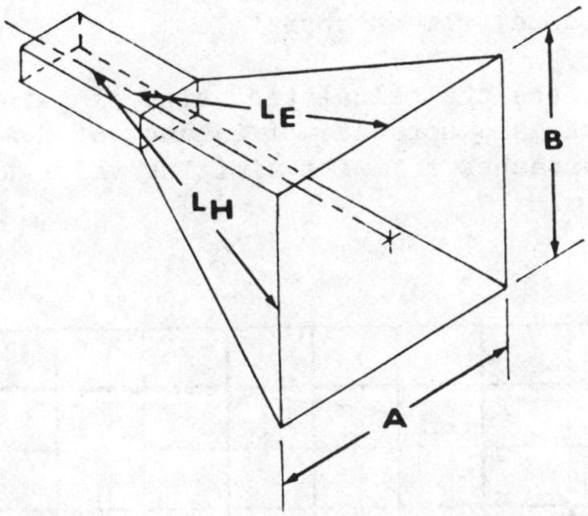

Figure 12. Standard gain horn dimensions used in computation of near-field gain [taken from Larsen (1979)].

Larsen has developed two equations which determine the gain reduction factors R_H and R_E, in dB. These are given by

$$R_H = (0.01\alpha)(1+10.19\alpha + 0.51\alpha^2 - 0.097\alpha^3) \tag{15}$$

due to the H-plane flare of the horn, and

$$R_E = (0.1\beta^2)\ (2.31 + 0.053\beta) \tag{16}$$

due to the E-plane flare of the horn. Larsen gives the theoretical gain of a horn as

$$G(dB) = 10 \log (AB) + 10.08 - R_H - R_E. \tag{17}$$

The net input power to the horn is determined through forward and reflected power measurements at the feed to the horn using a bi-directional coupler and the field intensity S is then computed using the gain provided in equation 17 as

$$S = \frac{P_T G}{4\pi R^2}$$

where

S = power density (W/m^2)
P_T = transmitted power (W)
G = absolute numerical power gain of antenna
R = distance from antenna (m)

Figure 13 illustrates the calculated value of gain for a Narda model 645 standard gain horn at a frequency of 2.45 GHz. Notice that the gain approaches a finite limiting value beyond a distance of about 2 m.

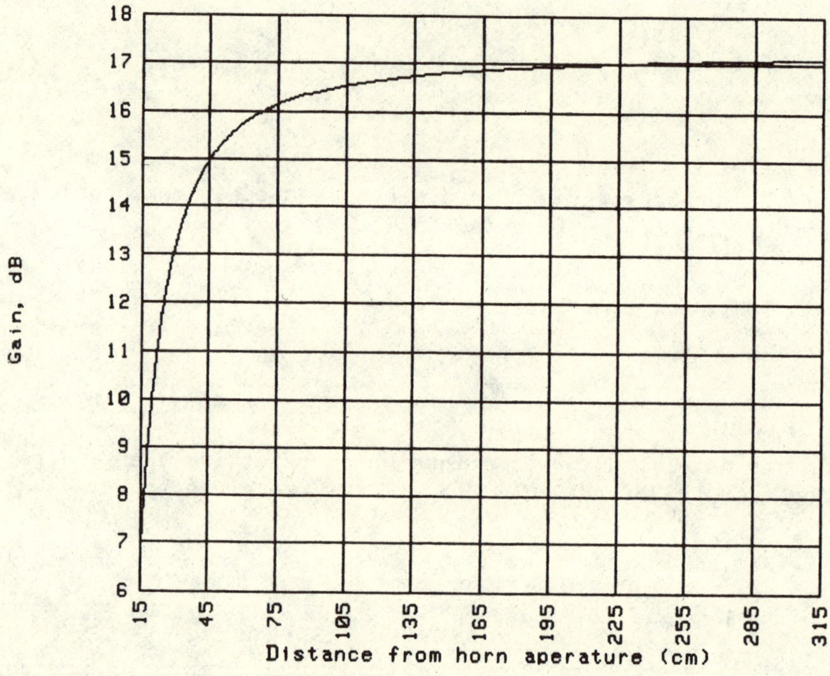

Figure 13. Calculated gain for a Narda Microwave Corporation model 645 standard gain horn at a frequency of 2.45 GHz using equations 14, 15, 16 and 17. Note that the gain approaches a finite limiting value beyond a distance of about 2 m.

<u>Compact Antenna Ranges</u>. Another method for achieving a plane wave irradiation field for calibration purposes consists of using the so-called compact antenna range. Such a device, produced by the Scientific Atlanta Company, facilitates the creation of plane wave fields at very short distances by reflecting a wave off of a curved surface. In this instance the field is most commonly determined via measurement with a suitable transfer probe which has

been previously calibrated via other means. This technique has found most application in the microwave frequency range above 1 GHz.

Antenna Gain by the Identical Antenna Method. White (1971) describes a method for experimentally determining the gain of an antenna. The method requires that two identical antennas be used; one is used to transmit a signal while the other is used to receive the signal. By measurement of the net power delivered to the transmitting antenna P_T and the net power delivered from the receiving antenna P_R the antenna gain of the antennas is given by

$$G = \frac{4\pi R}{\lambda}\sqrt{\frac{P_R}{P_T}} \tag{18}$$

Where R is the distance between the antennas and λ is the free-space wavelength. Appendix B illustrates how to relate the gain of an antenna to antenna factor for use in field strength measurements.

Transfer Probe Methods

Standard Gain Receiving Dipole Antennas. Taggart and Workman (1969) describe the use of standard gain receiving dipole antennas by the National Bureau of Standards for use in calibrating other antennas. These antennas are based on the accurately calculable theoretical gain of a resonant half-wave dipole. Each dipole is physically cut to a resonant length and the induced radiofrequency voltage at the feed point of the dipole is measured after detection by a semi-conducting diode as a dc voltage. A small filtering network is used to remove radiofrequency currents from the leads which go to a high impedance dc voltmeter. A direct calibration of the diode detector assembly is accomplished by applying a balanced and accurately known radiofrequency voltage across the diode and measuring the dc voltage output. Since the gain of a resonant half-wave dipole is known to be 1.64, the dc output voltage from the dipole, when it is illuminated by a plane wave field, can then be accurately related to the incident electric field strength. The ultimate accuracy of this technique is dependent on the ability to accurately calibrate the diode response by way of a balanced voltage source and the reflections which are inherent to conducting antenna calibrations on a range. Antennas are calibrated via a substitution process, substituting the antenna to be calibrated for the standard dipole and measuring its response to the known field. In practice the use of such calibrated dipoles in outdoor situations results in ultimate accuracies of about ±1 dB.

Establishing Known Magnetic Fields. Taggart and Workman (1969) discuss a method for calibrating loop receiving antennas. The method consists of placing the loop being calibrated on the axis of a single-turn, unshielded, balanced transmitting loop of known radius carrying a known current. The magnitude of the field produced by the single-turn circular loop is given by

$$E = \frac{60\, r_1^2\, I}{(d^2+r_1^2+r_2^2)^{3/2}} \sqrt{1 + \left(\frac{2\pi d}{\lambda}\right)^2} \tag{19}$$

where

E = equivalent free-space electric field strength in rms
r_1 = radius of transmitting loop (m)
r_2 = radius of receiving loop (m)
d = axial spacing between the coaxial loops (m)
I = transmitting loop current (A)
λ = free-space wavelength (m)

Note that equation 19 finds the equivalent E field and assumes that E/H = 377 ohms. Thus the H field may be determined as well. Equation 19 is only valid for determining the field strength where r_1, r_2, and d are electrically small compared to λ. The loop spacing should be a minimum of four times the radii of the larger of r_1 or r_2 for equation 19 to be valid within one percent.

Guided Wave Techniques. Guided wave calibration techniques are mostly used at lower radiofrequencies up to about 1 GHz. The term guided wave is defined here to apply to any method of establishing a known electric and/or magnetic field by way of propagating a wave through some form of transmission line. Transmission lines may include open parallel plane lines, transverse electromagnetic cells, and rectangular waveguides.

Rectangular waveguides are appropriate for use in the 500 MHz to 1 GHz frequency range. In practice power is propagated through the waveguide to a matched absorptive load. The upper frequency in the guide is limited to that in which operation is in the dominant TE_{10} mode. For the TE_{10} mode the direction of the electric field vector is across the narrow face of the guide as shown in Figure 14. Larsen (1979) describes a method for calculating the strength of the electric E and magnetic H fields within the guide. According to Larsen the E-field amplitude is constant in the y direction but varies sinusoidally in the x direction. Propagation is in the z direction. The lowest "cutoff" frequency which will propagate in the guide (f_{co}) is given by

$$f_{co} = \frac{1.5 \times 10^8}{a} \tag{20}$$

where f_{co} is in Hertz and a is the guide width in meters. The largest or cutoff wavelength is given as

$$\lambda_{co} = 2a. \tag{21}$$

The wavelength inside the guide (λ_{wg}) for these conditions is given by:

$$\lambda_{wg} = \frac{1}{\sqrt{\left[\frac{1}{\lambda_o}\right]^2 - \left[\frac{1}{\lambda_{co}}\right]^2}} \tag{22}$$

The intrinsic impedance of the wave travelling in the guide Z_w is

$$Z_w = \frac{-Ey}{H_x} = Z_o \left[\frac{\lambda_{wg}}{\lambda_o}\right] = \frac{Z_o}{\sqrt{1 - [\lambda_o/2_a]^2}} \text{ ohms.} \tag{23}$$

The E and H fields at the center of the rectangular waveguide are, according to Larsen (1979), given by

$$E_y = \sqrt{\frac{2\ Z_w P_z}{ab}} \quad \text{and } H_x = \sqrt{\frac{2P_z}{Z_w ab}} \tag{24}$$

where

E_y = rms magnitude of the maximum E field at the center of the guide (V/m)
H_x = rms magnitude of the H field in the guide center (A/m)
P_z = total power flow in the guide (watts)
ab = cross section area of waveguide (m^2) = $\frac{1}{a^2}$

Aslan (1979) illustrates the actual method of performing the calibration in the waveguide. A longitudinal slot is cut in one side of the guide and a broadband measurement probe to be calibrated is inserted through the slot and positioned at the center of the guide in the maximum of the E field. The net power propagated through the waveguide is determined using a bi-directional coupler at the input end of the guide. Due to the imperfect impedance match of the waveguide to coax adapters, a slight standing wave exists in the guide and the probe being calibrated is moved along the length of the waveguide while the probe response is measured. The average value of the probe response is used to minimize the uncertainty introduced by reflections. Alternately a tuner may be employed between the waveguide and the load to remove the slight standing wave. A theoretical evaluation of possible field perturbation caused by the slot in the side-wall has not been accomplished.

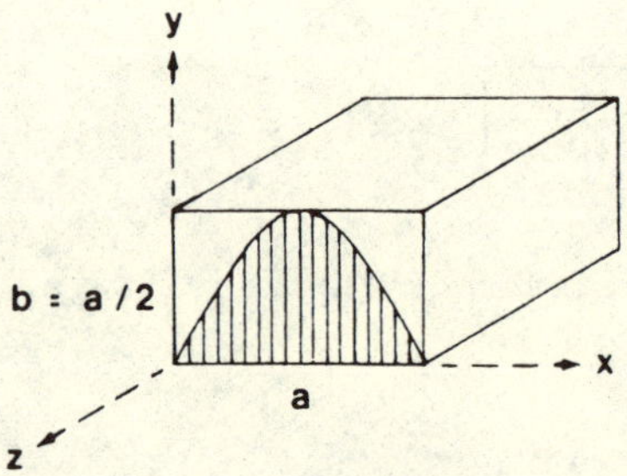

Figure 14. Waveguide illustration showing dimensions and electric field variation across the guide [taken from Larsen (1979)].

Major advantages of using the waveguide technique are (a) the ability to create very intense fields with relatively low power generators and (b) the containment of the field, i.e., except for very small leakage from the slot, the signal is not radiated into space thereby reducing the probability of causing interference. The major disadvantages are (a) difficulty in establishing the uncertainty in the exact field strength in the guide because of reflections and (b) the possibly inconvenient introduction of the test probe due to physical size of the probe. Aslan (1975) claims that an uncertainty of about ±0.5 dB can be achieved using the averaging technique he describes. John (1975) discusses in detail possible errors in the waveguide technique depending on the size of the probe relative to the waveguide dimensions.

<u>Parallel Plane Transmission Lines</u>. White (1971) provides details on the use of parallel plane transmission lines for creating known field intensities for electromagnetic susceptibility testing of electronic equipment. Mild (1980) described a form of open coaxial line, i.e., a TEM type of transmission line but one without sides.

A more common approach developed recently is the use of so-called transverse electromagnetic (TEM) cells.

Transverse Electromagnetic (TEM) Cells. The TEM cell, has been treated extensively by Crawford (1974). The TEM cell consists of a large, rectangular, coaxial transmission line typically constructed to have a nominal characteristic impedance of 50 ohms. Two major advantages of the TEM cell are (a) the enclosed nature of the cell which makes a closed, non-radiating system and (b) the property of the cell to produce a TEM mode of wave propagation, when used at suitably low frequencies for a given physical size. The TEM mode of propagation is equivalent to the electromagnetic wave propagated in the far field in front of a standard gain horn; i.e., the wave impedance is 377 ohms. At frequencies sufficiently low so that only the TEM mode propagates through the cell, a uniform and calculable electromagnetic field is established. Under TEM conditions, the electric field at a point midway between the center conductor and either the top or bottom of the cell is given by

$$E = \frac{V}{d} = \frac{\sqrt{Z_c P}}{d} \tag{25}$$

where E = electric field strength (V/m)
V = radiofrequency voltage between the center conductor and outer cell wall (V)
d = distance from center conductor to the outer wall (m)
P = power transmitted through the cell (W)
Z_c = effective cell impedance at calibration position within the cell (nominally, the characteristic impedance of the TEM cell or 50 ohms)

In practice it is common to use simply the cell's characteristic impedance for Z_c rather than the actual input impedance looking toward the load from the plane of calibration (normally the longitudinal midpoint of the cell). Determination of the actual impedance at the cell midpoint may be determined from calculation by knowledge of the cell's characteristic impedance, the terminating load impedance, and the electrical length from the load to the midpoint. When used for calibrating broadband electromagnetic field measurement probes, a convenient method of measuring the transmitted power is to use a high-power attenuater on the output end of the cell and direct connection of a power meter. At low frequencies, nominally less than 10 MHz, it is commonly more accurate to measure the radiofrequency voltage on the center conductor of the cell at either the input or output end.

TEM cells may be used to establish calibration fields with an uncertainty of ±1 dB with little trouble; uncertainties of ±0.5 dB are achievable using reasonable care. TEM cells may be used at frequencies up to beyond 1 GHz but in a practical sense, because of size constraints for calibrating broadband probes, they are normally employed only to about 300-500 MHz. The smaller the cell, the higher the upper frequency at which a TEM mode may still be achieved. Also, it is common practice to limit the vertical dimension of the object to be inserted in the cell to no more than one-third of the separation distance between the central conductor and the outer wall. Thus, a compromise exists between the useable upper frequency and physical size for introduction of probes. Access to the TEM cell is made either through one of the doors in the side wall or a small opening in either the top or bottom.

Selected Applications

Tell and Mantiply (1980) reported results of an extensive series of environmental radiofrequency field measurements made in 15 US metropolitan areas. These measurements were performed using the semi-automated measurement system shown in Figure 7. The measurements were primarily restricted to the domestic broadcast bands within the US consisting of the AM radio standard broadcast band (0.54 - 1.6 MHz), the low VHF television band (channels 2-6; 54 - 88 MHz), the FM radio broadcast band (88 -108 MHz), the high VHF television band (channels 7-13; 174 - 216 MHz), and the UHF television band (channels 14-83; 490 -890 MHz). Using population weighted measurement sites, measurements were made of all broadcast signals throughout a given city. Based on the measurement data, propagation models were constructed to compute the expected field intensity at many locations throughout the metropolitan area. Each computation point conformed to a census enumeration district (CED), a small geographical cell used for census purposes and within which the population and centroid coordinates are known. Upon calculation of the fields at each CED the accumulative fraction of the population exposed to various intensities of electromagnetic fields (the power density equivalent of all incident broadcast signals) was determined. Figure 15 provides the results obtained for the 15 cities. Note that the median exposure level, i.e., that to which 50 percent of the study population were exposed, was about 5 nW/cm^2. Also, it was found that approximately 1 percent of the population were exposed to fields with intensities greater than 1 $\mu W/cm^2$.

These results suggest that most of the population are not exposed to fields thought to be biologically harmful and that most measurement emphasis should be placed on selected, specific exposure situations to better define the population exposed to the highest intensity fields.

Tell et al. (1979) have also gathered data on the maximum electric field strength values measurable near the base of broad-

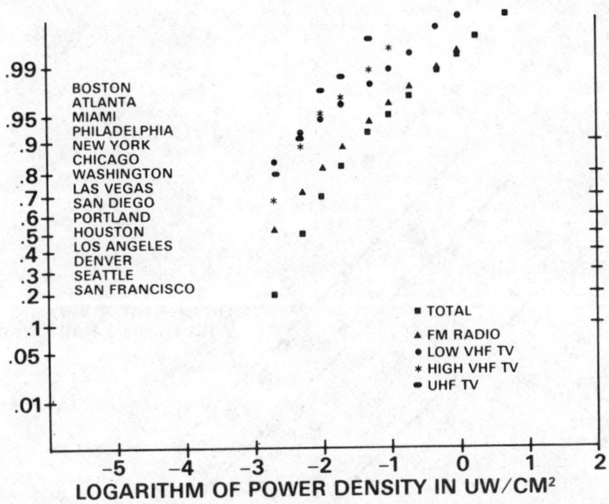

Figure 15. Accumulative fraction of population in 15 US cities exposed to electromagnetic fields $\leq$ indicated values of power density [taken from Tell and Mantiply (1980)].

cast towers supporting FM radio broadcast antennas. These measurements, performed with a broadband electric field sensor, were prompted by the observation of relatively intense grating lobes (undesired, downward lobes of radiation) beneath FM antennas (Tell and Janes; 1975; Tell, 1978). Figure 16 gives the measurement results after the electric field strength was normalized to a common effective radiated power of the station of 1 kW. Most measurements were made within 35 m of the tower.

Based on these measurements Tell et al. (1979) estimated the number of FM radio stations in the US which would produce various electric field strengths at ground level in their immediate vicinity. The analysis involved an evaluation of the height of FM radio station antennas and effective radiated power for approximately 40 FM radio stations. The results suggested that there are a few FM installations with ground level fields greater than 194 V/m, the current radiofrequency safety guide used in the US. It was estimated that about 8 percent of all FM stations could

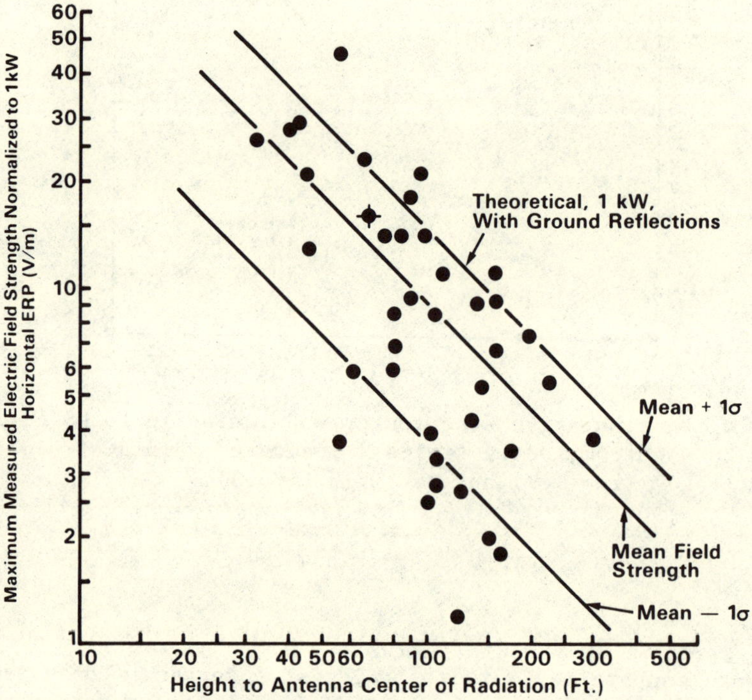

Figure 16. Maximum measured electric field strength for 1 kW horizontal polarized effective radiated power at ground level near 40 FM radio stations in the State of California, USA [taken from Tell et al. (1979)].

produce field strengths of up to 61 V/m, the newly proposed American occupational safety standard. The results pointed out that virtually all stations could exceed the Soviet safety guide for the population.

INSTRUMENTATION FOR MEASUREMENT OF ELECTROMAGNETIC FIELDS: EQUIPMENT, CALIBRATIONS AND SELECTED APPLICATIONS PART II - EXTREMELY-LOW-FREQUENCY (ELF) FIELDS

Introduction to the ELF Measurement Problem

The ELF spectrum of practical interest seems to extend from dc to about 100 Hz. Within this region the principal source of everyday exposure to ELF fields is the ac electric power system which operates at 50 or 60 Hz depending upon the country. Certainly man's predominant ELF exposure is to these fields which seem to permeate the environment even in very remote areas but are, relative to other sources, very intense in most urban, suburban, and residential locations. Other sources of man-made ELF fields are also widespread and include such diverse areas as dc driven rapid transit train systems (Fraser-Smith and Coates, 1978), new geophysical exploration devices (Morrison et al., 1978), and transient impulses originating on telephone lines. The use of ELF to communicate with deeply submerged submarines has been studied for a long time (Burrows and Niessen, 1972; Wait, 1972; Bernstein et al., 1974; IEEE Transactions, 1974).

Although there is no convincing evidence in the biological effects literature that harmful effects may be induced in experimental animals subjected to ELF fields with field strength magnitudes in the range found in the environment, some research results seem to imply that man may in fact be influenced in some way by ELF fields. It is for this reason, and the fact that man's experience with these fields is so new, that it is of interest to measure the intensity of ELF exposure.

As in the case with the radiofrequency spectrum, the two basic field parameters of interest are the electric E and magnetic H field strength magnitudes. Both broadband and narrowband types of instruments exist for ELF measurements.

Broadband Instruments. The available broadband instruments are designs primarily intended for the measurement of the electric and/or magnetic field strength of 60/50 Hz fields associated with electric power systems. The IEEE (1978) has suggested two classifications of these broadband measuring instruments: (a) the self-contained or free-body meter, which measures the 60/50 Hz current flowing between two halves of an isolated conductive body in an electric field and (b) the ground reference type of meter, which measures the current to ground from a probe introduced into an electric field. Since ground reference meters can only be used under special conditions of a known ground reference, they are not suitable for most survey-type measurements.

Free-body type field meters consist of a pair of electrodes which can take the form of parallel flat metallic plates or two metallic split shells which actually form a case for the electronics contained inside them. The probe and detector circuitry are supported by an insulated handle to remove the meter as far as practical from the operator's body thereby minimizing perturbation of the ambient field. Metering electronics measure the displacement current which is induced to flow between the two electrodes. This displacement current is then related to the charge induced on each electrode and ultimately, through a geometry dependent function, to the electric field strength.

The detector circuitry consists of diode rectification of the ac current flowing between the electrodes and, because of the detector's non-linear characteristics, will not necessarily, accurately measure a 60/50 Hz field which has significant harmonic distortion. Instruments are calibrated to read the rms value of the field. Most meters are quite accurate when compared to the accuracy of radiofrequency measuring instruments and commonly may have uncertainties of less than 5 percent.

Bracken (1976) described a Soviet version of a portable free-body type of field meter designated as a Type II 3-1. This instrument was assessed to have a nonlinear meter circuit and to be subject to corona formation in high strength fields because of the right angle design of the case. Spiegel et al. (1979) describe the development of an optically isolated ELF electric field sensor.

It should be stressed that the above described instruments are intended for application in electric power line fields. Were the meters to be used at other frequencies a calibration should be accomplished at the specific frequency of interest. Also, these instruments are designed to be responsive to one field polarization component and must be reoriented to measure more than one component of the field. An evaluation of the polarization response for commercial meters and other factors influencing measurement accuracy has been accomplished by Kotter and Misakian (1977).

The IEEE (1979) has developed a set of recommended practices for measurement of electric and magnetic fields from ac power lines which incorporates much of the work of Kotter and Misakian (1977).

Narrowband instrumentation - Broadband 60/50 Hz instruments are by their intended application typically fairly high level measurement devices; i.e., they are most useful for determining the strength of electric fields that are most likely to be of concern from a hazard point of view. However, if the amplitude of relatively weak electric and magnetic fields are to be measured, a different approach to the problem is needed. In this case the use of narrowband measurement techniques are employed making use of tuneable field strength receivers, real-time spectrum analyzers, and assorted and specialized kinds of ELF field pick-up devices such as rod antennas and loops. In each case when using a pick-up device for sensing of the ELF field its calibration must be appropriately applied to the instrument reading to obtain the intensity of the field in question.

A more convenient method to assess ELF spectra makes use of so-called real-time spectrum analyzers. The term real-time refers to the relatively high speed at which the analyzer can display the signal amplitude vs frequency. At ELF to attain high frequency resolution, swept techniques require extremely long measurement times because of the effective response time of the very narrow filters. As an alternative to a swept analyzer, parallel bank-of-filter analyzers have been developed which use a large number of filters operated in parallel; i.e., the input frequency spectrum is applied simultaneously to a set of filters thereby providing essentially true real-time response. The disadvantage is that the filters are usually fixed at specific frequencies and such instruments are large because of the number of filters required.

Another approach to real-time analysis is the use of the fast Fourier transform (FFT) to convert time data to the frequency domain. This approach samples the input signal in the time domain, similar to a digital oscilloscope, and then through the mechanism of an automatic, hardwired FFT algorithm, computes the frequency spectrum of the input signal. The instrument provides a calibrated display, in either logarithmic or linear units of input voltage, as a function of frequency and offers a variety of built-in signal averaging modes of operation.

By combining a real-time spectrum analyzer with an appropriate pick-up device, data on electric or magnetic field intensities at ELF can be acquired in a relatively short time. Figure 17 illustrates a typical magnetic field detection system. A pick-up loop consisting of 50,000 turns of wire on a ferrite core is tuned to resonance at the desired frequency of maximum sensitivity by means of a capacitor across the coil winding. Magnetic fields fluxing through the coil induce a current to flow in the windings. The output voltage of the coil is delivered to a high input impedance dc amplifier which contains filtering circuits to remove or greatly reject 60 Hz signals induced by electric power line fields. When examining ELF spectra the presence of the typically larger 60 Hz signals from power systems can saturate the amplifier electronics leading to reduced sensitivity in the frequency region of interest. The output of the dc amplifier is then presented to either a tuned receiver or spectrum analyzer for detection, analysis, and display.

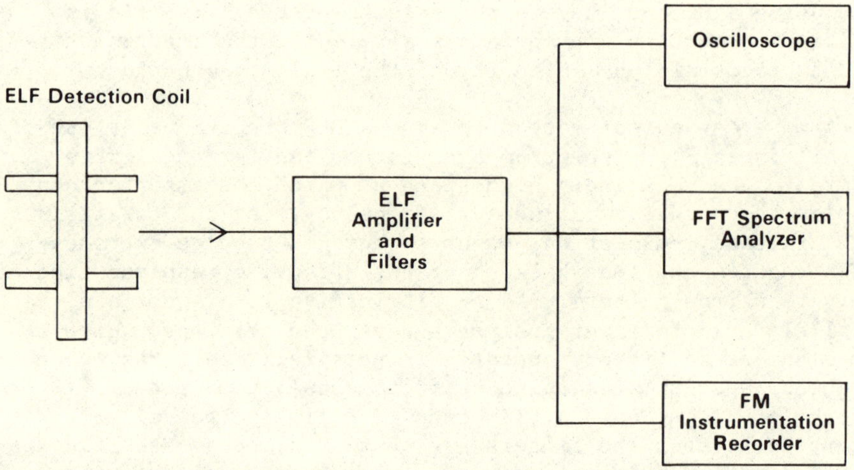

Figure 17. Block diagram of an extremely low frequency magnetic field detection system. The magnetic field produces a voltage drop across the terminals of the coil which is amplified, filtered and presented to recording and analysis equipment.

Overall system sensitivity is of course a function of the size of the pick-up loop, the resonant frequency of the loop, the dc amplifier gain and noise floor, and the sensitivity of the receiver or spectrum analyzer. It is fairly straight forward to obtain magnetic field sensitivities of about 10n Gauss rms at 10 Hz when used with a spectrum analyzer resolution bandwidth of 0.3 Hz with a signal to noise ratio of 10 dB.

By automating the spectrum analyzer with a small computer the frequency response of the entire coil-electronics system may be removed from the final displayed data and spectral data may be plotted in terms of absolute magnetic field amplitude.

The measurement of ELF electric fields is best accomplished by the use of active, vertically polarized rod antennas. An illustrative antenna of this type, designed specifically for applications at ELF is very sensitive and can provide useable response down to less than 3 Hz. A problem with such antennas is that they must typically be operated in areas removed from ambient 60

Hz power line fields greater than about 1 V/m to achieve their full performance potential.

Calibration of ELF Instrumentation

Electric field and magnetic field measuring instruments require different methods for calibration. Electric field strength calibrations are most readily accomplished by use of a pair of large parallel plates with a known ac voltage impressed across them. Magnetic field strength calibrations are commonly accomplished with either loops or Helmholtz coil assemblies.

The IEEE (1978) outlined a technique using parallel plates to calibrate power line field survey meters. Two parallel, square metallic plates separated by a distance d are driven by an ac voltage source. The electric field strength magnitude E at the midplane of the setup is given by

$$E = V/d \tag{26}$$

where V is the voltage impressed across the plates (V).

Considerable work on analyzing the spatial variation of the unperturbed electric field between the plates has been accomplished. Fringing field effects at the periphery of the plates tends to modify the field which would be expected to occur at the center point of the plates. Shih, DiPlacido and Ware (1977) calculated the variation in electric field as a function of plate spacing compared to plate dimension for square plate electrodes. For a pair of parallel plates 1 m square each and spaced by 50 cm, the variation in field magnitude was found to be less than one percent from the simply computed value at the center on the midplane. This suggests that for practical calibrations, a relatively simple method exists for evaluating survey meters. For maximum accuracy the harmonic content of the applied voltage should emulate that of the field to be ultimately measured. A total overall uncertainty of about 5 percent is a practically realizable goal.

To further increase the field homogeniety some workers have made use of guard rings to grade the field at the perimeter of the structure. This process tends to provide isolation from surrounding perturbations caused by the local environment.

The evaluation of field meter frequency response may be determined by (a) changing the frequency of the voltage applied to the parallel plates or (b) direct injection of different frequency ac currents onto the meter electrodes (IEEE, 1978).

Both single loops and Helmholtz coils have been used for calibrating loop pick-up devices. The use of single square loops is outlined by the IEEE (1978). Single loops are simpler to make and it is easy to achieve magnetic field uniformity of about one percent. In practice a known current is driven through the calibrating loop and the magnetic field is computed at the location of calibration.

It is found that for a 1 m x 1 m square calibrating loop the variation in magnetic field strength over a 6 cm square region centered in the loop is less than 2 percent.

For a simple circular coil of wire the magnetic flux density B and field strength H are given by Winch (1963) as

$$B = \frac{\mu_o NI}{2a} 10^4 \text{ Gauss} \; ; \; H = \frac{NI}{2a} \quad \text{A/m.} \tag{27}$$

For a circular Helmholtz coil system Winch (1963) gives the magnetic flux density and field strength as

$$B = \frac{8 \mu_o NI}{5^{3/2} a} 10^4 \text{ Gauss} \; ; \; H = \frac{8 NI}{5^{3/2} a} \quad \text{A/m.} \tag{28}$$

where

N = number of turns in each coil
I = current flowing in coils (A)
a = radius of coil (m)

The computed magnetic field is for a point midway between the two Helmholtz coils which are spaced a distance apart equal to their radii.

Selected Applications

Tell et al. (1977) reported results of extensive calculations and measurements of electric field strengths near ground level under extra-high-voltage (EHV) electric power lines. Figure 18 taken from their work illustrates the vertically polarized electric field strength under a 765 kV transmission line. Both calculated and measured data are given showing the good agreement obtained between the two methods. Nominal maximum values of electric field of about 10 kV/m can exist beneath 765 kV lines at 1 meter above ground. Wigdor (1980) has extended the computed results of electric field strength for 115 and 230 kV transmission lines. An investigation of the effects of different measurement techniques to determine electric and magnetic field strength under EHV overhead power transmission lines is described by Lambdin (1978).

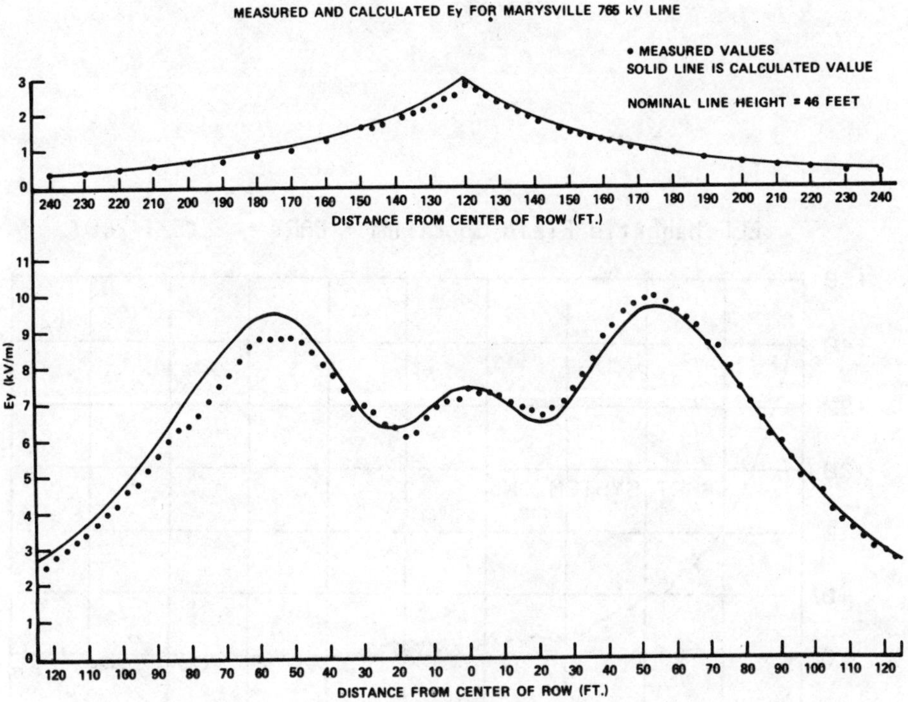

Figure 18. Vertically polarized electric field strength under a 765 kv electric power transmission line. Dots represent measured values and solid curve represents computed field strength [taken from Tell et al. (1977)].

The Environmental Protection Agency (unpublished data) has recently made measurements of the 60 Hz electric and magnetic fields found in Las Vegas residences due to the electric wiring within the structures. A total of 25 homes were studied. Measurements were made at typically five locations within each room of the residence and averaged. It was found that for all of the homes, taken as a group, the average electric field strength was 5.8 V/m with a range of 2.0 - 12.7 V/m and the average magnetic field flux was 2.5 mGauss with a range of 0.6 - 7.8 mGauss.

An interesting observation of ELF magnetic fields using a narrowband detection system was made in Oakland, California, at a measurement site over one of the tracks of the Bay Area Rapid

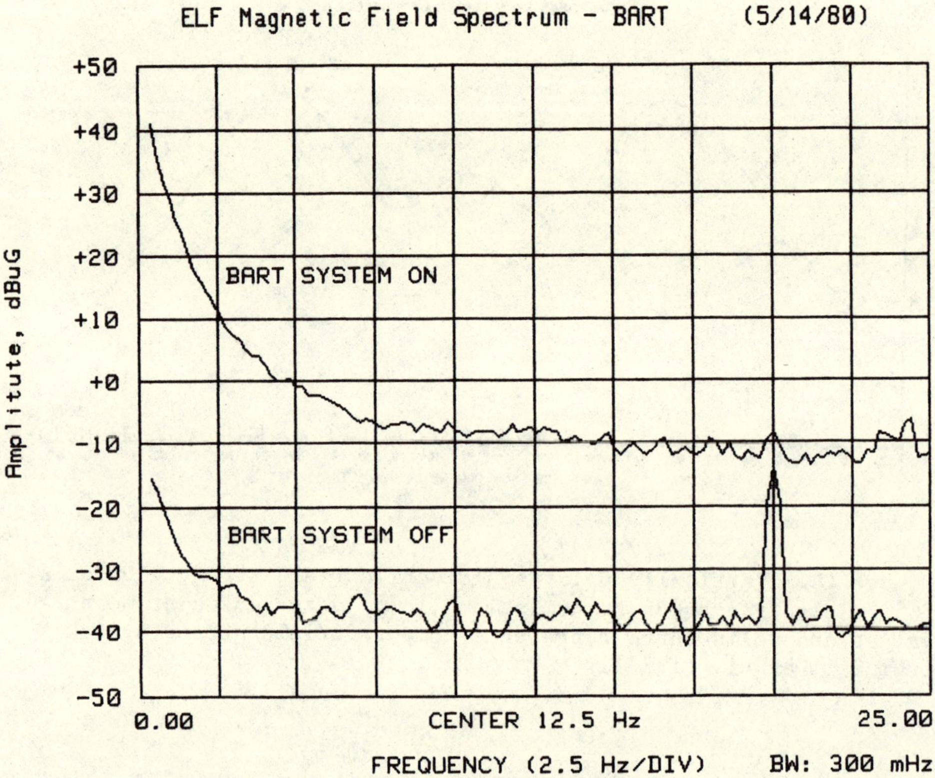

Figure 19. Measured magnetic field flux (dBμG) obtained near Bay Area Rapid Transit System train station in Oakland, California, USA, during daytime operation and quiet period in early morning hours.

Transit system (BART) which serves the San Francisco-Oakland Bay metropolitan area. The BART system employs dc driven motor trains with the current provided via the track rails. The measurements were made with a 50,000 turn loop, a high-gain dc amplifier and a spectrum analyzer, to observe the variation in magnetic field flux amplitude with frequency. Figure 19 is a computer plot of some of these measurement data obtained by the Environmental Protection Agency; the data have been corrected for the frequency response of the measuring system such that the ordinate values are in terms of absolute magnetic field flux (dBμG). The graphs show the difference between times when the BART trains are running, during most of the day, and a period in the early morning hours, approximately 0300 - 0500 local time, when the system is quiet. These data are similar to those of Fraser-Smith and Coates (1977) and show very measurable differences in the magnetic field amplitude during hours of operation of the BART system.

APPENDIX A

Conversion of dBm to dBμV in a 50 ohm system.

The voltage associated with a 0dBm (1 mW) signal in a 50 ohm impedance system is

$$V = \sqrt{50P} = \sqrt{50\Omega \times 0.001\ \text{W}}$$

$$= 0.224 \text{ volt} = 224{,}000\ \mu\text{V}$$

$$\text{Since dB}\mu\text{V} = 20 \log \frac{V(\mu V)}{1\ \mu V}$$

$$V = 20 \log \frac{224{,}000\ \mu V}{1\ \mu V} = 106.99\ \text{dB}\mu\text{V}$$

Thus 0 dBm = 107 dBμV
+10 dBm = 117 dBμV
-10 dBm = 97 dBμV

APPENDIX B

The antenna factor (AF) may be related to antenna gain (G) through the following derivation.

$$E = V(AF) \quad \text{and} \tag{1}$$

$$A_e = \frac{G\lambda^2}{4\pi} \tag{2}$$

where

E = electric field strength (V/m)
V = induced antenna voltage delivered to detector (V)
AF = antenna factor (m^{-1})
A_e = effective area of antenna (m^2)
G = antenna gain
λ = wavelength (m)

The power collected by the antenna is

$$P = S\,A_e \tag{3}$$

where

P = power collected by antenna

S = incident power density illuminating antenna (W/m^2)

Since $P = \frac{V^2}{50}$ for the 50 ohm detector and $S = \frac{E^2}{377}$ for the incident field,

$$\frac{V^2}{50} = \frac{E^2}{377} \cdot \frac{G\lambda^2}{4\pi} = \frac{E^2}{377} \cdot \frac{G}{4\pi} \left(\frac{300}{F}\right)^2 \tag{4}$$

where $\lambda = \frac{300}{F}$; F = frequency (MHz)

Thus $$E = V\,\frac{0.0324\ F}{\sqrt{G}} = V(AF) \tag{5}$$

The term $\frac{0.0324\ F}{\sqrt{G}}$ is the antenna factor. For a half-wave dipole G = 1.64 and AF = 0.025 F. It is clear that as frequency is increased, the antenna factor will increase linearily as seen in Figure 6. Differences between values of AF computed by equation 5 and those actually measured for half-wave dipoles are due to losses inherent to the matching network which exists between the antenna and the receiver.

REFERENCES

Aslan, E. (1972), Broadband isotropic electromagnetic radiation monitor. IEEE Transactions on Instrumentation and Measurement, Vol. IM-21, No. 4, November, pp. 411-424.

Aslan, E. (1975), Simplify leakage probe calibration. Microwaves, December, pp. 52-54, 57.

Aslan, E. (1976), A low-frequency H-field radiation monitor. In Biological Effects of Electromagnetic Waves, Vol. II, selected papers of the USNC/URSI annual meeting, Boulder, Colorado, October 20-23, 1975, ed. C. C. Johnson and M. L. Shore. U.S. Department of Health, Education, and Welfare, Public Health Service, Bureau of Radiological Health report (FDA) 77-8011, December, pp. 229-238, NTIS accession number PB 268 095.

Aslan, E. (1979), The maturing of electromagnetic radiation hazard instruments. Microwave Journal, May, pp. 83- .

Bassen, H. (1977), Internal dosimetry and external microwave field measurements using miniature electric field probes. In Symposium on Biological Effects and Measurement of Radio Frequency/Microwaves, proceedings of a conference held in Rockville, Maryland, February 16-18, 1977, USDHEW publication (FDA) 77-8026, pp. 136-151.

Bassen, H. and R. Peterson (1976), Complete measurement of electromagnetic fields with electro-optical crystals. In Biological Effects of Electromagnetic Waves, Vol. II, selected papers of the USNC/URSI annual meeting, Boulder, Colorado, October 20-23, 1975, ed. C.C. Johnson and M. L. Shore. U.S. Department of Health, Education, and Welfare, Public Health Service, Bureau of Radiological Health report (FDA) 77-8011, December, pp. 310-323, NTIS accession number PB 268 095.

Belsher, D. (1975), Development of near field electric energy density meter model EDM-2. U.S. Department of Health, Education, and Welfare report NIOSH 75-140, March.

Bendix Corporation Research Laboratories (1970), Development of liquid crystal microwave power density meter. U.S. Department of Health, Education, and Welfare, Public Health Service, Bureau of Radiological Health report BRH/DEP 70-8, May, 14 p., NTIS accession number PB 191 396.

Bernstein, S. L., M. L. Burrows, J. E. Evans, A. S. Griffiths, D. A. McNeill, C. W. Niessen, I. Richer, D. P. White, and D. K. Willim (1974), Long range communication at extremely low frequencies. *Proceedings IEEE*, Vol. 62, No. 3, pp. 292-312.

Bowman, R. R. (1970), Quantifying hazardous electromagnetic fields: practical considerations. National Bureau of Standards Technical Note 389, April, 15 p.

Bowman, R. R. (1974), Some recent developments in the characterization and measurement of hazardous electromagnetic fields. In *Biologic Effects and Health Hazards of Microwave Radiation*. Proceedings of an International Symposium, Polish Medical Publishers, Warsaw, pp. 217-227.

Bowman, R. R., E. B. Larsen, D. R. Belsher, and P. F. Wacker (1970), Second progress report, *Electromagnetic hazards project*, unpublished NBS report, September.

Bracken, T. D. (1976), Field measurements and calculations of electrostatic effects of overhead transmission lines. *IEEE Transactions on Power Apparatus and Systems*, Vol. PAS-95, March/April, pp. 494-504.

BRH (1970), The effect of instrument averaging time on microwave power density measurements. U.S. Department of Health, Education, and Welfare, Public Health Service, Bureau of Radiological Health report BRH/DEP 70-12, June, 25 p., NTIS accession number PB 192 322.

Burrows, M. L. and C. W. Niessen (1972), ELF communication system design. In *Ocean '72*: IEEE International Conference on Engineering in the Ocean Environment, IEEE publication 72 CHO 660-10CC, pp. 95-109.

Cheung, A., H. Bassen, M. Swicord, and D. Witters (1976), Experimental calibration of a miniature electric field probe within simulated muscular tissues. In *Biological Effects of Electromagnetic Waves*, Vol. II, selected papers of the USNC/URSI annual meeting, Boulder, Colorado, October 20-23, 1975, ed. C. C. Johnson and M. L. Shore. U.S. Department of Health, Education, and Welfare, Public Health Service, Bureau of Radiological Health report (FDA) 77-8011, December, pp. 324-337, NTIS accession number PB 268 095.

Conover, D. L. (1971), Evaluation of lithium fluoride for microwave dosimetry applications. U.S. Department of Health, Education, and Welfare, Public Health Service, Bureau of

Radiological Health report BRH/DEP 71-6, April, 25 p., NTIS accession number PB 198 406.

Crapuchettes, P. W. (1970), Microwave leakage instrumentation. In Biological Effects and Health Implications of Microwave Radiation, USDHEW publication BRH/DBE 70-2, pp. 210-216.

Crawford, M. L. (1974), Generation of standard EM fields using TEM Transmission cells. IEEE Trans. Electromagnetic Compatibility, Vol. EMC-16, November, pp. 189-195.

Ely, T. (1958), Field trial of Richardson microwave dosimeter. In Proceedings of the Second Tri-service Conference on Biological Effects of Microwave Energy, ed. E. G. Pattishall and F. W. Banghgart, Astia document AD 131 477.

Fletcher, K. and D. Woods (1969), Thin-film spherical bolometer for measurements of hazardous field intensities from 400 MHz to 40 GHz. Non-Ionizing Radiation, Vol 1, September, p. 57.

Fraser-Smith, A. C. and D. B. Coates (1978), Large-amplitude ULF electromagnetic fields from BART. Radio Science, Vol. 13, No. 4., August, pp. 661-668.

Hagn, G. H., S. C. Fralick, H. N. Shauer, and G. E. Barker (1971), A spectrum measurement/monitoring capability for the Federal government. Final report on contract OEP-SE-70-102 prepared for Office of Telecommunications Policy by Stanford Research Institute, SRI project 8410, May.

Herman, W. A. and D. M. Witters (1980), Microwave hazard instruments: an evaluation of the Narda 8100, Holaday, and Simpson 380M. U.S. Department of Health and Human Services, Public Health Service, Bureau of Radiological Health report HHS publication (FDA) 80-8122, June, 37 p.

Hewlett Packard (1974), Spectrum analysis, spectrum analyzer basics. Hewlett Packard application note 150, April, 50 p.

Hopfer, S. (1972), An ultra-broadband probe for RF radiation measurements. In CPEM Digest 1972, proceedings of Conference on Precision Electromagnetic Measurements, June 26-29, 1972, Boulder, Colorado, pp. 64-66.

Hopfer, S. and Z. Adler (1980), An ultra broad-band (200 kHz - 26 GHz) high sensitivity probe, IEEE Transactions on Instrumentation and Measurement, Vol. IM-29, No. 4, December, pp. 445-451.

IEEE (1974), Special issue on extremely low-frequency communications, guest ed. J. R. Wait. _IEEE Transactions on Communications_, Vol. COM-22, No. 4, April.

IEEE (1978), Measurement of electric and magnetic fields from alternating current power lines. _IEEE Transactions on Power Apparatus and Systems_, Vol. PAS-97, No. 4, July/August, pp. 1104-1114.

IEEE (1979), IEEE recommended practices for measurement of electric and magnetic fields from ac power lines. IEEE standard 644-1979, New York.

Iskander, M. F., C. H. Durney, and D. L. Jaggard (1980), The development of a microwave personnel dosimeter. Presented at Bioelectromagnetics Society symposium, San Antonio, Texas, September 14-18. Abstract in _Bioelectromagnetics_, Vol. 1, No. 2, p. 238.

John, W. (1975), The calibration problem of dipole probes for near-field measurements at microwave-radiators, _Nachrichtentechn. Z._, Vol. 28, No. 3, pp. 89-92.

Kanda, M., F. X. Ries, and D. R. Belsher (1979), A broadband, isotropic, real-time, electric-field sensor (BIRES) using resistively loaded dipoles. NBS publication NBSIR 79-1622.

Klein, H. F., M. L. Swicord, D. G. Brown, and R. L. Moore (1970), Investigation of the response of the Microlite 287 probe to microwave fields, U.S. Department of Health, Education, and Welfare, Public Health Service, Bureau of Radiological Health report BRH/DEP 70-20, August, 44 p., NTIS accession number PB 193 223.

Kornberg, H. A., M. M. Stevenson, T. D. Bracken, S. Bortniak, and C. A. Annestrand (1980), Health effects of occupational exposure to ELF fields. Presented at Bioelectromagnetics Society symposium, San Antonio, Texas, September 14-18. Abstract in _Bioelectromagnetics_, Vol. 1, No. 2, p. 238.

Kotter, F. R. and M. Misakian (1977), AC transmission line field measurements. NBS technical report HCP/T-6010/E1, November.

Kucia, H. R. (1972), Accuracy limitation in measurements of HF field intensities for protection against radiation hazards _IEEE Transactions on Instrumentation and Measurements_, Vol. IM-21, No. 4, November, pp. 412-415.

Lambdin, D. L. (1978), A comparison of measurement techniques to determine electric fields and magnetic flux under EHV overhead power transmission lines. USEPA technical report ORP/EAD 78-1, March, 14 p., NTIS accession number PB 292 067.

Langlet, I. (1978), Investigation of some RF meters. National Institute of Radiation Protection report SSI: 1978-023, S-104 01 Stockholm, Sweden, July, 17 p.

Larsen, E. G. (1979), Techniques for producing standard EM fields from 10 kHz to 10 GHz for evaluating radiation monitors. In Electromagnetic Fields in Biological Systems, proceedings of a symposium held in Ottawa, Canada, June 27-30, 1978, published by the International Microwave Power Institute, publication 78CH1438-1 MTT, pp. 96-112.

Levine, H. and R. L. Moore (1970), Microwave oven test load evaluation and determination of internal microwave energy distribution. U.S. Department of Health, Education, and Welfare, Public Health Service, Bureau of Radiological Health report BRH/DEP 70-23, August, 25 p., NTIS accession number PB 193 804.

Matheson, R. J. (1977), A radio spectrum measurement system for frequency management data IEEE Transactions on Electromagnetic Compatibility, Vol. EMC-19, No. 3, August, pp. 225-230.

McMahon, J. H. (1973), Capability of the FCC mobile monitoring van. In Proceedings of the IEEE Vehicular Technology Conference Record, Cleveland, Ohio, December 3-5.

Mild, K. H. (1980), Occupational exposure to radiofrequency electromagnetic fields. Proceedings of the IEEE, Vol. 68, No. 1, January, pp. 12-17.

Minin, B. A. (1974), Microwaves and human safety. Translated from Russian by Joint Publications Research Service, report JPRS 65506-1, 20 August 1975, available from National Technical Information Service, pp. 232-254.

Moore, R. L., S. W. Smith, R. L. Cloke, and D. G. Brown (1970), A comparison of microwave detection instruments. U.S. Department of Health, Education, and Welfare, Public Health Service, Bureau of Radiological Health report BRH/DEP 70-7, April, 9 p., NTIS accession number PB 191 395.

Morrison, H. F., N. E. Goldstein, M. Hoversten, G. Oppliger, and C. Riveros (1978), Description, field test and data analysis of a controlled-source EM system (EM-60). Lawrence Berkeley Laboratory Report LBL-7088, October.

Rudge, A. W. and R. M. Knox (1970), Near-field instrumentation. U.S. Department of Health, Education, and Welfare, Public Health Service, Bureau of Radiological Health report BRH/DEP 70-16, July, 69 p., NTIS accession number PB 194-748.

Ruggera, P. S. (1976), E-and H-field instrumentation and calibration below 50 MHz. In Biological Effects of Electromagnetic Waves, Vol. II, selected papers of the USNC-URSI annual meeting, Boulder, Colorado, October 20-23, 1975, ed. C. C. Johnson and M. L. Shore. U.S. Department of Health, Education, and Welfare, Public Health Service, Bureau of Radiological Health report (FDA) 77-8011, December, pp. 281-296, NTIS accession number PB 268 095.

Ruggera, P. S. (1977), Near-field measurements of RF fields. In symposium on Biological Effects and Measurement of Radiofrequency-Microwave (ed. D. G. Hazzard). U.S. Department of Health, Education, and Welfare, Public Health Service, Bureau of Radiological Health report (FDA) 77-8026, July, pp. 104-116, NTIS accession number PB 272 906.

Shih, C. H., J. DiPlacido, and B. J. Ware (1977), Analysis of parallel plate simulation of the transmission line electric field as related to biological effects laboratory studies. IEEE Transactions on Power Apparatus and Systems, Vol. PAS-96, No. 3, May/June, pp. 962-968.

Spiegel, R. J., E. H. Cooper, E. L. Bronaugh, and D. R. Kerns (1979), An improved optically isolated ELF electric field sensor. Presented at IEEE International Symposium on Electromagnetic Compatibility, in IEEE publication 79CH1383-9 EMC, pp. 429-434.

Swicord, M. L. (1971), Microwave measurements and new types of detectors for evaluation of health hazards. U.S. Department of Health, Education, and Welfare, Public Health Service, Bureau of Radiological Health report BRH/DEP 71-1, January, 33 p., NTIS accession number PB 197 715.

Swicord, M. L., H. Bassen, W. Herman, J. Dugg, and J. Bing (1976), Methods and instrumentation for the evaluation and calibration of microwave survey instruments. In Biological Effects of Electromagnetic Waves, Vol. II, selected papers of the USNC/URSI annual meeting, Boulder, Colorado, October 20-23, 1975, ed. C. C. Johnson and M. L.

Shore. U.S. Department of Health, Education, and Welfare, Public Health Service, Bureau of Radiological Health report (FDA) 77-8011, December, pp. 297-309, NTIS accession number PB 268 095.

Taggart, H. E. and J. L. Workman (1969), Calibration principles and procedures for field strength meters (30 Hz to 1 GHz). NBS Technical Note 3370, March.

Tell, R. A. (1978), Near-field radiation properties of simple linear antennas with applications to radiofrequency hazards and broadcasting. USEPA technical report ORP/EAD 78-4, June, NTIS accession number PB 292 647.

Tell, R. A., N. N. Hankin, J. C. Nelson, T. W. Athey, and D. E. Janes (1976), An automated measurement system for determining environmental radiofrequency field intensities II. In Proceedings of NBS symposium on Measurements for the Safe Use of Radiation, March 1976, NBS publication NBS SP 456 (ed. S. P. Fivozinsky), pp. 203-213.

Tell, R. A. and D. E. Janes (1975), Broadcast radiation: a second look. In Biological Effects of Electromagnetic Waves, ed. by C. C. Johnson and M. L. Shore (selected papers of the USNC-URSI 1975 annual meeting, Boulder, Colorado, October), 2 volumes, USDHEW publication (FDA) 77-8011, NTIS accession number PB 268 095.

Tell, R. A., D. L. Lambdin, R. E. Brown, and E. D. Mantiply (1979), Electric field strengths in the near-vicinity of FM radio broadcast antennas. Presented at 1979 IEEE Broadcast Symposium, Washington, D.C., September 21.

Tell, R. A. and E. D. Mantiply (1980), Population exposure to VHF and UHF broadcast radiation in the United States. Proceedings of the IEEE, Vol. 68, No. 1, January, pp. 6-12.

Tell, R. A. and J. C. Nelson (1974), RF pulse spectral measurements in the vicinity of several air traffic control radars. USEPA technical report EPA-520/1-74-005, May, 45 p., NTIS accession number PB 235 733.

Tell, R. A., J. C. Nelson, D. L. Lambdin, T. W. Athey, N. N. Hankin, and D. E. Janes (1977), An examination of electric fields under EHV overhead power transmission lines. USEPA technical report EPA-520/2-76-008, April, 39 p., NTIS accession number PB 270 613.

White, D. R. J. (1971), EMI test instrumentation and systems, Vol. 4 of A Handbook Series on Electromagnetic Interference and Compatibility, published by Don White Consultants, Gainesville, Virginia.

Wigdor, M. (1980), Electric fields under power lines (supplement to an examination of electric fields under EHV overhead power transmission lines). USEPA technical report ORP/EAD 80-1.

Winch, R. P. (1963), Electricity and magnetism. Prentice-Hall, Inc., Englewood Cliffs, New Jersey.

DOSIMETRY OF RADIO FREQUENCY AND MICROWAVE RADIATION: THEORETICAL ANALYSES

Maria A. Stuchly

Radiation Protection Bureau
Health and Welfare Canada
Ottawa, Ontario K1A 0L2

INTRODUCTION

Theoretical dosimetry concerns the determination by calculations of the electric field distribution or the specific absorption rate (SAR) distribution in models of humans and animals exposed to electromagnetic (EM) waves. The calculations are performed by solving Maxwell's equations for a given configuration approximating the exposed object (an animal, a human being, a part of a human body), and for given exposure conditions (e.g. plane wave at a given frequency, incident from a given direction). Whenever the model is a close approximation of a biological body, the equations become nearly prohibitively complex and difficult to solve. However, even analyses of greatly simplified models provide valuable information for quantifying interactions of EM waves with biological systems. The results obtained from simple models often provide valuable insight and qualitative understanding that can facilitate the analysis of more complex models. Theoretical dosimetry is closely linked with experimental dosimetry, since progress in one area of dosimetry frequently stimulates further development and progress in the other.

Early recognition and development of theoretical dosimetry is due to Schwan, Anne, and their colleagues[1-13]. The last decade witnessed rapid progress and many impressive achievements in theoretical dosimetry as recently reviewed by Durney[4] and compiled in the handbooks[5,6]. Several different models were analyzed, including spherical[7-13], cylindrical[14-16], prolate spheroidal[17-18], ellipsoidal[19-20], block models composed of cubical cells arranged to simulate the human body[21-25]. Analyses of these models were performed for exposures to the plane wave. More recently simple near-field exposures [26-28] were also treated. Various analytical and numerical techniques were employed.

In this contribution a brief review of the techniques used in theoretical dosimetry is given, a detailed treatment can be found in the original publications. The emphasis is placed on the results obtained and the general picture that has emerged, that relates the average SAR and its distribution to various exposure conditions.

METHODS OF CALCULATION

Models

The models analysed theoretically are of various shapes. The electrical properties (the permittivity) of the materials used to construct models are selected in one of the following ways:

- homogeneous; equal to the average tissue properties,
- layered; a core having the properties of muscle, surrounded by a layer having the properties of fat, surrounded by a layer of skin, or other relevent combinations, e.g. skin-bone-brain tissue,
- non-homogeneous; consisting of cubes having homogeneous properties.

Long-Wavelength Approximation

The long-wavelength approximation can be used at frequencies where the largest dimension of the object is small compared with a free space wavelength (less than 0.2λ, λ is the free space wavelength). With this assumption the perturbation theory is used and a semi-static solution obtained (the fields are only slightly different than the static fields). The basis of the perturbation theory is the expansion of incident, scattered and interior (inside the body simulating a human or an animal) fields in a power series in k, where k is the free-space propagation constant. Only the first-order term of the power expansion is taken into account.

The long-wave approximation was first employed for a spheroid model of man and animals [17,18], later for an ellipsoidal model[19,20] and subsequently data was obtained for models of humans of various sizes, a squirrel monkey, a baboon, a dog, a rabbit, a guinea pig, rats of various sizes, mice of various sizes[29], all exposed to the plane wave. Recently, the long-wave approximation method was used in the near-field[30].

Extended Boundary Condition Method

The extended boundary condition method is a matrix formulation based on an integral equation[31]. The method is exact within the limits of numerical computation capabilities. Presently, the method is used to about 80 MHz for the prolate spheroidal model of man, and up to higher frequencies for smaller size models, exposed to the plane wave[5]. It is also used for calculation of the near-field exposures to a short electric dipole[27] and a small loop[28].

Moment Method

This method is based on solving numerically a tensor integral equation for the electric field inside the absorbing body[32]. The integral equation is transformed into a matrix equation, and a solution is obtained by matrix inversion. The model is composed of a number of cubical blocks arranged to form a human-like shape. This method was used to calculate the average SAR and the SAR distribution for man in free space[21,23,32] and standing on a ground plane[22]. A detailed calculation of the SAR in the human head[24] was also conducted. Very recently this method was used to solve a near-field exposure problem[26].

Cylindrical Approximation

In the frequency range where the wavelength in free-space is very short compared with the dimensions of the object, a cylinder rather than a spheroid is a good approximation of a human body. An analysis of a cylinder is certainly much simpler than of a spheroid. For human models, this approximation is valid in the frequency range 400 MHz - 7 GHz[16].

Geometrical Optics Approximation

In this technique it is assumed that the wavelength in free space is short enough that the radiation can be described in terms of rays[16]. It is assumed, that the rays are totally absorbed, not reflected from internal discontinuities.

Empirical Techniques

These techniques utilize antenna theory and curve fitting[4] to the experimental or calculated (by another method) results. As a final product of these techniques a simple formula is obtained for calculating the average SAR for given exposure conditions and model dimensions[5,33,34].

Summary

The combination of the methods outlined before has allowed the calculation of the average SAR for the plane-wave exposure over the whole range of RF and MW as illustrated in Fig. 1. The distribution of the SAR has also been obtained.

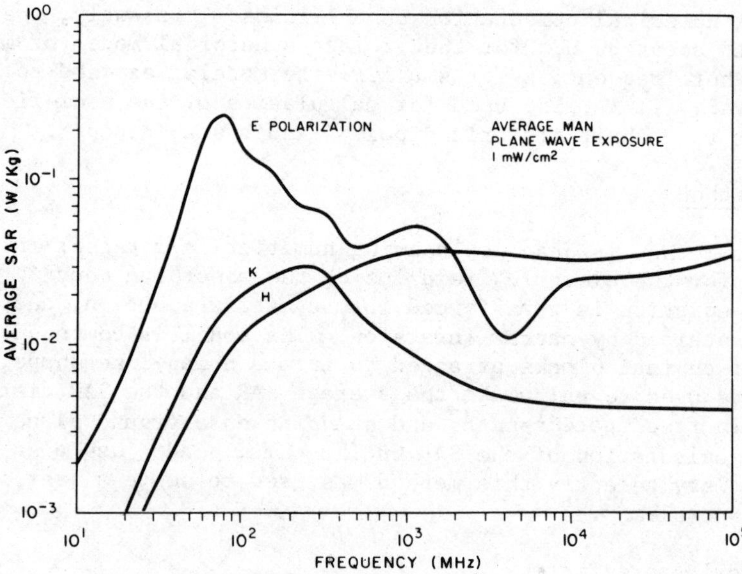

Figure 1. Average specific absorption rate vs. frequency.

EXPOSURE TO A PLANE WAVE

Polarization

In determining the average SAR and its distribution in various models of human-beings and animals to a plane wave, the wave polarization (the orientation of the wave vectors E, H and k with respect to the body) plays an essential role. For prolate spheroidal models, three polarizations can be distinguished (Fig. 2), while for ellipsoidal models six different configurations of the field vectors with respect to the object are possible. Since for elipsoids having the semi-axis lengths not substantially different ($b \approx c$), (which is the case for the ellipsoids representing most of the biological bodies), the SAR for two polarizations are very close, further discussion will be limited to spheroidal models and three polarizations. Any arbitrary polarization can be obtained from a combination of the three standard polarizations.

The average SAR for circularly polarized waves, with the k vector perpendicular to the long axis of the spheroid, a, is equal to a half of the sum of the average SARs for E and H polarized

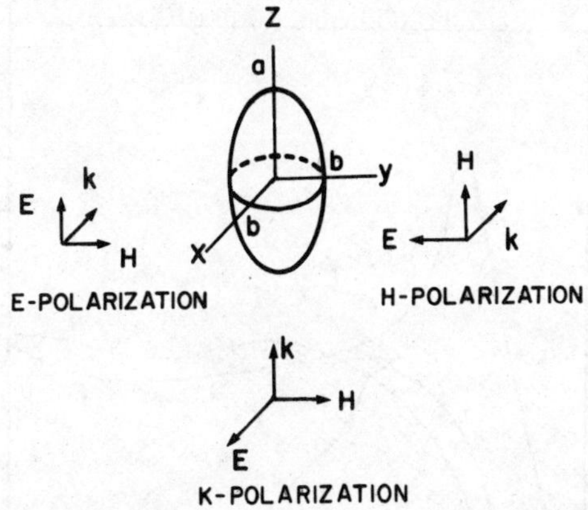

Figure 2. Configurations of the electromagnetic fields and the prolate spheroidal model.

waves with the same incident power density[5].

$$SAR_C = \tfrac{1}{2}(SAR_E + SAR_H) \tag{1}$$

where SAR_C is the SAR produced by a circularly polarized wave with broadside incidence, SAR_E is the SAR produced by an E-polarized wave, and SAR_H is the SAR produced by an H-polarized wave. For circularly polarized waves with end-on incidence, the SAR is a sum of the two linearly k-polarized incident plane waves. For elliptically polarized waves incident waves the SAR can be calculated as an appropriate combination of non-equal amplitude incident linear plane waves.

Average SAR - Frequency and Polarization Dependance

The average specific absorption rate depends on the frequency and polarization of the plane wave. The results obtained by theoretical analysis of the spheroidal and cylindrical models and confirmed experimentally are shown in Figs. 3 and 4 for various species. In all cases the incident power density is 1 mW/cm^2. From these data the following conclusions can be drawn:

- the average SAR is a function of frequency,
- the average SAR depends on the wave polarization, and is greatest for the E-polarization except at higher frequencies, where it is slightly greater for the H-polarization,
- the average SARs for the E and k polarization exhibit

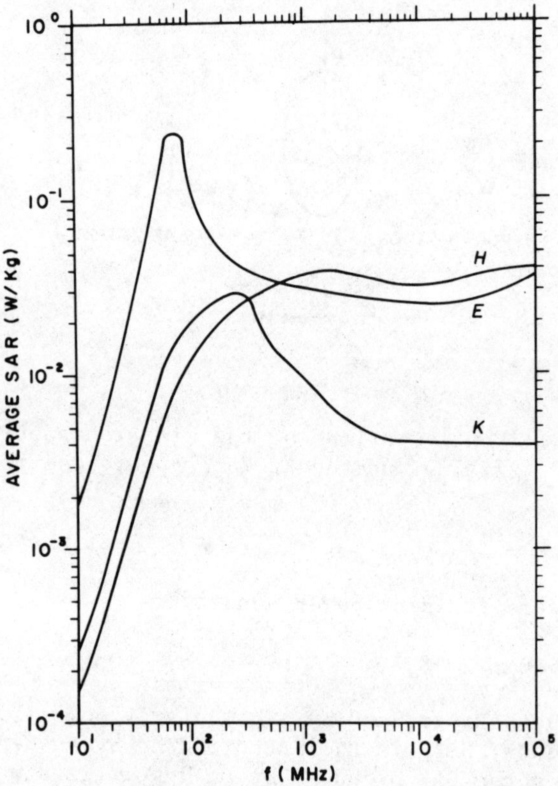

Figure 3. Average SAR in a prolate spheroidal model of an average man. The incident power density 1 mW/cm^2.

a maximum at certain frequencies, called the resonant frequencies. The resonant frequency depends on the size of the model. For the E-polarization the resonant frequency[35] is approximately equal to:

$$f_r = 11.4/L_{(cm)} \quad (GHz) \tag{2}$$

where L is the longest dimension of the model (in cm),

- below resonance for all polarizations, the average SAR decreases rapidly with frequency, approximately as f^2 (f is the frequency),
- above the resonance for the E and k polarization, the average SAR decreases initially as 1/f, and later reaches a nearly constant value (determined by so called optical absorption cross-section equal about one half of the physical cross-section[35]). Furthermore, the average SAR at resonance is a function of the body dimensions as illustrated in Fig. 4, which shows the SAR for the E-polarization for three species. The maximum average SAR (at resonance) for a small

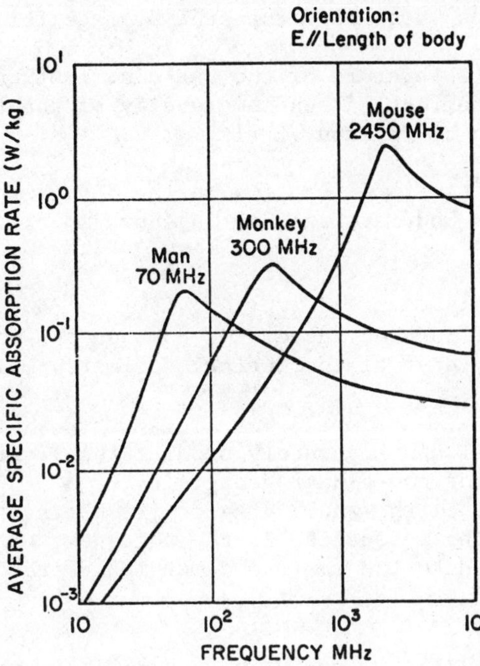

Figure 4. Average SAR for prolate spheroidal models of man, monkey and mouse. The incident power density 1 mW/cm^2.

mammal (mouse) is greater than for larger animals (monkey and man).

SAR Distribution

It was early recognized that the distribution of the SAR within biological bodies is highly non-uniform and theoretical solutions were sought for simple models, as well as experimental investigations were conducted on scaled models. The theoretical treatment of the realistic-block model of man provided more accurate information about the SAR distribution. What is particularly important is the fact that in this model the electrical properties of various parts of the body are selected to simulate the actual properties. The average SAR for the whole body, the head and the neck are shown in Fig. 5, for the E polarized wave of a power density of 1 mW/cm^2 incident from the front. An interesting insight can be gained from these curves. For instance, the absorption in the head is substantially greater at about 350 MHz than at the whole-body resonant frequency of about 80 MHz. Similarly, the absorption in the neck exhibits three "resonances", and in each case the absorption is greater than the average for the whole body.

A more detailed picture of the SAR distribution at the resonant frequency and the effect of non-homogeneity of the tissue are given in the publication by Hagmann et al[23].

The effect of the polarization on the SAR of the head as compared to the whole body average SAR is shown in Fig. 6.

Tissue Layering

Importance of layered instead of homogeneous models was recognized in the early days of theoretical dosimetry[1], later it was shown that[15,15]:

- a planar model can accurately predict the layering resonance frequencies for non-planar geometries;
- the resonance of the whole body or its parts are independent of the layering resonance, if the thickness of the layers is small compared to the maximum dimension of the body or the parts;

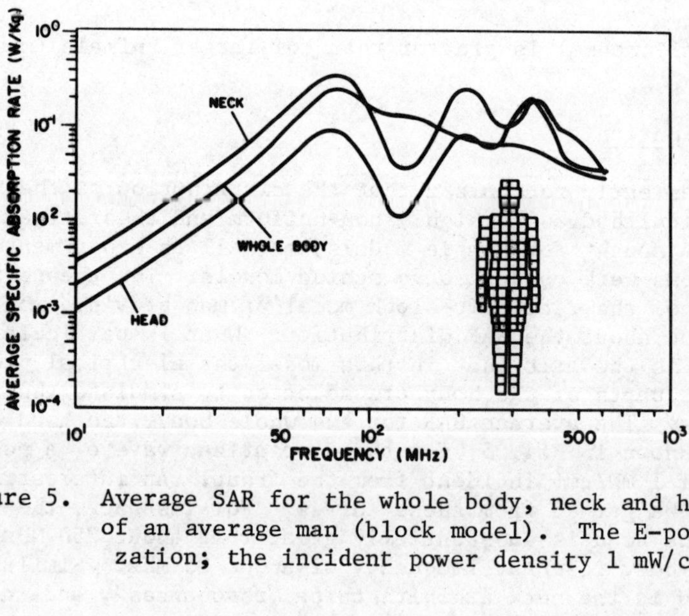

Figure 5. Average SAR for the whole body, neck and head of an average man (block model). The E-polarization; the incident power density 1 mW/cm^2.

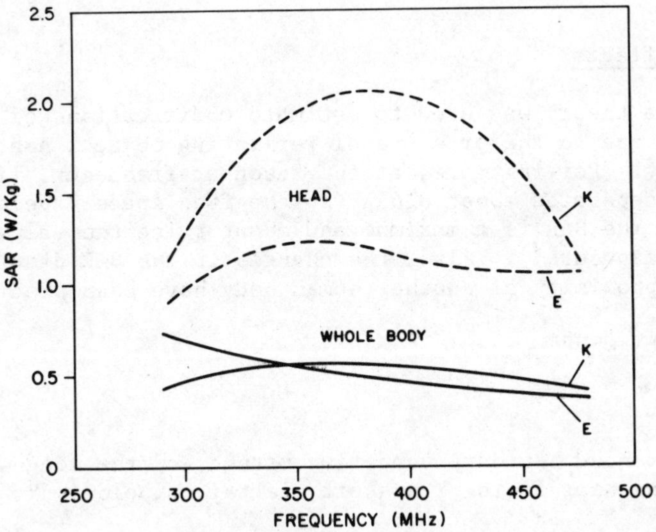

Figure 6. Whole-body average SAR and head average SAR for a block model of an average man. The incident power density 10 mW/cm^2.

- for a model of an average man the layers affect the average SAR in the frequency range 0.4 - 8 GHz. The maximum increase in the SAR occurs at approximately 2 GHz. The SAR at that frequency is about twice that for the homogeneous model;
- the frequency of the layering resonance does not depend on the wave polarization.

The effect of clothing was also investigated employing the layered model[15]. It is concluded that for frequencies below 2 GHz, the clothing has very little effect on the average SAR.

<u>Ground-Plane</u>

An increase in the average SAR at resonance and a shift of the resonant frequency when an exposed body is in contact with a ground plane was predicted from an approximate analysis based on antenna theory[37] and observed experimentally[38]. Exact calculations were subsequently made for a block model of man[34]. The SAR curves for a man in contact with a ground plane and for free space exposure are shown in Fig. 7. The distribution of the SAR within the body is also affected by the ground plane[34]. The effect of a finite distance between the ground plane and the body has also been investigated[4].

Multibody Effects

Antenna theory was used to estimate modifications of the average SAR due to the presence of reflecting objects near the exposed body. For instance, at the resonant frequency, if the two bodies are separated about 0.65λ (λ -the free space wavelength) the increase in the SAR is a maximum and about twice the value for the free space exposure[35]. Also, the changes in the SAR distribution due to the proximity of another human body have been predicted[34].

NEAR-FIELD EXPOSURE

Short Dipole

The extended boundary condition method and the long-wavelength models in the near field of a short electric dipole[27,30]. In all

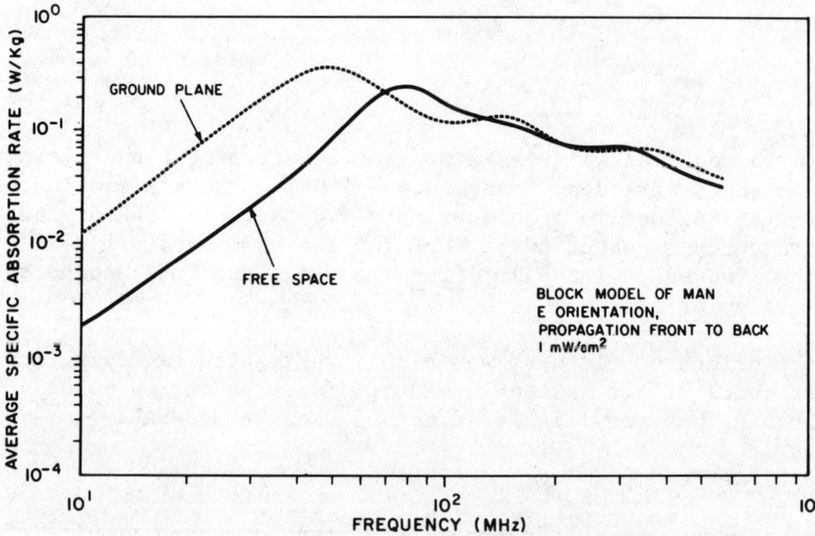

Figure 7. Average SAR for an average man in free space and on the ground plane.

the calculations, the value of the dipole moment is selected such that when the dipole is located far away from the spheroid, the radiated power is equal to that for the plane-wave irradiation. Since the far-field radiated power is inversely proportional to the square of the distance from the spheroid, the normalization constant proportional to the square of the distance is employed. This normalization involves equating the energy flux of the dipole within a solid angle determined by the spheroid and the total energy of the plane-wave crossing the surface area of the spheroid perpendicular to the direction of propagation. This allows one to compare the near-field exposure with the far-field exposure.

The normalized average SAR for an average man for three dipole locations corresponding the E-, k- and H-polarization and a $(\lambda/d)^2$ relationship were calculated[6]. A comparison between the average SARs for the plane-wave and the short dipole indicates that when the dipole is located at distances greater than about 0.35λ from the spheroid, the average SARs are the same. The steady increase in the average SAR for distances less than 0.15λ is observed. It is due to the strong reactive near-field components. The SAR distribution significantly varies in the near-field from the far-field only when $d/\lambda < 0.5$.

Small Loop

The analysis was performed employing the extended boundary condition method[26]. The solution is valid for loops having a circumference $2\pi a_1 < 0.1\lambda$, where λ is the free space wavelength. The loop current is normalized so that the power values at large distances are equal to those obtained from plane-wave of 1 mW/cm^2. The average SAR varies approximately as $(\lambda/d)^4$ for distances greater than 5λ. It oscillates around the $(\lambda/d)^4$ for smaller distances, with an increase for $d/\lambda < 0.4$. The distribution of the SAR is highly non-uniform with the greatest values at the surface of the spheroid.

Aperture Fields

The average SAR and its distribution were calculated for a block model of man exposed to a prescribed vector electric field closely approximating the field generated by RF sealers at 27 MHz[26]. The incident field was expressed in terms of an angular spectrum of plane-waves. The method of moments was then used to calculate the electric fields in the 180 cells of the model. The SAR values approach those for the plane-wave as the width of the aperture approaches one wavelength. The SARs in all parts of the body are less than for the corresponding plane-wave incident fields[26].

CONCLUSIONS

Theoretical dosimetry together with experimental dosimetry plays an essential role in quantifying the results of the experiments with animals exposed to RF and MW fields, and in evaluating potential hazards of the human exposure to these fields. It has been unequivocally established, that the interactions of RF and MW fields with living systems depend on the distribution of the electric field within the exposed body rather than on the intensity of the external exposure field. The presently available methods provide quantitative data on the average specific absorption rate and in many cases limited data on the SAR distribution for various exposure conditions of models of mammals exposed to plane waves in a broad frequency range, from kHz up to 300 GHz. Only limited data is available for exposures in the near-field.

Further research is needed in dosimetry, developing and employing both theoretical analyses, and experimental techniques. One of the important problems to be addressed is determination of the average SAR and its distribution for bodies exposed in the near-field to the radiators coupled (interacting) with the exposed bodies. Evaluation of the field (SAR) distribution in more realistic (shape, dielectric properties) models of mammals is also of a great importance.

REFERENCES

1. H.P. Schwan and K. Li, Hazards Due to Total Body Irradiation. Proc. IRE, Vol. 44, pp. 1572-1581 (1956).
2. A. Anne, M. Saito, O.M. Salati and H.P. Schwan, Relative Microwave Absorption Cross Section of Biological Significance, in "Tri-Service Conf. on Biological Effects of Microwave Radiation", M.F. Peyton, ed. (1961).
3. H.P. Schwan, Interaction of Microwave and Radio Frequency Radiation with Biological Systems, IEEE Trans., Vol. MTT-19, pp. 146-152 (1971).
4. C.H. Durney, Electromagnetic Dosimetry for Models of Humans and Animals: A Review of Theoretical and Numerical Techniques. Proc. IEEE, Vol. 68, pp. 33-40 (1980).
5. C.H. Durney, C.C. Johnson, P.W. Barber, H. Massoudi, M.F. Iskander, J.L. Lords, D.K. Ryser, S.J. Allen and J.C. Mitchel, Radiofrequency Radiation Dosimetry Handbook, Second Edition, USAF School of Aerospace Medicine, Report No. SAM-TR-78-22 (1978).
6. C.H. Durney, M.F. Iskander, H. Massoudi, S.J. Allen and J.C. Mitchell, Radiofrequency Radiation Dosimetry Handbook, Third Edition, USAF School of Aerospace Medicine, Report No. SAM-TR-80-32 (1980).
7. A.R. Shapiro, R.F. Lutomirski and H.T. Yura, Induced Fields and Heating Within a Cranial Structure Irradiated by an

Electromagnetic Plane Wave, IEEE Trans., Vol. MTT-19, pp. 187-196 (1971).

8. H.N. Kritikos and H.P. Schwan, Hot Spots Generated in Conducting Spheres by Electromagnetic Waves and Biological Implications, IEEE Trans. on Biomed. Engn., Vol. BME-19, No. 1 (1972).
9. J.C. Lin, A.W. Guy and G.H. Kraft, Microwave Selective Brain Heating, J. Microwave Power, Vol. 8, pp. 275-286 (1973).
10. W.T. Joines, and R.J. Spiegel, Resonance Absorption of Microwaves by Human Skull, IEEE Trans. Biomed. Engng., Vol. BME-21, pp. 46-48 (1974).
11. C.M. Weil, Absorption Characteristics of Multilayered Sphere Models Exposed to UHF/Microwave Radiation. IEEE Trans. Biomed. Eng., Vol. BME-22, pp. 468-476 (1975).
12. H.N. Kritikos and H.P. Schwan, The Distribution of Heating Potential Inside Lossy Spheres. IEEE Trans. Biomed. Eng., Vol. BEM-22, pp. 457-463 (1975).
13. A. Hizal and Y.K. Baykal, Heat Potential Distribution in an Inhomogeneous Spherical Model of a Cranial Structure Exposed to Microwaves Due to Loop or Dipole Antennas, IEEE Trans. Microwave Theory Techn., Vol. MTT-26, pp. 607-612 (1978).
14. H.E. Bussey and J.H. Richmond, Scattering by a Lossy Dielectric Circular Cylindrical Multilayer, Numberical Values, IEEE Trans. of AP, Vol. AP- , pp. 723-725 (1975).
15. H. Massoudi, C.H. Durney, P.W. Barber and M.F. Iskander, Electromagnetic Absorption in Multilayered Cylindrical Models of Man, IEEE Trans. Microwave Theory Techn., Vol. MTT-27, pp. 825-830 (1979).
16. H. Massoudi, C.H. Durney and C.C. Johnson, Geometrical - Optics and an Exact Solution for Internal Fields in and Energy Absorption by a Cylindrical Model of Man Irradiated by an Electromagnetic Plane Wave, Radio Science, Vol. 14(65), pp. 35-42 (1979).
17. C.H. Durney, C.C. Johnson and H. Massoudi, Long-Wavelength Anslysis of Plane Wave Irradiation of a Prolate Spheroid Model of Man, IEEE Trans., Vol. MTT-23, pp. 246-253 (1975).
18. C.C. Johnson, C.H. Durney and H. Massoudi, Long-Wavelength Electromagnetic Power Absorption in Prolate Spheroid Model of Man and Animals, IEEE Trans. on Microwave Theory Technique, Vol. MTT-23, pp. 739-747 (1975).
19. H. Massoudi, C.H. Durney and C.C. Johnson, Long-Wavelength Analysis of Plane Wave Irradiation of an Ellipsoidal Model of Man. IEEE Trans. Microwave Theory Techn., Vol. MTT-25, pp. 41-46, (1977).
20. H. Massoudi, C.H. Durney and C.C. Johnson, Long-Wavelength Electromagnetic Power Absorption in Ellipsoidal Models of Man and Animals. IEEE Trans. Microwave Theory Techn., Vol. MTT-25, pp. 47-52, (1977).
21. K.M. Chen and B.S. Guru, Internal EM Field and Absorbed Power Density in Human Torsos Induced by 1-500 MHz EM Waves,

IEEE Trans. Microwave Theory Techn., Vol. MTT-25, pp. 746-756 (1977).

22. M.J. Hagmann and O.P. Gandhi, Numerical Calculation of Electromagnetic Energy Deposition in Models of Man with Grounding and Reflector Effects. Radio Science, Vol. 14(6S), pp. 23-30 (1979).

23. M.J. Hagmann, O.P. Gandhi and C.H. Durney, Numerical Calculation of Electromagnetic Energy Deposition for a Realistic Model of Man, IEEE Trans. Microwave Theory Techn., Vol. MTT-27, pp. 804-809 (1979).

24. M.J. Hagmann, O.P. Gandhi, J.A. D'Andrea and I. Chatterjee, Head Resonance: Numerical Solutions and Experimental Results. IEEE Trans. Microwave Theory Techn., Vol. MTT-27, pp. 809-813 (1979).

25. S. Rukspollmuang and K.M. Chen, Heating of Spherical Versus Realistic Models of Human and Infrahuman Heads by Electromagnetic Waves. Radio Science, Vol. 14(65), pp. 51-62 (1979).

26. I. Chatterjee, M.J. Hagmann and O.D. Gandhi, Electromagnetic Energy Deposition in an Inhomogeneous Block Model of Man for Near Field Irradiation Conditions. IEEE Trans., Vol. MTT-28, pp. 1452-1459 (1980).

27. M.F. Iskander, P.W. Barber, C.H. Durney and H. Massoudi, Irradiation of Prolate Spheroidal Models of Humans in the Near Field of a Short Electric Dipole, IEEE Trans. Microwave Theory Techn., (to be published) (1981).

28. A. Lakhtakia, M.F. Iskander, C.H. Durney and H. Massoudi, Irradiation of Prolate Spheroidal Models of Humans and Animals in the Near Field of a Small Loop Antenna, (to be published) (1981).

29. C.C. Johnson, C.H. Durney, P.W. Barber, H. Massoudi, S.J. A Allen and J.C. Mitchell, Radiofrequency Radiation Dosimetry Handbook. USAF School of Aerospace Medicine, Report No. SAM-TR-76-35 (1976).

30. H. Massoudi, C.H. Durney and M.F. Iskander, Long-Wavelength Analysis of Near-Field Irradiation of Prolate Spheroidal Models of Man and Animals. Electron. Lett., Vol. 16, pp. 99-100 (1980).

31. P.C. Waterman, Symetry, Unitarity, and Geometry in Electromagnetic Scattering. Phys. Rev., Vol. 3, pp. 825-839 (1971).

32. D.E. Livesay and K.M. Chen, Electromagnetic Fields Induced Inside Arbitrarily Shaped Biological Bodies. IEEE Trans. Microwave Theory Techn., Vol. MTT-22, pp. 1273-1280 (1974).

33. O.P. Gandhi, Dosimetry - The Absorption Properties of Man and Experimental Animals, Bull. New York Acad. Sci., Vol. 55, pp. 999-1020 (1979).

34. O.P. Gandhi, M.J. Hagmann and J.A. D'Andrea, Part-body and Multibody Effects on Absorption of Radio Frequency Electromagnetic Energy by Animals and by Models of Man, Radio Science, Vol. 14(6S), pp. 15-22 (1979).

35. O.P. Gandhi, State of Knowledge for Electromagnetic Absorbed

Dose in Man and Animals. Proc. IEEE, Vol. 68, pp. 24-32 (1980).

36. P.W. Barber, O.P. Gandhi, M.J. Hagmann and I. Chatterjee, Electromagnetic Absorption in a Multilayered Model of Man. IEEE Trans. Biomed. Engn., Vol. BME-26, pp. 400-403 (1979).
37. O.P. Gandhi, Conditions of Strongest Electromagnetic Power Deposition in Man and Animals, IEEE Trans. Microwave Theory Techn., Vol. MTT-23, pp. 1021-1029 (1975).
38. O.P. Gandhi, Polarization and Frequency Effects on Whole Animal Absorption of R.F. Energy. Proc. IEEE, Vol. 62, pp. 1171-1175 (1975).

MOLECULAR INTERPRETATION OF THE DIELECTRIC BEHAVIOUR OF BIOLOGICAL MATERIAL

E. H. Grant

Physics Department, Queen Elizabeth College
University of London
London, United Kingdom

INTRODUCTION

The dielectric behaviour of biological tissue depends ultimately upon the properties of the molecules comprising it. The interpretation of the dielectric properties of biological material can therefore be made at a molecular level, although it is sometimes more convenient and appropriate to consider them in terms of cells and membranes. This is particularly so when _in vivo_, rather than _in vitro_, situations are being discussed.

The relationship between the bulk dielectric behaviour of biological tissue and its cellular or membrane structure is considered by Schwan[1] elsewhere in this book. The present paper will be devoted to the interpretation in terms of molecular structure and properties although there are, of course, certain situations where there is some overlap between the two areas.

Biological material consists of water, proteins plus numerous other biological macromolecules in various concentration. The water molecule is polar and possesses a dipole moment (μ) of around 2 Debye units. Although not an SI unit the Debye (D) is convenient in size and is roughly equal to the dipole moment produced by one electron and one positron separated by 2nm. To convert to coulomb-meters (the SI unit of dipole moment) it is necessary to multiply by 3.3×10^{-30}. Small biological molecules such as amino-acids or the lower peptides typically possess a dipole moment of value in the range 10 - 40D but as the complexity of the molecule increases there is no regular relationship between dipole moment and size, the overriding consideration being the number of charged groups and the way they are distributed throughout the molecule. Thus haemoglobin and bovine serum albumin, both of molecular weight 68000, have dipole moments of around 400D and 200D, respectively. In contrast to this lack of relationship between dipole moment and molecular weight, the dielectric relaxation time τ is directly dependent upon it and increases fairly regularly with it, although for larger molecules shape is also important. Thus water has a relaxation time of 10ps at 20°C, triglycine (molecular weight 189) has τ = 200ps and the relaxation time of both haemoglobin and serum albumin is around 10^5ps.

The molecules in a biological solution at 37°C will be fluctuating in motion owing to the thermal energy of 1/2kT associated with each degree of freedom. This is accompanied by the breaking and reforming of hydrogen bonds. If an electric field E is applied, the molecules are subject to field energy μE as well as thermal energy kT, and the resulting motion will depend upon a combination of the two factors. To obtain some idea of the relative contribution let us calculate the effect of an electric field E = 0.2kV/m on a myoglobin molecule of dipole moment μ = 150D. The value of kT is 4×10^{-21}J, which is a factor of around 10^5 larger than μE. For a plane wave in free space of power density 10mW/cm^2 the value of the electric field is 0.10kV/m. In tissue it would be lower than this. Thus at these values of E the thermal energy completely dominates the energy due to the electric field and it follows therefore that field strengths of around 10^4kV/m are required to produce a significant degree of molecular orientation. This prediction has been verified experimentally by the observation[2] that dielectric saturation occurs for poly-benzyl-L-glutamate at 50kV/cm. Hence at field strengths corresponding to power densities being considered for current Protection Guides there are no field induced effects in respect to macromolecules. Whether or not they occur with cells or other biological structures depends upon the cell size and other factors.[1]

The dielectric dispersion curve of a typical solution of polar biological macromolecules in water is shown in Figure 1. By convention the dispersion regions are termed β, δ and γ in ascending order of frequency, where the symbols refer respectively to the contributions from the solute, the water of hydration and the bulk water. This will be considered in more detail later. For compact biological macromolecules such as globular proteins the β dispersion is due to dielectric relaxation of the molecules, behaving as permanent dipoles. However, mechanisms other than dipolar orientation can also give rise to a β dispersion. The mere presence of heterogeneity in

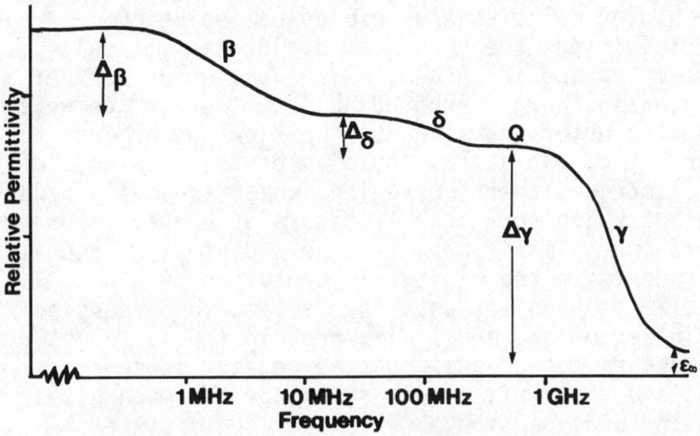

Fig. 1 Dielectric dispersion of an aqueous solution of biological macromolecules

the system means that Maxwell-Wagner type processes can occur, with consequent fall in relative permittivity with frequency of the form indicated in Figure 1. Another alternative mechanism is proton fluctuation, i.e. the motion of protons on and off the macromolecule. The theoretical aspects of these and other possibilities have been considered elsewhere;[1,3] the present article is concerned more with the applications.

Dipolar relaxation and proton fluctuation are commonly observable in respect to globular proteins and smaller molecules such as amino acids and peptides. Maxwell-Wagner phenomena tend to be observed with a higher level of organization, such as occurs in the case of lipoproteins, where the molecular weight is in excess of two million. Some authorities doubt the wisdom of referring to such structures as molecules and prefer the term particle or complex. However, for the purpose of this paper systems like lipoproteins in an aqueous environment will be considered as biphasic solutions at a molecular level, in order to distinguish them from whole tissues and phenomena involving cells and membranes, which are discussed by Schwan.[1] For these latter systems the β dispersion is very large and is typically associated with a fall in permittivity from several thousands or tens of thousand, to below one hundred. As with lipoprotein molecules the underlying mechanism is Maxwell-Wagner in character, but the presence of the cell membranes causes much larger polarization.[1]

In any biological tissue or biological solution numerous ions of various types are present. Biological molecules, whether freely moving in an aqueous solvent or as part of a membrane, contain charges protruding from the surface which, in turn, attract counterions. Counterion flow can produce a very large polarization and is responsible for the existence of another dielectric dispersion region, which typically occurs below 1kHz but which occasionally occurs at higher frequencies. This dispersion region is known as the α dispersion and is the mechanism underlying the dielectric behaviour of DNA at low frequencies.[4] It also accounts for dielectric dispersion observed[5] in serum low-density lipoprotein (LDL). Counterion relaxation occurs, of course, just as readily in cell suspensions and whole tissue and is one of the mechanisms underlying the α dispersion observed for these systems.[1]

Having indicated in the INTRODUCTION the broad features of dielectric behaviour of biological material, and its general interpretation at a molecular level, the rest of the paper will be concerned with examining specific cases and with explaining the kind of information which can be obtained. It must be re-emphasized that with whole tissue the magnitude of the α and β dispersions caused by the presence of cells and membranes is so large that effects due to the properties of individual molecules are obscured. Therefore with <u>tissue</u>, information at a molecular level can be obtained from observations made on the γ dispersion, or at the high frequency end of the β dispersion where the effect of the dispersion has ceased, but not at lower frequencies. In contrast, with accurately prepared aqueous solutions of biological molecules the molecular properties of the solute can be examined directly without any interfering background effects.

DIELECTRIC PROPERTIES OF AMINO ACIDS, PEPTIDES AND PROTEINS

The dielectric behaviour of this group of substances can be considered, in most cases, as an example of dipolar relaxation of the individual molecules.

Amino acids and peptides

An amino acid can be represented structurally as an amino group NH_2 and a carboxyl group COOH attached to a carbon atom, with the other two bonds from the carbon being made to a hydrogen atom plus another grouping which is characteristic of the particular amino acid. In an aqueous environment ionization takes place and the amino and carboxyl groups become NH_3^+ COO^-, respectively, the molecule in this case being termed a zwitterion. The charge on each group is numerically equal to that on the electron. The dipole moment (μ) of an amino acid molecule lies between 15 – 30D, the important deciding factor being the distance between the charged groups. Thus for glycine, where the amino and carboxyl groups are attached to the same carbon atom, $\mu \sim 19D$, whereas for ε – aminocaproic acid (five carbon atoms between the amino and carboxyl groups) $\mu \sim 30D$. The relaxation time τ increases with the molecular weight: for glycine (MW=75) in water at 20°C the relaxation time is 50ps but for ε – aminocaproic acid (MW=131) it is more than five times greater. Bearing in mind that the relaxation time of water at 20°C is 10ps and that a dielectric dispersion region (Figure 1) typically occupies at least two decades of frequency it is apparent that the amino acid and water dispersion regions overlap considerably especially when the former has a relatively low molecular weight. Therefore to obtain accurate information from a dielectric study on an amino acid solution it is necessary to measure permittivity and conductivity (or dielectric loss) at many frequencies in the appropriate range in order to obtain an unambiguous interpretation about the nature of the dispersion of the amino acid and the water content individually. The curve in Figure 1 refers to a protein solution, where of course, the effects of solute and solvent are well separated. When the dielectric increment Δ_S, of the solute (amino acid) has been obtained the molecular dipole moment μ can be calculated[3] using Kirkwood's theory of polar dielectrics. The relaxation time can be related to temperature according to the theory of rate processes, and therefore from the knowledge of the change in τ with temperature, the potential barrier surmounted during dielectric relaxation can be calculated. This may be identified with the strength of the solute-solvent bonds which, from a dielectric study of amino acids in solution[3] are found typically to have a value of around 17kJ/mole; this correlates well with the energy of a hydrogen bond and is thus consistent with the hypothesis that such a bond is broken in dielectric relaxation.

Peptides are formed from the bonding together of two or more amino acids. The dipeptide diglycine, comprising two glycine molecules, is a zwitterion but, with the amino and carboxyl groups now further separated, the dipole moment is 29D compared with the 19D for glycine. The dipole moment of triglycine is 37D, and so on for the higher peptides. Since the principal factor determining the molecular dipole moment (μ) is the separation of the charged groups, all zwitterionic dipeptides would be expected to have similar values of μ. This is borne out by the facts, for example diglycine, glycylalanine and analylglycine all have values of μ lying in the range 30 ± 1D. The relaxation time of peptides, as with amino acids, increases with molecular weight although the shape of the molecule also becomes an important factor with these larger molecules. The form of the variation of relaxation time with temperature for peptides in an aqueous environment can be interpreted in terms of the breaking of a solute-solvent hydrogen bond. This observation of an activation enthalpy for dielectric relaxation of around 15-20kJ/mole has been observed not only for amino acids and peptides in aqueous solution but for other polar, although not zwitterionic, molecules of biological importance including ATP, urea and various sugars.[3] The same value of activation enthalpy as the above also occurs in respect of proteins in solution and in pure water itself. It therefore appears as though the solute-solvent hydrogen bonds are the dominating factor underlying dielectric relaxation of biological molecules in water for a wide range of biological media.

Proteins in aqueous solution

As the size and complexity of biological molecules increase the distribution of the charged groups within the molecule departs markedly from the simple zwitterionic form experienced with molecules such as amino acids and peptides. With a protein molecule there will generally be numerous basic and acidic groups protruding from the surface each of which will contribute to the dipole moment. Moreover the sign of the charge will depend upon the pH of the environment. Apart from these surface charges there will be contributions to the overall dipole moment from the backbone of the molecule, which may have the form of a chain or an α-helix. In addition to this there will be a mean square dipole produced by protons fluctuating on and off the side groups. For proteins of known structure these contributions may be assessed separately[7] but in any event it is a fairly formidable exercise to give a detailed account of molecular dipole moment in terms of structure. However, although it may at first sight appear paradoxical, there is another sense in which interpreting dielectric data on protein solutions is easier than for smaller molecules such as amino acids and peptides. This is because the protein molecule is so much larger in relation to the solvent (water) molecules that it can be considered to behave as a macroscopic spheroid rotating in a continuum. The highly directional solute-water bonds average out over the surface of the macromolecule because so many water molecules are involved, and the orientation can be considered as being well approximated by a suitable hydrodynamic model such as the rotation of a ball-bearing in oil. This concept was adopted by Debye[8] in one of the earlier theories of dielectric relaxation, and its relevance to protein molecules orienting in water was exploited by Oncley[9] in the first comprehensive investigation of a series of biological molecules by dielectric methods.

The dielectric behaviour of a protein solution is indicated in Figure 1. To a first approximation the permittivity curve can be represented by

$$\varepsilon = \varepsilon' - j\varepsilon'' = \varepsilon_\infty + \frac{\Delta_\beta}{1 + j\omega\tau_\beta} + \frac{\Delta_\delta}{1 + j\omega\tau_\delta} + \frac{\Delta_\gamma}{1 + j\omega\tau_\gamma} \quad (1)$$

where Δ and τ are the dielectric increment and the relaxation time of the dispersion in question. The form of equation (1) assumes that all three dispersion regions may be represented by the Debye equation with a single relaxation time. For the γ dispersion (bulk water) this is a good approximation but for the δ dispersion (water of hydration) the assumption is unlikely to be so valid. These dispersions will be considered later in the paper. For the β dispersion (protein) the assumption of a single relaxation time would be true for a spherical molecule but will become increasingly invalid for asymmetric molecules. The variation of the form of the relaxation function is rather outside the scope of this paper but is considered in detail elsewhere.[3,9] In the present article it will be convenient to illustrate the principles involved by taking the case of a molecule whose shape does not depart too greatly from spherical, e.g. haemoglobin. For such a case equation (1) is a good approximation to the observed dielectric behaviour. If the complex permittivity of a protein solution such as that of haemoglobin is measured over a wide frequency range and the data fitted to equation (1) the six unknown quantities can be obtained. It is assumed that ε_∞, the relative permittivity at very high frequencies is around 5: its precise magnitude is unimportant.

The molecular dipole moment μ can then be evaluated[6] from

$$\mu^2 = \frac{2\varepsilon_0 MkT\Delta_\beta}{Nc} \quad (2)$$

where ε_0 is the permittivity of free space, M is the molecular weight of the protein, N is the Avagadro constant and c the concentration of protein. Thus from a dielectric investigation carried out on haemoglobin solution[10] the molecular dipole moment was found to be 400D. From the relaxation time $_\beta$ the radius of the hydrated molecule r can be calculated from

$$\tau_\beta = 4\pi r^3 \frac{\eta}{kT} \quad (3)$$

where η is the viscosity. This equation is based on the Debye theory.[8] From the same dielectric investigation[10] on haemoglobin r was calculated from the measured value of τ_β and found to be 3.29nm, which is around 0.5nm greater than the radius of the molecule in the anhydrous state. This difference may be attributed to a layer of 'bound' water which is so tightly attached to the protein that it rotates with it as one unit at these frequencies (around 1MHz). Therefore this is one method of measuring bound water (water of hydration) and must be considered alongside the other two methods to be discussed later.

In summary it can be stated that the following parameters of interest can be obtained from the study of the dielectric dispersion curve of an aqueous solution of dipolar biological molecules; molecular dipole moment, size of the hydrated molecule when in an aqueous environment, quantity of water of hydration and nature of intermolecular bonding. To this list may be added molecular shape if the molecules are either particularly elongated or particularly flattened. The case of biological solutions whose dielectric behaviour is not determined principally by the molecules behaving as a permanent dipole will now be considered. In general these are much larger and more complex molecules, and frequently two clearly identifiable dispersion regions (rather than one as seen for protein solutions) are observed. As mentioned in the INTRODUCTION the lower frequency dispersion (α) may be attributed to motion of counterions and the higher frequency region (β) to a Maxwell-Wagner mechanism arising from the heterogeneity of the system. Either of the two examples quoted in the INTRODUCTION, DNA or serum lipoproteins, would serve as a good model to illustrate the principles involved. For the present purpose the second alternative will be chosen.

Serum low density lipoproteins (LDL)

LDL may be defined as that group of lipoproteins having a density range 1.006 - 1.063 and a flotation rate of 0-20 Svedberg units. In human plasma LDL is the most abundant lipoprotein present and carries the cholesterol, which is strongly related to the incidence of coronary heart disease.

Dielectric measurements carried out on an aqueous solution of LDL at 20°C show the presence of four dispersion regions; an α dispersion with a relaxation frequency of 500kHz, a β dispersion centered around 5MHz, a small δ dispersion lying in the range 0.2 - 0.5GHz and the usual γ dispersion with a relaxation frequency of 17GHz. The relaxation frequency is the reciprocal of the relaxation time multiplied by the reciprocal of 2π. Examination of the parameters describing the α dispersion showed[5] the dielectric increment Δ_α to be independent of solution pH and only slightly dependent on temperature. The relaxation frequency was shown also to be independent of these solution parameters, and to have a temperature dependence corresponding to an activation enthalpy of only around 4kJ/mole. The absolute value of this relaxation frequency and those of the other three dispersions was shown to be several orders of magnitude higher than that which would be required to account for the data assuming dipolar rotation. These conclusions taken together all point to the interpretation as being due to a counterion mechanism of the type proposed by Schwarz.[11] Moreover the assumption of a counterion mechanism enables the surface charge on the lipoprotein molecule to be calculated and the value obtained in this particular study[5] was $2X10^{-18}C$, which agrees well with that determined independently from electrophoresis experiments. Dielectric dispersion experiments therefore are a useful alternative means of determining molecular surface charge. The counterion hypothesis was further checked by removing[12] certain surface groups in a known manner by the action of the enzyme trypsin, which results in an increase of the negative surface charge by 70 percent. This correlated with the observed[12] change in the measured amplitude of the dispersion.

Interpretation of the β dispersion was carried out assuming a Maxwell-Wagner mechanism and by using the Pauly-Schwan equations.[13] This interpretation predicted values of dielectric increment and relaxation time in excellent agreement with those observed experimentally. However, the interior of the LDL molecule was required to be relatively conducting in its behaviour which, on initial consideration, would appear to place some of the protein (known to be a good conductor) at the centre and the lipid (known to be a good insulator) surrounding it. The rest of the protein would be on the outside of the molecule. The former requirements would be at variance with conclusions from X-ray studies which infer that the lipid is at the centre of the molecule. Owing to the ignorance surrounding the structure of LDL this apparent contradiction is not yet completely resolved but one possible compromise would be if the lipid were in the centre but were surrounded by a shell of ions which would give it conducting properties. The dielectric and X-ray methods are complementary in that the former is more sensitive to the properties of the centre of the molecule whereas the strength of the latter technique is in the information which it can provide on the structure of the exterior.

So far the present paper has been concerned with showing how the molecular properties of the non-aqueous part of a biological solution determine its overall dielectric behaviour and with explaining the ways by which measurements of complex permittivity can be used to measure various molecular parameters of biological and biophysical interest. In the next section the behaviour of the water will be considered and it will be shown how water structure and properties in biological material can be obtained from dielectric measurements.

DIELECTRIC PROPERTIES OF WATER IN BIOLOGICAL MATERIAL

Pure water

Before considering water in biological material it will be convenient to summarize first the dielectric behaviour of pure water. This has been the subject of a considerable amount of experimental investigation over the past forty years and as a result the form of the dielectric dispersion curve is well understood in the frequency range from DC up to around 30GHz. To a good approximation the dielectric properties of water in this region can be represented by the equation

$$\varepsilon = \varepsilon' - j\varepsilon'' = \varepsilon_\infty + \frac{\varepsilon_s - \varepsilon}{1 + j\omega\tau} \tag{4}$$

This is of course the same form as the final term of equation (1) but with the dielectric increment Δ_γ being written in full as $\varepsilon_s - \varepsilon_\infty$ where ε_s is the static permittivity of the pure liquid and ε is the plateau value to which ε' would fall at frequencies much higher than τ^{-1} assuming that no further dispersion occurs. Measurements carried out within the past few years[14,15] show, however, that further dispersion <u>does</u> occur in the far infrared, and that therefore ε_∞ has no physical signifcance but is merely a mathematical parameter chosen in order to give a good fit to equation (4) for measured permittivity data on water at frequencies from DC up to around 30GHz. The value of $\varepsilon_s - \varepsilon_\infty$ is proportional to the square of the molecular dipole moment but the precise relationship is uncertain owing to ignorance concerning the local structure and short range intermolecular forces existing in liquid water.

An interesting observation is that a very good linear relationship is observed between τ and η despite the fact that the structure of liquid water is such as to invalidate the model assumed in the original derivation[8] of equation (2). Although empirical attempts have been made[16] to explain this at a molecular level the precise nature of the observed linearity is surprising and has not been properly accounted for. One sure fact that does stand out, however, is that the processes of viscosity and dielectric relaxation are just as strongly related for pure water as they are for the solutions of biological macromolecules in water. The variation of relaxation time with temperature for pure water is consistent with an activation enthalpy of around 16kJ/mole which, as for the biological solutions discussed above, indicate that hydrogen bond breakage is the rate determining step in dielectric relaxation.

Bound water and free water

In biological material the influence of the biological macromolecules on the water must be such as to change the dielectric behaviour of the latter from that of pure water. The question to be decided is the nature and extent of this influence, and in the endeavour to cope with this situation it has been traditional to divide the aqueous content into 'free' water and 'bound' water. These are, of course, purely relative words and, in retrospect, it would probably have been better to have chosen some other terminology. Since however these and other terms are now firmly entrenched in the literature it is important to try to give them some sort of quantitative meaning.

It has already been mentioned above that in pure water a hydrogen bond has to be broken before a molecule can rotate in dielectric relaxation. For water molecules adjacent to a biological macromolecule the solute-solvent bonds would in general be stronger than the hydrogen bond in liquid water, and therefore the influence of the macromolecule is such as to restrict the rotation of these adjacent water molecules. Since the relaxation time is a measure of the freedom of molecular rotation in the electric field it would be expected that this would be lengthened in relation to the relaxation time of those water molecules at some distance away from the macromolecule. According to this picture, therefore, bound water is water exhibiting its dispersion region at frequencies somewhat lower than that of free water. Provided the relaxation frequencies are sufficiently far apart the dispersion regions of the two forms of water would be separately observable experimentally. In fact this direct observation of the bound water dispersion was first made by Schwan[17] for haemoglobin and confirmed later for egg albumen[18] and serum albumen;[19] it is designated the δ dispersion and its position in the spectrum is shown in Figure 1. The γ dispersion is then due to all the rest of the water present, and may be referred to as the free water or, better, the bulk water. An alternative term to bound water would be water of hydration which has a distinguished history in physical biochemistry, being first coined by Cohn and Edsall[20] to describe water 'carried through the solution by unit weight of protein in sedimentation, diffusion and electrophoresis experiments'. Whichever definition or concept is used, however, it is important to realize that the assumption of the existence of just two forms of water in biological material is no more, and no less, than a convenient means of interpreting the various sets of available experimental data within the given resolution and experimental error. Thus experimental data gained by using a wide variety of independent techniques - sedimentation, diffusion, polarization of fluorescence, nuclear magnetic resonance, low angle X-ray scattering, viscosity, electrophoresis and dielectric measurements can all be well interpreted in terms of a model whereby the hydrated macromolecule is regarded as a core surrounded by a shell of water about two molecular layers in width which behaves differently from the rest of the water in the system. This is what may be described as bound water or water of hydration.

Another question which is often discussed is the proportion of the water in a biological material which exists as water in hydration. The problem can be looked at from the point of view of the intermolecular forces which are likely to be present. The surface of the macromolecule contains hydrophilic, ionic and hydrophobic groups, and the nature of the solute-water bonds can be considered accordingly. Hydrogen bond and electrostatic forces fall off rapidly with distance and molecules beyond the second, or at the very furthest, the third layer away from the macromolecule would not be affected. Hydrophobic bonds are more difficult to assess, and longer range effects may be a possibility. However, any long range ordering would appear to make a minimal contribution to the water of hydration as defined above and as measured by the various experimental techniques listed. The relative amounts of bulk water and water of hydration must depend upon the nature of the biological material being considered for concentrated suspensions of relatively small biological molecules all the water would be affected. For media containing a low concentration of large macromolecules most of the water would be unaffected, i.e. the water would have the same dielectric properties as pure liquid water.

Experimentally the relative proportion of bound and bulk water can be obtained by comparing the increments of the δ and γ dispersions (Figure 1). The numerical value of the ratio $\Delta_\delta/\Delta_\gamma$ gives a very rough indication of the relative amounts of bound and free water present in any given tissue or biological material and to obtain a more accurate value it is necessary to employ an appropriate dielectric mixture theory. For example in previous work[21] on the dielectric properties of myoglobin it was found for an aqueous solution of concentration 161mg/ml that $\Delta_\delta = 5.1$ and $\Delta_\gamma = 63$, giving a ratio of 0.08. Interpreting the data rigorously gave a hydration factor of 0.23g water for 1g of myoglobin which corresponds to a volume of 4mls of bound water in the presence of around 80mls of bulk water, i.e. a ratio of around 0.05. Deducing the water of hydration from measurements made on the amplitude of the dispersion gives good values provided that allowance is made, if appropriate, for any other possible mechanisms such as side chain rotation[22] or proton fluctuation.[23]

As mentioned above an alternative method of studying hydration using dielectric techniques is to measure the relaxation time of the β dispersion and to calculate from this the volume of the hydrated macromolecule. The quantity of water or hydration can then be obtained by deducting the volume of the non-hydrated molecule, which is obtainable from the literature or by using other techniques. It should be noted that the hydration obtained using this method corresponds to water carried around with the molecule as it rotates in a radiofrequency electric field. It could be thought of as water having a viscosity much greater than that in the continuum. This concept of hydration is not identical with the picture of water molecules having their rotation restricted such that dielectric relaxation occurs at frequencies an order of magnitude less than those of free water: this is the concept underlying the explanation of the δ dispersion. Therefore the quantity of bound water deduced from observations on the δ dispersion should not be expected to be precisely the same as that calculated from the β dispersion although in practice the values deduced for a given biological macromolecule normally agree to within experimental error.

A third method of measuring hydration using dielectric techniques is less accurate than the other two in an absolute sense but does have the great advantage that it can be used in respect of whole tissue as well as with aqueous solutions. It was pointed out in the INTRODUCTION that, for tissue, the contribution of the macromolecules on an individual basis to the β dispersion is unresolvable owing to the dominating influence of the cell membranes. By the same token the δ dispersion is obliterated as a separate entity. Thus an alternative means of measuring hydration is very useful, and the method to be described is based on the original proposal in 1952 of Buchanan, et al.[24] If the permittivity is measured at a frequency a little below the low frequency limit of the γ dispersion (point Q on Figure 1) it may be assumed that the only form of molecular rotation able to take place is due to the bulk water molecules. The permittivity at Q (ε_Q) will then be less than the static permittivity of pure water (ε_W) by an amount which depends upon the volume of the non-aqueous content of the tissue (ν) plus the volume of the water of hydration. Similar arguments can be presented[25] for the effect on conductivity measured at this frequency. By assuming an appropriate dielectric mixture formula the volume of the hydrated macromolecules present in the tissue can be calculated and the hydration obtained by deduction of ν. A suitable mixture relationship is based on a formula derived by Maxwell

$$\frac{\varepsilon_Q - \varepsilon_w}{\varepsilon_Q + 2\varepsilon_w} = \nu \frac{\varepsilon_p - \varepsilon_w}{\varepsilon_p + 2\varepsilon_w} \tag{5}$$

where ε_p is the permittivity of the protein at these frequencies (~5). Recent work[26] on human and rabbit lens material in which measurements were made over the frequency range 0.1 - 6GHz using a Time Domain Spectrometer[27] has shown that around 20 percent of the total water content exists as water of hydration in the nuclear zone of the lens of the human and the rabbit. In contrast the amount of bound water in the cortical zone could not be distinguished from zero to within experimental error, for both species.

The method has two weaknesses. The first is that the parameter to be experimentally determined is $\varepsilon_w - \varepsilon_Q$, which is a small difference between large quantities. Therefore considerable effort must be made to reduce experimental error in ε_Q to a minimum. The second shortcoming is the use of equation (5) for a system of hydrated macromolecules, bearing in mind that this was devised originally for a suspension of macroscopic spheroids in a continuum. For biological macromolecules there are, however, typically between 10^3 and 10^4 water molecules in the first two shells. Therefore the macroscopic type of model of a core surrounded by a layer of bound water is probably not too removed from the true configuration of a hydrated protein molecule. Uncertainties due to both of these objections, experimental and conceptual, are reduced considerably if the method is used to compare hydrations between similar molecules rather than to measure hydration absolutely. Systematic errors then disappear. Situations where comparative values are useful are when it is required to contrast the bound water content between two parts of the same tissue, or between the same region of tissue in different species (as in the examples given above). This may include the case when molecules from pathological tissue exhibit a different hydration from the same type of molecule present in normal tissue, as was observed[5] for serum low density lipoproteins present in patients with genetically determined coronary disease when compared with controls.

REFERENCES

1. H.P. Schwan, this volume.

2. G.P. Jones, M. Gregson and M. Davies, Total dielectric saturation observed in a dipolar system, Chem. Phys. Letters 4: 33 (1969).

3. E.H. Grant, R.J. Shepphard and G.P. South, "Dielectric behaviour of biological molecules in solution", Oxford University Press, Oxford (1978).

4. S. Takashima, Study of dielectric behaviour of DNA in shear gradient, Biopolymers 12: 145 (1973).

5. C.G. Essex, E.H. Grant, R.J. Sheppard, G.P. South, M.S. Symonds, G.L. Mills and J. Slack, Dielectric properties of normal and abnormal lipoprotins in aqueous solution, Ann. N.Y. Acad. Sci. 303: 142 (1977).

6. J.G. Kirkwood, Dielectric polarisation of polar liquids, J. Chem. Phys. 7: 911 (1939).

7. G.P. South and E.H. Grant, Dielectric dispersion and dipole moment of myoglobin in water, Proc. Roy. Soc. Lond. A. 328: 371 (1972).

8. P. Debye, "Polar Molecules", Reinhold, New York (1929).

9. J.L. Oncley, Reference 20, Chapter 22.

10. E.H. Grant, G.P. South, S. Takashima and H. Ichimura, Dielectric dispersion in aqueous solutions of oxyhaemoglobin and carboxyhaemoglobin, Biochem. J. 122: 691 (1971).

11. G. Schwarz, A theory of the low frequency dielectric dispersion of colloidal particles in electrolyte solution, J. Phys. Chem. 66: 2636 (1962).

12. G.S. Chana, M.J. Chapman, R.J. Sheppard, G.L. Mills, S. Goldstein and E.H. Grant, A comparative dielectric study of human serum low density lipoprotein before and after partial digestion by trypsin, J. Supramol. Struct. 13: 47 (1980).

13. H. Pauly and H.P. Schwan, The impedance of a suspension of spherical particles surrounded by a shell, Zs. f. Naturforshung 14B: 125 (1959).

14. M.N. Afsar and J.B. Hasted, Measurements of the optical constants of liquid H_2O and D_2O between 6 and 450 cm^{-1} J. Opt. Soc. Am. 67: 902 (1977).

15. E.H. Grant, S. Szwarnowski and R.J. Sheppard, Dielectric properties of water in the microwave and far infrared regions, "Biological Effect of Nonionizing Radiation". American Chemical Society Symposium Series 157: 47 (1981).

16. E.H. Grant, Relationship between relaxation time and viscosity for water, J. Chem. Phys. 26: 1575 (1957).

17. H.P. Schwan, Electrical properties of tissue and cell suspensions, in "Advances in Biological and Medical Physics", J.H. Lawrence and C.A. Tobias, eds., Academic Press, New York (1957).

18. E.H. Grant, Electric behaviour of egg albumen solutions at ultra-high frequencies, Nature 196: 1194 (1962).

19. E.H. Grant, Dielectric dispersion in bovine serum albumen, J. Mol. Biol. 19: 133 (1966).

20. E.J. Cohn and J.T. Edsall, "Proteins, Amino-Acids and Peptides", Reinhold, New York (1942).

21. E.H. Grant, B.G.R. Mitton, G.P. South and R.J. Sheppard, An investigation by dielectric methods of hydration in myoglobin solutions, Biochem. J. 139: 375 (1974).

22. B.E. Pennock and H.P. Schwan, Further observations on the electrical properties of haemoglobin bound water, J. Phys. Chem. 73: 2600 (1969).

23. G.P. South and E.H. Grant, The contribution of proton fluctuation to dielectric relaxation in protein solutions, Biopolymers 12: 1937 (1973).

24. T.J. Buchanan, G.H. Haggis, J.B. Hasted and B.G. Robinson, The dielectric estimation of protein hydration, Proc. Roy. Soc. Lond. A213: 379 (1952).

25. K.R. Foster, J.L. Schepps, R.D. Stoy and H.P. Schwan, Dielectric properties of brain tissue between 0.01 and 10GHz, Phys. Med. Biol. 24: 1177 (1979).

26. A.W.J. Dawkins, C. Gabriel, R.J. Sheppard and E.H. Grant, Electrical properties of lens material at microwave frequencies, Phys. Med. Biol. 26: 1 (1981).

27. A.W.J. Dawkins, R.J. Shepphard and E.H. Grant, An on-line computer based system for performing time domain spectroscopy. 1. Main features of the basic system, J. Phys. E. Sci. Instrum. 12: 1091 (1979).

DIELECTRIC PROPERTIES OF BIOLOGICAL TISSUE AND CELLS AT RF- AND MW-FREQUENCIES

Herman P. Schwan

Max-Planck-Institut für Biophysik
Frankfurt a.M., Germany
and
Department of Bioengineering/D3 *
University of Pennsylvania
Philadelphia, Pennsylvania 19104, U.S.A.

The electrical properties are important for our understanding of the mechanism of interaction of electromagnetic fields with biological systems, including biopolymers, membranes and cells. Our knowledge of dielectrical properties is rather advanced[1,2]. I shall first summarize the state of our present knowledge of such properties. Then, in the last lecture which I present in this course, I draw conclusions about possible mechanisms of interactions.

PRINCIPLE MECHANISM

The two electrical properties which define the electrical characteristics are the dielectric constant or permittivity relative to free space ε and the conductivity σ. These properties change with temperature and strongly with frequency. As the frequency increases from a few Hertz to Gigahertz, the dielectric constant of tissues such as muscle decreases from several million to only a few units and the conductivity increases from a few mMho/cm to nearly a thousand.

---

* Permanent Address

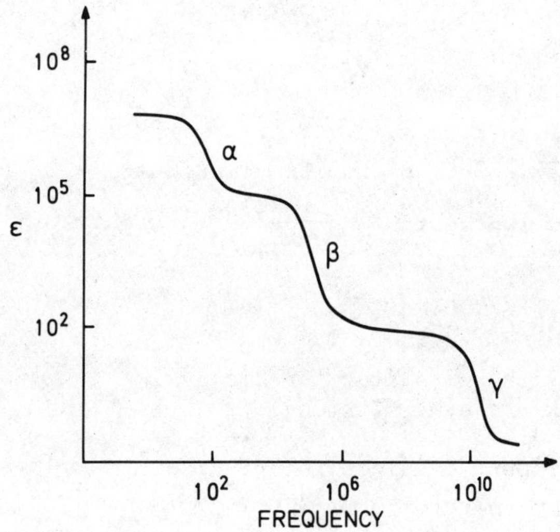

Fig. 1. Dielectric constant ε of tissues of high water content as function of frequency.

Figure 1 indicates the dielectric behavior of practically all tissues of high water content. Two remarkable features stand out: unusually high permittivity values at low frequencies and three relaxation regions α, β, γ at low, medium and very high frequencies. Each of these relaxation regions is in its simplest form characterized by equations of the Debye type

$$\varepsilon = \varepsilon_\infty + \frac{\varepsilon_o - \varepsilon_\infty}{1 + (\omega T)^2} \quad ; \qquad \sigma = \sigma_o + (\sigma_\infty - \sigma_o)\frac{(\omega T)^2}{1 + (\omega T)^2} \qquad (1)$$

where ω is angular frequency, the constants are determined by the values at the beginning and end of the dispersion change and T is a time constant. If properties change with frequency as indicated by these equations, we name such properties "dispersive" and the phenomena of frequency dependance itself a "dispersion". Mechanism which give cause for such a dispersive behavior are called "relaxation" mechanism. It can be shown that the Fourier transformed equivalent behavior in the time domain is an exponential of time, indicating the relaxation of the system from one state to another under the influence of a sudden step in potential or current.

This is indicated in figure 2. The dielectric displacement D, i.e. the charge per unit area, changes usually as a function of time as a step potential is applied to the sample of interest. This is indicated in the upper part of the figure. In the simplest case this time dependence is exponential

$$D = a + b\,(1 - e^{-t/T}) \tag{2}$$

Then the frequency dependence is of the type given by the equations (1). σ_o represents an additional conductivity contribution due to other mechanism. It accounts for a finite low frequency conductance term not demanded by the exponential time dependence of D in the frequency domain.

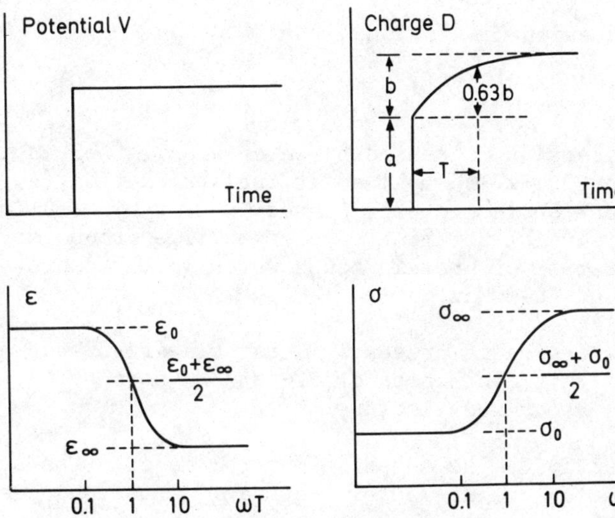

Fig. 2. Dielectric behavior in time- and frequency- domain. Upper: Typical response of D to a step potential versus time. Lower: Corresponding frequency dependence of ε and σ.

The mechanisms responsible for these three relaxation regions are indicated in Table 1. Inhomogeneous structure causes the β-dispersion, i.e., the polarization resulting from the charging membranes through intra- and extracellular fluids. Rotation of molecules having a permanent dipole moment such as water and proteins is responsible for the γ-dispersion (water). A small addition to the tail of the β-dispersion causes a corresponding β_1-dispersion of proteins. And tissue proteins elevate somewhat the high frequency tail of the β-dispersion. The β_1-effect caused by tissue proteins is small compared to the Maxwell-Wagner effect and occurs at somewhat higher frequencies. Subcellular structures, such as mitochondria, cell nuclei and other subcellular organelles also contribute to the β-dispersion. These structures are smaller in size than the surrounding cell. Therefore their relaxation frequency is higher, but their total dielectric increment smaller. Hence they contribute another addition to the tail of the β-dispersion (β_1).

Table 1. Electrical Relaxation Mechanism for Tissues with High Water Content

Mechanism	Dispersion
Cellular Structures (Maxwell-Wagner, induced dipoles)	β
Permanent Dipole Rotation (Debye)	γ, β-tail
Counterion Relaxation	α
Membrane Relaxation	α

The γ-dispersion is caused by water and its relaxational behavior near 20 GHz. A small additional relaxation (δ) between β and γ-dispersion is probably caused in part by rotation of amino acids, partial rotation of charged side groups of proteins and the relaxation of protein bound water which occurs somewhere between 300 and 2000 MHz.

The α-dispersion is presently least clarified and shall not concern us in this discussion of RF- and MW-properties. It will be discussed in our next lecture.

The conductivity increases in several major steps symmetrical to the changes of the dielectric constant. These changes are in accord with the theoretical demand

$$- \sigma_o = \frac{\varepsilon_o - \varepsilon_\infty}{T} \varepsilon_r \qquad (3)$$

which can be derived from the Kramer-Kronig equations which describe dispersive behavior. ε_r is the dielectric constant of free space $8{,}84 \cdot 10^{-14}$ F/cm.

Table 2. Characteristic Frequencies Observed with Biological Material for α-, β- and γ- dispersion Effects (approximate ranges)

Dispersion	Frequency Range (Hz)
α	$1 - 10^4$
β	$10^4 - 10^8$
δ	$10^8 - 10^9$
γ	2.10^9

Table 2 indicates the variability of the characteristic frequencies for the various mechanisms α, β, γ and δ from one biological object to another. Clearly there exists considerable variation depending on cellular size and other factors. However the γ-dispersion is sharply defined at the same frequency range.

Table 3 attempts to summarize at what level of biological complexity the various mechanisms occur. Electrolytes display only the γ-dispersion characteristic of water. Biological macromolecules in water add to the water's γ-dispersion a δ-dispersion. Proteins and nucleic acids in particular add further dispersions in the β and α-range as stated above. Suspensions of cells free of protein and vesicles display a Maxwell-Wagner β-dispersion and the γ-dispersion of water. If they contain proteins, a weak β-dispersion caused by the polarity of proteins is added and a δ-dispersion. If the cells carry a net charge, an α-mechanism caused by counter ion relaxation is added and if their membranes relax on their own an additional α-mechanism may appear.

I shall first concentrate on supporting evidence and its implications for the β-mechanism since it dominates tissue properties from low RF-frequencies to about 1 Ghz. Dr. Grant will consider the dielectric properties of electrolytes, tissue water and biopolymers (γ-effect). And in my last lectures, I shall more closely examine the various factors which govern the α-dispersion and implications with regard to ELF- and RF-field sensitivities. However I shall not deal with macroscopic biophysical (bioengineering) principles, such as RF and MW penetration values, relative absorption cross sections, averaged and local SAR-values and resultant temperature elevations. Presumably, Dr. Guy will deal with these topics in these Proceedings.

Table 3. Electrical Relaxation Effects of Various Biological Systems

Water and Electrolytes	γ
Biological macromolecules	
amino acids	$\delta + \gamma$
proteins	$\beta + \delta + \gamma$
nucleic acids	$\alpha + \beta + \delta + \gamma$
Cellular systems	
Vesicles, no surface charge	$\beta + \gamma$
with surface charge	$\alpha + \beta + \gamma$
Cells, free of protein	$\beta + \gamma$
with protein	$\beta + \beta$ tail $+ \gamma$
with surface charge	$\alpha + \beta + \gamma$
with relaxing membranes	$\alpha + \beta + \gamma$
with organelles only	
(connecting with outer membrane)	$\alpha + \beta + \gamma$
(not connecting)	$\beta + \beta$ tail $+ \gamma$

RF-DISPERSION

Membranes are responsible for the dielectric properties of tissues and cell suspensions at RF's. Many cells and cellular organelles have been extensively investigated by many investigators, including Fricke[3], Cole[4], and Schwan[1,2]. This work led to a detailed understanding of the role of cell membranes in the polarization processes of biological cells and tissues in the RF range. The principal mechanism responsible for dielectric polarization is the accumulation of charges at membranes from extra and intracellular fluids.

The pertinent mathematical theory is based on generalizations of equations already derived by Maxwell for spherical cells and Raleigh for cylindrical cells perpendicular to the direction of the field. Both Maxwell and Raleigh derived their equations for direct current. However their solutions can be extended to the AC-case by replacing the DC-boundary conditions at the interfaces by corresponding demands for continuity in the AC-case. The general solutions for a suspension of spherical particles surrounded by a shell as given by Maxwell can be shown to reduce to the equations (1), if the shell or membrane thickness is rather small compared to the radius R. This is usually the case for biological cells. Equations for the parameters in the equations (1) and (2) are then obtained. For spherical particles, the following equations were derived[1]

$$\varepsilon_o - \varepsilon_\infty = \frac{9}{4\varepsilon_r} \frac{\rho RC_m}{\left(1 + RG_m(\rho_i + \frac{1}{2}\rho_a)\right)^2} \rightarrow \frac{9}{4\varepsilon_r} \rho RC_m \qquad (4)$$

$$\sigma_o = \sigma_a \left\{ 1 - 1.5\rho \frac{1 + RG_m(\rho_i - \rho_a)}{1 + RG_m(\rho_i + \frac{1}{2}\rho_a)} \right\} \rightarrow \sigma_a(1\text{-}1.5\rho) \qquad (5)$$

$$\sigma_\infty = \sigma_a \left\{ 1 + 3\rho \frac{\sigma_i - \sigma_a}{\sigma_i + 2\sigma_a} \right\} \qquad (6)$$

for the limit values of the simple dispersion which characterizes the frequency dependence. The time constant is

$$\tau = \frac{RC_m}{2\frac{\sigma_a\sigma_i}{\sigma_i + 2\sigma_a} + RG_m} \rightarrow RC_m\ (\rho_i + 0.5\ \rho_a). \qquad (7)$$

In these equations C_m and G_m are capacitance and conductance per cm^2 of the cell membrane, R is the cell radius, ρ the cellular volume fraction assumed to below, $\sigma_i = 1/\rho_i$, and $\sigma_a = 1/\rho_a$ are the conductivities of the cell interior and suspending medium. More elaborate closed form expressions have been developed for cases when the stated assumptions are no longer valid[5,6]. An exact representation of the dielectric properties of a suspension of shell surrounded particles as a sum of two dispersions is available. lable[7]. For typical membrane conductances equations (4,5) reduced to the simple forms to the right of the arrows.

Equations (1, 7) can be represented by the equivalent circuit shown in figure 3, which displays the same frequency response. The membrane capacitance per unit area C_m appears in series with the access impedances ρ_i and $\rho_a/2$, while the term $\sigma_a(1\text{-}1.5\rho)$ provides for the conductance of the shunting extracellular fluid. The time constant τ which determines the frequency where the impedances $1/\omega C_m R$ and $(\rho_i + \rho_a/2)$ are equal is given by equation (7). For typical values of σ_i, $\sigma_a \sim 0.01$ mho/cm, $C_m = 1$ F/cm^2, R = 10 μm and p = 0.5, equation (4) shows that dispersion magnitude $\varepsilon_o - \varepsilon_\infty$ is exceptionally high. From the circuit in figure 3 it is apparent that at low frequencies the total potential applied to the cell develops across the membrane capacitances C.

At very high frequencies however the total potential is consumed by the cell interior. The switch over occurs at a frequency

$$f_c = 1/2\pi\tau \qquad (8)$$

where τ is given in equation (7). For the example chosen before, it has a value of 1.1 MHz. A precise Laplacian calculation of the maximum membrane potential induced at the cellular poles in the field direction gives therefore

$$\Delta V = \frac{1.5ER}{\sqrt{1 + (\omega\tau)^2}} \qquad (9)$$

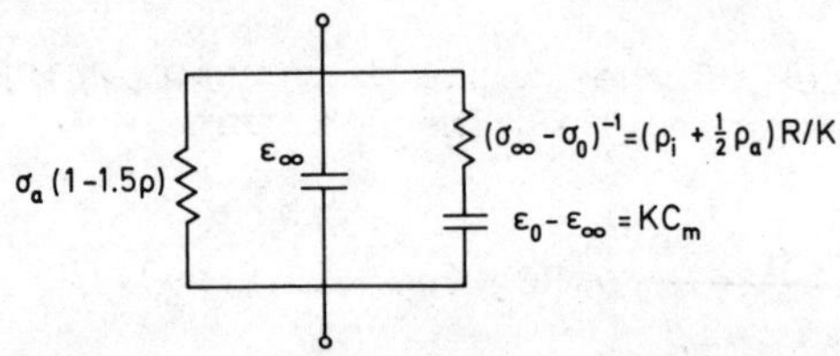

Fig. 3. Equivalent circuit for a suspension of spherical cells. The constant K is equal to $9\rho/\varepsilon_r$ for small p.

MICROWAVE DISPERSION

Dielectric studies of cell suspensions and tissues have been extended well into the microwave frequency range. Data up to 8500 MHz have been summarized by Schwan already in 1957[1]. More recently dielectric studies have been extended up to 18 GHz on muscle tissue[8]. It immediately became apparent that the dielectric behavior of tissues and cell suspensions in the microwave frequency range is largely determined by the strongly dispersive behavior of water. Indeed, from the analysis of the RF-properties summarized above, it follows that cell membranes impose no hindrance on the flow of electricity through the cell interior for frequencies above 100 to 300 MHz. Consequently it is apparent that as far as dielectric properties are concerned, tissues of high water content and cells simply behave as water containing some 20% proteins. This predictive model served well to describe numerically the dielectric properties observed at frequencies from about 100 MHz to many GHz. This approach tacitly assumes that the dielectric properties of tissue water are identical with those of normal water. Furthermore the availability of dielectric data for the cellular protein solutions is assumed. These two items are summarized now. They will be discussed in greater detail by Grant in these Proceedings.

Water and Tissue Water

The dielectric properties of pure water have been well established from DC up to microwave frequencies, approaching the infrared[9]. For all practical purposes they are characterized by a single relaxation process centered near 20 GHz at room temperature. Static and infinite frequency permittivity values are, at room temperature, close to 78 and 5, respectively. Hence the microwave conductivity increase predicted by equation (1) is close to 0.8 mho/cm above 20 GHz, much larger than typical low-frequency conductivities of biological fluids which are about 0.01 mho/cm. The dielectric properties of water are independent of field strength up to fields of the order 100 kV/cm.

The dielectric properties of electrolytes are almost identical to those of water with the addition of a σ_o term in Eq. (1) due to the ionic conductance of the dissolved ion species. The static dielectric permittivity of electrolytes of usual physiological strength (0.15 N) is about two units lower than that of pure water, a negligible change.

Hoeber[10] had already obtained a value for the conductance of the red cell interior. The work of Fricke[3] and that of Cole[4] provided additional data with no indication that tissue water might be differently structured from normal water. Earlier data frequently had to rely on extrapolations to higher frequencies where membrane properties no longer affect dielectric properties. But such extrapolations are difficult since tissue properties in the RF range include secondary dispersion phenomena caused by mitochondria, cell nuclei, and biopolymers. A direct and more precise determination of internal conductance values requires frequencies near 100 MHz, high enough to short-circuit and thereby eliminate membrane contributions and yet low enough to exclude conductance contributions from the rotation of water molecules. We measured the dielectric properties of various tissues and cell suspensions over the frequency range from 100 to 1000 MHz[11]. The results may be described as follows:

1. The dielectric constant of tissues of high water content and blood are identical to that of normal water if allowance is made for the space occupied by tissue proteins and hemoglobin.

2. The conductance values are approximately comparable to those calculated from the concentrations of ionic species. But there appears to be a systematic deviation with experimental values smaller than calculated ones. A detailed study was conducted with erythrocytes and ghosts containing varying amounts of Hb[12]. In the ghosts, agreement between theory and experiment was achieved at Hb concentrations less than half normal. At high concentration levels internal friction with proteins reduces the mobility of ions noticeably. This effect, if adequately considered, entirely removes the discrepancy between theory and experiment. No comparable analysis has yet been conducted for tissues and other cell suspensions.

3. Dielectric data for tissues and blood from 1000 to 8500 MHz[13] strongly indicated that the relaxation frequency for tissue water and normal water are identical even though the range of observation did not extend to the relaxation frequency of normal water.

Thus it appears that dielectric constants near 100 MHz, ion mobilities obtained from the conductance data, and tissue water relaxation compare well with properties characteristic of normal water if we correct for the small volume taken by protein bound water. However, this point of view has been challenged. Ling and his colleagues[14] stated that tissue water is differently structured from normal water, a view shared by a small but active group of biophysicists. Drost-Hansen also believes that the identification of tissue water with normal water is naive and has developed his own concepts of structured water[15]. Hovey at al[16] attempted to determine the internal conductance of aplysia cells and derived values which simply could not be understood unless one assumed vastly different properties of cellular and normal water. However, in a subsequent paper[17] this earlier work was corrected and the original internal conductance values were replaced by values supportive of our views stated above. Then there appeared a series of papers by Masszi et al[18,19] stating that the relaxation frequency of tissue water is appreciably shifted from that of normal water. Their work was carried out at a frequency of 2.45 GHz and based on an evaluation of conductance data. At this frequency the Debye contribution to the low frequency conductivity is already appreciable and sensitive to the value of the relaxation frequency. But in a more recent detailed analysis of available tissue data we could not find a confirmation of this conclusion[20].

Techniques have recently become available in our laboratory which extend the range of observation to 18 GHz, close to the relaxation frequency of normal water at room temperature and twice that of 9°C water. We decided to check the previously unpublished data by Herrick[13], which had been made available to us, to extend tissue data to 18 GHz, and to review the question of tissue water with the precision microwave techniques now available using a microwave network analyzer. The dielectric properties of barnacle muscle were investigated first, concentrating on the relaxation frequency of tissue water[8]. Two approaches were chosen. The first one is based on an evaluation of the Cole-Cole circle in the complex dielectric phase. The static dielectric constant obtained is as one might predict using Maxwell's mixture equation to account for the protein volume. The peak of the circle gives the relaxation frequency and is identical to that of free water. The second approach evaluates conductance data alone and is an adaptation of a technique used by us before[21]. The conductance is plotted versus a normalized conductance axis. The result is a straight line as may be seen from the relaxation equation (1) for the conductance and its slope is given by the relaxation frequency and thus provides f_c. At high frequencies values were obtained for the slope providing a relaxation frequency identical with that of normal water. But at lower frequencies the slope changes for the 37°C curve. This analysis demonstrates that this change is caused by a subsidiary protein UHF dispersion. For a more detailed discussion, see[8].

We conclude therefore that Masszi's results, obtained at much lower frequencies, were in error since he did not appropriately correct for the UHF-dispersion effect unrelated to tissue water and probably caused by proteins[22, 23, 24].

More recently, Jenin and Schwan[25] have pointed out how to determine the time constant of cell water from lower frequencies data. Again, a time constant was noted which compared well with that of normal water. At the same time the dielectric properties of the hemoglobin solution inside the red cell were noted to be identical with those of a solution of hemoglobin in normal water of equal concentration.

We therefore conclude that cellular water is, at least from a dielectric point of view, identical with normal water.

Protein Solutions

The dielectric properties of proteins and nucleic acids have been extensively reviewed[26, 27]. Protein solutions exhibit three major dispersion ranges. One occurs at RF's and is believed to arise from molecular rotation in the applied electric field. Typical characteristic frequencies range from about 1 to 10 MHz, depending on the protein size. Dipole moments are of the order of 200-500 Debyes and low-frequency increments of dielectric permittivity vary between 1 and 10 units/g protein/100 ml of solution. The high-frequency dielectric permittivity of this dispersion is lower than that of water because of the low dielectric permittivity of the protein leading to a high-frequency decrement of the order of 1 unit/g protein/100ml. This RF dispersion is quite noticeable in pure protein solutions, but in tissues and cell suspensions it only contributes slightly to the large β-dispersion found in these materials.

At microwave frequencies the dielectric properties of tissues are dominated by the water relaxation centered near 20 GHz. The magnitude of this water dispersion in tissues is typically diminished by some 20 dielectric units due to the proteins which displace a corresponding volume of water.

Between these two readily noticeable dispersions is a small one, termed the δ-dispersion by Grant. It was first noted for hemoglobin[22] and then carefully examined for hemoglobin[23] and albumin[24]. This dispersion is characterized by a fairly broad spectrum of characteristic frequencies extending from some hundred to some thousand MHz. Its magnitude is considerably smaller than that of the other two dispersions, and it is thought to be caused by a corresponding dispersion of the protein bound water and/or partial rotation of polar subgroups. Its contribution to the dielectric properties of cell suspensions and tissues is therefore small.

ELECTRICAL PROPERTIES OF TISSUES

The dielectric properties of tissues have been several times reviewed by Schwan[1, 2] and by Johnson and Guy[28]. A more recent summary of data has been given by Stuchly[29].

RF-data of electrical conductivity and resistivity are largely based on results by Rajewsky and his colleagues[30]. However the techniques employed sensed only the impedance magnitude. At that time, it was assumed that the reactive component could be neglected. Furthermore tissue samples were minced in order to accomodate the sample chamber. For this reason Stoy et al[31] collected tissue data in the RF-range with nearly identical results for the conductivity data. Osswald[32] investigated dielectric properties of a variety of tissues from 25 to 100 MHz for 20°C and 37°C. His results were obtained with excised tissue samples.

ELF-data were measured in vivo by Schwan and Kay[33, 34, 35]. Microwave data were obtained by many authors as reviewed by Schwan[1]. Two more extended efforts were those by Schwan and Li[11] investigating the electrical properties of many tissues from 100 to 1000 MHz and Herrick et al[13] from 1 to 8.5 GHz. But Herrick's data were never published by herself and are only available through information made available by her to this writer and reported in above cited reviews. For this reason and in order to extend the frequency range well above 8.5 GHz Foster et al more recently carried out measurements up to 18 GHz[8, 36]. All these data were obtained with excised material and at several temperatures. They are also internally consistent, i.e. they establish rather smooth continuous variations over the total frequency range investigated i.e. from RF-frequencies below 100 MHz to almost 20 GHz. No attempt will be made here to assemble all these data again and reference is made to the reviews listed above.

Applications of all these data depend on the frequency range investigated. Low frequency data have been useful in theoretical electrocardiography and impedance plethysmography, i.e. the study of blood flow by electrical means. RF- and MW-data have been a prerequisite for dosimetry studies and developments of more advanced diathermy techniques. Furthermore all these data have been essential in discussions of biohazards caused by exposure to electromagnetic fields with frequencies ranging from DC to many GHz. Dielectric studies with cell suspensions have been of great fundamental interest as indicated in the first lecture of these Proceedings. Fundamental mechanism which are the cause of observed data and their characteristic frequency dependancies are directly relevant to the mode of action of such fields on biological systems.

Living and Dead Tissues

Rajewsky et al[30] were probably the first to study how the conductivity of tissues changes with time. The magnitude of the β-dispersion decays slowly over a period of several days. Concurrent metabolic studies revealed that ceasing cellular functions and membrane breakdown are the responsible mechanism. Only few studies have been conducted on this topic at ELF frequencies. Schwan's[37] data suggest that the α-dispersion may disappear within a few hours for reasons not yet clarified. Theoretical considerations and a few experimental data suggest on the other hand that the γ-dispersion should not be affected by tissue death. The γ-dispersion is not altered by membrane breakdown since membranes do not contribute to it as was stated above. Furthermore the properties of water are not anticipated to change with death, nor does the magnitude of the volume taken by the proteins change. Figure 4 attempts to summarize these observations.

Linearity

At ELF tissue properties appear to be independent of the magnitude of the applied signal for field strength values below approximately 1 V/cm[33]. Corresponding current density values are near 1 mA/cm^2.For higher field strength and current density levels stimulation of excitable tissues results in altered tissue structure and configuration and can be expected to cause nonlinear behavior. These phenomena are not anticipated at RF- and MW frequencies. Hence linearity should extend to much higher field strength levels and current densities provided that the tissue temperature can be kept constant. No studies of the limits of linearity of tissue properties have been conducted sofar at these frequencies.

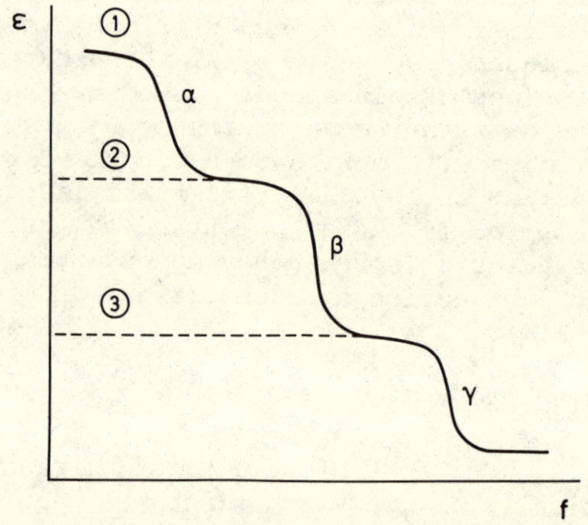

Fig. 4. Frequency dependance of the dielectric constant of tissues with high water content. The schematic diagram attempts to summarize time dependence after death. Curve 1 exists in vivo, but deteriorates within a few hours for unknown reasons. Curve 2 deteriorates to curve 3 in a few days due to membrane breakdown processes.

Normal vs. Abnormal

Cancerous tissues should change their dielectric properties at low frequencies where cellular structure can affect these properties strongly as explained above. Indeed Fricke observed such changes at or near 20 KHz. Data at microwave frequencies are apparently solely determined by water and macromolecular content as noted above. Hence abnormality should only cause dielectric changes if these quantities are affected. The few available data appear to support this conclusion, but can not be reviewed here.

Anisotropy

Cellular structure suggest anisotropy of dielectric properties at ELF and low RF data. But since cell structure does not affect microwave data, such data are anticipated to be isotropic. A few studies at ELF and RF and not reviewed here support this conclusion. But no systematic work has been sofar conducted over the total frequency range.

ACKNOWLEDGMENT

Support by the Alexander von Humboldt-Stiftung, which provided a Senior U. S. Scientist Award is gratefully acknowledged.

REFERENCES

1. H. P. Schwan, Electrical properties of tissue and cell suspensions, in "Advances in Biological and Medical Physics", Vol. V, Academic Press, Inc., New York (1957).
2. H. P. Schwan, Electrical properties of cells: principles, some recent results and some unresolved problems, in "The Biophysical Approach to Excitable Systems: Proc. Symp. Honoring K. S. Cole's 80th Birthday", W. J. Adelman and D. E. Goldman, eds., Plenum Press, New York (1981).
3. H. Fricke, Phys. Rev. 21:708 (1923).
4. K. S. Cole, "Membranes, Ions and Impulses", University of California Press, Berkeley, Cal. (1972).
5. H. P. Schwan and H. J. Morowitz, Electrical properties of the pleuropneumonia-like organism A 5969, Biophys. J. 2:395 (1962).
6. H. P. Schwan, S. Takashima, V. K. Miyamoto and W. Stoeckenius, Electrical properties of phospholipid vesicles, Biophys. J. 10:1102 (1970).
7. H. Pauly and H. P. Schwan, The impedance of a suspension of spherical particles surrounded by a shell, ZS. f. Naturforschung 14b:125 (1959).

8. K. R. Foster, J. L. Schepps and H. P. Schwan, Microwave dielectric relaxation in muscle, Biophys. J. 29:271 (1980).
9. M. N. Afsar and J. B. Hasted, J. Opt. Soc. Amer. 67:902 (1977).
10. R. Höber, Eine methode die electrische leitfähigkeit im innern von zellen zu messen, Arch. ges. Physiol. 148:189 (1912).
11. H. P. Schwan and K. Li, Capacity and conductivity of body tissues at ultra-high frequencies, Proc. of I.R.E. 41:1735 (1953).
12. H. Pauly and H. P. Schwan, Dielectric Properties and Ion mobility in erythrocytes, Biophys. J. 6:621 (1966).
13. J. F. Herrick, D. G. Jelatis and G. M. Lee, Personal communication as cited in Ref. 1.
14. G. N. Ling, C. Miller and M. M. Ochsenfeld, The physical state of solutes and water in living cells according to the association induction hypothesis, Ann. New York Acad. Sci. 204 C. F. Hazlewood Ed., (1973).
15. W. Drost-Hansen, Water and biological interfaces: Structural and functional aspects, Phys. Chem. Liq. 7:243 (1977)
16. M. M. Hovey, A. F. Bak and D. O. Carpenter, Low internal conductivity of aplysia neuron somata, Science 176:1329 (1972).
17. K. R. Foster, J. M. Bidinger and D. O. Carpenter, The electrical resistivity of cytoplasm, Biophys. J. 16:991 (1976).
18. G. Masszi, A. Szuarto and P. Grof, Investigations on the ion- and water-binding of muscle by microwave measurements, Acta Biochim. Biophys. Acad. Sci. Hung. 11:129 (1976).
19. G. Masszi, Dielectric relaxation and water structure in gelatin solutions, Acta Biochim. Biophys. Acad. Sci. Hung. 7:349 (1972).
20. H. P. Schwan and K. R. Foster, Microwave dielectric properties of tissue: Some comments on the rotational mobility of tissue water, Biophys. J. 17:193 (1977).
21. H. P. Schwan, R. J. Sheppard and E. H. Grant, Complex Permittivity of water at 25°C, J. Chem. Phys. 64:2257 (1976).
22. H. P. Schwan, Electrical properties of bound water, Ann. New York Acad. Sci. 125:344 (1965).
23. B. Pennock and H. P. Schwan, Further observations on the electrical properties of hemoglobin bound water, J. Phys. Chem. 73:2600 (1969).
24. E. H. Grant, The structure of water, neighbouring proteins, peptides and amino acids as deduced from dielectric measurements, Ann. New York Acad. Sci. 125:418 (1965).

25. P. C. Jenin and H. P. Schwan, Some Observations on the dielectric properties of hemoglobin's suspending medium inside human erythrocytes, Biophys. J. 30:285 (1980).

26. S. Takashima, Dielectric properties of proteins. 1. Dielectric relaxation, in:"Physical Principles and Techniques of Protein Chemistry", J. S. Leach, ed., Academic Press, New York (1969),

27. S. Takashima and A. Minikate, Dielectric behavior of biological macromolecules, in: "Digest of Dielectric Literature", National Research Council, Washington, D.C. 37:602 (1975).

28. C. C. Johnson and A. W. Guy, Nonionizing electromagnetic wave effects in biological materials and systems, Proc. IEEE 60:692 (1972).

M. A. Stuchly, J. of Microwave Power (1980).

30. B. Rajewsky, Ultrakurzwellen, Ergebnisse der biophysikalischen Forschung, Bd. 1 Georg Thieme, Leipzig, Germany (1938).

31. R. D. Stoy, K.R. Foster and H. P. Schwan, Dielectric properties of mamalian tissues from 0.1 to 100 MHz. A summary of recent data, Submitted for publication.

32. K. Osswald, Messung der Leitfaehigkeit und dielektrizitaetskonstante biologischer gewebe und fluessigkeiten bei kurzen wellen, Hochfrequenz. Elektroakustik 49:40 (1937).

33. H. P. Schwan and C. F. Kay, Specific resistance of body tissues, Circulation Research 1V:664 (1956).

34. H. P. Schwan and C. F. Kay, Capacitive properties of living tissues, Circulation Research 5:439 (1957).

35. H. P. Schwan and C. F. Kay, Conductivity of living tissues, Annals N. Y. Acad. of Sci. 65:1007 (1957).

36. K. R. Foster, R. D. Stoy and H. P. Schwan, Dielectric properties of brain tissue between 0.01 and 7 GHz. Physics in Med. and Bio. 24:1177 (1979).

37. H. P. Schwan, Electrical propeties of muscle tissue at low frequencies, ZS. F. Naturforschung 9b:245 (1954).

BIOPHYSICS OF THE INTERACTION OF ELECTROMAGNETIC ENERGY WITH CELLS AND MEMBRANES

H. P. Schwan

Department of Bioengineering*
University of Pennsylvania
Philadelphia, Pennsylvania 19104

and

Institut für Biophysik der
Universität des Saarlandes
Boris Rajewsky Institut
Homburg/Saar, West Germany

INTRODUCTION

Appropriate consideration of the mechanism of interaction of electrical fields outside and inside a living being requires discussions of macroscopic "field coupling" effects and the effects of fields on cellular structures as well as molecular effects. We shall present here these coupling considerations as they pertain to potentials which are induced across membranes and inside cells for the various dielectric dispersion ranges α, β, γ discussed before[1, 2]. In addition, we consider field interactions with cells as a whole, i. e. field induced cellular force effects. But we will not consider field effects on macromolecules. Macromolecular properties have been summarized in detail by Grant[3] in this volume. Theoretical predictions based on the Langevin-equation and experimental evidence indicated that significant interactions with single macromolecules require substantial field strength levels well above those of interest here[4]. We shall also not summarize "subtle" interactions since they are discussed by Adey in this volume[5] and

---

* Permanent Address

by us previously[6, 7]. Their mechanism remains unknown and it is not clear if they occur at the molecular or cellular level or are caused by more macroscopic transduction phenomena.

COUPLING CONSIDERATIONS

Two coupling considerations are of prime importance in assessing the effects of electrical fields outside the human body on biological cell membranes: First, how do fields external to the human body translate in in-situ field strength values? Second, how do fields in-situ and fields outside biological cells translate into membrane potentials and field strength values inside the cells?

Transformation of External Fields into In-situ Fields

Equation (1) lists the relationship between external and internal fields for the case of a spherical particle with isotropic properties as indicated in figure 1.

$$E_i = \frac{3E_o K_o}{K_i + 2K_o} \tag{1}$$

Here K_o and K_i are the complex specific admittances

$$K = \sigma + j\omega\varepsilon\varepsilon_r \tag{2}$$

where σ conductivity, ε dielectric constant relative to free space and $\varepsilon_r = 8.84\times10^{-14}$ Farad/cm. The equation follows from an appropriate solution of the Laplace equation for the potential distribution inside and outside the sphere. If the surrounding medium is air and the sphere has tissue like electrical properties

$$K_o = j\omega\varepsilon_r \quad ; \quad |K_i| > |K_o| \tag{3}$$

then

$$E_i = \frac{\rho f E_o}{6\cdot10^{10}} \quad ; \quad j_i = \frac{f E_o}{6\cdot10^{10}} \tag{4}$$

with j_i internal current density (A/cm), f frequency (Hz) and specific resistance (Ohm-cm). For example for 10 Hz ρ is about 600 Ohm-cm for tissues such as muscle and consequently $E_i = 10^{-7} E_o$. We conclude:

For ELF-frequencies the internal field is very small compared to the external field strength.

For microwave frequencies internal and external fields

compare in order of magnitude.

The internal field strength changes proportional with the external field strength.

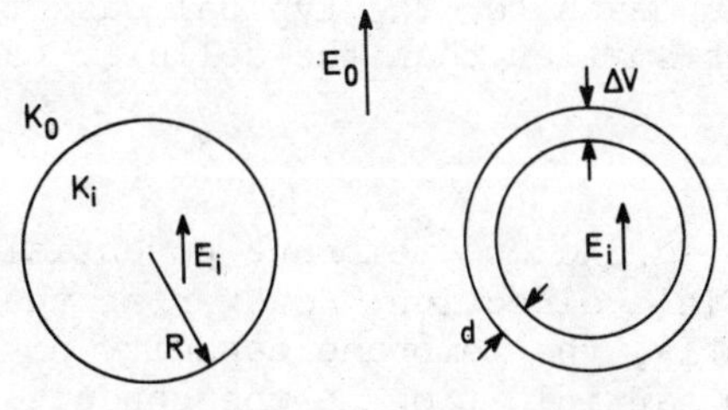

Fig. 1. Solid and shell (membrane) surrounded sphere exposed to an alternating electrical field E_o.

The derivation of equations (4) is valid as long as the dimensions of the sphere are small compared to the wavelength, an assumption no longer valid above 100 MHz. Detailed dosimetry studies revealed that at higher frequencies rather complex field distributions exist as discussed by Guy[8] and by Stuchly[9] in this volume. However in spite of this complexity, internal and external field strength values compare in order of magnitude at frequencies between 0.1 and a few GHz. At still higher frequencies, internal field values again decrease except for the body surface where they continue to be comparable to external fields.

Transformation of In-situ Fields into Membrane Potentials

The Laplacian treatment of the case of a solid homogeneous isotropic sphere can also be applied to the case of a cell surrounded by a conducting extracellular fluid. Equation (1) becomes then more complex. However for low frequencies it is valid to assume that cells are poor conductors. This may be readily recognized from the β-dispersion mechanism discussed in reference[1] in these Proceedings. At low frequencies the cell capacitors block the interior from participation in the conduction process and all electrical transport is practically restricted to the small extra cellular space. Then equation (1) reduces to

$$E_1 = 1.5\ E_o \tag{5}$$

We note that the external field perturbation can not differentiate between a homogeneous poorly conducting cell and a cell with a poorly conducting cellular membrane which surrounds a highly conducting interior. Hence, and from the circuit of figure 3 of reference [1] we conclude that the potential equation (5) is E_i integrated over the dimension of the cell, but only applied to the membranes. This means for the typical case that the membrane thickness d is much smaller than the cellular radius R

$$\Delta V = 1.5 E_o R \tag{6}$$

where ΔV is the field induced membrane potential at the "poles" indicated by the field direction. However as the frequency increased significantly, the membrane capacity no longer blocks the cell interior from participation in the conduction process. In this case the more general solution

$$\Delta V = \frac{1.5 E_o R}{\sqrt{(1 + \omega T)^2}} \tag{7}$$

is readily derived from the circuit in figure 3 of reference 1 and T is the time constant of the β-dispersion

$$T = RC_m\ (\rho_i + \frac{1}{2}\rho_a) \tag{8}$$

For high frequencies $f > 1/2\ \pi T$ combination of equations (7) and (8) results in

$$\Delta V = \frac{1.5 E}{C_m\ (\rho_i + \frac{1}{2}\rho_a)} \tag{9}$$

i. e., the induced membrane potential becomes independant of the radius R.

Consider in situ fields of the order of 1 V/cm and a cellular radius of 10 μm and specific resistances ρ_i and ρ_a near 100 Ohm-cm. Then the induced membrane potential at low frequencies is 1.5 mV and the cut-off frequency is near 1 MHz and the 1 GHz membrane potential about 1.5 μV.

In figure 2 the frequency dependance of ΔV is presented together with the time dependance of this potential in response to a potential step. We conclude:

Cells integrate at low frequencies the external potential over their dimension and apply it to the membranes;
Cells act as high pass filters as far as the induced membrane potential is concerned;
The "cut-off" frequency f_c is equal to $1/2\pi T$ with T the time constant which characterizes the center of the β-dispersion[1].
For microwave frequencies cellular membranes receive only a very small fraction of the extracellular field. Typically at 1 GHz transmembrane potentials are 1000 fold smaller than potentials below the cut-off frequency for a given in-situ extracellular potential.

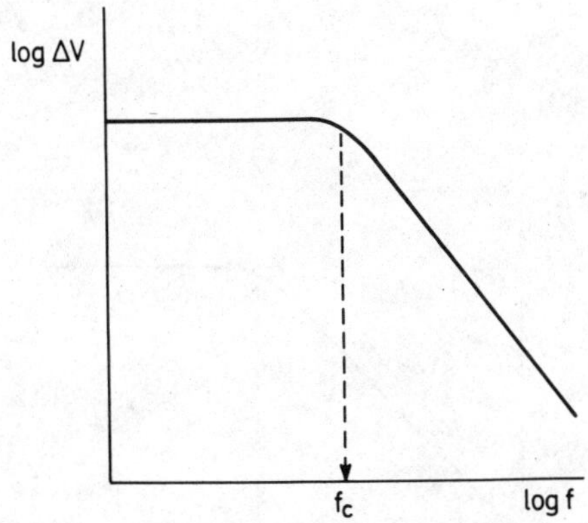

Fig. 2. Frequency dependance of induced membrane potential for a constant extracellular field strength.

Above considerations can be readily extended to more complex cellular shapes such as ellipsoids and cylinders. The principal conclusions drawn remain valid.

External Field and Membrane Potential

We next replace the assumption of a frequency independant extracellular potential by the more realistic assumption of a frequency independant potential in air, i. e., outside the human body. This we achieve by combining equations (4) and (7). Then

$$\Delta V = \frac{R\rho f E_o}{4 \cdot 10^{10} \sqrt{1 + (\omega T)^2}} \tag{10}$$

which reduces for frequencies above $f_c = 1/2\pi T$ to

$$\Delta V = 4 \cdot 10^{-12} \frac{\rho E_o}{C_M(\rho_i + \frac{1}{2}\rho_a)} \tag{11}$$

and for frequencies below to

$$\Delta V = 25 \cdot 10^{-12} R\rho E_o f \tag{12}$$

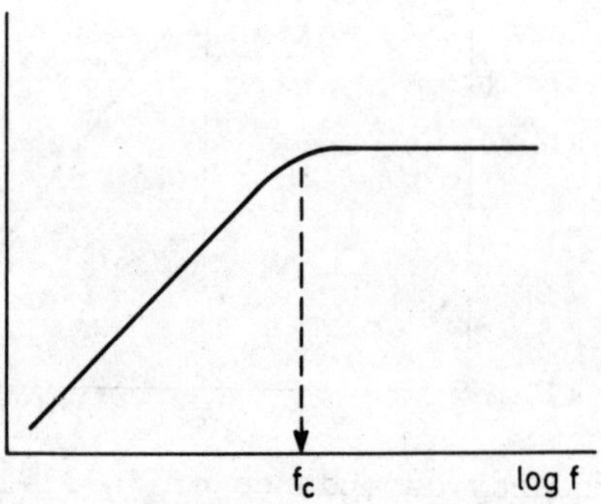

Fig. 3. Frequency dependance of induced membrane potential for a constant field strength outside the human body (air).

The frequency dependance of equation (10) is shown in figure 3. Now the induced membrane potential is independant of frequency above the cut-off frequency and decreases linearly below it as the frequency declines. For typical biological parameters $C_m = \mu F/cm^2$ and resistivities ρ_i and ρ_a for intra- and extra-cellular space near 100 Ohm-cm we calculate from equation (8)

$$T = 1.5 \cdot 10^{-4} R \tag{13}$$

For a cellular size of 100 μm the cut-off frequency is 100 KHz. The induced membrane potential above the cut-off frequency is

$$\Delta V = 2.6 \cdot 10^{-6} E_o \tag{14}$$

It is independant of radius R and frequency f and the resistivities since ρ becomes comparable to ρ_i, ρ_a if the cell membranes are short circuited (i. e. for $\omega T >> 1$). This means that induced membrane potentials are for external field strength levels of some V/cm vanishing small compared with cellular resting membrane potentials. They are also very small compared with potentials which are needed to stimulate nervous and muscular tissues.

Magnetic and Electric Fields

Above discussions neglect the magnetic component demanded by Maxwell's equations for alternating fields. This problem may be discussed for the case of a tissue sphere exposed to an external electrical field. Then, from an equation derived by Lin et al[9], we calculate the ration of the total heat H_M which is generated magnetically by Eddy currents to that developed by the electrical field H_E. It is

$$\frac{H_M}{H_E} = 0.44 \left(\frac{R}{\lambda} \right)^2 \left(\varepsilon_1^{\,2} + \varepsilon_2^{\,2} \right) \tag{15}$$

with R radius of tissue sphere, λ wavelength in air and ε_1, ε_2 real and imaginary part of the complex dielectric constant $\varepsilon^x = \varepsilon_1 - j\varepsilon_2$ of tissue. For most of the frequency range ε_1 is small compared to ε_2, reference 10. Therefore equation (15) reduces to

$$\frac{H_M}{H_E} = 1580(R\sigma)^2 \tag{16}$$

with σ electrical conductivity in Mho/cm and the radius R in cm. For $\sigma = 10^{-2}$ Mho/cm and $\sigma = 10^{-3}$ Mho/cm, values H_M/H_E of 158 and 1.58 are obtained respectively for a radius of 31 cm. The σ-values of 10^{-2} and 10^{-3} are typical for low microwave frequencies near 100 MHz and ELF frequencies below 10 KHz respectively. We recognize therefore that at ELF frequencies the magnetic component does not significantly alter above stated results. However at microwave frequencies induced membrane potentials for typical body dimensions may be considerably enhanced by the magnetic component. This is particularly true near the exposed surface of the body since Eddy currents are there most pronounced.

Further Cellular Coupling Considerations

Above stated results are based on a simple model of the cell as indicated above. What happens to more complex models with subcellular organelles is indicated in fugure 4. A nucleus, half the size of the cell, is assumed inside the cell with an internal resistivity equal to that of the interior of the cell and its exterior. Both the cellular and the nuclear membranes are assumed to have a capacity of 1 $\mu F/cm^2$. Then, from equation (8), the nuclear time constant has half the value of the cellular time constant. The induced membrane potential below cut-off would also be half that of the cell, if the nucleus would be exposed to a frequency independant field E_o. Above the cut-off frequency, equation (9), the membrane potential is independant from the radius and hence equal for a nucleus and the cell if individually exposed to the same field. Below the cellular cut-off frequency the nucleus in the cell is shielded by the outer cellular membrane and therefore its membrane potential decreases proportional with the field in the cell cytoplasma. Taking all these factors into consideration results in the nuclear membrane potential induced as indicated in figure 4. Clearly, the nuclear membrane receives a potential equal to that of the cellular membrane at frequencies above the nuclear cut-off frequency. Only between the two cut-off frequencies of the cell and the nucleus is this induced potential independant of frequency. The nuclear membrane potential therefore displays the characteristics of a bandpass filter with the two cut-off frequencies given by the cellular and nuclear cut-off frequencies f_c and f_n.

Similar conclusions pertain to other organelles such as mitochondria. However some subcellular systems connect to the outer membranes, such as the endoplasmic reticulum or the tubular system. They contribute to the α-dispersion as discussed before, reference 11. Below the characteristic frequency of this dispersion membrane potentials for both outer cellular and subcellular membranes are equal since the access resistance to the subcellular system is small compared to the reactance of the connecting mem brane capacitance[11]. But above the characteristic frequency of this α-dispersion contribution, this no longer is true and only the outer membrane is polarized. Hence the potential across connecting membrane systems behave as a low pass filter with a cut-off frequency equal to the characteristic frequency of the α-dispersion to the extent that it is caused by subcellular membranes connecting with the outer membrane system. A more detailed discussion should also consider the potential drop outside the cellular membrane due to the counter ion surface admittance and its frequency dependance[11]. An independantly conducted discussion of cellular potentials has been presented by Drago and Ridella[12, 13], also stressing the highly frequency specific dependance of induced membrane potentials and cytoplasmic field strength values. These latter potentials are of course important if one considers fields acting on the macromolecular components inside cells.

We conclude: The actual frequency dependance of cellular membrane potentials and internal fields is highly frequency specific, including cut-off frequencies extending from less than 100 Hz to many MHz. Therefore one would anticipate that any mechanism of interaction of EM-fields with cellular systems must also be rather frequency specific. However, we wish to stress that these specific responses are not those of rather sharp resonances.

Internal Fields

Similar considerations as stated above for the membrane potential yield field strength values inside cells and subcellular organelles. These field strength values are important since they act on suspended macromolecular components such as proteins and nuclear acids. The principle to be used to calculate upper limits for the internal field strength values E_i may be expressed by the equations

$$(E_i R)^2 + (\Delta V)^2 = (1.5 E_o R)^2 \tag{17}$$

$$E_i = \frac{1.5E}{\sqrt{1 + (1/\omega T)^2}} \tag{18}$$

Equation (17) states that the sum of the potential drop in the cellular or subcellular interior and the potential drops across the membrane must equal the potential applied to the cell over its dimension if all terms are sqd. Equation (18) is readily obtained from equations (7) and (17). Equation (17) is readily derived from the circuit in figure 3, reference 1. Equation (17) assumes that the radius R is large compared to the membrane thickness d, an assumption valid for biological cells. It furthermore assumes that the effective specific admittance $\Delta_i = \sigma_i + j\omega\varepsilon\varepsilon_r$ of the cell is small compared to that of the suspending medium. However, as the frequency increases this is no longer true since the cell membranes become short-circuited and the interior participates in the electrical conduction process. In the limit $\omega \rightarrow \infty$ the cell's specific admittance becomes identical with that of the interior which is known to be about half that of the suspending medium. For this limit we obtain from equation (1)

$$E_i = 1.2 E_o \tag{19}$$

Thus the potential drop across the cell is simply $1.2 E_o \cdot R$ instead of $1.5 E_o \cdot R$. The equation (17) is therefore slightly over-emphasizing the field strength inside the cell but may be used as a good approximation.

We conclude that the internal field strength increases from zero to a constant level 1.5 E as the membrane potential decreases. This change occurs at frequencies comparable to the cellular cut-off frequency for the membrane potential.

Table I. Membrane polarization and exposure of the interior of cells and subcellular organelles for various frequency ranges. Different conditions exist for cells and for organelles which connect or do not connect with the outer cell membrane. Frequency ranges are listed in ascending order: (a) from low values up to the α-dispersion range, (b) from there to the cellular β-dispersion range, (c) further up to the β-dispersion of the subcellular component and (d) above all β-dispersion frequencies for cells and organelles.

	(a)	(b)	(c)	(d)
Frequency Ranges	α-Disp. < 0.1 KHz	To Cell. β-Disp. 0.1 KHz $\rightarrow f_c$	To Subcell. β-Disp. $f_c \rightarrow f_o$	Above $> f_c, f_o$
Cells				
Membranes	Polarized	Partially polarized	Not Polar.	Not Polar.
Interior (Proteins etc.)	Double Shielded	Shielded	Exposed	Exposed
Organelles:				
Membranes	Not Polar.	Not Polar.	Polarized	Not Polar.
Interior (Nucleic acids)	Double Shielded	Double Shielded	Shielded (Partial)	Exposed
Connecting Organelles:				
Membranes	Polarized	Not Polar.	Not Polar.	Not Polar.
Interior	Not Exp.	Exposed	Exposed	Exposed

Application of above stated principles yields the results summarized in table 1. Here we differentiate between various frequency ranges. They are:

Below the α-dispersion;
Between α-dispersion and cellular β-dispersion;
Between β-dispersions of cells and subcellular particles;
Above the cut-off frequencies for cells and organelles.

Between the stated frequency regions transitions occur from one stated condition to the next. The term "shielded" refers to conditions where the surrounding membrane consumes the total potential and no internal field therefore can exist. The term "double shielded" indicates that not only the cell membrane but also the membrane surrounding the subcellular organelle protect the interior of the organelle. The term "polarized" indicates that the membrane is charged and the term "exposed" indicates the existence of internal fields. For example, the interior of the cell nucleus is double shielded from low frequency extracellular fields by both the cellular and the nuclear membrane. Its membrane is polarized as indicated in figure 4, between the two cut-off frequencies of cellular and nuclear membrane. At still higher frequencies both membrane systems are no longer polarized by the external field and cellular and nuclear interior are exposed to the field.

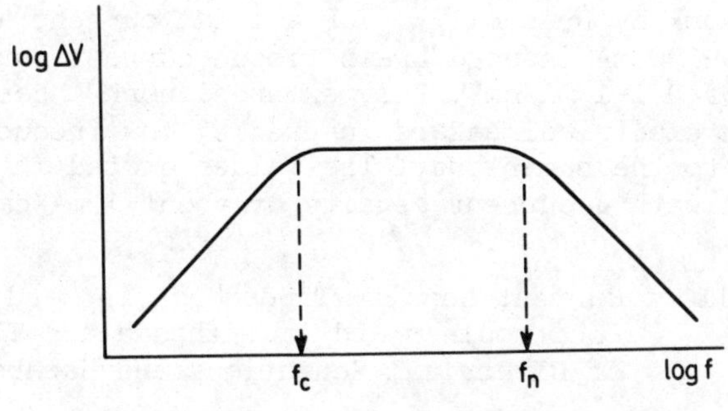

Fig. 4. Frequency dependance of the induced membrane potential of a cell nucleus for a constant extracellular field strength.

The frequency sensitivities reported above can not explain the results reported by Grundler[14] in this volume. Nor do they explain the modulation sensitive results reported by Adey[5, 6]. But they demonstrate that valuable insight is gained about the highly frequency specific distribution of field induced membrane potentials and potentials acting on macromolecules from an analysis of the dielectric properties of cell suspensions and tissues.

SIGNIFICANT MEMBRANE POTENTIALS

In the previous section, we have discussed how to translate external fields into in situ fields and membrane potentials. We have not indicated however what membrane potentials appear to be biologically significant. Surprisingly, but little work appears to have been conducted over an extended frequency range which relates to this topic. However there are numerous data available which are indicative in this regard. Table 2 summarizes some of this material and has been discussed before in greater detail[7]. It appears from this that current density levels of the order of 1 mA/cm^2 and field strength values in situ near 1 V/cm are needed to cause biological significant responses such as excitation of nervous or muscular tissues. The quoted values vary however considerably with some values more than ten-fold lower than those just stated. Extended experience exists with pacemakers and threshold values range about 0.1-10 mA/cm^2, depending on electrode size and other parameters[15]. In electrohypnosis, electrosleep and electrical anaesthesia total currents applied are about 10 to 100 mA. Corresponding current densities in the brain may be estimated based on the work by Driscoll[16]. For a total current applied to the head of 10-100 mA induced brain tissue current densities are of the order of 0.1-1 mA/cm^2. Very extended work[17] has been carried out on electrical hazards caused by low frequency potentials applied to the human body. The values quoted in the table are consistent with a current density of about 1 mA/cm^2.

Table II. Current Density Thresholds in Cardiology, Electrosleep and Anaesthesia and Threshold of Electrical Sensations and Hazards.

Pacemaker, Threshold	0.03 - 10 mA/cm^2
Electrosleep and Anaesthesia	10 - 100 mA
Electro-Hazards:	
Sensation	1 mA
"Let Go"	10 mA
Fibrillation	100 mA

The quoted values are probably only valid for frequencies below 1 or 10 KHz. At higher frequencies responses diminish, presumably as a consequence of above discussed relationships between in situ field strength values and evoked membrane potentials. An additional reason is therefractory period of some msec, which characterizes the time dependance of the action potential and the membranes ability to respond to repeated stimuli.

Much higher sensititivities than those reported above have been stated. No attempt is made here to summarize these results since this topic is summarized by Adey[5, 6] in this volume. A question however remains: Are these subtle biological responses indicatice of responses to very small evoked membrane potentials of the order of less than 1 μV across the membrane or are they caused by other mechanism not yet identified?

FIELD INDUCED FORCES

Electric fields can directly interact with matter and create forces that can act on molecules as well as on cellular and larger structures. Most of these interactions are reversible and do not necessarily have demonstrable biological effects. An example is the movement of ions in an AC field, which is inconsequential, provided that the field is weak enough to prevent undue heating from molecular collisions (e.g., below about 1 V/cm, corresponding to 1 mA/cm^2 in a physiological medium). Another example is the orientation of polar macromolecules. For field strength values of interest here, only a very partial preferential orientation with the field results. Complete orientation and consequent dielectric saturation requires field strength of thousands of volts per centimeter. Changes of this magnitude do occur in membranes on depolarization. Hence, field-induced orientation and changes in orientation of membrane molecules appear possible. Corresponding tissue current densities would be in milliamperes per square centimeter, as discussed above.

The simplest example of the forces which are generated by electrical charges is the attraction of the two plates of a capacitor. The force is given by

$$F\ (\text{dyn/cm}^2) = 10^7\ QE = 10^7\ Cd\ E^2 \qquad (20)$$

Here Q is the charge in Asec, C is the capacity in Farad, E the field strength (V/cm) and d the plate distance (cm). We note that the force is proportional to the square of the field strength. Hence there exists also an effective force if an AC potential is applied. If a particle is transported into the field between the capacitor plates, it acquires a potential energy. Work has to be performed to accomplish the transport from the free field space into the field. Corresponding forces have been known for some time as ponderomotoric forces, but only considered for DC fields. We shall discuss these forces for biological media and state that they become significant at field strength levels or only slightly above those required for significant thermal effects to occur.

They are therefore of concern to those interested in possible non-thermal biological effects of EM-fields.

Table 3 summarizes observed manifestations of field-generated forces. The field effects may manifest themselves as orientation of particles in the direction of the field or perpendicular to it. Or "pearl chain" formation, i.e., the alignment of particles in the field direction may occur. This has long been considered a mysterious demonstration of microwave induced biological effects. Deformation or destruction of cells can be achieved with fields. The movement of cells in inhomogeneous electrical fields can be affected.

Table III. Summary of Various Phenomena Caused by Alternating Electrical Fields.

"Pearl Chain" Formation

Orientation of Nonspherical Cells

Movement (Dielectrophoresis)

Deformation of Cells

Destruction of Cells

Fusion of Cells

Zimmermann et al.[18] have observed the destruction of red cells and ghost formation. Neumann and Rosenheck[19] studied the effects of fields on chromaffin vesicles. Friend et al.[20] as well as Goodman[21,22] studied the effects of fields on fairly large cellular organisms. Orientation effects have been observed by Teixeira-Pinto et al.[23] by Sher[24] and by Novak[25]. Pohl[26] developed "dielectrophoresis" as a tool of separating cells in inhomogeneous fields. Elul et al.[27] observed cell destruction phenomena and cell chape changes. No attempt is made here to summarize the total literature on this topic and additional discussions have been presented elsewhere[28,29]. Some of these field-generated force effects can be very startling and dramatic, especially near the tip of small electrodes. Of a similar nature is the movement of magnetostatic bacteria recently reported by Blakemore[30] in magnetic fields of fairly low intensity. Apparently, these bacteria are equipped with magnetic properties and are therefore significantly oriented by the magnetic field and motivated to move in the field direction.

We postulate that ponderomotoric forces become noticable if associated potential energy changes become comparable or greater than thermal energies KT (K Boltzman constant, T absolute temperature). Consider for example the case of a spherical particle. Its induced dipol moment has a value

$$\mu = R^3 E_o \frac{\varepsilon_1^* - \varepsilon_2^*}{\varepsilon_1^* + 2\varepsilon_2^*} \tag{21}$$

where ε_1^*, ε_2^* are complex dielectric constants $\varepsilon^* = \varepsilon - j\sigma/\omega$ of the particle and surrounding medium respectively and R is its radius. The potential energy of this induced dipol, defined by the work which must be performed to move a dipol of this value into the field E, may be estimated by multiplication of $|\mu|$ with E_o and the absolute dielectric constant of the suspending medium ε_2. By equating this dipol energy with KT a "threshold" field strength E_{th} is then defined

$$\varepsilon_2 E_{th}^2 R^3 \left| \frac{\varepsilon_1^* - \varepsilon_2^*}{\varepsilon_1^* + 2\varepsilon_2^*} \right| = KT \tag{22}$$

In this argument the field strength E appears only squared. Hence it should not matter if we consider DC or AC-fields, provided that in the case of AC-fields appropriate dielectric parameters are introduced. The equation (22) states that the threshhold field strength E_{th}, for given dielectric properties of the system, obeys the relationship

$$E_{th}^2 R^3 = \text{const.} \tag{23}$$

We furthermore note that the magnitude of the complex part of the induced dipol is in most cases either equal to 1 or 1/2. Thus with $KT = 4 \cdot 10^{-21}$ Joules at room temperature and an electrolyte as the exterior medium with $\varepsilon = 78$

$$E_{th} R^{1.5} = 2.4 \cdot 10^{-5} \text{ Vcm}^{-1/2} \quad \text{for } |\varepsilon_1^*| > |\varepsilon_2^*| \tag{24}$$

$$3.4 \cdot 10^{-5} \quad \text{for } |\varepsilon_1^*| < |\varepsilon_2^*| \tag{25}$$

A more detailed derivation for the phenomena of pearl chain formation[31] gives values of 6.4 and $9.6 \cdot 10^{-5}$ $\text{Vcm}^{-1/2}$. Experimental evidence appears to support this approach. The phenomena of pearl chain formation has been studied extensively in our laboratory. A perusal of the results of Sher[24] and Schwan and Sher[32] gives a value of $E_{th} R^{1.5}$ of 6.6 $\text{Vcm}^{1/2}$, Kresch's results[33] indicate 8.6 and Takashima and Schwan[34] a value of 11. An additional survey of data obtained with erythrocytes, silicone particles and E.coli conducted by this author gives 8.0 $\text{Vcm}^{-1/2}$. For the case of orientation of E.coli a somewhat smaller value of 3.2 $\text{Vcm}^{-1/2}$ is obtained[32]. Choosing an everage value of $8 \cdot 10^{-5}$ $\text{Vcm}^{-1/2}$ we note that for E = 1V/cm the radius R is close to 20 µm.

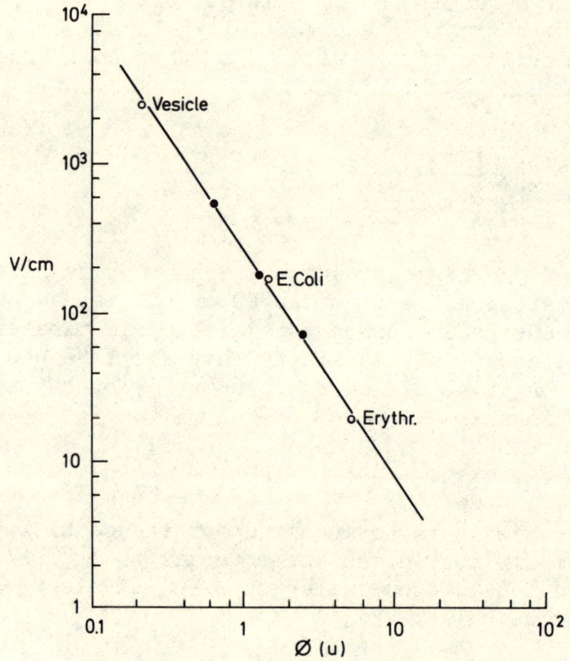

Figure 5. Threshold field strength for pearl chain for mation as a function of particle size. The open circles represent results obtained with biological cells as indicates and the full circles data with silicone particles. The data fit the theoretical demand indicted by the solid line and appear to be insensitive to the dielectric properties of the particles.

All sorts of biological particles of different effective complex dielectric constants behave similar in an electrolyte medium as demanded by above outlined theory. Figure 5 illustrates this fact. Neumann and Rosenheck's results on chromaffin vesicles[19] are combined with data for E.Coli and erythrocytes and silicon particles (full circles) obtained by Sher[24]. The total material fits convincingly the solid line of slope -1.5 which is demanded by the theory. The line is drawn to fit the data with a constant $E_{th} R^{1.5} = 8 \text{ Vcm}^{-1/2}$.

We conclude that significant force effects may exist at the cellular level at field strength levels of some V/cm. But at the molecular level necessary field strength values are very high compared to field levels of interest at this meeting.

The emergence of significant field force effects for structures larger than 10 or 20 μm at field strength values of about 1 V/cm invites comparison with threshold field levels which are thermally significant or are known to cause excitation at lower frequencies. 1 V/cm in situ has been cited above for low frequencies as a very approximate number characterizing the onset of significant membrane responses. The base metabolic rate for man, if expressed in electrical units, corresponds to the heat created in tissues by current densities comparable to 1.2 mA/cm^2 at low frequencies. However man's ability to tolerate an additional heat input comparable to the base metabolic rate is excellent and no significant temperature rise is expected. Furthermore, if such heat deposition is only locally administered, the rest of the body serves as an excellent cooling reservoir. We conclude therefore that significant nervous membrane responses at low frequencies and field induced cellular responses over the total frequency range have comparable threshold levels. Significant temperature elevations in man require somewhat larger field strength levels.

ACKNOWLEDGMENT

Support by the Alexander von Humboldt-Stiftung, which provided a Senior U.S. Scientist Award, and by the Office of Naval Research is gratefully acknowledged.

REFERENCES

1. H. P. Schwan, Dielectric Properties of Biological Tissue and Cells at RF- and MW-Frequencies in: "Advances in Biological Effects and Dosimetry of Low Energy Electromagnetic Fields", this volume (1981).
2. H. P. Schwan, Dielectric Properties of Biological Tissues and Cells at ELF-Frequencies in: "Advances in Biological Effects and Dosimetry of Low Energy Electromagnetic Fields", this volume (1981).

3. E. H. Grant, Dielectric Properties of Biological Material: Molecular Considerations in: "Advances in Biological Effects and Dosimetry of Low Energy Electromagnetic Fields", this volume (1981).
4. H. P. Schwan and K. R. Foster, RF-Field Interactions with Biological Systems: Electrical Properties and Biophysical Mechanisms, Proc. IEEE 68:104 (1980).
5. W. R. Adey, Biological Effects on the Central Nervous System in: "Advances in Biological Effects and Dosimetry of Low Energy Electromagnetic Fields", this volume (1981).
6. W. R. Adey, Overview on the Biological Effects of ELF: Fundamentals-1 in: "Advances in Biological Effects and Dosimetry of Low Energy Electromagnetic Fields", this volume (1981).
7. H. P. Schwan, Classical Theory of Microwave Interactions with Biological Systems in: "The Physical Basis of Electromagnetic Interactions with Biological Systems", L. S. Taylor and A. Y. Cheung, Eds., Proc. Workshop at Univ. of Maryland, College Park (1977).
8. H. P. Schwan, Dielectric Properties of Biological Tissues and Biophysical Mechanisms of EM-Field Interaction, in: "American Chemical Soc. Symp. Series" (1981).
9. J. C. Lin, A. W. Guy and C. C. Johnson, Power Deposition in a Spherical Model of Man Exposed to 1-20 MHz Electromagnetic Fields, IEEE Trans. Microwave Theory MTT-21 (12):791 (1973).
10. H. P. Schwan, Determination of Biological Impedances in: "Physical Techniques in Biological Research", W. L. Nastuk, ed., Academic Press, New York Vol. 1963).
11. H. P. Schwan, Electrical Properties of Cells: Principles, Some Recent Results, and Some Unresolved Problems, in: "The Biophysical Approach to Excitable Systems", W. J. Adelman, Jr. and D. E. Goldman, eds., Plenum Pub. Corp., New York (1981).
12. G. P. Drago and S. Ridella, Bioelectromagnetics, 1:216 (1980).
13. S. Ridella, Personal Communication (1981).
14. W. Grundler, Biological Effects of RF and MW Energy at Molecular and Cellular Level-II, in: "Advances in Biological Effects and Dosimetry of Low Energy Electromagnetic Fields", this volume (1981).
15. O. Z. Roy, J. R. Scott and G. C. Park, IEEE Trans. (1976).
16. D. A. Driscoll, An Investigation of a Theoretical Model of the Human Head with Application to Current Flow Calculations and EEG Interpretation, Ph.D. Thesis, Univ. of Vermont, (1970).

17. H. P. Schwan, Biological Hazards From Exposure to ELF Electrical Fields and Potentials, NWL Tech. Rpt. TR-2713, USNWL, Dahlgren (1972).
18. U. Zimmermann, G. Pilwat and R. Riemann, Biophys. J. 14:881 (1974).
19. E. Neumann and K. Rosenheck, J. Memb. Biol., 10:279 (1972).
20. A. W. Friend, E. D. Finch and H. P. Schwan, Science, 187:357 (1974).
21. E. M. Goodman, B. Greenebaum and M. T. Marron, Effects of Extremely Low Frequency Electromagnetic Fields on Growth and Differentiation of Physarum Polycephalum; Tech. Report Phase 1 (Continuous Wave), Univ. of Wisconsin (1975)..
22. E. M. Goodman, B. Greenebaum and M. T. Marron, Effects of Extremely Low Frequency Electromagnetic Fields on Physarum Polycephalum; Tech. Report, ONR, Contract N-00014-76-C-0180, Univ. of Wisconsin (1976).
23. A. A. Teixeira-Pinto, L. L. Nejelski, J. L. Cutler and J. H. Heller, Exp. Cell Res., 20:548 (1960).
24. L. L. Sher, Mechanical Effects of AC Fields on Particles Dispersed in a Liquid: Biological Implications, Ph.D. Thesis, Univ. of Penna., Phila. (1963).
25. B. Novak and F. W. Bentrup, Biophysik, 9:253 (1973).
26. H. A. Pohl, J. Biol. Phys., 1:1 (1973).
27. R. Elul, J. Physiol., 189:351 (1967).
28. S. M. Bawin and W. R. Adey, Brain Interactions with Weak Electric and Magnetic Fields, Neurosci. Res. Prog. Bull., MIT Press, 15 (1977).
29. H. P. Schwan, Field Interactions with Biological Matter in: "Electrical Properties of Biological Polymers, Water and Membranes", eds. S. Takashima and H. M. Fishman, Annals of N.Y. Acad. of Sci., New York Vol. 303 (1977).
30. R. Blakemore, Science, 190:377 (1975).
31. M. Saito and H. P. Schwan, The Time Constants of Pearl Chain Formation in: "Biological Effects of Microwave Radiation", M. F. Peyton, ed., Plenum Press, New York (1961).
32. H. P. Schwan and L. D. Sher, Alternating Current Field Induced Forces and Their Biological Implications, J. Electrochem. Soc., 116:170 (1969).
33. L. D. Sher, E. Kresch and H. P. Schwan, On the Possibility of Nonthermal Biological Effects of Pulsed Electromagnetic Radiation, Biophys. J., 10:970 (1970).
34. S. Takashima and H. P. Schwan, unpublished.

BROADBAND MM-WAVE SPECTROSCOPY ON BIOLOGICAL SAMPLES

F. Kremer

Max-Planck-Institut für Festkörperforschung
7000 Stuttgart 80
Fed. Rep. Germany

INTRODUCTION

During the initial phase of broadband mm-wave spectroscopic investigations on biological samples, one is faced with serious and very different problems: On the one side biological cells like E.c. or yeast usually live in an aqueous solution, so that the absorption of the cells is probably totally masked by the strong absorption of the aqueous solution itself. If one dries the cells, then the cells are often no longer living. (Of course there exist some special biological systems which can live without outer water; the brine shrimp Artemia salina for instance, or spores). On the other side, the absorption of biological macromolecules is very weak, so that quite sensitive methods are necessary. Often samples such as DNA, RNA or lysozyme are most conveniently obtained in a powder form which is more or less inhomogeneous. This complicates the situation again. I would like to introduce the methods we developed in Stuttgart, to solve or to circumvent these problems.

But first let me describe very briefly the conventional techniques which are used in mm-wave-spectroscopy and ask how applicable they are for biological samples. Perhaps the main spectroscopic technique is the cavity perturbation technique. The principle is as follows: In a cavity with typical dimensions of a few wavelengths, a field of known distribution is generated. Inserting a sample at a certain place inside the cavity, so that the perturbation of the modes is negligible, changes the eigenfrequency and the width of the resonance curve. From that the complex index of refraction can be calculated. This technique is widely used up to frequencies of about 70 GHz . With increasing frequency it becomes more and more difficult because of the strongly decreasing waveguide and cavity dimensions. Furthermore, this method is very narrow-band and from that standpoint not convenient for broadband spectroscopy.

Another waveguide method is reflectometry in which the measurement of phase and amplitude of a reflected wave is used to determine the complex index of refraction. This method was used by a group of Professor Grant in London to measure for the first time the dielectric properties of water at 70 GHz /1/. It is also narrowband.

A method, which is in principle broadband, is a quasi-optical set-up. In Stuttgart we have a transmission spectrometer /2/ of this type which is quite suitable for absorption measurements of strongly absorbing and homogeneous samples. It is not applicable for scattering and inhomogeneous samples, because of the extinction due to scattering. For weakly absorbing samples like dry biomolecules, the technique is also not useful because one needs such thick samples, that lens effects in the sample occur. Furthermore, standing waves between the optical components and especially within the sample are very disturbing. To circumvent the above mentioned difficulties and to have the possibility to measure the complex index of refraction in the broadband range from 40 - 170 GHz, we have developed a resonator, based on the principal of an untuned cavity.

THE MULTIMODE RESONATOR

An approximately isotropic and homogeneous field is created inside a high-Q, greatly oversized resonator by supplying radiation from an appropriate tunable source. The Q of such a multimode resonator is only slightly dependent on the frequency as long as the wavelength remains very small relative to the cavity dimensions. The isotropy and homogeneity of the field can be enhanced by use of a mechanical mode stirrer, and/or by dithering the source frequency over an excursion small compared to the spectral resolution required of the instrument. The sample to be measured is introduced into the cavity and the resultant change in Q can easily be measured with good precision /3/.

When the sample is a gas that fills the entire cavity the absorption coefficient can be accurately deduced from the Q measurements. This was done by Becker and Autler /4/ and by Lamb /5/ in 1946 to measure the absorption of water vapor at a wavelenth range between 0.7 cm and 1.7 cm. In the case of a solid or liquid dielectric sample which fills only a portion of the cavity volume, reflections at the sample surfaces complicate the procedure and may compromise its accuracy. One of the principal advantages of the untuned resonator technique for such samples is that radiation reflected or scattered back into the unoccupied portion of the cavity does not contribute to the Q-loss which is measured. However, multiple reflections inside the sample can produce standing waves and thus make it difficult to determine the effective absorption pathlength, and hence, the absorption coefficient.

Heretofore only low-loss dielectrics like polyethylene and Teflon have been measured, and an empirical factor has been employed to correct for the effects of reflections at the sample surfaces. The dependence of the correction factor on the refractive index in such samples is quite small and has therefore been neglected /6/. These measurements were carried out by Llewellyn-Jones et al. in 1980. By considering lamellar dielectric samples for which the Maxwell-equation boundary-value problem can be solved analytically we show here that interference effects resulting from multiple reflections make it possible in some circumstances to determine both the real and imaginar parts of the complex index of refraction from a series of Q measurements with samples of different thickness /7/. Surprisingly, these interference effects are observable in spite of the fact that radiation is incident on the sample from all directions and that a detector placed inside the cavity to perform the Q measurement sees only the space- and time-averaged field.

Q-Value of the Cavity

It is convenient to associate a quality factor Q with each of the principal cavity loss mechanisms. The Q-factor is defined generally by the following relationship

$$Q^{-1} = \frac{\text{rate of loss of photons from cavity}}{\omega \cdot \text{number of photons stored in cavity}} \quad . \qquad (1)$$

Here ω is the angular frequency of the radiation in the cavity. The Q-factor associated with absorption in the sample, which it will be convenient to denote by Q_S, can be evaluated by comparing the absorption loss to the loss of photons in a sample of known dielectric properties. The Q-factor associated with that calibration sample will be denoted by Q_C. It is also useful to associate a factor Q_R with the remaining resonator losses, which include absorption in the cavity walls and losses through the aperture that is used to feed radiation into the cavity.

In practice the radiation field inside the cavity is sampled by one or more detectors which produce signals proportional to the photon density in the cavity. It is therefore convenient to employ rate equations formulated explicitly in terms of the number of photons in the cavity. The cavity is constructed with dimensions of the order of 100 times the wavelengths at which measurements are to be made. As a consequence the cavity modes are very closely spaced in frequency, and when radiation from a narrow-band source is fed into the cavity, the individual modes are excited at essentially equal rates. In addition, the whole ensemble of cavity modes is continuously shifted back and forth in space by use of a mechanical mode stirrer whose period is small compared to the integration time of the detector system. Under these conditions the radiation field is highly homogeneous and isotropic throughout the cavity, and the photon density averaged over the detector integration time and all of the excited modes has the constant value N/Ω where N is the total number of photons and Ω is the cavity volume.

If the cavity contains an absorbing sample a source feeding radiation into the cavity at an average rate M will establish a stationary photon population N which satisfies the following equation:

$$\frac{dN}{dt} = 0 = M - \ell_R N - \ell_S N. \tag{2}$$

Here the loss coefficients ℓ_R and ℓ_S correspond to photon losses inherent in the cavity structure and absorption in the sample respectively. Each of the loss rates, $\ell_R N$ and $\ell_S N$, can also be expressed in the form $\ell N = \omega N/Q$. The summation of the individual loss rates in eq. 2 to obtain the total cavity loss rate is then seen to correspond to summation of the reciprocal of the corresponding Q-factors and produces the reciprocal of the total cavity Q.

In order to determine the loss coefficient ℓ_S, which characterizes the sample absorption, the measurements corresponding to the following set of conditions are made while the source power is held constant.

i) no sample in cavity $\quad M = \ell_R N_O \quad$ (3)

ii) calibaration sample in cavity $\quad M = \ell_R N_C + \ell_C N_C \quad$ (4)

iii) unknown sample in cavity $\quad M = \ell_R N_S + \ell_S N_S \quad$ (5)

If the linear range of the detection system is not exceeded, the signal measured at each step of the procedure is proportional to the corresponding value of N. The necessity of evaluating the constant of proportionality (i.e. the detector responsivity) can be avoided by employing only ratios of detector signals measured under the various cavity conditions. We denote $R_C = N_C/N_O$ and $R_S = N_S/N_O$. R_C and R_S are then equal to the ratios of the corresponding detector signals, and simultaneous solution of eqs. 3-5 yields the following expressions for ℓ_R and ℓ_S.

$$\ell_R = \ell_C \frac{R_C}{1 - R_C} . \tag{6}$$

$$\ell_S = \frac{R_C}{R_S} \frac{1 - R_S}{1 - R_C} \ell_C . \tag{7}$$

By calculating the rate ℓ_C at which photons are absorbed in the calibration sample (s. next chapter) one determines the Q-value of the resonator.

Calculation of Absorption Coefficient

Lamb treats the radiation field inside the cavity as a photon gas and calculates the number of photons per second which strike a hole and hence escape from the cavity. To do this the number of photons approaching the hole at a given incidence angle Θ is reckoned and this quantity is then integrated over Θ. To the extent that the homogeneity of the field inside the cavity is left unperturbed by the presence of either the hole or the thin flat sample, the number of photons which strike such a sample at a given incidence angle can be obtained by simply multiplying Lamb's corresponding expression by two; i.e., whereas the hole is single sided as seen from the cavity, photons strike the sample with equal probability from both sides. Contrary to the hole, which, apart from the varying aspect angle it presents to photons arriving at various angles, displays an angle-independent transmission towards the exterior, the absorbing sample has angle-dependent reflection and transmission coefficients. These coefficients are also functions of the wavelength λ, the sample thickness d, and the dielectric constant of the sample.

It is convenient to express the dielectric properties of the sample in terms of the complex index of refraction, $\tilde{n} = n + ik$. The real part n is just the refractive index of Snell's law, and the absorption coefficient in Lambert's law is related to k by $\alpha = 2\omega k/c$. The sample reflection coefficient, which specifies the fraction of the radiation incident at angle Θ that is reflected from the sample back into the cavity field, will be denoted by $R = R(\Theta,n,k,d,\lambda)$. The transmission coefficient, which is defined in analogous fashion, will be denoted by $T = T(\Theta,n,k,d,\lambda)$. These quantities are indicated in Figure 1.

Both coefficients are also polarization dependent, and polarizations perpendicular and parallel to the plane of incidence will be denoted respectively by subscripts σ and π. The fraction A of the photons striking the sample that is absorbed is given in terms of R and T by the energy conservation relationship

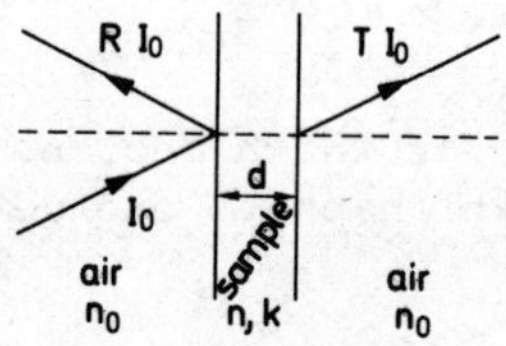

Fig. 1 Sample geometry

R + T + A = 1 (Fig. 2). Since the radiation field in the cavity is unpolarized, the total absorption coefficient for the lamellar sample is obtained by averaging over the two perpendicular polarization components. Incorporation of these considerations into Lamb's Derivation yields

$$\ell_S N_S = \frac{A_S C N_S}{\Omega} \int_0^{\pi/2} A_T(\Theta,n,k,d,\lambda)\,\sin\Theta\cos\Theta d\Theta. \qquad (8)$$

Here $A_T = (A_\sigma + A_\pi)/2$, and A_S is the area of each side of the sample.

Finally, combination of eqs. 7 and 8 yields

$$I(n,k,d,\lambda) = \int_0^{\pi/2} A_T(\Theta,n,k,d,\lambda)\sin\Theta\cos\Theta d\Theta = \frac{A_C}{A_S}\frac{R_C}{R_S}\frac{1-R_S}{1-R_C} \qquad (9)$$

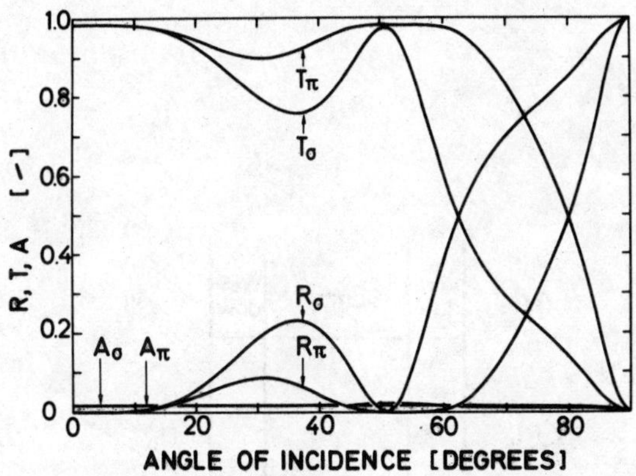

Fig. 2 Reflection, transmission and absorption factor for a lamellar sample with $n_o = 1$, $n = 1.5$, $k = 0.0005$, $d = 1$ cm and $\nu = 70$ GHz.

To avoid problems associated with absolute calibration of the detector is expedient to employ only ratios of detector signals. A procedure which proves to be very convenient is to intercompare lamellar samples of the same surface area but different thickness. Under some conditions the accuracy of the final results can be enhanced by also comparing samples of the same thickness but different surface area /3/. As a first step we consider only the comparison of two samples of different thickness. Denote quantities corresponding to the first sample by appending a subscript 1, and use subscript 2 for the second sample. Application of eqs. 8 and 9 to the two samples in succession then leads to the following result:

$$\frac{\ell_{S1}}{\ell_{S2}} = \frac{R_{S2}}{R_{S1}}\,\frac{1-R_{S1}}{1-R_{S2}} \quad \text{or} \quad \frac{I_1(n,k,d_1,\lambda)}{I_2(n,k,d_2,\lambda)} = \frac{R_{S2}(1-R_{S1})}{R_{S1}(1-R_{S2})} \; . \qquad (10)$$

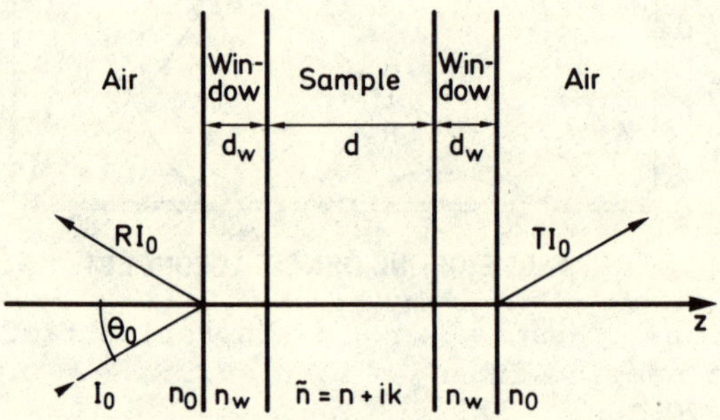

Fig. 3 Schematic diagram of sample with windows. All of the interfaces are normal to the z-axis.

Lamellar sample with windows

To measure liquid samples one has to solve the appropriate Maxwell-boundary value problem, schematically shown in Fig. 3.

The window material is taken to be lossless and hence its refractive index is real. It will be denoted by n_w and the window thickness, which is the same for both windows will be denoted by d_w. The refractive index of the surrounding medium will be denoted by n_o.

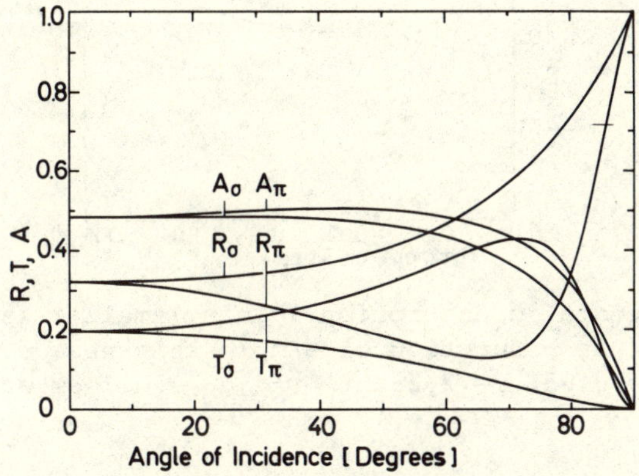

Fig 4 Reflection, transmission and absorption factors calculated for $n^- = 3.88$, $k = 2.26$, $d = 0.01$ cm and $\nu = 70$ GHz. For the windows $n_w = 2$ and $d_w = 0.1$ cm.

We have used a matrix method described by Abelès /8/ and widely used for the treatment of thin film optical filters to calculate reflection and transmission factors for the lamellar sample with windows.

The structure of the R, T and A curves for a very strongly absorbing lamellar sample is illustrated in Fig. 4.

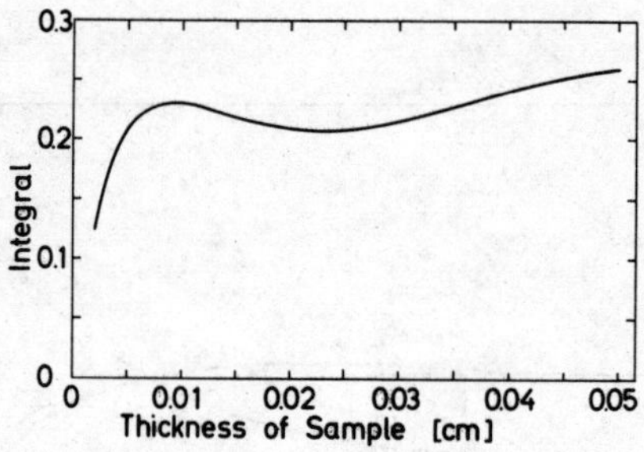

Fig. 5 The integrated absorption I in a lamellar sample with windows as a function of sample thickness d. Calculated for n = 3.88, k = 2.26, n_w = 2, d_w = 0.1 cm and ν = 70 GHz.

The n, k values used in the calculation correspond to H_2O at 20°C and were measured at 70 GHz by Szwarnowski et al., who used a waveguide technique /1/. The value of n_w used in the calculations is approximately correct for fused quartz at 70 GHz /9/.

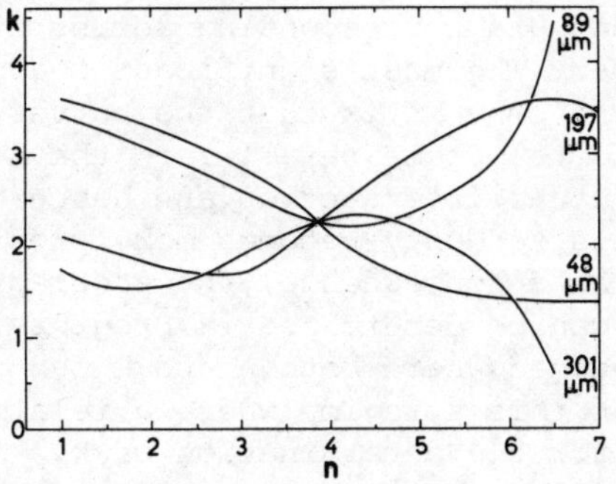

Fig. 6 Calculated loci of n, k values which produce a constant value of I_d/I_∞ for several sample thicknesses: a) d = 48 µm; b) d = 89 µm; c) d = 197 µm; d) d = 301 µm. Here again n_w = 2 and d_w = 0.1 cm.

In Fig. 5 the integral defined in eq. (9) is plotted for the same sample. Note that interference effects cause a 100 µm sample to absorb more strongly than one that is 200 µm thick. Additional, gradually decreasing undulations occur for values of d somewhat larger than those shown here. Finally at still larger values of d, absorption in the sample becomes complete, the undulations die out, and I approaches a constant value determined only by reflection at the first sample surface. We will denote this final constant value of I by I_∞.

Fig. 6 illustrates the behaviour of the locus of points in n, k space which corresponds to a constant ratio I_d/I_∞, for each of a series of different sample thickness d. In an experiment the constant I_d/I_∞ ratios would be determined by the detector ratios on the right hand side of eq. (10). In the preparation of Fig. 6 these values were determined from Fig. 5. The sample thicknesses for which curves are given correspond to values used in the experimental verification of the procedure.

In Figs. 7, 8 and 9 a corresponding series of graphs is shown for a weaker absorber. The most significant feature of these graphs in the present context is that the curves in n, k space shown in Fig. 9 tend to become parallel to the n-axis in the vicinity of their mutual intersection and hence have very shallow crossing angles. This tendency becomes more pronounced as k is decreased further. As a consequence, the accuracy with which the intersection point can be determined is progressively decreased until a point is reached where both n and k can no longer be determined. It is in this k regime where a relatively crude estimate of n suffices for the determination of k.

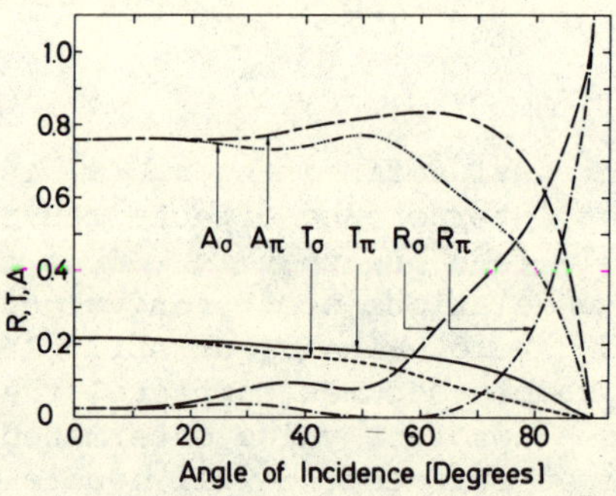

Fig. 7 Reflection, transmission and absorption factors calculated with n = 1.5, k = 0.05, d = 1 cm, n_w = 2, d_w = 0.1 cm and ν = 70 GHz.

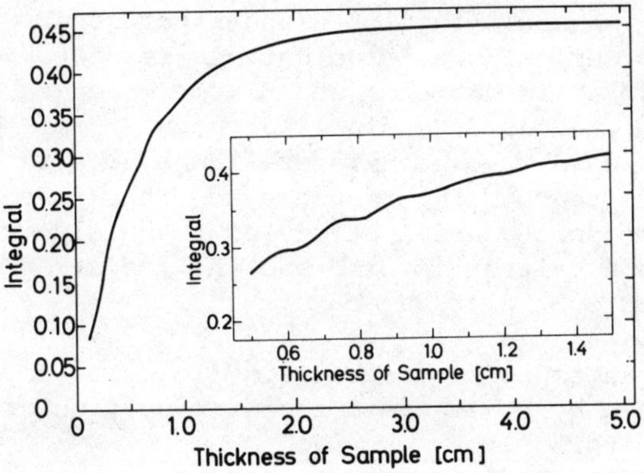

Fig. 8 I as a function of sample thickness for $n = 1.5$, $k = 0.05$, $n_w = 2$, $d_w = 0.1$ cm and $\nu = 70$ GHz.

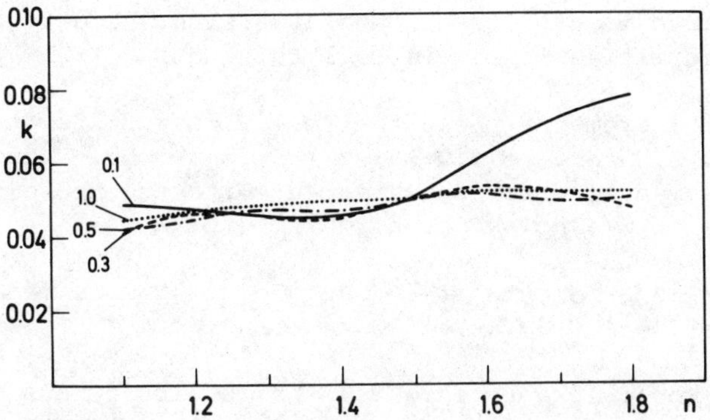

Fig. 9 n, k space loci of constant I_d/I_∞ for several sample thicknesses: a) $d = 0.1$ cm, b) $d = 0.3$ cm, c) $d = 0.5$ cm, d) $d = 1.0$ cm. The curves have a common intersection at $n = 1.5$ and $k = 0.05$.

EXPERIMENTAL

Preliminary measurements of n and k for water and glycerin have been made at 70 GHz using a large untuned resonator. The resonator is a cylinder 40 cm in diameter and 80 cm in length. Its gold-plated inner-surface is textured to minimize specular reflections. The source is a backward wave oscillator. The source intensity and the intensity inside the cavity are measured with crystal detectors. To enhance the homogeneity and isotropy of the field inside the cavity a mechanical mode stirrer is used and the radiation source is frequency modulated over a 15 MHz band.

The Q of the empty resonator is $\sim 2 \cdot 10^5$. The detector signal ratios designated by R_S in the preceeding section are only reproducible to within ±1%.

The sample containers used for these measurements were made for fused quartz. They had windows with a nominal thickness of 0.1 cm, and the thickness of the sample space varied between nominal values of 50 µm and 0.1 cm. The cells were 5 cm in diameter. Unfortunately the cells were not very uniform in thickness and had maximum deviations from the mean value of about ±10%.

In Figure 10 the n, k loci determined by using the measured detector ratios in eq. 10 are shown. The solid lines correspond to the average value of the measured detector ratios. Associated with each such curve is a cross-hatched area with the detector drift and the non-uniformities in sample cell thickness.

These measurements yield the following results at 70 GHz for water at $\sim 20^{o}C$: n = 3.91 ± 0.16; k = 2.33 ± 0.09. These values are within experimental error in agreement with the above mentioned measurements of Swarnowski et al.

Similar measurements at 70 GHz and $\sim 20^{o}C$ were made on glycerine, yielding n = 4.6 ± 0.2, k = 1.00 ± 0.05.

Next I would like to show you the results of absorption measurements on dried biomolecules like RNA, collagene and lysozyme. The samples were placed inside teflon containers which had a wall thickness of 6 mm and an inner diameter of 46.6 mm. The inner edges of the containers were covered with a thin foil of aluminium in order to reflect radiation there. This is necessary because in the calculation the model of thin infinite sheets of material is used. To measure the absorption also at low temperatures the sample cells could be placed inside a cryostat, which was temperature-controlled by a stream of nitrogen gas. The results are shown in Tab. 1.

The room temperature values of the absorption differs by a factor of 5 - 10 from the values at -150°C. That could be caused by freezing out adsorbed water on the molecules. Compared to water - the absorption of the molecules is smaller by a factor of 100 - 500 for room temperature and by a factor of more than 1000 at -150°C. From these data one can conclude, that one has hardly a chance to find a possible mm-wave resonance of the molecules as long as they are solved in water. Presumably that is also true for spectroscopic studies on whole cells.

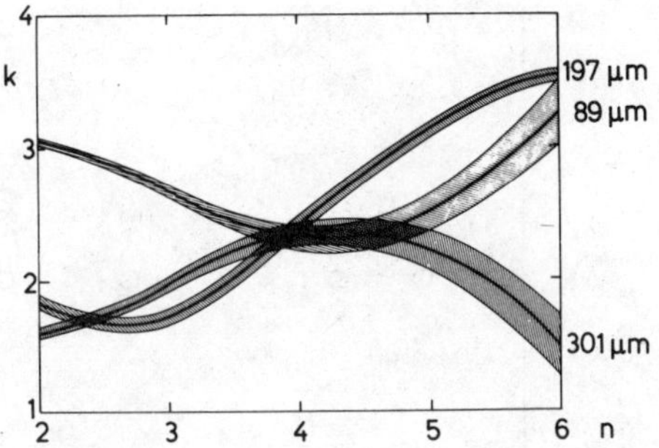

Fig. 10 n, k loci derived from experimental measurement at 70 GHz on water at ~20°C. The shaded area common to all of the cross-hatched uncertainty bands determines the accuracy limits on the measured values of n and k.

CONCLUSION

Let me come to the end: I introduced you to the technique of the broadband multimode resonator, which provides the possibility to measure the complex index of refraction of strongly absorbing samples ($K \geq 0.1$) and the absorption coefficient of low absorbing samples in the broadband range from 40 - 170 GHz. Especially for scattering samples like powders the presented method seems to be the only way possible for dielectric measurements in the mm- und submm-wave regime, and could perhaps therefore be very useful for studies on biological objects like macromolecules and cells. This work was done in close collaboration with Prof. J.R. Izatt, Prof. Genzel and Dr. Keilmann.

Tab. 1 Absorption of RNA, collagene and lysozyme at 70 GHz at room temperature and at $-150^{\circ}C$. The samples were placed inside of teflon-containers, which had an inner diameter of 46.6 mm and an inner height of 10 mm.

Sample	Thickness [mm]	Temperature [$^{\circ}C$]	R_S	I	α [cm^{-1}]
RNA (γ=0.224 g/cm^3)	10	25	0.88	0.0526	0.16±0.01
		-150	0.97	0.0118	0.035±0.002
Collagen (γ=0.222 g/cm^3)	10	25	0.66	0.2023	0.48±0.02
		-150	0.95	0.0189	0.034±0.002
Lysozyme (γ=0.172 g/cm^3)	10	25	0.739	0.1389	0.31±0.02
		-150	0.932	0.0287	0.057±0.002

Tab. 2 As table 1 with the calculated values of k assuming n.

<u>Absorption measurements at 70 GHz:</u>

Sample	Thickness [mm]	Temperature °C	R_S	I	Calculated $k \cdot 10^{-3}$ for n assumed to be: 1.3	1.4	1.5	1.6
RNA (γ=0.224 g/cm^3)	10	25	0.88	0.053	5.38	5.56	5.30	5.86
		-150	0.97	0.012	1.14	1.18	1.11	1.25
Collagen (γ=0.222 g/cm^3)	10	25	0.66	0.2033	15.9	16.8	16.5	17.1
		-150	0.95	0.0190	1.10	1.21	1.12	1.23
Lysozyme (γ=0.172 g/cm^3)	10	25	0.739	0.1389	10.1	10.6	10.8	11.0
		-150	0.532	0.0287	1.83	1.97	1.87	2.00

REFERENCES

1. S. Szwarnowski, R.J. Sheppard, Precision Waveguide Cells for the Measurement of Permittivity of Lossy Liquids at 70 GHz, J. of Physics E: Scientific Instruments 10, 1163 (1977).

2. H.R. Chandrasekhar, L. Genzel, Millimeterwave Spectra of Some Superionic Conductors, Zeitschrift für Physik B35, 211 (1979).

3. F. Kremer, J.R. Izatt, Millimeterwave Absorption Measurements in Low-Loss Dielectrics Using an Untuned Cavity, accepted for publication in International Journal of Infrared and Millimeter Waves (1981).

4. G.E. Becker, S.H. Autler, Water Vapor Absorption of Electromagnetic Radiation in the Centimeter Wave-Length Range, Phys. Rev. 70, 300 (1946).

5. W.E. Lamb, Jr., Theory of a Microwave Spectroscope, Phys. Rev. 70, 308 (1946).

6. D.T. Llewellyn-Jones, R.J. Knight, P.H. Moffat and H.A. Gebbie, New Method of Measuring Low Values of Dielectric Loss in the Near Millimetre Wavelength Region Using Untuned Cavities, Proc. IEE, 535 (1980).

7. J.R. Izatt, F. Kremer, Millimeter-Wave Measurement of Both Parts of the Complex Index of Refraction Using an Untuned Cavity Resonator, accepted for publication in Applied Optics (1981).

8. F. Abelès, Chapter 5 in "Advanced Optical Techniques", edited by A.C.S. van Heel, North Holland Publ. Co., (1967).

9. C.M. Randall, R.D. Rawcliffe, Refractive Indices of Germanium, Silicon and Fused Quartz in the Far Infrared. Applied Optics 6, 1889 (1967).

THEORY OF RESONANT EFFECTS OF RF AND MW ENERGY

Friedemann Kaiser

3. Institut für Theoretische Physik
Universität Stuttgart
Pfaffenwaldring 57, 7000 Stuttgart - 80

INTRODUCTION

1.1 "What one usually expects"

The absorption of non-ionizing electro-magnetic radiation is predominantly determined by the bulk dielectric properties (bulk complex permittivity $\varepsilon(\omega)$ and bulk attenuation function $\alpha(\omega)$) of the irradiated system. Since water represents a most important constituent of biological systems, microwaves, and particularly millimeter waves, are strongly absorbed in these systems.

The very importance of water can be demonstrated when one looks at some characteristic features of MW electromagnetic wave propagation in tissue[1]. In tissues of high water content (e.g. muscles, skin) one finds wavelengths, penetration depths and electric resistivities which are far below the values one can measure for the same frequencies in tissues of low water content (e.g. fat, bone). In both types of tissue one gets, in addition, a decreasing penetration depth with increasing frequency and an increasing conductivity. Furthermore, the state of water in the tissue components is very important. At room temperature for example, the rotational relaxation frequency of water (τ_r^{-1} = 17 G Hz) is far above that of bound water, which lies in the 100 MHz region.

A detailed knowledge of the frequency dependent dielectric properties of tissue and the role of water in MW absorption is required to understand the radiation induced biological effects[2,3].

To first order $\alpha(\omega)$ and $\varepsilon(\omega)$ are determined by the rotational relaxation of both, free and bound water. As a consequence, when irradiated by nonionizing electromagnetic waves the temperature of the biological material is raised and temperature-dependent processes are influenced. The complex problem of biological effects of MW and RF* radiation must be evaluated in the light of modern physics, including all possible interactions of the radiation with living systems.

Besides water related mechanism, other processes of energy absorption do exist, ranging from submolecular to cellular levels. These processes include rotational relaxations, translational vibrations and tunneling on a molecular level. Within this "classical picture", local chemical processes, ion and molecular transport, molecular deformations, orientations and excitations can occur. Furthermore, rotational torques of permanent or induced dipole moments of molecules or of parts of them are conceivable.

1.2. "Beyond what one usually expects"

The creation of direct effects of the electric field of RF and MW radiation in biological systems would require unrealistically high intensities. Any direct change of a system under the influence of electric fields lies beyond the region of linear response and cannot be calculated using properties of the dielectric function.

In table 1 we have presented some measured or calculated "in situ" electric fields. It should be stressed that the external fields change as the wave enters a dielectric medium with complex structure.

Strong electric fields and the related high intensities can lead to irreversible biological effects due to strong heating. However, besides heating effects, well documented biological effects exist, which arise from an irradiation at very low intensities (e.g. below 10 mW/cm^2), where thermal effects can be excluded. In addition a strong frequency dependence of the effects has been found[4-6].

It seems obvious to link these frequency dependent biological effects of a resonance type to absorption bands in certain biomolecules, but it has turned out that such resonances are properties of the whole system. It can easily be shown that common quantum effects (e.g. narrow band resonances) in the RF and MW region are rather unlikely. Up to about 100 GHz no significant population differences within a set of quantum states are present, consequently the black body radiation is well above the saturation power density[7].

* RF and MW frequencies and wavelengths:
RF: 300 KHz - 300 MHz → 1 km — 1m;
MW: 300 MHz - 300 GHz → 1 m — 1 mm.

Table 1. Order of magnitude of some electric fields used in experiments ("in situ" fields,measured or calculated),compared with fields,occuring in nature.The low intensity experiments exhibit a specific frequency dependence,vid.ref.15 .

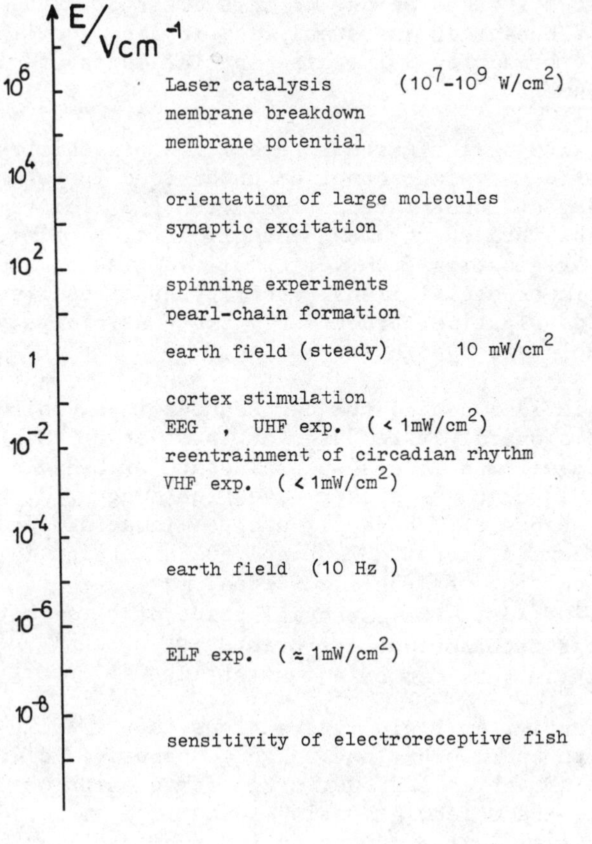

However, these conclusions are not valied if parts of the system are not in thermal equilibrium. Multiple quantum transitions and highly nonlinear effects are required for this situation to occur.

II CONSEQUENCES

A description of those absorption mechanisms of RF and MW radiation that cannot be explained in terms of heating or by direct high intensive processes requires new concepts. It is well-known in modern physics that an energy input must not necessarily lead to a thermalization of the supplied energy, consequently the temperature of the system does not increase. A well-known example exhibiting this behaviour is the Laser. Systems of this type are nonlinear and open ones, which are stabilized far from thermal equilibrium by a suitable energy input. They are capable of a behaviour, which is completely absent in the regime of linear dynamics.

Biological systems belong to this class of systems. At least some modes of behaviour are stabilized in a nonequilibrium state. This can only be achieved if these special modes are isolated from their environment.

Nonlinear dynamic systems reveal the possibility to describe biological effects which cannot be understood in terms of heating or through direct local interactions with the electromagnetic fields. Though the absorbed energy may be negligible, specific effects may be created, originating from very small volumes of the system. Besides nonlinear oscillations, other types of nonlinear behaviour (so-called "dissipative structures") are possible, e.g. non oscillating bistable steady states.

The basic idea behind the new concept is as follows: parts of the active biological system are, at least at certain periods of biological development, in a special state of behaviour. Some modeling approaches for these states have been suggested, we mention the possible existence of coherently excited large dipole oscillations in membranes and of metastable highly polar states in enzymes (a detailed discussion of Fröhlich's ideas may be found in two recent review articles[8,9]. The essential point of these models is that only nonlinear interactions can create these highly nonthermal states, which in turn can only be stabilized by energy input.

Consequently, em field interactions in the 10^{10} - 10^{12} Hz region are assumed to operate by long range cooperative molecular interactions within membranes. Thus, oscillating parts of biological membranes are the "molecular" basis of coupling em fields to other biological entities, i.e. coherent internal oscillations (e.g. of electric nature) couple to external fields. Since membranes contain a considerable number of proteins and other molecules, frequencies below and above the 10^{10} - 10^{12} Hz region are possible.

From a mathematical point of view, nonlinear stable oscillations are special solutions of nonlinear dynamic systems. These oscillations store most of the energy required for the relevant processes; the role of an external perturbation only consists in triggering the occurrence of a particular effect.

From a biological point of view this means that internal (i.e. metabolic) energy is responsible for the special active state whereas the RF or MW energy acts only as a trigger signal to create a biological response.

In the present paper we want to restrict ourselves to a discussion of temporal dissipative structures (nonlinear oscillations of limit cycle type). They seem to be the most important ones, at least with respect to the behaviour one finds when nonlinear systems are perturbed by external periodic fields. At the very beginning we want to describe different types of resonantly excited systems of both, linear and nonlinear systems.

III RESONANCES IN LINEAR AND NONLINEAR OSCILLATIONS

Oscillations can exhibit a special frequency and intensity dependent behaviour of resonance type. We start with a very brief discussion of some simple and well-known oscillator models. With the aid of these models we become acquainted with the principal types of oscillations and their specific responses to a periodic stimulation.

3.1. Free Oscillations

3.1a Conservative Oscillations

We begin with a well-known example of a nonlinear, conservative oscillating system, the physical pendulum. Its equation of motion reads

$$\Theta\, d_{tt}\varphi + m\, g\, l \sin\varphi = 0 \tag{1}$$

(Θ = moment of inertia, m g = weight, $d_t X \equiv \frac{d}{dt} X \equiv \dot{X}$)

For a small angle φ Eq. (1) can be linearized,

$$\Theta\, d_{tt}\varphi + m\, g\, l\, \varphi = 0 \tag{1a}$$

The latter equation describes a harmonic motion, representing a continuum of closed trajectories in the φ - $\dot{\varphi}$ plane (phase-plane).

For increasing values of φ the motion gets anharmonic, its dynamics is given by Eq. (1). However, the trajectories still remain closed. The actual state of oscillation is completely determined by the total initial energy, E_o, which is "constant of motion". For $E_o > m\,g\,l$ the oscillation (libration) changes into a rotation.

Both, linear and nonlinear conservative oscillations are rather crude idealizations of real systems. At least linear damping mechanism (dissipative processes) are always present. Furthermore, conservative systems do not possess structural stability and the trajectories are not asymptotically stable. Both types of stability are highly desirable for all models in order to be within a realistic description. We do not want to present here details of stability theoretical methods, they may be found in excellent standard text books[10-12].

3.1b Oscillations with Dissipation

As an example of linearly damped oscillators we take the damped harmonic oscillator

$$d_{tt}\, X + \gamma\, d_t\, X + X = 0 \tag{2}$$

or its nonlinear extension

$$d_{tt}\, X + \gamma\, d_t\, X + X - \alpha\, X^3 = 0 \tag{3}$$

(X = normalized coordinate, γ = measure for damping strength).

The only stable solution is the nonoscillating steady state $X_s = 0$ for $\gamma > 0$ ($\gamma < 0$ is completely unstable). An additional nonlinear term (e.g. $-\alpha X^3$) does not change the overall behaviour. The most famous nonlinearly damped oscillating system is the Van der Pol oscillator[13]:

$$d_{tt}\, X + \mu(X^2 - 1)\, d_t\, X + X = 0 \tag{4}$$

For large values of X, it corresponds to a damped, linear oscillator. With $X^2 \rightarrow A^2$ one gets

$$d_{tt}\, X + \mu\, A^2\, d_t\, X + X = 0 \tag{4a}$$

and for $X \rightarrow 0$ an unstable damped linear oscillator results,

$$d_{tt}\, X - \mu\, d_t\, X + X = 0 \tag{4b}$$

The solution of Eq . (4) can easily be understood, since it must lie between the two limiting cases (4a) and (4b). As a result one gets one single and unique closed trajectory , the so-called limit cycle. This trajectory is the only one, where the "total damping per period" is zero. The limit cycle amplitude X can be obtained by multiplying Eq. (4) with $\dot{X}$. After an integration over the unknown period T, one is left with

$$< \mu(X^2 - 1)\, \dot{X}^2 >_T = 0 \qquad (4c)$$

From this equation, the steady state limit cycle $X_{LC} \equiv a = 2$ follows, if a harmonic approximation, $X = a \cos t$ is assumed. $X > 2$ and $X < 2$ correspond to a positive (negative) damping; losses ($\mu X^2 \dot{X}$ for $X = 2$) are compensated by gain processes ($-\mu \dot{X}$). A physical definition of a limit cycle is straightforward: a limit cycle is a periodic oscillation which is built up at the expense of a nonperiodic, internal source of energy. Furthermore, both, the frequency and amplitude of a limit cycle are completely determined by the internal parameters and the nonlinear dynamics within the system. This type of oscillation is called self-sustained, since in spite of dissipative processes the internal oscillation does exist without an external energy input.

The very importance of self-sustained oscillations compared to other types can be demonstrated when one applies an external periodic field to the internal oscillation. This will be discussed in the following chapter.

The principal behaviour of oscillations like that described by Eqs. (1-4) have been drawn in figure 1. Both, the oscillation diagrams (amplitude X as a function of time t) and the phase-plane diagrams (amplitude X as a function of velocity $\dot{X}$) have been presented.

3.2 Forced Oscillations

To understand the different possible types of externally driven oscillators we divide the unperturbed oscillators into two classes: self-sustained and non self-sustained oscillators. The class of non-self sustained oscillations consists of linear and nonlinear conservative oscillating systems and nonconservative linear and nonlinear systems with only a linear dissipative term. Self-sustained oscillators (i.e. limit cycles) are nonconservative systems with nonlinear dissipative processes.

3.2a Externally Driven Non Self-Sustained Oscillators

The action of an external periodic force shows the well-known resonance behaviour. The amplitude of the resulting oscillation increases in the resonance regime, i.e. when the external frequency λ approaches the internal one, $\omega_0 = 1$ (vid. Fig. 1). Without damping the system is destabilized ("resonance catastrophy"). This behaviour is, for example, exhibited by the harmonic oscillator (vid. Eq. 1a)

$$\ddot{X} + X = F_o \cos \lambda t \qquad (5)$$

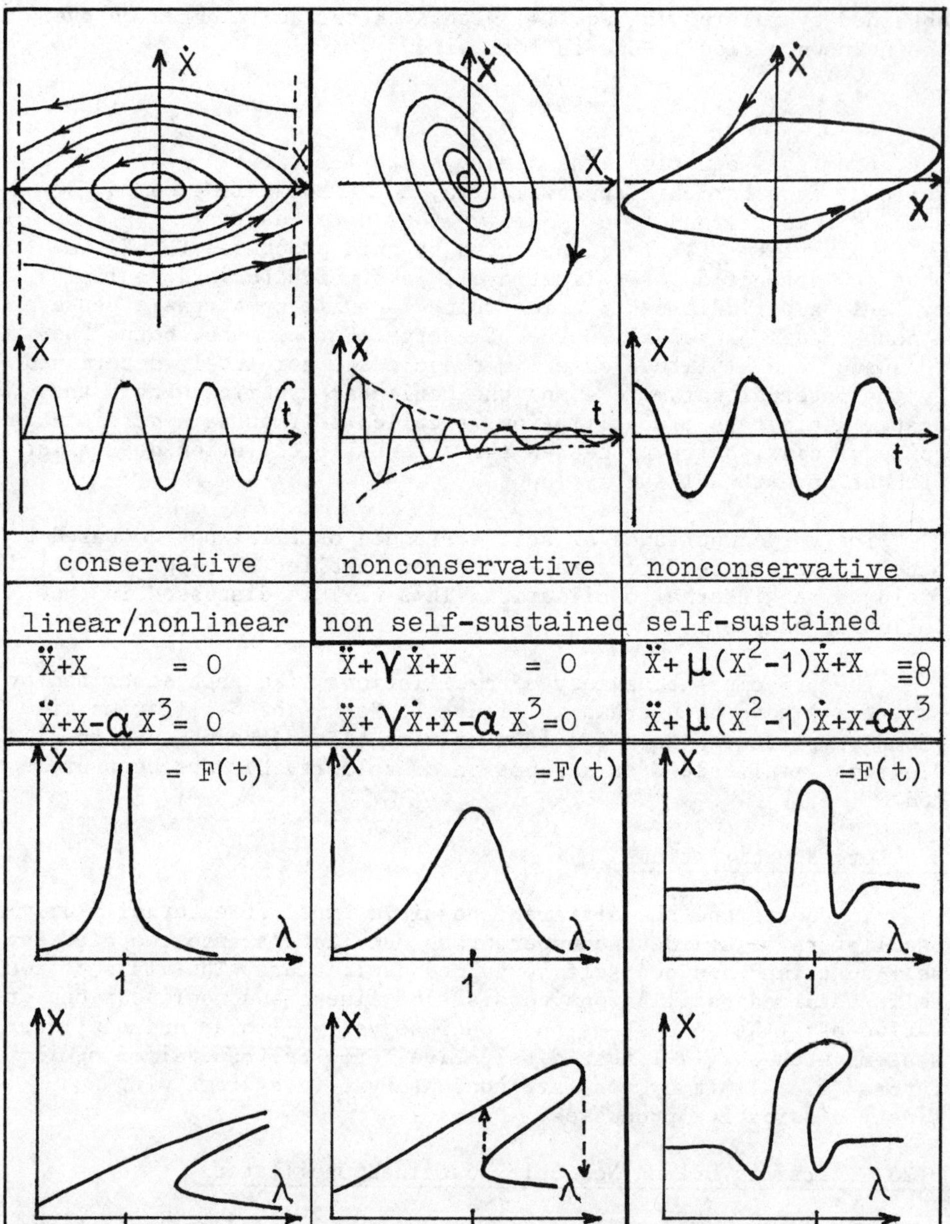

Figure 1: Phase-plane behaviour and oscillations (velocity $\dot{X}$ as a function of amplitude X and amplitude X as a function of time t) for some very simple oscillators (upper part). Frequency response curves of the same oscillators, with an external drive $F(t) = F_o \cos \lambda t$.

and the anharmonic oscillator

$$\ddot{X} + X - \alpha X^3 = F_o \cos \lambda t \tag{6}$$

($F(t) = F_o \cos\lambda t$ is an external harmonic field).

An additional linear damping term stabilizes the resonant oscillation. Well-known examples are the damped harmonic oscillator (vid. Eq. 2)

$$\ddot{X} + \gamma \dot{X} + X = F_o \cos \lambda t \tag{7}$$

and the Duffing oscillator (vid. Eq. 3)

$$\ddot{X} + \gamma \dot{X} + X - \alpha X^3 = F_o \cos \lambda t \tag{8}$$

The resulting motion is a superposition of transients (which are damped out) with an oscillation, which is determined by the external parameters, i.e. the frequency λ and the field strength F_o. For Eq. (7), this solution reads

$$X(t) = e^{-\frac{1}{2}\gamma^2 t} (a\, e^{i \Lambda t} + b\, e^{-i \Lambda t})$$

$$+ F_o \left[(1 - \lambda^2)^2 + \lambda^2 \gamma^2 \right]^{-1/2} \cos (\lambda t - \Psi)$$

with $\lambda^2 = 1 - \frac{1}{4}\gamma^2$; $\tan \Psi = \frac{\gamma \lambda}{1 - \lambda^2}$

With increasing t, the first two terms on the r.h.s. of Eq. (9) vanish, the system oscillates with the external frequency and an amplitude, which is directly proportional to F_o. With $\gamma \to 0$ the solution of Eq. (5) can be obtained. In this case one gets for $t \to \infty$ $X(t) \to \infty$, when λ approaches the internal frequency $\omega_o = 1$. The nonlinear terms-αX^3 in Eqs. (6) and (8) lead to additional contributions, in particular to a nonlinear superposition of higher harmonics. It causes the occurence of multi-stability and of jumps from low amplitude oscillations to higher ones. The frequency response curves of oscillations (5-8) have been drawn in figure 1.

Neglecting conservative oscillations and transitions of damped oscillations (both of which are not realistic in actual steady state situations), non self-sustained oscillators exhibit a behaviour, which is completely determined by the external parameters F_o and λ. For $F_o \to 0$ no oscillation can exist; only in the resonance regime, considerable amplitudes of oscillation are present.

3.2b Externally Driven Self-Sustained Oscillators

Instead of treating general systems for which the algebra is involved, we treat again a simple system that exhibits the essential ideas. We will briefly discuss the Van der Pol oscillator, subject to an external periodic force. From Eq. (4) we get

$$d_{tt} X + \mu(X^2 - 1) d_t X + X = F_o \cos \lambda t \tag{9}$$

Eq. (9) has been investigated in great detail[14]. The techniques how to do these investigations will be presented in the next chapter, where some more general model systems will be discussed. In the present chapter it is sufficient to give some essential results. The frquency response curve of Eq. (9) is shown in figure 1. Remarkable is the very sharp resonance. Small external fields are sufficient to cause a strong increase in the amplitude. In the resonance region the system oscillates with the external frequency λ, whereas the internal frequency ω_o is completely suppressed. This region shows a synchronized behaviour, it is called entrainment.

On both sides of the entrainment region, the amplitude of the oscillation is partially suppressed to values, which are below those of the free oscillation with amplitude X_o ("peak-dip shape" of resonance curve, vid. Fig. 1). Quasi-periodic and aperiodic ("chaotic") oscillations with varying amplitudes and frequencies occur. Examples of these types of oscillations are given in the following chapters (vid. Figs. 10, 11, 16, and 17). They demonstrate the competition (nonlinear superposition) between free internal and forcing external oscillations. These extraordinary oscillations are largely restricted to self-sustained, externally driven oscillators.

Far away from the entrainment region only the free oscillation with frequency ω_o and amplitude X_o can exist.

In the preceeding discussion we have restricted ourselves to primary resonances (i.e. resonance behaviour in the region $\lambda \approx \omega_o$). However, for both, self-sustained and non self-sustained oscillations, secondary and higher resonances do exist. This means that subharmonic ($\lambda \approx n\, \omega_o$) and superharmonic ($\lambda \approx \frac{1}{n}\, \omega_o$) oscillations with n = 2, 3... are possible. The very difference of these resonances with respect to self-sustained and nonself-sustained systems is shown in figure 2. The latter systems can only oscillate with multiples or submultiples of the frequency ω_o, supposing that the external force is sufficiently strong in order to bring the system into the resonance regions. Outside these regions no oscillation can exist.

Limit cycle systems, on the contrary, can exhibit a more pronounced behaviour: sub- and superharmonic entrainment, free oscillations just between these regions and quasi-periodic and a-periodic oscillations very close to the entrainment regions (vid. Fig. 2).

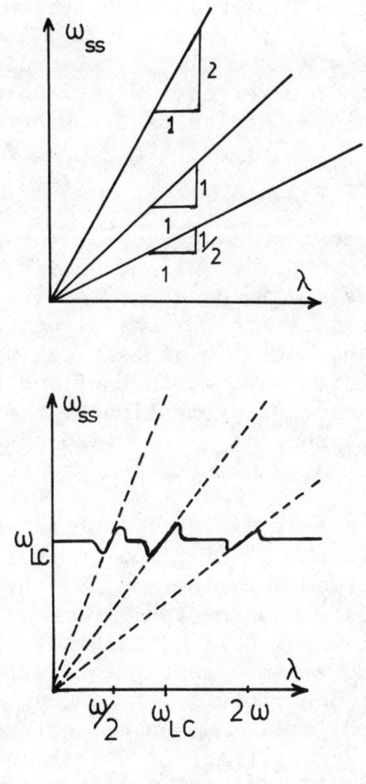

Figure 2. Steady state frequency ω_{ss} for a driven oscillator (qualitative behaviour) :
a. non self-sustained oscillator,
b. self-sustained oscillator.
Only harmonics and second sub- and superharmonics, i.e. primary and secondary resonances have been drawn.

3.3 Significance and Importance of Limit Cycles

In general, externally driven limit cycles can exhibit a great variety of oscillating behaviour, the details of which are rather sensitive to the frequency and intensity of the external stimulus.

Furthermore, nonlinear oscillations of limit cycle type reveal a possible explanation of the experimentally found specific sensitivities of biological systems to a weak external stimulus[15]:

> only a small amount of external energy is necessary to create a response since the inherently stored limit cycle energy will build up the signal (trigger effect of the external em fields).

Oscillatory phenomena in macroscopic dimensions are frequently observable in the living world. Well-known examples of rhythmic behaviour are spontaneous and induced periodicities of bioelectric nature (e.g. propagation of excitations along nerve membranes), slow oscillations in the activity of cortical neurons (i.e. EEG activity) etc. In addition, a multitude of endogenous rhythms (e.g. circadian rhythms) deserve being mentioned. Some of these oscillations have been discussed in[9], where also examples of nonlinear oscillations from physics, chemistry and biochemistry can be found.

In conclusion, there are several aspects which make limit cycles and outstanding tool in the description of oscillating phenomena in biological systems. We summarize some of the properties though most of them have already been quoted:

1. LC can only exist in nonlinear, dissipative systems[10],
2. externally driven LC exhibit an extremely specific frequency and intensity dependent behaviour[9],
3. externally driven LC can cause a nonlinear response, which is internally created (trigger effect of external fields)[16-18],
4. internally or externally driven LCs are a suitable description of circadian rhythm[19].

Only a few references have been added. They might introduce the reader into further work on these subjects.

Finally, it should be emphasized on the basis of the above ideas that both, oscillations in biological systems and their interactions with external fields can be described by externally driven limit cycles[20]. With this concept the existence of specific nonlinear resonant effects in irradiated biological systems is conclusive.

It is the purpose of the present paper to restrict to resonances of externally driven self-sustained oscillations. With this restriction we only deal with those resonances which are properties of the whole system or at least of its oscillating parts. Hence, direct resonances on a microscopic basis are excluded. This procedure seems reasonable, since only low intensity effects will be described, which can not be explained within the conventional interaction mechanism.

The limit cycle concept ought to be viewed as a reasonable hypothesis for the understanding of nonthermal effects. This general scheme stresses both, the importance of self-sustained oscillations and their possible realization by electric vibrations in biological systems. In addition, the concept presented here agrees well with and is embedded in more general concepts. These are known as "self-organization in nonequilibrium system"[21] and "Synergetics"[22], to mention the most promising developments within the last years.

IV MODELS

To give an interpretation of our concept, we want to present some model systems. These models are examples of a typical nonlinear behaviour and they might perhaps serve as an explanation of some specific effects found in experiments (vid. refs. 5-9, 15). It should be emphasized that the models are rather speculative. However, they are based on both, the physical properties and the relevant physical laws, which determine the dynamics of the system under consideration.

4.1 Generalized Van der Pol Oscillator (MI)

The Van der Pol oscillator is a well-known and best studied example of a limit cycle oscillation. It has its origin in nonlinear electric circuits, an example of which is shown in Figure 3. Applying Kirchhoff's rules, the following equation for the voltage can easily be derived:

$$L\,C\,d_{tt}\,v + (R\,C - M\,S(v))\,d_t\,v + v = 0 \tag{10}$$

In reduced variables, this equation reads

$$d_{tt}\,X + \mu(1 - S(X))\,d_t\,X + X = 0$$

The nonlinear dissipative Term $\mu(1 - S(X))$ describes the competition between a purely Ohmic damping process and nonlinear feedback processes within the circuit.

We want to discuss a special type of Eq. (10a) which to the author's knowledge has not yet been discussed in the literate. We choose

$$d_{tt}\,X + \mu(-1 + X^2 - \alpha X^4 + \beta X^6)\,d_t\,X + X = F_o \cos \lambda t \tag{11}$$

where, in addition, an external periodic force has been taken into account (r.h.s. of Eq. 11).

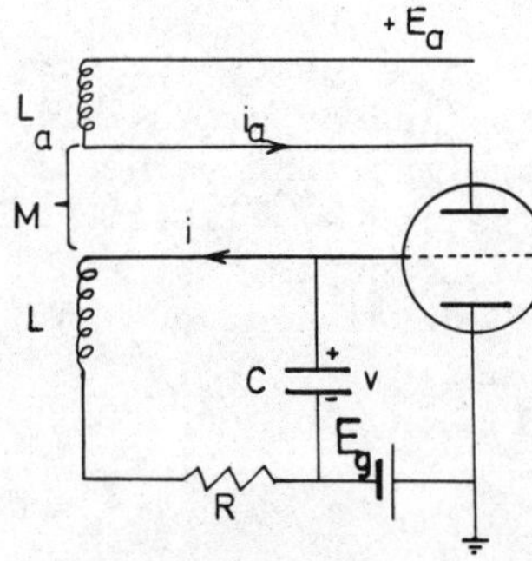

Figure 3. Circuit diagram: valve generator with the resonant circuit in the grid circuit. M leads to a nonlinear inductive feedback e.m.f.

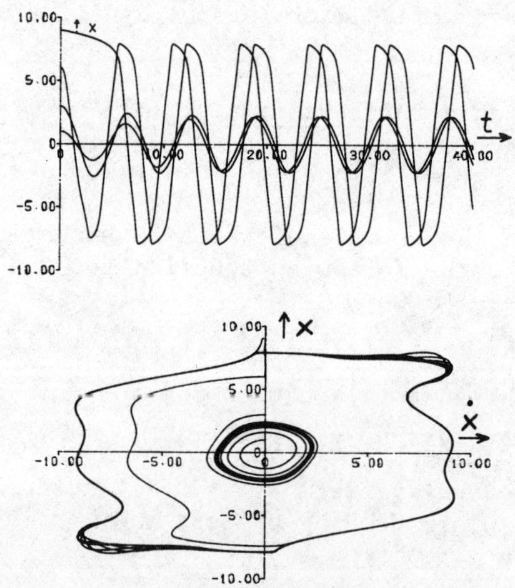

Figure 4. Phase plane ($\dot{X}$ - X) and oscillation (X - t) diagrams of the free oscillation of MI (for 4 different values of the initial conditions)

Eq. (11) has been analysed by both, approximate analytical methods and numerical integration procedures. The details of these investigations will be omitted. It suffices to mention that in the resonance region, an asymptotic solution of the form

$$x(t) = a(t) \cos (\lambda t - \varphi(t)) \tag{12}$$

and outside this region

$$x(t) = a(t) \cos (t - \varphi(t)) + \frac{F_o}{1 - \lambda^2} \cos \lambda t \tag{13}$$

have been assumed. Both solutions reflect the essential characteristics of the fundamental oscillations of Eq. (11).

When Eq. (12) or Eq. (13) is combined with Eq. (11), one obtains rather complicated equations for the amplitude a(t) and the phase $\varphi(t)$, which will not be given here. In addition, a stability theoretical investigation for the steady state solutions must be performed in the usual way[10]: One linearizes the differential equations for a(t) and $\varphi(t)$ around their steady states. The eigenvalues of the related Jacobi matrix determine both, the type of steady state and its stability.

The results of the rather lengthy calculations and of the numerical procedures are shown in a series of diagrams:

1. Without the external field, two stable oscillations with frequencies ω_1 and ω_2 and amplitudes X_1 and X_2 exist; an unstable LC is situated between the two LCs. The stable oscillations are given in figure 4.

2. The different regions of stability are shown in figure 5. Stable nodes (SK) and stable foci (SF) in the Van der Pol plane (i.e. Fig. 5) correspond to stable oscillating solutions of Eq. (11). All other regions are unstable.

3. For a time-independent external stimulus ($F(t) = F_o$), oscillating and nonoscillating regions are possible. The transition from the small to the large amplitude oscillation is separated by a stable non-oscillating state. For $F_o > F_3$ both oscillations are suppressed (vid. Fig. 6).

4. By time-dependent external means and by parameter variations the system can be driven from one stable oscillation to the other one. Furthermore, the external field can lead to a complete collapse of the small amplitude oscillation. The closer the external frequency λ is to the internal one, ω_1, the smaller is the critical field strength F_{oc}, which is necessary for the breakdown of the small oscillation and the subsequent transition to the other one. For $F_o > F_{oc}$, the system can only exist in the large amplitude state. In figure 7, the steady state frequencies and

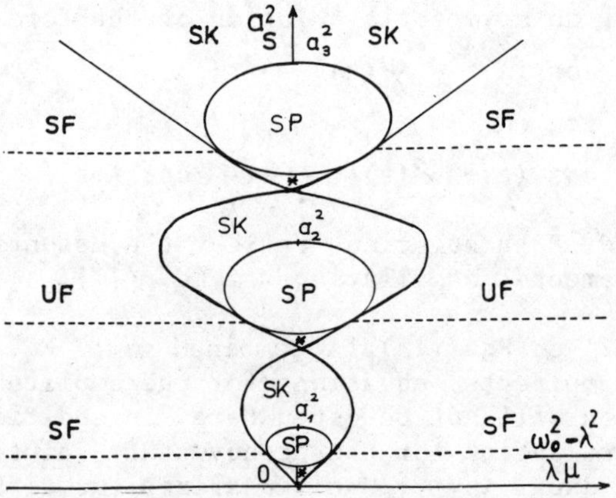

Figure 5. Stability diagram (Van der Pol plane). Regions of stable and unstable amplitudes a_s as a function of the detuning parameter σ for the externally driven oscillator (MI).
SP = saddlepoint; UK, UF = unstable node, focus;
SK, SF = stable node focus.

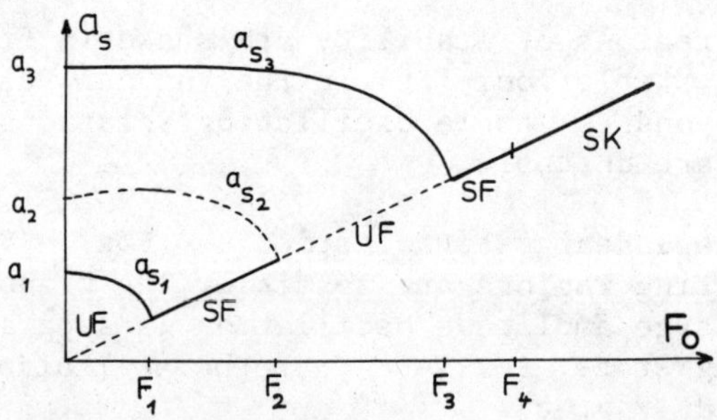

Figure 6. Steady state amplitudes a_s of the externally driven oscillator (MI) for $F(t) = F_o$.
——— stable solutions, SF and SK are non-oscillating ones,
------- unstable solution.
a_1, a_2 and a_3 are the amplitudes for $F(t) = 0$.

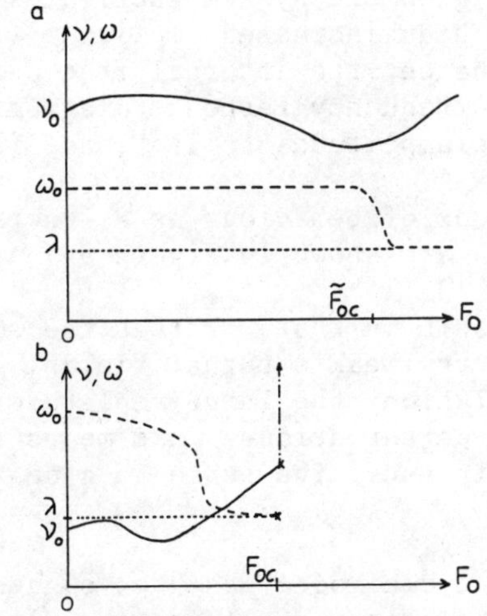

Figure 7. Steady state amplitude ν and steady state frequency ω as a function of the external field strength F_o for $F(t) = F_o \cos \lambda t$ (λ fixed).
a. large amplitude limit cycle,
b. small amplitude limit cycle (gets unstable).
ν_o, ω_o are the corresponding values of the free oscillation. ———— ν, -------- ω, ········· λ.

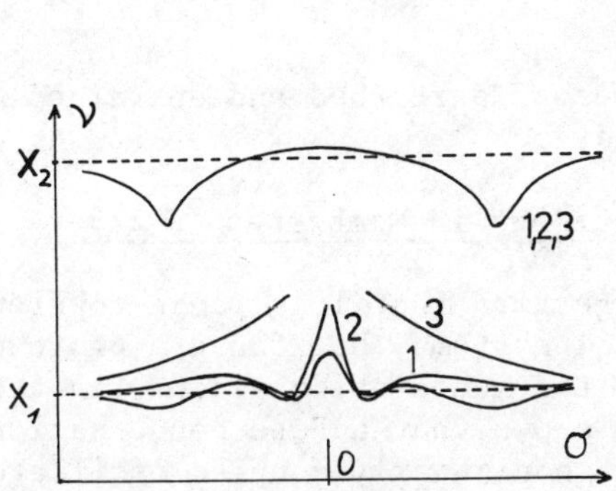

Figure 8. Frequency response diagram (resonance diagram) of MI. Steady state amplitude ν as a function of the detuning parameter for three different values of F_o ($F_{o1}<F_{o2}<F_{o3}$). Remarkable is the instability region of the small oscillation.

amplitudes have been drawn as a function of F_o for an arbitrary frequency λ.

5. In the resonance region the system oscillates with the external frequency λ and with an increased amplitude (entrainment region). Far away from resonance, the internal free oscillations are present. The complete frequency response diagram for both, the small and the large amplitude oscillations, is given in figure 8.

6. The different regions of behaviour as a function of the external parameters F_o and λ are shown in figure 9.

The important result is that, whereas the small oscillation can be influenced by very weak external fields, leading to a total collapse of the oscillation, the large amplitude oscillation is rather stable against perturbations. This means that the system can be driven from a highly sensitive state to a nearly unperturbable one.

A multiple limit cycle model has been suggested[23] to explain some rather interesting experimental results with respect to Ca^{2+}-efflux measurements in the ELF- and MW-irradiated brain[24, 25]. On the basis of the generalized Van der Pol oscillator, two stable oscillating calcium states would exist. With regard to the frequency and intensity specific behaviour of this model, both, the frequency and intensity windows (which are the dominant features of the experiments) receive a possible explanation. However, a physical basis for our mathematical model is still lacking. Work towards this direction is going on, it has been started on the basis of Grodsky's membrane model[26].

Typical examples of perturbed and entrained oscillations are given in figures 10a, b.

4.2 Coherent Oscillations in Membranes (M II)

Fröhlich's suggestion that long range coherence might be important in biological systems, has found a profound demonstration and verification in two model calculations. In the coherent oscillation model he has shown that a Bose condensation-like excitation results, if a set of nonlinearly coupled oscillators is pumped by external energy supply above a certain threshold[27]. In the high-polarization model he has been able to show that metastable highly-polarized oscillating states can exist in dielectric materials of suitable properties. Both, a few rather exciting experimental results and some model calculations on a strongly physical basis seem to support these ideas (vid. Refs. 8, 9 and 28 for details).

Recently Fröhlich has extended his ideas to give a possible explanation of the extraordinary high sensitivity of certain bio-

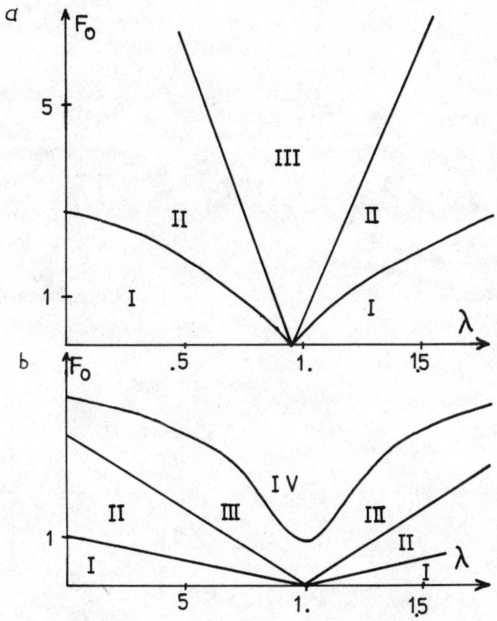

Figure 9. The regions of different behaviour of the externally driven limit cycle (MI):
I free oscillations (LC with ω_o)
II quasi-periodic oscillations
III entrainment (LC with λ)
IV unstable region (transition to the large amplitude oscillation).
a. large amplitude oscillation
b. small amplitude oscillation

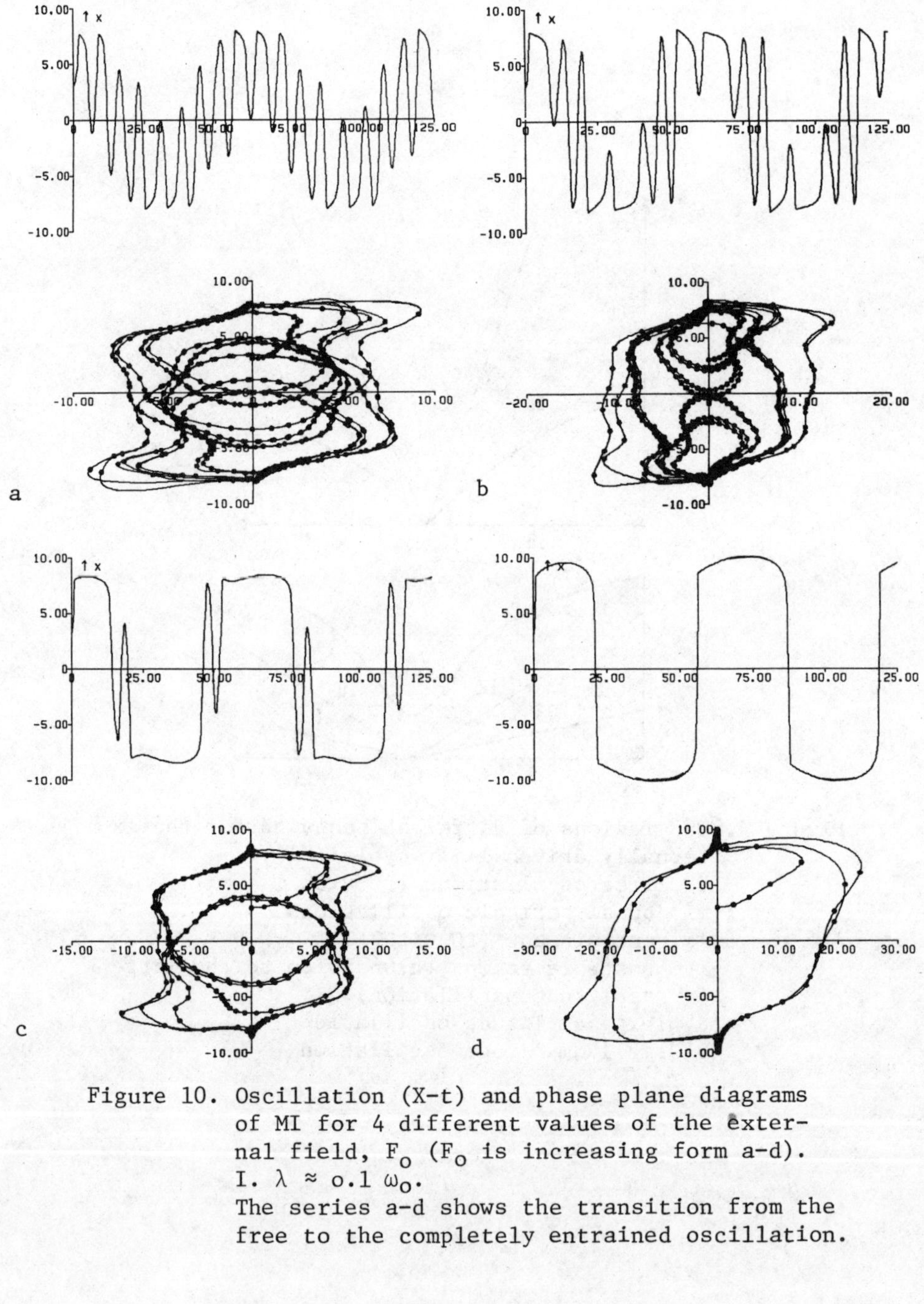

Figure 10. Oscillation (X-t) and phase plane diagrams of MI for 4 different values of the external field, F_o (F_o is increasing form a-d). I. $\lambda \approx 0.1\ \omega_o$.
The series a-d shows the transition from the free to the completely entrained oscillation.

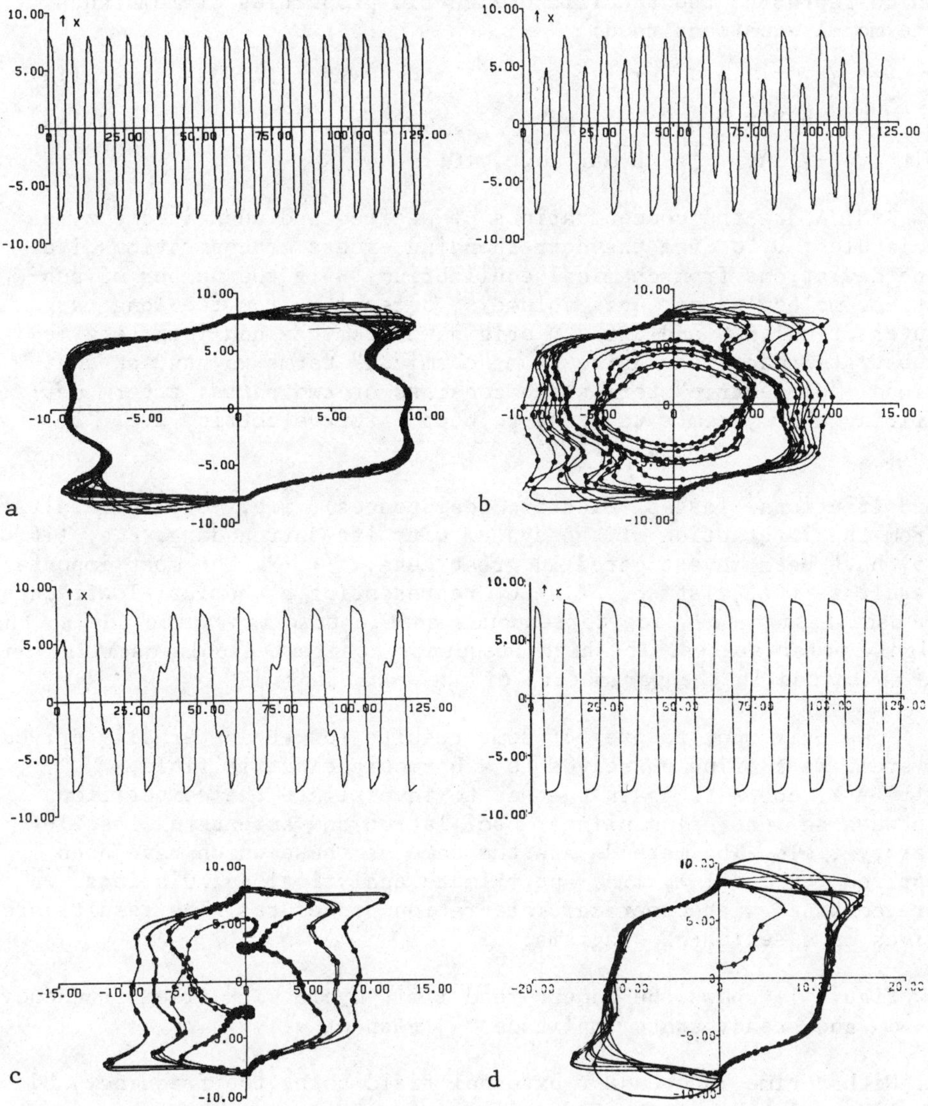

Figure 10. (Continued)
II. $\lambda \approx 0.5\ \omega_o$.
The series a-d shows the transition from the free to the completely entrained oscillation.

logical systems to very weak external electric and magnetic signals. The model is a combination of both, a nonlinear chemical reaction, which is based on long range interactions, and a ferroelectric terms, which represent the specific dielectric properties of membranes. The model equations read:

$$\dot{\nu} = \gamma\,\sigma + \alpha\,A\,\sigma\,\nu + (c^2\,e^{-\Gamma^2\,\nu^2} - d^2)\,\nu + F(t) \tag{14}$$

$$\dot{\sigma} = -\,\beta\,\nu - \alpha\,A\,\sigma\,\nu \tag{15}$$

with $\nu = N - \gamma | \alpha A$, $\sigma = S - \beta | \alpha A$, $\alpha, \beta, \gamma > 0$.

N, A are the concentrations of excited and unexcited enzyme molecules; ν, σ are the corresponding excess concentrations, i.e. the deviations from chemical equilibrium. S is the number of substrate molecules per unit volume. $\gamma\,\sigma$ results from the long range interaction, $\beta\,\nu$ and $\alpha\,A\,\sigma\,\nu$ originate from the nonlinear enzyme-substrate reactions. Aside from "chemical" terms we have an additional "dielectric" term which consists of two parts: a term describing the system's tendency to become ferroelectric, i.e.

$$c^2\,e^{-\Gamma^2\,\nu^2}\,\nu \tag{16}$$

and frictional losses (electric resistences), i.e. $-d^2\nu$. F results from the interaction of the system with its surrounding. Eqs. (14, 15) have been investigated in great detail[17, 18]. The most important result is the existence of a LC, representing a chemical lowfrequency oscillation to which corresponds an electric vibration due to the highly polar states. The high frequency coherent dipole oscillation is contained in the parameters of the equations.

We only want to present some results for the externally driven system. We confine ourselves to a harmonic electric field, $F(t) = F_o \cos \lambda t$. Again one has to investigate the competition between an internal nonlinear oscillation and an external oscillatory field. The methods are the same as those which have been applied for model I, i.e. approximate analytical calculations, which are combined with numerical integration procedures. The results are given in a series of diagrams:

1. Figure 11 shows the unperturbed limit cycle with fixed frequency ω_o and steady state amplitude ν_o, respectively.

2. With a time-independent external field both, the frequency and the amplitude of the free oscillation decrease as a function of an increasing field strength F_o. For $F_o > F_c$, a stable nonoscillating steady state is build up, no oscillating solution can exist. This behaviour is shown in figure 12.

3. A time-dependent external field ($F(t) = F_o \cos \lambda t$) leads to a competition between the driving and the free oscillation. In figure 13 both, the resulting steady state amplitude and the

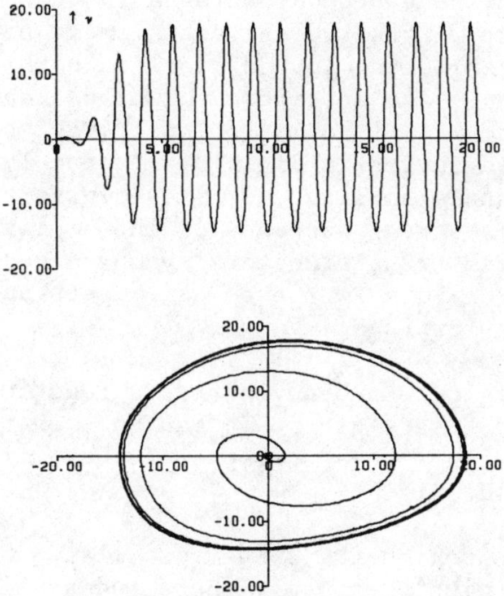

Figure 11. Oscillation (X - t) and phase plane ($\dot{X}$ - X) diagram of the free oscillation (MII).

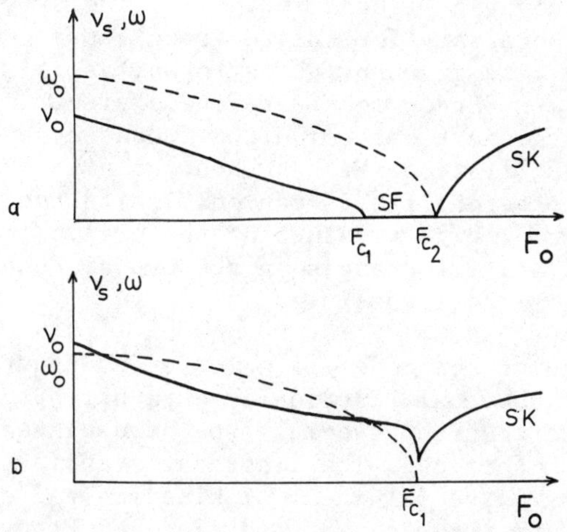

Figure 12. Steady state amplitude ν_s and frequency ω as a function of F_o (MII with $\dot{F}(t) = F_o$) for 2 different parameter sets (ν_o, ω_o are the free amplitude and frequency, respectively).
a. $c^2 - d^2 - \beta^2 < o$; ———————— ν_s
b. $c^2 - d^2 - \beta^2 > o$; ------------ ω.

related frequency have been drawn as a function for the external frequency λ. Near ω_0 the typical entrainment behaviour (nonlinear resonances) is exhibited. In addition, on both sides of entrainment quasi-periodic and aperiodic solutions lead to variations of ω_λ and ν_λ from $\omega_{\lambda,max}$ to $\omega_{\lambda,min}$ and $\nu_{\lambda,max}$ to $\nu_{\lambda,min}$, respectively (dashed curves in Fig. 13). In the lower part of Fig. 13, the steady state amplitude ν_λ is shown as a function of F_o. Remarkable is the strong decrease of the amplitude. This behaviour reflects the transition to a synchronized oscillation (entrainment). For $F_o = F_c$ the solution gets unstable, no oscillation can exist for $F_o > F_c$.

4. The different regions of behaviour as a function of the external parameters λ and F_o are given. It can be seen that the smallest value F_o, which leads to a collapse of the limit cycle, lies below $\lambda = \omega_0$ (vid. Fig. 14).

5. In the resonance region the system oscillates with the external frequency λ and with a strongly increased amplitude. Again the characteristic "peak-dip shape" of self-sustained and driven oscillations is present. The complete frequency response diagram has been drawn in figure 15. Contrary to the large amplitude oscillation of Model I, the resonance curve gets unstable for large excitations.

6. Typical examples of perturbed oscillations (quasi-periodic, entrained) are shown in figures 16 and 17. The critical strength F_{oc}, which is necessary for the LC to collapse and to create a response signal, is given by the external as well as by the internal parameters. Predominant are the dielectric ones (c^2, d^2), since these parameters determine the frequency and amplitude of the internal oscillation. We have been able to show that pulsed and modulated external fields can only shift the instability point towards smaller or higher values of the critical field strength per cycle. Qualitative changes in the overall behaviour of the driven LC system are impossible.

The relevance of the model is a matter of controversal discussions. Though the chemical reaction is a rather speculative one, one should realize that the special type of nonlinear reaction can be replaced by an other one. The important step is the combined existence of both, a special chemical kinetics and a related electric behaviour. Both terms can be modified, but they must be based on physical laws and the extraordinary dielectric properties of the material.

V CONCLUSIONS

The models considered exhibit a behaviour which is typical and well-known for nonlinear oscillations. In addition, an external

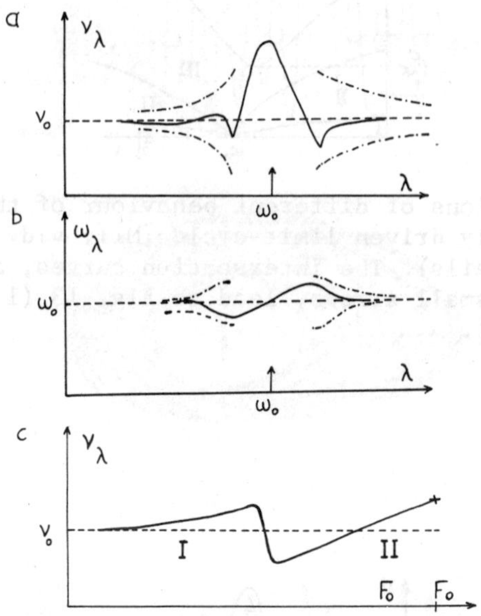

Figure 13. Steady state amplitude ν_λ (a) and steady state frequency ω_λ (b) as a function of the external frequency λ and ν_λ as a function of F_o for an arbitrary frequency λ (c).
(ω_o, ν_o are the frequency and amplitude of the free oscillation).
-·-·-·-·-·-·-: upper and lower limit for ω and ν in the quasi-periodic region. Remarkable is the sharp transition when λ reaches the entrainment region (limit of entrainment).
c. I quasi-periodic oscillations,
II complete entrainment.
For $F_o = F_c$, the system gets unstable.

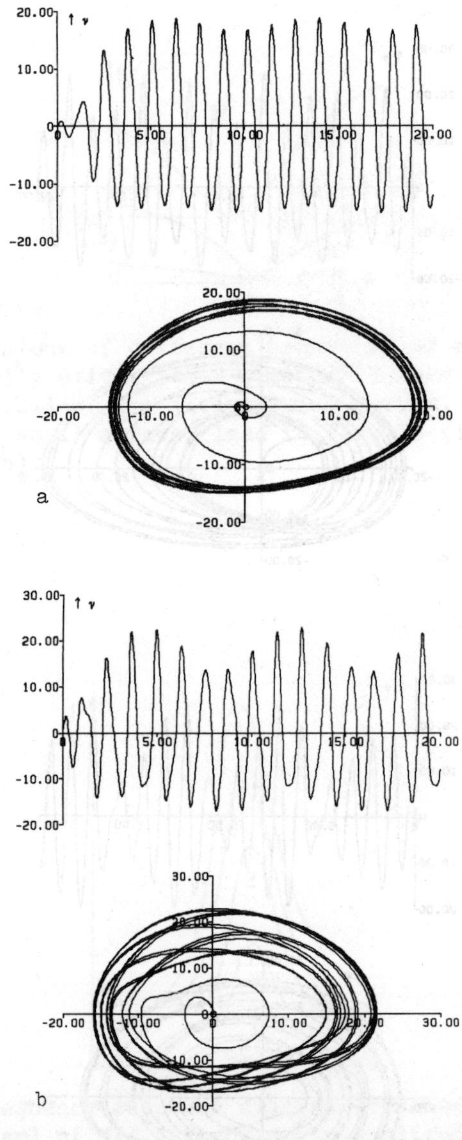

Figure 17. Oscillations and phase plane diagrams (vid. Fig. 16) for 5 different values of F_o (F_o increases from a - e), λ is fixed ($\lambda \approx 9/5\ \omega_o$). One recognizes the transition from the free to the forced oscillation (figs. a - d) and the onset of instability (fig. e).

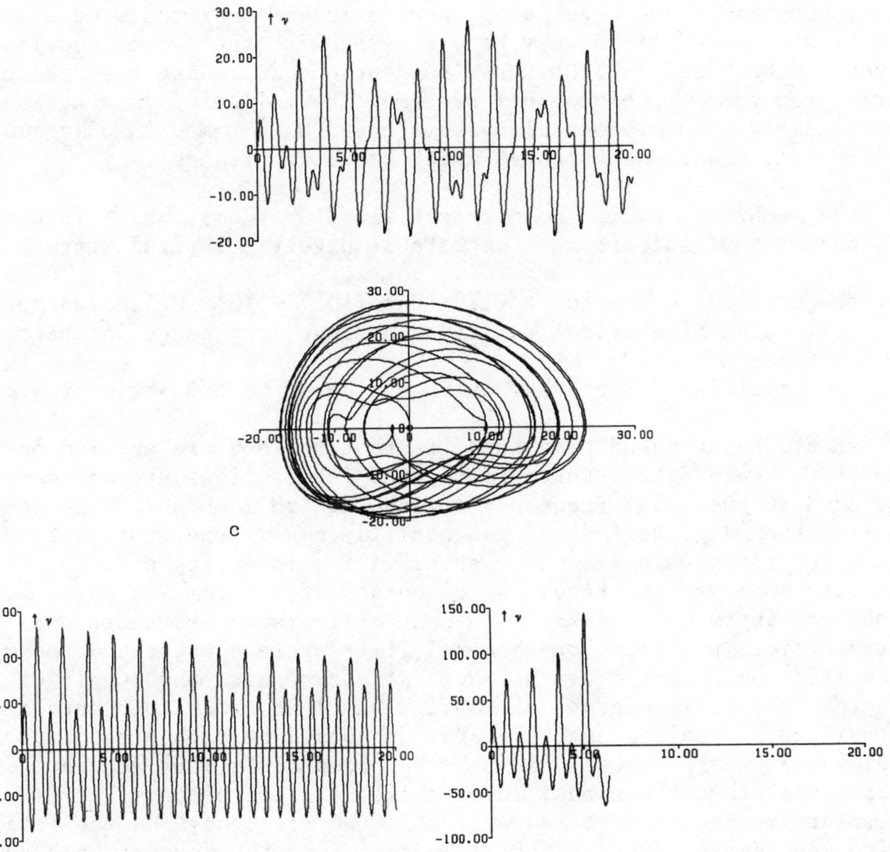

Figure 17 (Continued)

periodic stimulus causes the specific effects of nonlinear resonances within self-sustained oscillators. Externally driven, both models (M I and M II) display a pronounced frequency and intensity dependent behaviour.

Details of the underlying interaction of an irradiated system with external em fields may be discussed with the aid of models. They may be based on Fröhlich's suggestions including the dielectric properties of biological systems. The following interaction mechanism within biological systems have to be taken into account [9,30,31], though many others might be of importance:

1. the membrane intrinsicelectric field (10^5 V/cm), which is perhaps responsible for the metastable highly polarized states,

2. the coherent electric oscillations (10^{10} - 10^{12} Hz), leading to collective biochemical reactions through long range interactions,

3. the resulting ELF branch, which may describe EEG activities.

It should be stressed that the different regions are not independent from each other. Furthermore, the interactions are not restricted to the above frequency regions and to membranes. The assumed existence of self-sustained oscillations is the essential point in order to explain frequency specific low intensity effects. These oscillations are the result of cooperativity in complex systems, they are intimately linked with nonequilibrium constraints and irreversibility. Both, the general limit cycle concept and the more specific concept of coherent oscillations require the supply of energy (metabolic energy, biological pump) in order to create and stabilize a specific active state. It should be emphasized that the relevance of the concept can only be checked by very accurate experimental investigations. To establish a clear picture, it is absolutely necessary to measure both, the frequency and the intensity dependence of the effects. In addition, the measurements should include the duration of irradiation and both, an increase and decrease in the applied field intensity to detect possible hysteresis effects.

From a theoretical point of view, one has to solve the problem of the onset of a propagating pulse after the LC collapse. This necessitates the introduction of space dependent variables and of appropriate boundary conditions. This problem has already been discussed for model 2[18].

APPENDIX

We have made a rather crude estimate to check whether the parameters of our models are within a reasonable order of magnitude with respect to the underlying physical ideas. For an electrically charged oscillating sphere in a liquid with Van der Pol dynamics, i.e.

$$m \ddot{X} + ß (X^2 - \gamma^2) \dot{X} + k X = N e E \cos \omega t$$

or in reduced variables

$$\ddot{X} + \mu (X^2 - 1) \dot{X} + X = F_o \cos \lambda t$$

one gets in the GHz region a resonance line width of 10 - 100 MHz which is about one hundreth of the oscillating frequency. The applied external field is in the region of V/cm, corresponding to intensities of some mW/cm^2. This rather oversimplified estimate is an indication that both, the parameters and the reduced variables of our models may lie within a reasonable physical range.

Literature Cited

1. S. Baransky and P. Czerski, "Biological Effects of Microwaves", Dowden , Hutchinson and Ross, Stroudsbourg (1976)
2. H. P. Schwan, "Dielectric properties of brain tissue between 0.01 and 10 GHz", Phys. Med. Biol. 24: 1177 (1979)
3. E. H. Grant, "The role of water in MW absorption by biological material with particular reference to MW hazards", Phys. Med. Biol. 24: 1168 (1979)
4. N. D. Devyatkov, "Influences of mm-band electromagnetic radiation on biological objects", Usp. Fiz. Nauk 110: 452 (1973)
5. J. Bertaud, M. Dardalhon, N. Rebeyrotte and D. Averbeck, "Action d'un rayonnement électromagnetique á longueur d'onde millimétrique sur la croissance bactérienne", C. R. Acad. Sci. 281D: 843 (1975)
6. W. Grundler and F. Keilmann, "Nonthermal effects of mm MW on yeast growth" Z. Naturforsch. 33c: 15 (1978)
7. F. Barnes, in: "Nonlinear Electromagnetics", P. L. E. Uslenghi ed., Academic Press, New York (1980)
8. H. Fröhlich, "The Biological Effects of MW and Related Questions", Advances in Electronics and Electron Physics, 53: 85-152 (1980)
9. F. Kaiser, "Nonlinear Oscillations (Limit Cycles) in Physical and Biological Systems", in: "Nonlinear Electromagnetics", P.L.E. Uslenghi ed., Academic Press, New York (1980)
10. A.A. Andronov, A.A. Vitt and S.E. Khaikin, "Theory of Oscillators", Pergamon Press, Oxford (1964)
11. M.W. Hirsch and S. Smale, "Differential Equations, Dynamical Systems, and Linear Algebra", Academic Press, New York (1974)
12. A.A. Andronov, L.A. Leontovich, I.I. Gordon and A.G. Maier, "Qualitative Theory of Second-order Dynamic Systems", J. Wiley, New York (1980)
13. B. Van der Pol "On relaxation oscillations", Phil. Mag. Ser. 7, 2: 978 (1926)

14. B. Van der Pol, "Forced oscillations in a circuit with nonlinear resistance", Phil. Mag. Ser. 7, 13: 65 (1972)
15. S.M. Bawin and W.R. Adey eds., "Brain interactions with Weak Electric and Magnet Fields", Neurosci. Res. Progr. Bull. 15: 1-107 (1977)
16. H. Fröhlich, in Ref. 15: 67-72
17. F. Kaiser, "Limit cycle model for brain waves", Biol. Cybernet. 27: 155 (1977)
18. F. Kaiser, "Coherent oscillations in biological systems", Z. Naturforsch. 33a: 294 (1978)
Z. Naturforsch. 33a: 418 (1978)
19. R. Wever, "The circadian system of man", Springer-Verlag, New York (1979)
R. Wever (private communication, 1981)
20. F. Kaiser, "Coherent modes in Biological Systems, perturbation by external fields", in: "Biological Effects of Nonionizing Radiation", K. Illinger ed., ACS Symp. Series, Washington (in print 1981)
21. G. Nicolis and I. Prigogine, "Self-organization in nonequilibrium systems", I. Wiley, New York (1977)
22. H. Haken, "Synergetics, an Introduction", Springer-Verlag, Berlin (1978).
23. F. Kaiser, Workshop on the "Mechanism of microwave biological effects", University of Maryland, May 1979 (unpublished) Summary in: workshop report, L.S. Taylor and A.Y. Chenng eds., University of Maryland (1980).
24. W.R. Adey, "Models of membranes of cerebral cells as substrates for information storage", Bio. Systems 8: 163 (1977)
25. S.M. Bawin and W.R. Adey in Ref. 15
26. I.T. Grodsky, "Neuronal membrane: A physical synthesis", Math. Biosci. 20: 191 (1976)
27. H. Fröhlich, "Long range coherence and energy storage in biological systems", Int. J. Quant. Chem. 2: 641 (1968)
28. F. Kaiser, "Boltzmann equation approach to Fröhlich's vibrational model", Z. Naturforsch. 34a: 134 (1977)
29. H. Fröhlich, in Ref. 15
30. K. Illinger, Workshop on the "Physical basis of electromagnetic interactions with biological systems", University of Maryland, June (1977)
31. F. Kaiser, Symposium on the "Biological effects of electromagnetic waves", Helsinki, Finland (1978) Radio Science (in print, 1980).

EXPERIMENTAL RF AND MW RESONANT NONTHERMAL EFFECTS

Fritz Keilmann

Max-Planck-Institut für Festkörperforschung
7000 Stuttgart 80
Fed. Rep. Germany

Introduction

There exist a few experiments which show a resonant response of biological systems to an applied radiofrequency or microwave irradiation. In other words, the effects observed in these cases vary distinctly with small changes of the irradiation frequency. Thus the important experimental question arises whether this resonant behavior is either inherent in the biological system, or whether it only reflects a resonant behavior of the employed irradiation system. Of course the latter is not of any fundamental interest. In this lecture I want to point out some theoretical and experimental criteria to solve this question.

A different but closely related problem is centered around the word "nonthermal". Its use without clear definition has sometimes brought confusion to scientific discussions. Let me here try to find its possible meaning, with two aspects in mind: (i) a possibly interesting specific interaction mechanism is invoked from any microwave irradiation effect which cannot be brought about by mere heating of the biological system; (ii) any irradiation of course results in heating of the biological system, but this might not be the most interesting consequence of the irradiation.

As long as the existence of nonthermal biological effects of microwaves stays disputed one should employ the utmost care in (i) keeping the irradiation-induced temperature rise to a minimum, (ii) measuring the temperature and (iii) measuring the temperature dependence of the biological parameter investigated. I will discuss some relevant experimental procedures which in any case will have to fit to the very important biological boundary conditions of cleaning, stirring, nutrition etc.

Microwave irradiation fields are strongly modified by the dielectric response of the biological systems investigated. In many objects it is not possible to obtain spatially resolved measurements of field strength, irradiation intensity and absorbed power density. Theoretical models then have to be employed, using dielectric parameters obtained from spectroscopy. Microwave fields incident on and scattered from biological objects can, however, be measured accurately, and standard procedures as well as methods for stabilizing and measuring frequencies will be mentioned.

Low-Level Electromagnetic Fields

High frequency electromagnetic fields are generally considered "low-level" when the intensities I are below about 10 mW/cm^2. A (plane wave) intensity I corresponds to an oscillating electric field strength $E = (2I/\varepsilon_0 nc)^{1/2}$, where ε_0 is the free space dielectric constant, n is the real part of the refractive index of the material, and c is the vacuum light velocity. Taking n = 9 (for water) we obtain E = 0.65 V/cm for I = 10 mW/cm^2. We can convince ourselves that indeed 10 mW/cm^2 represent a critical intensity if we consider two different types of interaction of the wave with biological matter.

At first we consider rectification of the wave at some hypothetical passive element in the biological object. The maximum d.c. voltage which could possibly be produced is given by $U = E \cdot l$ where l is the effective antenna length associated with the rectifying element. In order to produce any biological action the rectified voltage should at least become comparable to the physiological voltages of 10 or 100 mV which are known to exist across nerve and other membranes, i.e. U > 1 mV /1/. On the other hand the length l is limited by the size of the biological object. If we insert here $l \leq 10$ µm for a typical cell size we come to the conclusion that for such cells it is only above 10 mW/cm^2 where one could imagine that a rectification mechanism could in principle apply.

A second interaction mechanism is heating. Any estimation of the possible temperature rise strongly depends both on the strength of absorption, and on the channels available for cooling. I will come to specific models later, but here I would like to state the production of a resting human adult which is about 70 W. It has been estimated that an additional external heating power of the same amount would increase the average body temperature by about 1^oC which surely is a significant temperature rise. Using 0.7 m^2 for the body surface this heating occurs at an (absorbed) intensity of 10 mW/cm^2.

Heat Loss Mechanisms

As ways of cooling we consider heat conduction and infrared emission. A third possibility would be cooling by evaporation of water which amounts to the substantial value of 10 mW cooling power for just 14 mg water evaporated per hour. Although this may be of considerable interest for special investigations, we rather like to avoid evaporation in well-controlled microbial experiments for its difficult assessment and further consequences. Still notice for reference that the evaporation of water from an open agar-filled petri dish in an incubator at $33^{o}C$ - as I estimate from /2/ - cools the agar surface at the "intensity" of 10 mw/cm^2.

Radiative cooling by infrared emission is governed by the temperature difference ΔT between the surface layer considered and the surroundings. At physiological temperatures the pertaining cooling intensity I is proportional to ΔT at least up to $\Delta T = 10^{o}C$, and also proportional to the infrared emissivity ε of the surface material. With a typical value of $\varepsilon = 0.8$ we have $I = 0.5$ mW/cm^2 ^{o}C. Turned around this means that the maximum temperature rise which can be induced in a biologic specimen (of ε=0.8) by an (absorbed) microwave intensity of 0.5 mW/cm^2 is just $1^{o}C$. If therefore biological effects are observed at incident powers of 10 μW/cm^2, as I will discuss below, we can safely say that the maximum microwave-induced temperature rise is at most $0.02^{o}C$.

A further mechanism is surface cooling by convection of air. In a windstill environment this heat loss is roughly 0.3 mW/cm^2 for a vertical surface $1^{o}C$ warmer than the surrounding air. The effect therefore is an even lower limit to the possible microwave-induced temperature rise just considered, to a value near $0.01^{o}C$.

Let me now turn to heat conduction which helps to equilibrate the temperature inside a biological body should a local heating occur, e.g. by microwave irradiation. I do not intend, however, to cover active mass transport e.g. blood flow and other thermoregulatory mechanisms of highly developed species. Let it suffice to consider as the minimum heat exchange the basic passive heat conduction. Simplifying to the one-dimensional problem with a thermal gradient $\Delta T/\Delta Z$ the heat flow is

$$I = \lambda \cdot \Delta T/\Delta Z \ . \qquad (1)$$

Here λ is the heat conductivity of the medium which is 0.006 W/cm^{o}C for water. Thus a 10 mW/cm^2 heat load on a water surface (e.g. by high frequency microwaves which are absorbed in a thin surface layer) requires a thermal gradient of $1.7^{o}C$ per cm of depth in order to be balanced in a steady state by heat conduction.

Biological materials surely have a different heat conductivity λ compared to water, but the difference is not large so that order-of-magnitude calculations are meaningful. The lowest possible heat conduction occurs in air (λ = 0.0002 W/cm ^{o}C) and materials with air-filled pores (λ = 0.0003 W/cm^{o}C for styrofoam). Any fully condensed medium has, however, a higher conductivity value ranging from 0.002 W/cm ^{o}C for disordered solids and organic liquids up to several W/cm ^{o}C for perfect crystals. Biological cells consist to a great percentage of water, and can ask whether the rest contributes to give a somewhat higher or a somewhat lower overall conductivity than that of pure water. My answer is a likelihood of an increased overall conductivity by the presence of proteins, membranes etc., since these represent well-ordered structures in close contact to water, plus they also are known to increase the degree of order in the solvent water ("bound" and "vicinal" water).

Microscopic Hot Spots (?)

Sometimes it has been hypothesized that "microthermal" mechanisms could play a role when microwave-induced biological effects occur at low irradiation intensities. Heat conduction, however, cools any microscopic hot spot the more efficient the smaller the spot size is. Thus the maximum possible temperature rise becomes extremely small /3/.

Let me illustrate this very important statement with numerical examples. First we assume that we have a microwave intensity I = 10 mW/cm^2. Next we assume that the irradiated biological system somewhere contains a very strong microwave absorber of spherical shape with diameter a. Imagine a cell (a = 1 μm) or a very large molecule (a = 100 Å). Now we assume that the absorbed heating power P quickly equilibrates within the spherical body, but steadily leaks out by heat conduction into the surrounding medium (assumed to be water with λ = 0.006 W/cm ^{o}C). With the arguments from the preceding paragraph we can neglect any thermal barrier effects at the interface, and thus have a simple formula /4/ for the steady-state overtemperature of the absorbing particle in respect to its surrounding

$$\Delta T = A \cdot a^2/(12\lambda) \qquad (2)$$

A is the specific absorption rate in W/cm^3 of the absorber. How high can this possibly be? Using $A = I \cdot \alpha$ where α is the absorption coefficient of the absorber we obtain

$$\Delta T = 0.14\alpha a^2 \qquad (3)$$

(where I = 10mW/cm^2 is already inserted). Let us now try to estimate an upper limit of α which could apply here. From microwave spectroscopy we know that biological molecules, membranes etc. absorb rather weakly, so that $\alpha = 100\ cm^{-1}$ as found for water at millimeter waves should be more than a safe upper limit. Still we add a safety factor of hundred and use $\alpha \leq 10000\ cm^{-1}$ to obtain $\Delta T \leq 1400\ a^2$, i.e. $\Delta T \leq 0.000014^0C$ for even a 1 μm sized entity.

Such ridiculous small temperature differences can not be physiologically significant. Thus I conclude that "microthermal" mechanisms play no role in the low-level microwave biological interactions.

Nonthermal Resonant Effect in Yeast

Out of several experiments showing nonthermal resonant action of microwave irradiation (reviewed in ref.5-7) I only briefly mention our yeast experiment /8/ which is discussed by W. Grundler in detail in chapter X of these proceedings. Here the growth of a liquid culture of 3 μm-sized yeast cells is registered photometrically. The growth rate is significantly influenced by irradiation with low-level microwaves in the (so far tested) frequency range 41.6 to 41.8 GHz, where the effect depends sharply on frequency. For example, we observe growth enhancement at 41.782 ± 0.001 GHz which falls off in a bell-shaped frequency dependence of 0.010 GHz base-line width. Furthermore, the effect does not seem to depend on the irradiation power in the range 3 to 23 mW total applied to about 2 cm^3 of suspension.

For several reasons we believe to have a non-thermal effect here: low-level intensity, efficient cooling by heat conduction, plus non-contacting (time- and spatially-resolved) thermometry using laser interferometry (see below). A further hint excluding simple thermal mechanisms is the occurrence of the very sharp frequency dependence.

We can exclude standing wave resonances in the irradiation system as factors contributing to the very sharp frequency dependence (see below). Further, the fact that the effects are widely independent of irradiation intensity strongly contradicts the assumption of a thermal mechanism in conjunction with standing wave resonances.

Of the constituents of the yeast suspension, water is by far the strongest microwave absorber, giving a penetration depth of 0.02 cm at 42 GHz. The spectral dependence of water absorption is absolutely flat on the scale of the observed growth resonances, so that the site of the resonant interaction has to be located somewhere in the biological (molecular) structure. A great mystery from the standpoint of solid state spectroscopy remains the extremely narrow linewidth of 10 MHz /6,7/; only non-linear oscillator models /7,9/ seem to allow for narrow (vibrational) resonances in condensed environments.

With the small penetration depth of 0.02 cm the irradiation field is strongly inhomogeneous in the yeast suspension. Even with the large antenna surface of about 10 cm^2 /8/ only 10% of the cells are nominally exposed to more than 1/e of the input intensity at a given time. Mechanical stirring, however, assures that each cell passes through a high field region every few seconds. It is very remarkable then that we observe a flat dependence of the effects on radiation intensity. This may point to the existence of a very small threshold intensity, as e.g. was observed in /10/ at 10 $\mu W/cm^2$. Note also that Webb's early experiment /11/ was done at 7 $\mu W/cm^2$.

Transmission Line Resonances

In an irradiation experiment waves can be partly reflected from the sample (reflectivity R_1) at one end, and at some element, e.g. the source itself, on the other end of the transmission line (R_2). The result is a partially standing wave which changes the power delivered to the sample by a factor up to $q = 1 + 4f^2/\pi^2$ where f is the finesse $f = \pi(R_1R_2)^{1/4}/(1-(R_1R_2)^{1/2})$. In our experiment /8/ we have as upper limits $R_1 < 0.6$ (from dielectric values of teflon and water), $R_2 < 0.1$ (mismatch at isolator), thus $f < 2.1$ and therefore a power enhancement factor of only $q < 1.8$. Furthermore, the power enhancement occurs over resonant widths of $\Gamma = c/2lf$ where c is the phase velocity and l the distance between the reflectors.

Such transmission line resonances can routinely be monitored with the help of directional couplers and detectors, as was done in our continuation of the earlier yeast experiments /8/. Resonant widths of $\Gamma < 100$ MHz were not detected in our apparatus. For single-frequency irradiation experiments the reflection of the sample can be greatly diminished by using a monomode transmission line and a matching transformer.

Frequency Measurement

The sharp frequency dependence such as observed in the yeast experiments /8/ calls for high precision in frequency stabilization and measurement. One of the prerequisites is sufficient isolation of the source to prevent frequency pulling effects from a changing load, i.e. reflection from the object irradiated. Usually a small part of the wave is coupled off for frequency measurement. The precision of tunable cavity frequency meters is not quite adequate /8/ and heterodyne methods have to be used. For the 42 GHz region we found that two types of sources, backward wave oscillators and klystrons, show large frequency drifts so that active frequency stabilization is required. Phase locking to a quartz standard is easily obtained with klystrons, yielding an absolute frequency stability of ± 1 kHz.

Backward wave tubes are less stable and only marginal locking is achieved, resulting in an output spectrum with up to 1 MHz width at 42 GHz.

Non-Contacting Laser Thermometry

Temperature measurement in the presence of microwave radiation is difficult since the fields become distorted e.g. by metallic or ionic conductors. Liquid crystal probes offer partial solution where relatively large spatial (~ 1 mm), temporal (~ 1 sec) and temperature resolution (~ 0.3^{o}C) are sufficient, and where the presence of an invasive probe causes no biological problems. Laser interferometry in contrast offers a higher resolution thermometry in respect to space, time and temperature /12,13/ with the great advantage of being non-contacting.

The method uses the temperature-dependent change of the optical refractive index, which is 10^{-4} $^{o}C^{-1}$ (at the wavelength 633 nm of the HeNe laser) for water near 30°C. An interferometric optical setup is employed to measure the phase of the transmitted light which directly relates to the average temperature along the line of sight. With the high sensitivity of light detectors the laser intensity can be kept small enough to avoid any heating even with coloured aqueous suspensions. The presence of light-scattering particles, e.g. yeast cells, in the suspension, and the rapid stirring of such a suspension does not hinder the optical phase measurement.

The laser thermometer is routinely used to monitor the temperature stability and the absorbed microwave power in our newly developed multichannel photometer-nephelometer /14/. This instrument allows measurement of microbial growth curves with high precision, on up to eight cultures simultaneously. A HeNe laser with a beam width of 1 mm is used to measure the optical transmission of stirred suspensions in standard photometer cuvettes. A small residual reflection at the two glass/suspension interfaces suffices to impose a faint optical standing wave interference on the transmitted beam. While this is too small to interfere with the transmission measurement, it can be suitably amplified to reveal the temperature of the suspension. An example with 1 cm of liquid pathlength, which gives a temperature resolution of about 0.01^{o}C, is shown in Fig. 1. Apart from just measuring the temperature this information can readily be used to monitor the actually absorbed microwave power; the method here even is self-calibrating since the thermal time constant of the cuvette can be directly read from the trace after the on or off points (Fig. 1).

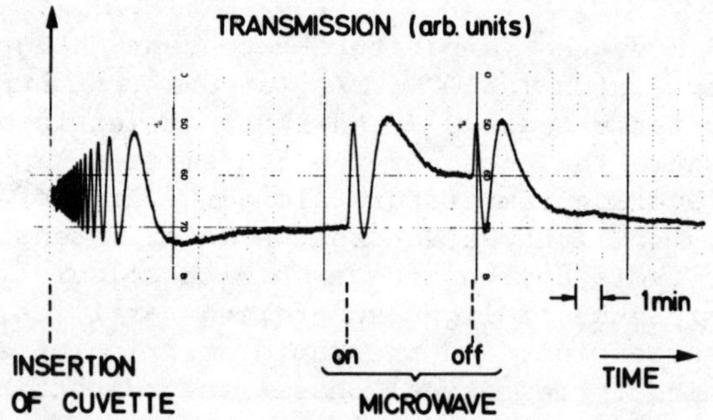

Fig.1. Non-contacting laser-interferometric thermometry on strongly stirred yeast suspension. The trace is the strongly expanded signal of the laser photometer showing optical interferences in accord to temperature changes (0.183°C/fringe). At first the temperature of the inserted cuvette stabilizes at the temperature of the photometer (31°C). Then c.w. microwave power is applied (81 mW absorbed) and leads to an enhanced steady-state temperature of 31.31°C fully reversible after switching off.

Inhomogeneous Intensity Distributions

With the strong absorption of high frequency microwaves in water a homogeneous irradiation intensity is only possible if one uses, e.g. a thin planar layer of suspension with a thickness somewhat smaller than one penetration depth (0.02 cm at 42 GHz). A practical design of such a cuvette was developed by us /13/, featuring a semipermeable membrane for gas exchange on one surface, and a single crystal sapphire wall for efficient thermal contact to a water bath on the other.

With the yeast experiment /8/ some field inhomogeneity was accepted in order to obtain access for the photometer beam and for the mechanical stirrer. Coupling of the microwave occurs through a fork-shaped teflon structure which has a surface of about 10 cm^2. Of course we cannot expect a constant irradiation intensity over this surface, but rather expect a certain partially standing wave pattern inside the teflon structure. Locally, up to about three times higher or lower intensities can be expected in respect to the average as calculated from a reflection coefficient $R_1 = R_2 = 0.5$. This pattern should, however, not vary noticeably on a tuning of the frequency over all our spectrum investigated /8/, i.e. 41.6 to 41.8 GHz, since the actual dimensions of our structure are rather small, of the order of a few wavelengths only.

The actual effective radiating interface can be visualized experimentally, again by laser interferometry. The principle is that after a short powerful microwave irradiation a two-dimensional interferogram is photographed. The temperature distribution obtained is identical with the initial microwave intensity distribution.

We verified the possibility of such a photography of an inhomogeneous field distribution with our teflon antenna of ref. /8/. As shown in Fig. 2, we used a Mach-Zehnder configuration, together with a HeNe laser and a polaroid camera. Fig. 3 shows the image (a) obtained without any microwave heating. In the central, 4 mm wide space between the teflon legs as well as in the left space between teflon and glass wall the field appears grey indicating neither totally destructive nor constructive interference of the sampling and reference light fields. The interference field is less uniform on the right side due to imperfect optics. Photograph (b) is taken after microwave exposure and clearly shows marked phase changes. With 1 cm pathlength in the water, one full interference fringe is expected for a temperature change of $0.63^{\circ}C$. Thus the maximum phase shift of roughly 1000° (2.8 fringes) has taken place just below the apex between the teflon legs, equivalent to a heating by $1.75^{\circ}C$. At a position of 6 mm below the apex, the heating is about $0.8^{\circ}C$ on the right and $0.6^{\circ}C$ on the left inner surface of the teflon leg.

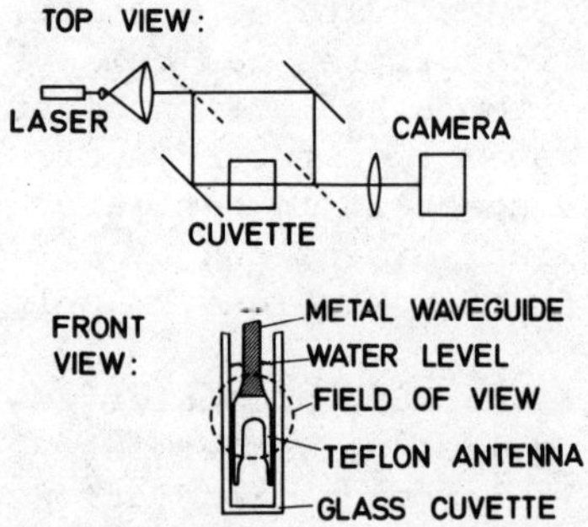

Fig.2 Schematic view of Mach-Zehnder interferometer capable of highly resolved temperature or irradiation intensity measurement. The arrow gives the orientation of the electrical field of the incoming microwave (Fig. 3b).

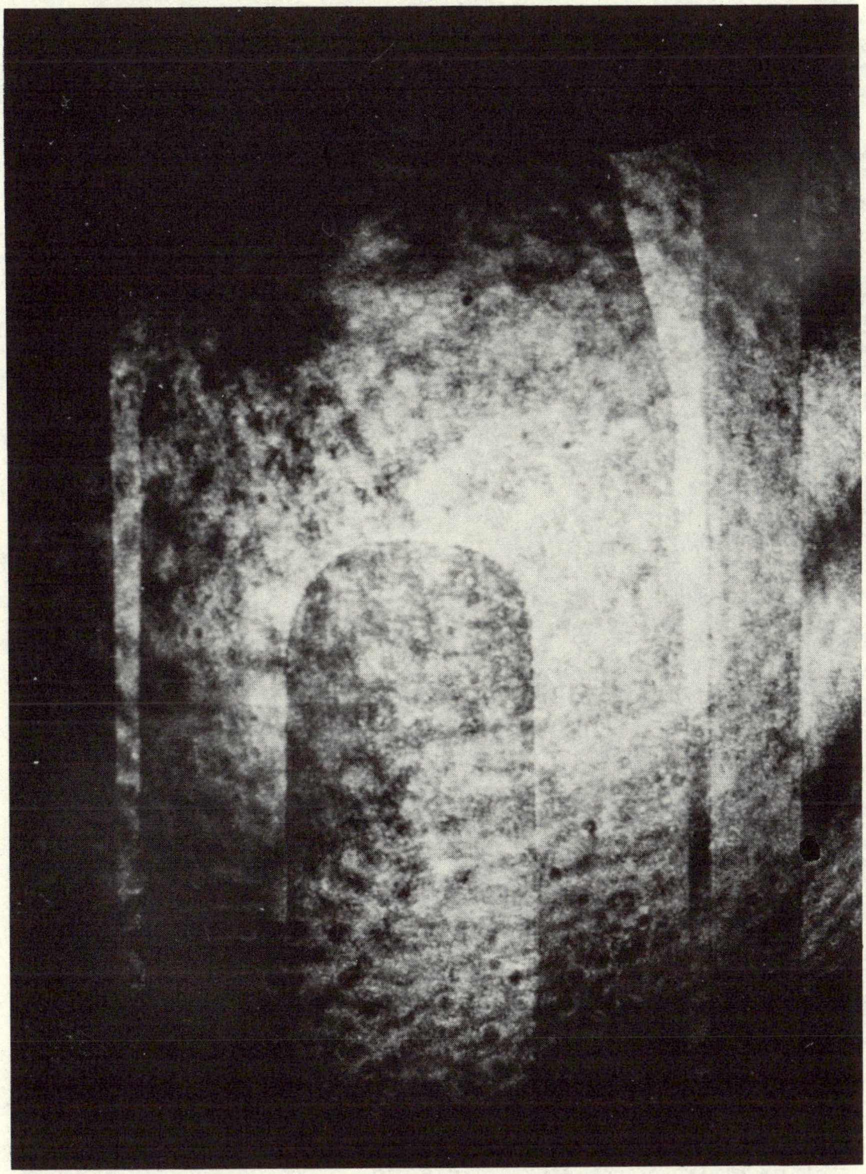

(a)

Fig. 3. Optical interferograms of water-filled glass cuvette without mechanical stirring. The teflon antenna is inserted as in the yeast experiments /8/. a - before irradiation. b - immediately after 3 sec of irradiation with a high-power klystron at 42 GHz, absorbed power 300 mW.

(continued)

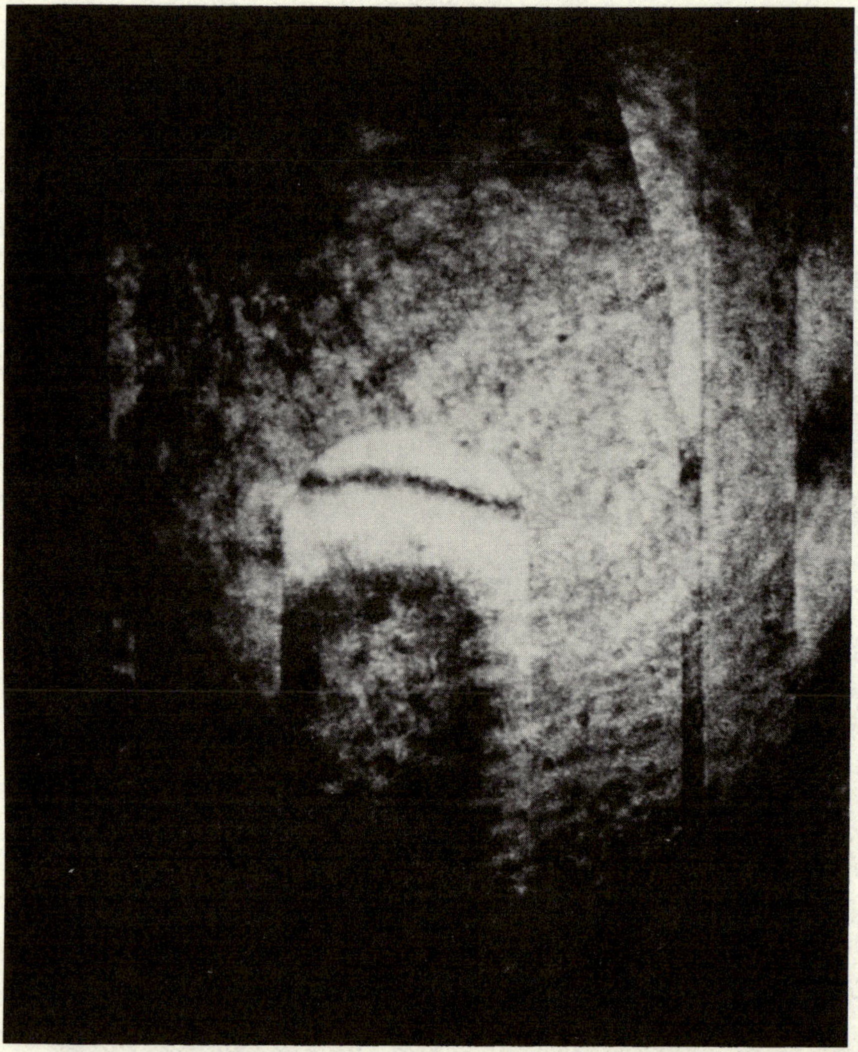

(b)

It is a pity that for these studies we did not have a still more powerful source at our disposal. For this reason we could not keep the microwave exposure time (3 sec here) shorter than the thermal time constant of about 0.1 sec with which thermal conduction diffuses an initial temperature gradient on the scale length of the microwave penetration depth (0.2 mm) in water. This means that the information on the original field distribution is lost, as far as the scale length of 0.2 mm is concerned. However, structures of at least 1 to 2 mm scale length are not fully smeared out by heat conduction in 3 sec. Therefore, the analysis of Fig. 3b can still give the very important information on how the intensity is distributed along the teflon/water interface. The result is indeed that sizeable irradiation occurs on any part of the interface, with no prominent hot spots visible. In our analysis we did not mention water convection. In fact this influence can not be fully neglected at 3 sec, as interferograms at longer exposures show: convection helps to raise the temperature just under the apex.

The same setup was used to measure possible temperature differences in the suspension with the mechanical stirring in action. The result is that no phase inhomogeneity remains observable at 300 mW power. From this we conclude that for usual conditions with 40 mW absorbed power, 0.02^{o}C is the maximum possible temperature difference between any points in the suspension, including the boundary layer at the teflon which we could observe with about 100 μm spatial resolution.

Acknowledgements

This work was developed in close collaboration with W. Grundler (Neuherberg) and the members of the microwave biology group in Stuttgart, F. Drissler, L. Genzel, F. Kremer and L. Santo. Financial support by the Deutsche Forschungsgemeinschaft is acknowledged.

Addendum

The non-contacting laser thermometry discussed in this paper was specifically developed for our millimeter-wave irradiation experiments of cell cultures. In addition, however, this method can be extended and probably find useful application in the general dosimetry of microwave exposure of laboratory animals and man.

In this field one desires to obtain a quantitative assessment of the distribution of absorbed power density or SAR within a model body. The proposal is now to construct such a model out of visibly transparent material, e.g. a water gel, and use a visible laser light to obtain holograms of this body just before and after microwave exposure. By optically subtracting these images all optical irregularities of the body are compensated, and one obtains an interference distribution solely given by the microwave induced heating. Such a hologram allows a convenient reading out of the microwave induced temperature rise at any desired point in the model body.

REFERENCES

1. F.S. Barnes and C.J. Hu, Model for Some Nonthermal Effects of Radio and Microwave Fields on Biological Membranes, IEEE Trans. MTT-25, 742 (1977).

2. M. Dardalhon, D. Averbeck and A.J. Berteaud, Determination of a Thermal Equivalent of Millimeter Microwaves in Living Cells, J. Micr. Power 14, 307 (1979).

3. F. Keilmann, Techniques in Microwave Studies, Collective Phen., 3, 169 (1981).

4. H.S. Carslaw and J.C. Jaeger, Conduction of Heat in Solids, Clarendon Press, Oxford 1971.

5. S.L. Arber, Cell and Molecular Effects and Mechanisms of Action of Microwave Electromagnetic Fields on Biological Systems, Electron. Obrab. Mater. USSR 3, 59 (1978), translated in Electrochem. Industr. Process. Biology.

6. F. Keilmann, Nonthermal Microwave Resonances in Living Cells, in Coherence in Spectroscopy and Modern Physics, F.T. Arecchi, R. Bonifacio, M.O. Scully eds., Plenum Corp., New York 1978.

7. H. Fröhlich, The Biological Effects of Microwaves and Related Questions, in Advances in Electronics and Electron Physics, Vol. 53, pp. 85-152 (1980).

8. W. Grundler, F. Keilmann and H. Fröhlich, Resonant Growth Rate Response of Yeast Cells Irradiated by Weak Microwaves, Phys. Lett. 62A, 463 (1977); W. Grundler and F. Keilmann, Nonthermal Effects of Millimeter Microwaves on Yeast Growth, Z. Naturforsch. 33c, 15 (1978).

9. F. Kaiser, Coherent Oscillations in Biological Systems, Z. Naturforsch. 33a, 294 and 418 (1978).

10. A.Z. Smolyanskaya and R.L. Vilenskaya, Effects of Millimeter-band Radiation on the Functional Activity of Certain Genetic Elements of Bacterial Cells, Sov. Phys.-Usp. 16, 571 (1974).

11. S.J. Webb and D.D. Dodds, Inhibition of Bacterial Cell Growth by 136 gc Microwaves, Nature 218, 374 (1968).

12. C.C. Davis and M. Swicord, Studies of Microwave Absorption in Liquids by Optical Heterodyne Detection of Thermally Induced Refractive Index Fluctuations, submitted to Radio Science (1979).

13. F. Keilmann and W. Grundler, Irradiation Systems for Studying Nonthermal Biological Effects of High Frequency Microwaves , Symp. Electromagnetic Waves and Biology, Jouy-en-Josas 1980.

14. F. Keilmann, D. Böhme and L. Santo, Multichannel Photometer-Nephelometer, Appl. Envir. Microbiology 40, 458 (1980).

BIOLOGICAL EFFECTS OF RF AND MW ENERGY AT MOLECULAR AND CELLULAR LEVEL

W. Grundler

Gesellschaft für Strahlen- und Umweltforschung mbH
Institut für Angewandte Physik
8042 Neuherberg, F.R. Germany

1. INTRODUCTION

Primary interaction between absorbed RF and MW energy and biological material takes place at the molecular and cellular levels. Biomolecules or assemblies of molecules are thought to be influenced by these external fields. These disturbances can be studied, for instance as effects on metabolism or regulation. The cell, as the smallest self reproducing unit, offers a great possibility for studying RF and MW effects as most biological mechanisms are involved in growth and cell division. Therefore, experimental studies on this level are both possible and necessary for investigating the basic mechanisms of biological interaction of ELM-wave energy.

The aim, however, of all investigations on objects ranging from cells to animals and humans seems to be to determine the causal chain from the primary energy absorption event through molecular, cellular and tissue reactions to the influence on a whole living body. But within this microscopic view of events and biomolecular reactions it is impossible - in my opinion - to bridge this gap at any time, as can be seen from the lack of this understanding in the field of ionizing radiation after 50 years of research. On the contrary, one should endeavour to establish general rules for the dependence of the biological test effect on the physical parameters used. If, for instance, the influence of a spectrum of frequencies or the behaviour of the effect in correlation to different power levels are known, a comparison to experiments of strongly varying biological levels is already possible. The knowledge of such macroscopic correlations is of important significance for both (i) the establishment and assessment of standards and (ii) the application and development of theoretical models, which in strong connection with experimental results may point the direction to the biological mechanisms involved.

In spite of many interesting RF and MW effects reported on the molecular and cellular level /1, 2, 3/, I will review only a few experiments, from which one can, to some extent, conclude a general aspect of the influence of the radiation. Then I would like to report on the present state of yeast experiments. Before starting, I have to comment on a second restriction concerning the running title of this lecture.

The majority of research performed in the past has concerned the effects of radiation fields of intensities which were high enough to produce heating in biological specimens. These mechanisms are well understood and documented /4, 5, 6, 7/. At present a very interesting branch of scientific work is developing in which low-intensity biological effects are investigated, especially within the microwave region of the ELM-wave spectrum /8, 9, 10, 11, 12/. Such effects, if different than expected from the temperature increase by the mean absorbed power, have to be tested in respect to the irradiation system and measuring system employed. Thus, the important question arises of whether this behaviour reflects either temperature inhomogenities within the experimental set-up or whether it is inherent in the biological system. The latter is, of course, of fundamental interest, in respect to the understanding of biology in a general sense. It may be that there is a key for solving questions concerned with biological organisation and information transport. The importance of such low level electromagnetic field experiments, on the other hand, concerns the lack of adequate physical laws for the description of this interaction. New models and theoretical considerations which are being developed /13, 14, 15, 16/ have to hold close contact to such experimental results.

Therefore, this lecture will report on molecular and cellular effects of low intensity microwaves, especially on the present state of yeast growth experiments.

2. EXPERIMENTS ON MOLECULAR AND CELLULAR BIOLOGICAL EFFECTS OF LOW INTENSITY MICROWAVES

The search for microwave biological effects, especially low level effects, should be accompanied by a systematic variation of the important independent parameters, like frequency, power flux density and irradiation time, because of (i) the possible discovery of common characteristics when investigating different biological endpoints and (ii) the existence of possibly further experimental facts for the determination of a "nonthermal" effect.

A strong frequency-dependent response, especially in a resonant form of the biological system points to special mechanisms not compatible with thermal origin. Such a dependence is not expected when the frequency-dependent absorption coefficient of water is taken into account, which shows an unstructured, flat behaviour in the millimeter wave region.

A non-linear dependence of the observed effects on intensity may also indicate an additional "non-thermal" influence. A microwave penetrating into a medium like water, the most absorbent component in a biological system, looses energy to it, which in the realm of linear response, is proportional to the intensity of the radiation. As a consequence, an increase in temperature must arise under stationary conditions proportional to the absorbed intensity.

2.1 Microwave biological effects on mammalian cells in vivo and in vitro

A great effort to determine low level microwave biological effects in the frequency range from 39 to 60 GHZ has been conducted in the USSR. Results have been reported on a dozen different experiments at different locations /10/. As an example, we reproduce the results by Sevastyanova and Vilenskaya /17/. The investigations deal with damage to bone marrow cells of mice arising from exposure to X-rays and the protecting effect of microwave irradiation. When prior irradiation with microwaves has taken place, then at certain frequencies and intensities the damage is vastly reduced.

In. Fig. 1 the reduction of X-ray damaged bone marrow cells from about one half to about 80 % survival by prior microwave irradiation of certain selected frequencies is demonstrated. No effect exists, however, at certain other frequencies.

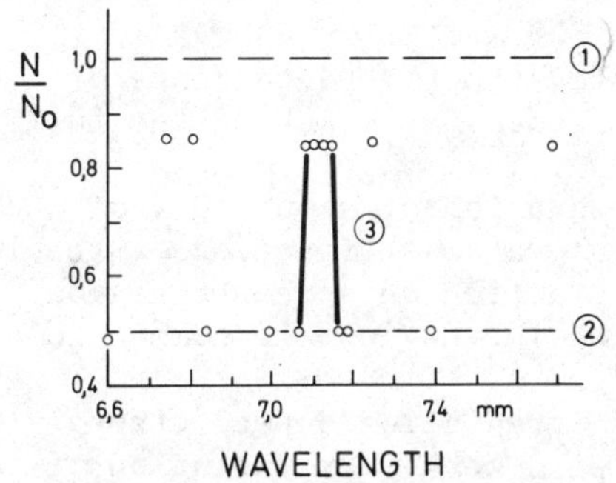

Fig. 1 Dependence of the relative number of bone marrow cells N/No on the wave length of the radiation. (N: number of surviving cells, No: number of cells without radiation; 1: control; 2: X-ray irradiated; 3: X-ray and millimeter wave irradiated) (Sevastyanova and Vilenskaya /17/)

Fig. 2 shows the dependence of this effect on intensity when microwave radiation of 7.1 mm wave length is applied. Below 9.9mW/cm^2 the effect is not be observed, at 10mW/cm^2 it reaches its maximum stepwise and remains constant for higher intensities up to a factor of 8.

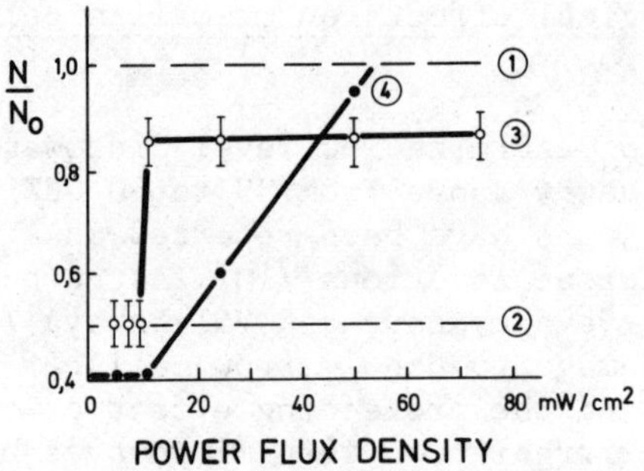

Fig. 2 Dependence of the relative number of bone morrow cells on the microwave power flux density (1: control; 2: relative number of X-ray irradiated cells; 3: when irradiated with X-ray and microwaves; 4: change Δt of skin temperature as function of millimeter wave intensity) (Sevastyanova and Vilenskaya /17/)

Fig. 3 demonstrates the time dependence of the effect. 60 min of irradiation are needed for reaching the full response.

Because of on absorption of about 70 % of the MW-irradiation by the skin /17/, only a small fraction of the 10mW/cm^2 will penetrate for direct action on a deeper region.

Similar experimental behaviour is common to a greater part of the results of /10/.

- The effects of irradiation depend strongly on frequency,
- the effects depend weakly on variation of power used through several orders of magnitude,
- the effects depend significantly on time of irradiation.

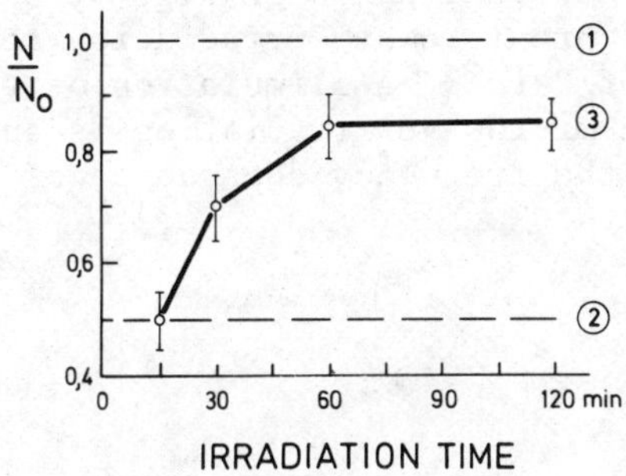

Fig. 3 Dependence of the number of bone marrow cells on the duration of MW-irradiation (1: control; 2: X-ray irradiated; 3: X-ray and millimeter-wave irradiated) (Sevastyanova and Vilenskaya /17/

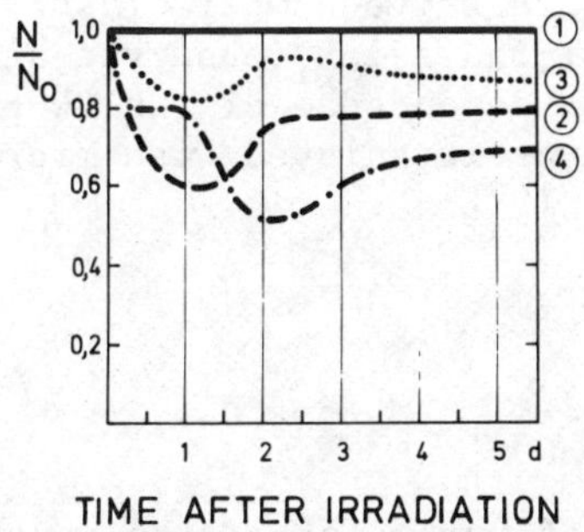

Fig. 4 Dependence of the relative number $\frac{N}{No}$ of bone marrow cells on time after X-ray irradiation (N: number of surviving bone marrow cells; No: number of cells without radiation; 1:control; 2: X-ray irradiation; 3: MW and X-ray irradiation; 4: X-ray and MW-irradiation)

A further in vivo experiment on bone marrow cells in mice is reported by Sevastyanova /18/ where the synergistic effects of X-rays or chemicals and MW-irradiation are analysed.

If one compares curves 2 and 3 in fig. 4, one recognizes a protecting effect of premicrowave irradiation to X-ray radiation damage by a factor of 2 to 3. A stimulation of the damage, however, can be observed when microwave irradiation is applied afterwards. Fig. 5 demonstrates the frequency dependence of the effects.

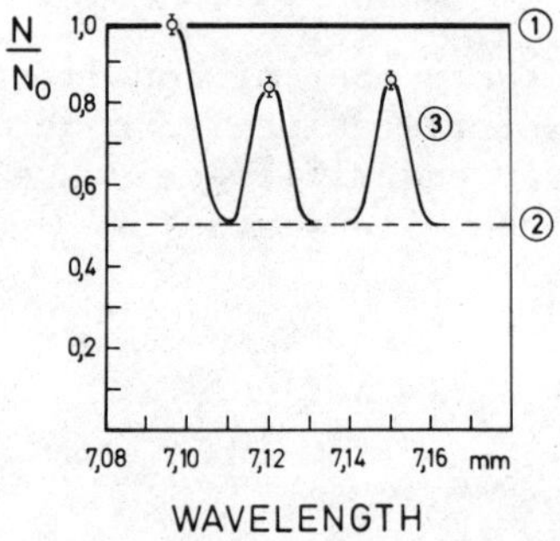

Fig. 5 1: control; 2: relative number of surviving bone marrow cells after X-irradiation (observed at a certain day after irradiation) 3: dependence of the MW-protecting effect on frequency when preirradiated with microwaves (Sevastyanova /18/)

A stepwise change of wavelength (step-width 0.01 mm) within the range of 7.095 mm to 7.16 mm, corresponding to a vacuum frequency interval from 42283 MHz to 41899 MHz, shows again a strong dependence of the protecting effect on frequency. The effect is observed at four frequencies, but vanishes at the four other ones producing a resonance-like structure.

Another interesting microwave effect at the molecular level in leukemia cells in vitro showing a strong low intensity dependence is reported by Chang, Huang and Joines (1980) /19/. They found a change in uptake and action of Methotrexate (MTX) after preirradiation of these cells by 1 GHz microwaves and a synergistic effect of microwave irradiation and MTX treatment, when testing the inhibition of DNA syntesis. In cancer chemotherapy, where MTX is

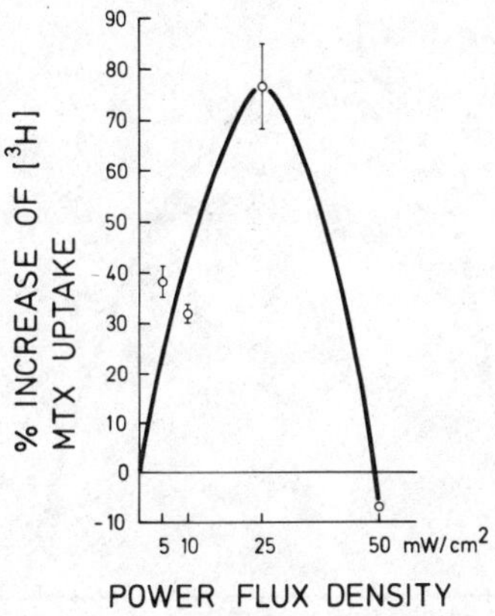

Fig. 6 Dependence of the relative increase of $|^3H|$MTX uptake of microwave irradiated and nonirradiated L 1210 leukemia cells on the power flux density of radiation; (bars: S.E. of 4 independent experiments). (From Chang et al., /19/)

used as an antitumor agent, toxicity to normal tissue should be relatively small. An alternative new approach could be the enhancement of the drug uptake by microwave preirradiation. MTX enters the cells by active transport and inhibits there the de novo DNA synthesis by affecting the conversion of desoxyuridine to thymidine before its incorporation into DNA.

MTX uptake is measured by determination of the absorbed radioactive content of the ^{3}H-labeled drug within irradiated and nonirradiated cells of an in vitro culture of leukemia cells harvested from a mouse.

The relative increase of $|^3H|$MTX uptake in dependence of different power densities used is seen in fig. 6.

The effect increases up to 78 % in an intensity range of 5 to 25^{mW}/cm^2. At the 50^{mW}/cm^2 level a decrease is observed, whereas the temperature of the suspension increases to 37.4° C, a value close to 37° C where the optimal condition for metabolic processes is achieved. The intensity dependence of MTX uptake shows the quite interesting behaviour of a window effect. To determine whether the same, observation holds for the proposed influence on DNA synthesis, the inhibition of $|^3H|$-labeled deoxyuridine uptake was tested afterwards and demonstrated in fig. 7.

Here the inverted-U relationship of the effect is demonstrated as the power density increased.

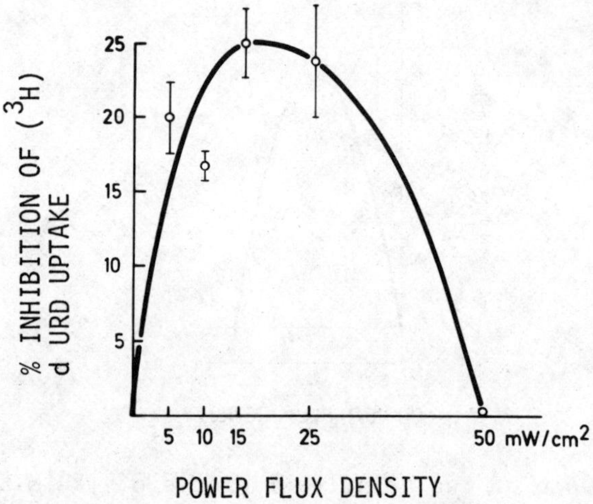

Fig. 7 Dependence of the relative inhibition of $|^3H|$dUrd uptake of microwave irradiated and nonirradiated L 1210 leukemia cells on the power flux density of radiation; (bars: S.E. of 4 independent experiments) (From Chang et al., /19/)

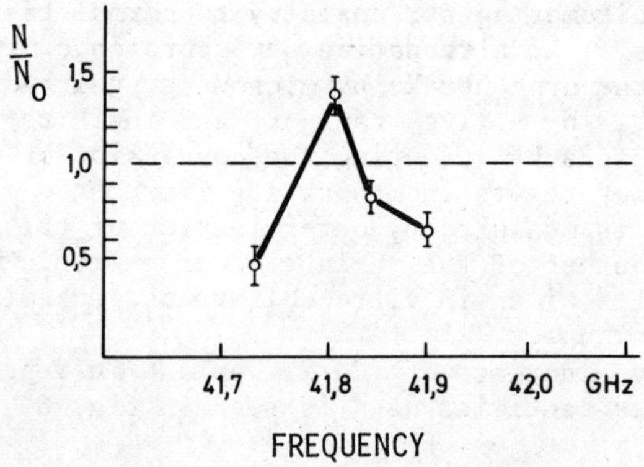

Fig. 8. Relative dependence of yeast cell growth rate on microwave frequency. From Devyatkov et al. /10/. Each point represents the mean of 10 experiments

Additionally, the authors report on a combined effect of drug and MW-radiation. DNA synthesis is reduced by a factor of nearly 0.8 compared with the control by MW-irradiation alone, by 0.6 due to MTX treatment and by 0.5 due to the combination of both.

2.2 Low intensity microwave effects on yeast cells

Entering this field some years ago, our experiment on yeast growth influenced by weak microwave radiation was suggested by results on yeast cells (*Rhodotorula rubra*) reported in /10/. Fig. 8 shows the influence of four different frequencies on cell division rate, where stimulation by one frequency and a depression by the other three points to a sharp frequency dependence of growth behaviour.

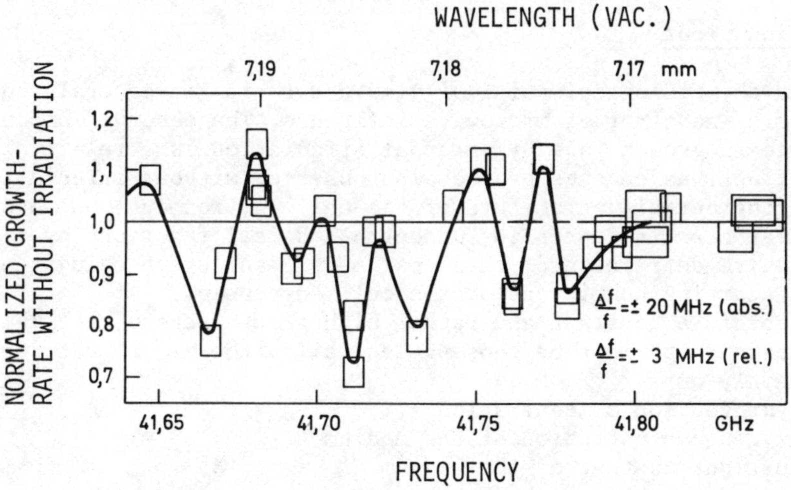

Fig. 9 Relative growth rate of yeast cells in dependence on microwave frequency. The full line is drawn by hand (Grundler and Keilmann /11/)

Due to these results we investigated growth rate dependence of *Saccharomyces cerevisiae* on frequencies near 41.8 GHz and found very remarkable effects (fig. 9). At certain frequencies the growth rate remains unchanged, others cause an increase of up to 12 % of the normalized and temperature corrected growth rate or a reduction of the effect up to 29 %. But the most interesting fact is the occurence of a multiplet of resonances between 41.64 and 41.79 GHz, each of them having a resonance linewidth of only about 10 MHz.

Because of the possibly far-reaching consequences of the existence of such low intensity microwave effects, it is important to confirm these experimental results. Before taking further steps in the analysis of certain relevant physical and biological parameters, we report here on our ongoing work of repeating the earlier experiments with higher precision. This report is also preliminary as some parameters which may influence the dependent variable observed have not yet been varied.

Before reporting our recent results, the experimental procedures should be roughly described in a way that techniques already reported /11/ are summarized and the improvements of the set-up are given in more detail. Growth behaviour of the cells, microwave technique and cell density measurements should be discused.

Growth behaviour

From the biological point of view growth is, in general, an inspecific indicator of microwave influence. The observed amount of change in growth rate by external irradiation is a relatively small effect. As changes can be also observed without irradiation by altering certain parameters of the cell environment, one has to take great care in depressing uncontrolled cell reactions by a quantitative definition of these parameters and by choosing the correct starting conditions of the cell suspension.

To obtain a constant and rather high growth rate μ, optimal growth parameters must be chosen. Generally, the growth rate depends mainly on

- hydrogen ion concentration
- oxygen concentration of the medium
- nutrient content of the medium
- temperature.

Yeast cells growing exponentially in a batch culture of glucose concentration used, change the hydrogen-ion concentration from pH = 6.1 to pH = 4.4 corresponding to the dissociation of keto-carbonacids produced by the cell during the disintegration of aminoacids. In our experiments this reduction stops at pH = 4.8. There is no uncontrolled influence on growth, because within a range of pH = 6.5 to pH = 4.5 growth rate rises to a maximum value and remains nearly constant.

Aerobically multiplying cells need oxygen. The respiration rate of the used strain is 2.5×10^{-16} mol/(cell · min). The oxygen intake was calculated to be 10^{-6} mol corresponding to a gas volume of 0.02 cm^3 per cm^3 of our aqueous culture growing exponentially for 5 h. Oxygen depletion was therefore not likely to be reached.

The nutrient content of the 2.5 ml medium offered by the measuring cuvette is sufficient for optimal growth conditions of the maximum number of 10^8 cells. Estimating the nutrient for these cells one needs (i) 0.16 ml medium for providing a sufficient amount of glucose and (ii) 0.27 ml medium for delivering the sufficient yeast extract, which acts as the growth limiting factor of the batch culture.

Dependence of the growth rate on temperature was defined without irradiation between 31° C and 34° C (fig. 10).

The result is a relative increase of 2.7 % per °C at T = 31° C, slowing down to 1.9 % per °C at T = 33° C.

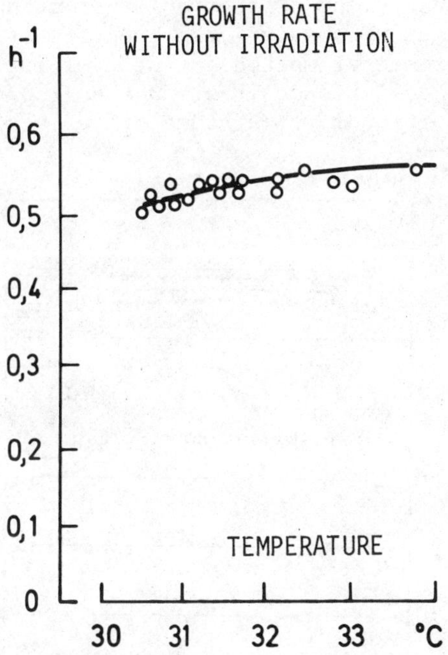

Fig. 10 Dependence of the growth rate of yeast cells on temperature.

Using thermostabilized cuvette housings in the photometers a long term temperature stability is achieved of both control cuvette within a range of 30.7 ± 0.1° C and the irradiated sample where the temperature rose up to 31° C at a maximum absorbed microwave power of 34 mW. The resolution of temperature measurements is better than 0.03° C (see fig. 11). Therefore, no additional temperature correction had to be performed.

<u>Microwave system</u>

A crystal controlled frequency standard holds for a very small systematic error in frequency (< 1 kHz) stabilizing a local oscillator, the third harmonic of which is mixed with the backward wave tube frequency (BWO 60, Siemens). A phase locked stabilisation by a Micro Now stabilizer results in a source wave stabilized at a constant frequency with an uncertainty of ± 1 MHz on an absolute scale (in /11/: ± 3 MHz on a relative and ± 20 MHz on an absolute scale).

The microwave power absorbed ranges now from 6 to 34 mW and can be measured by two methods: (i) as the difference between the power of the wave running forward and backward in the waveguide and (ii) by determining the small increase in temperature (up to 0.5° C), caused by microwave heating within the sample cuvette built as a calorimeter and thermostatted by water. The thermal coupling of the irradiated cuvette is made in such a way that it allows the exact measurement of the radiation induced temperature rise without giving up a comparatively good temperature long term stability. The experimental method for determining both the temperature of the two cell suspensions and the absorbed power by registrating a proportional temperature difference τ shows fig. 11.

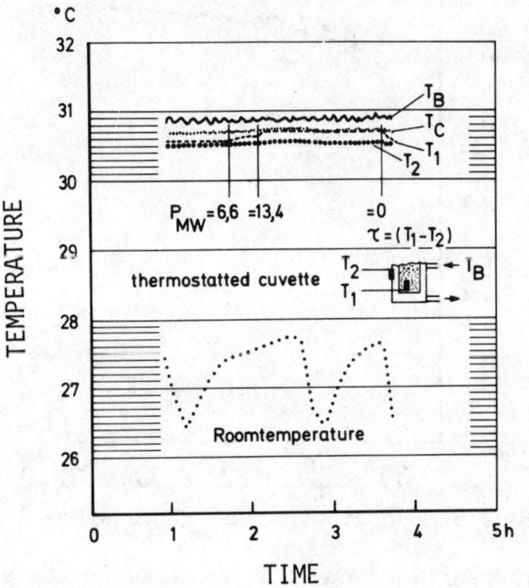

Fig. 11 Plotter trace of differently registrated temperatures. (T_B:thermostatted bath; Tc: control cuvette; T_1: surface of the irradiated cuvette; T_2: cuvette housing; $\tau=(T_1-T_2)$ is proportional to the absorbed microwave power)

The mean absorbed power is achieved by $P_{abs} = 84 \cdot \tau$ |mW| if τ in °C is inserted and the temperature of the irradiated cell suspension is defined by $T = T_2 + 1.32 \cdot \tau$. The numerical factors are achieved by special cooling experiments. It should be noted that this method allows the direct recognition of standing wave resonances.

The coupling of the microwave occurs through a submerged dielectric antenna (teflon), fork-shaped, which has a surface of about 10 cm^2 for maximizing the irradiated volume. The intensity distribution by this antenna and correlated problems are discussed by F. Keilmann in detail in a further chapter of these proceedings.

Measurements of growth

Light scattering is used to measure the growing cell concentration by observation of the extinction of a transmitted light beam of 550 nm wavelength. By this method the cell number is quite well measured as long as the volume distribution of the cells remains constant. In comparison to the former reported technique /11/ for achieving a higher accuracy we use two photometers, where irradiation and control experiments can now be performed simultaneously rather than sequentially. In both double-beam photometers two glas cuvettes of (1x1) cm^2 internal cross section were inserted, one filled by medium (2.5 ml) and the other one by the cell suspension. Extinction due to the presence of yeast cells was then defined by $E = -\log I/I_o$, where I is the transmitted light intensity and I_o the incident one. Figure 12a shows a typical recorder trace of the yeast cells extinction vs time. By the use of a logarithmic amplifier the well known growth curves are replotted on

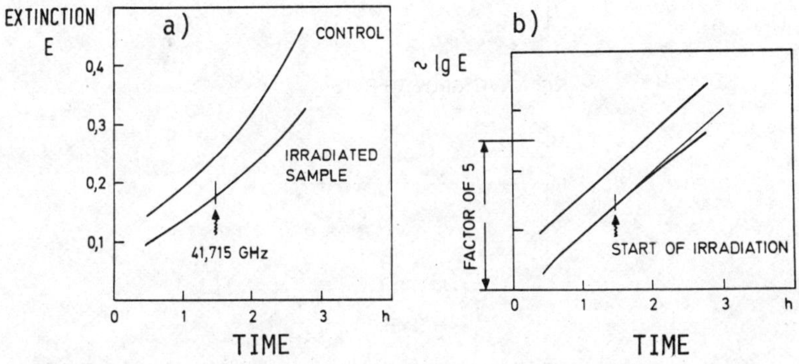

Fig. 12 a) Recorder trace of yeast cell extinction vs time of unirradiated and microwave irradiated cells;
b) logarithmic plot.

a logarithmic scale as shown in fig. 12b. The slope of the straight line of the traces represents the growth rate μ, where $\ln E \sim \ln N(t) = \mu t$ ($N(t)$ is the cell density at time t). The upper trace serves for control. Also that part of the logarithmic extinction curve, which is recorded before the time of switching on the microwave power, serves for control purpose. A parallel slope of both traces indicates the absence of disturbing influences so as infection or chemical poisoning.

Results and Discussion

In order to investigate microwave irradiation effects within the frequency range of 41640 MHz and 41835 MHz we performed 83 growth experiments. We received a group of control data (fig. 13) and of growth rate values influenced by the irradiation (fig. 14). The growth rates of the unirradiated controls (measured within a temperature interval of ± 0.1° C) were found to be reproducible with a small scatter of ± 4 % on a relative scale i.e. when the

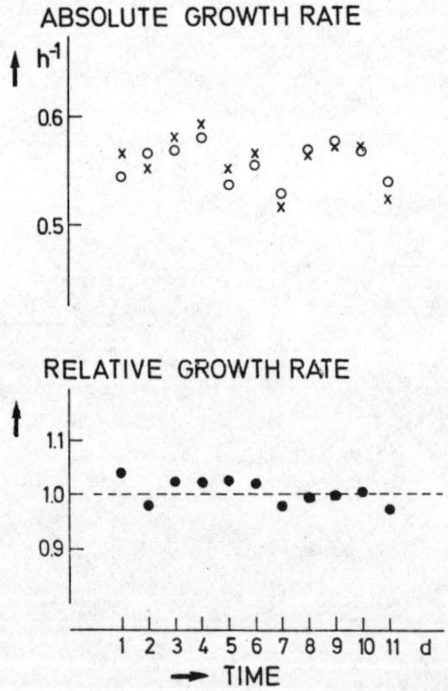

Fig. 13 Absolute and relative growth rate μ of a series of control experiments using both photometers (x,o). The normalization is defined as μ_x/μ_o

results of identical runs in both photometers are compared (see fig. 13b) without applied radiation. This is illustrated by the vertical error bar in figure 14. The absolut uncertainty of controls increases to ± 10 % taking into account systematic changes of some biological parameters, as the use of a new medium (different in age) or when new cells are taken from the stock culture (fig. 13).

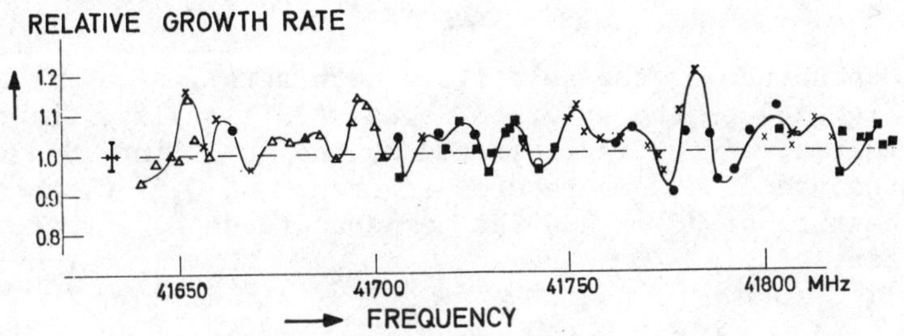

Fig. 14 Relative growth rate of yeast cells in dependence on microwave frequency. The different symbols refer to different experimental series. The full line is drawn by hand.

The relative growth rates of the irradiated samples and the corresponding controls can be seen in figure 14. The values vary between 89 % and 120 %. This fine tuning study shows again a strong frequency dependence. Furthermore a line width of nearly 10 MHz indicates a resonance-like behaviour. A strong comparison with the former results reported /11/ cannot be done directly because one has to take into account the absolute frequency scale uncertainty of ± 20 MHz of the first publication. In general, however, the former effects are reproduced by the use of a set-up improved in many aspects.

In addition, it should be pointed out that there is no correlation of the recently observed effects to the microwave power used within the range of 6 mW to 34 mW. This can be seen in figure 15, where the microwave power is shown vs normalized growth rates of fig. 14.

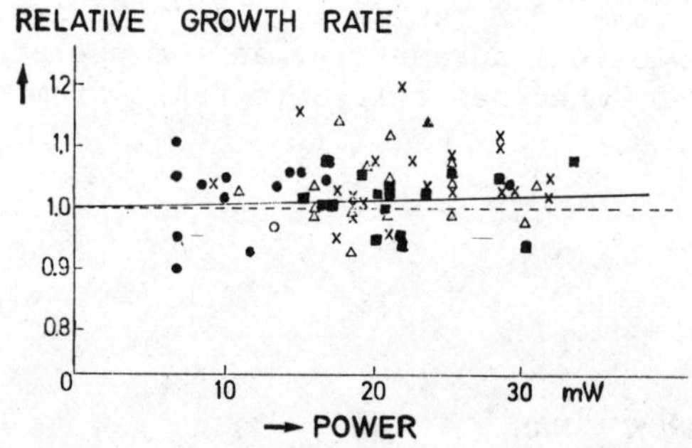

Fig. 15 Dependence of the relative growth rate (values from fig. 14) on the absorbed power. Additionally, the expected thermal effect is indicated by the full line, deduced by the use of a temperature difference of 0.5° C caused by heating of 30 mW and the temperature dependent growth rate of fig. 10

The experimental values are distributed on both sides of the full line (fig. 15), especially at low intensities positive effects are measurable and at high intensities negative effects. The dependence of the effects on frequency and the absence of any correlation to intensity used can not be explained by a simple thermal mechanism.

The most remarkable effects have been measured within the frequency range of 41770 and 41795 MHz (fig. 14). To test their reproducibility and to define the fine structure of a resonance we have performed a further set of 30 runs. The results are demonstrated in fig. 16. In spite of the relatively broad scatter at the minima indicating the influence of an until now unknown physical or biological parameter, the existence of a "resonance" structure of 10 MHz is confirmed once again.

At a frequency of 41782 MHz a well established positive growth effect seems to exist. Therefore, additional measurements have been performed with reduced power flux densities. Our first attempt to measure dependence of a growth effect on the intensity can be seen in fig. 17.

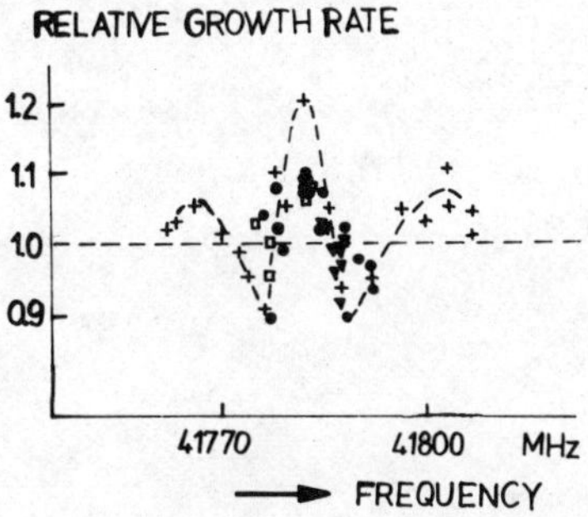

Fig. 16 Dependence of the relative growth rate on frequency. Additionally to the results of fig. 13 (+), the values of four further runs are drawn.

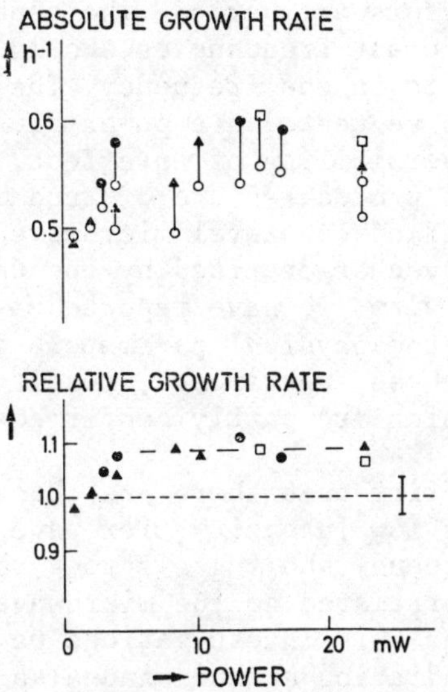

Fig. 17 Dependence of the absolute and relative growth rates at 41782 MHz on the power flux density. (o controls)

The results indicate that the effect remains constant although the power is increased by a factor of 4. Such a saturation effect is not explainable in terms of simple thermal response.

3. SUMMARY

For the interpretation of biological effects of RF and MW energy there is a need of more generalized results. Then, experiments with very different biological endpoints can be compared more easily and these data are more reasonably to be used in theoretical models. This contribution should suggest further experiments, where the independent parameters are varied. The dependence of one biological effect on different frequencies should be investigated rather than many effects on one frequency. The other important physical parameters to be tested are power flux density, duration of irradiation and reversibility of an effect.

These experimental procedures are of fundamental importance, especially on the field of low level microwave effects where such an effect can be mainly characterized by the definition of these dependencies. In this view, we have reported a few experiments, where in some respect the physical parameters are varied. Common to a greater part of these experiments, results on this generalized level are observed, which are partly confirmed by our yeast experiments.

In summary we reaffirm that there are changes in the yeast growth rate, caused by low intensity microwave irradiation. These effects depent on frequency showing a strong resonance-like behaviour and are not correlated to the microwave power in the range 6 to 34 mW. To continue this investigations we plan to use other geometries of the irradiation antenna and also a further dependent variable indicating a specific biological behaviour both in order to achieve stronger indication of the influence of the physical parameters and a better understanding of the resulting biological reactions.

REFERENCES

1. P.E. Tyler, ed., Biologic Effects of Nonionizing Radiation, New York Academy of Sciences, New York, Ann. N.Y. Acad. Sci. (1975).

2. S.F. Cleary, Biological Effects of Microwave and Radiofrequency Radiation, CRC Crit. Rev. Environ. Control, 121, June (1977).

3. S.M. Michaelson, Microwave Biological Effects: An Overview, Proceedings of the IEEE 68, 1: pp. 40-49 Jan. (1980).

4. H.P. Schwan, Interaction of Microwave and Radiofrequency Radiation with Biological Systems, IEEE Trans. Microwave Theory Tech. MTT-19: 146-152 (1971).

5. A.W. Guy, Analyses of Electromagnetic Fields induced in Biological Tissues by Thermographic Studies on Equivalent Phantom Models. IEEE Trans. Microwave Theory Tech. MTT-19: 205-214 (1971).

6. S.M. Michaelson, Human Exposure to Nonionizing Radiant Energy-Potential Hazards and Safety Standards, Proceedings of the IEEE, Vol. 60, No. 4, April (1972).

7. C.C. Johnson, A.W. Guy, Nonionizing Electromagnetic Wave Effects in Biological Materials and Systems, Proceeding of the IEEE, Vol. 60, No. 6, June (1972).

8. S.J. Webb and A.D. Booth, Absorption of Microwaves by Microorganismus, Nature 222: 1199 (1969).

9. A.J. Berteaud, M. Dardalhon, N. Rebeyrotte et D. Averbeck, Action d'un Rayonnement Electromagnétique á Longueur d'Onde Millimétrique sur le Croissance Bactérienne , C.R. Acad. Sc. Paris 281: D843 (1975).

10. N.D. Devyatkov, et al., Scientific Session of the Division of General Physics and Astronomy, USSR Academy of Sciences, Sov. Phys. -Usp. (Translation) 16: 568 (1974).

11. W. Grundler, F. Keilmann and H. Fröhlich, Resonant Growth Rate Response of Yeast Cells Irradiated by Weak Microwaves , Phys. Lett., 62A: 463 (1977); W. Grundler and F. Keilmann, Nonthermal Effects of Millimeter Microwaves on Yeast Growth , Z. Naturforsch. 33c: 15-22 (1978).

12. L.S. Taylor, Athermal Microwave Biological Effects: A Recapitulation, in: "The Mechanisms of Microwave Biological Effects", L.S. Taylor, A.Y. Cheung, ed., Report on a Workshop Univ. of Maryland, May (1979).

13. H. Fröhlich, The Biological Effects of Microwave and Related Questions, in: "Advances in Electronics and Electron Physics", Vol. 53: pp. 85-152 (1980).

14. F. Kaiser, Coherent Oscillations in Biological Systems, Z. Naturforsch. 33a; 294 and 418 (1978).

15. E.W. Prohofsky, Inducing soft mode transitions by interaction with radiation fields and possible relevance to microwave effects in biological materials; Phys. Lett., 63A: 179 (1977).

16. K.H. Illinger, Millimeter wave and far infrared Absorption in Biological Systems. Proceedings of "The Physical Basis of ELM Interactions with Biological Systems". L.S. Taylor and A.L. Cheung, Bureau of Radiological Health, Rockville, Maryland 20857: 43-66 (1978).

17. L.A. Sevastyanova, R.L. Vilenskaya, A Study of the Effects of Millimeter-Band Microwaves on the Bone Marrow of Mice, Sov. Phys. -Usp. (Engl. Transl.) 16: 570 (1974).

18. L.A. Sevastyanova, Properties of the Biological Action of mm-Radiowaves and their Application in Medicine, Vestn. Akad. Med. Nauk. SSSR (Germ. Transl.) pp. 65-68 (1979).

19. B.K. Chang, A.T. Huang, W.T. Joines, Inhibition of DNA Synthesis and Enhancement of the uptake and Action of Methotrexate by Low-Power-Density Microwave Radiation in L 1210 Leukemia Cells. Cancer Res., 40, 1002-1005 (1980).

INTERACTIONS OF ELECTROMAGNETIC FIELDS WITH LIVING CELLS AND MOLECULAR SYSTEMS

André-Jean Berteaud

Centre National de la Recherche Scientifique
Groupe de Recherche "Organisation Moléculaire et Macromoléculaire" (GR 35)
2, rue Henry Dunant
94320 THIAIS (France)

INTRODUCTION

The number of experimental data accumulated during the past few years, even if many of them are presently hypothetical, tend to reinforce the idea and the hypothesis that low intensity microwave and r.f. fields can produce alterations of certain biological processes in living matter. Indeed, this does not mean these alterations must be extended to human beings because the difference in scaling law between man and small animals which are generally used. Moreover, living system alterations are generally observed as small and reversible.

In order to obtain a better understanding of biological effects of these non ionizing waves, the scientific community must provide information on the basic physical and biological mechanisms involved in the interaction of fields with living systems as the general public is now very concerned with various domestic and industrial applications of these waves which are characterized by a strong dimensional coupling with any human neighbouring system.

The understanding of the mechanisms justifies the fact that research was developped several years ago at cellular and molecular levels.

THE SCATTERING PROPERTIES OF THE MICROWAVE ENERGY IN LIVING MATTER

Dielectric relaxation

The ultimate stage of the interaction between the r.f. electric field E and the living matter is a scattering process which transforms the e.m. energy into heat losses. This dispersion takes place by two different mechanisms, i.e. free charge oscillations (leading to conduction losses) and polar molecule rotation or reorientation (leading to dielectric rotationnal losses). This reorientation mechanism is highly specific of r.f. and microwaves frequencies and corresponds to a direct dipolar interaction of the electric field E with the permanent dipole moment of small molecules or fragments of biopolymers.

In the r.f. and microwave frequency bands, it is well known that the water molecule interaction with the r.f. electric field E (ω) is the dominant process by which the e.m. energy is transformed into heat loss. Microscopic heat loss results from the following considerations: water molecules are submitted to the field $E(\omega)$ (see figure 1) and experience a non coherent orientation (continuous or jump) in the field.

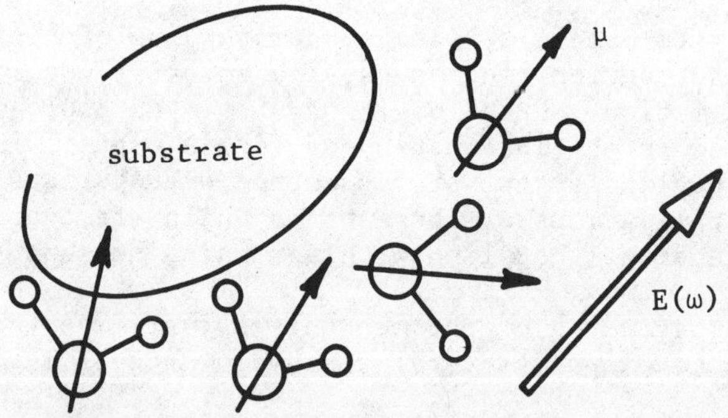

Fig. 1 - Four water molecules near substrate surface incoherently oscillate in $E(\omega)$ with $\omega \cong \omega r$. Mechanical vibration is converted to heat.

In the gas phase, water molecules are weakly coupled to each other and the energy losses are negligeable. In the liquid phase, molecules are strongly coupled to neighbouring water dipoles and if the frequency ω of the field $E(\omega)$ is near the dielectric relaxation frequency ωr, molecules experience reorientation forces and oscillate with a phase shifting between the neighbouring molecule dipoles which creates dielectric relaxation losses.

For field frequencies lower than the relaxation frequency ωr, the dipolar oscillation of the whole water molecules in the field $E(\omega)$ is coherent at short distance and losses become very small compared to other loss sources.

For field frequencies higher than ωr (particularly millimeter waves) the main relaxation losses decrease because water molecules become randomly oriented. However, a second Debye relaxation process with a lower intensity was generally observed which might be regarded as arising from orientation in the field $E(\omega)$ of those molecules which are free to do so without breakage of a hydrogen bond.

Chemical bonds

Another fundamental aspect of water molecules is the high sensitivity of their relaxation frequency to chemical bonds of water when they are scattered inside a complex material such as living matter. Between free water molecules for which ωr is near 17 GHz at 25°C and strongly bound molecules resulting from cooperative hydrogen bonds as in ice structure for which ωr is near 5 kHz, there exists a wide relaxation frequency spectrum for water according to the intensity of various chemical interactions. From data given by HASTED |1| one can represent the situation by plotting the dielectric loss variations as a function of frequency for water molecules with different chemical bonds at 25°C (see figure 2). Actually, for biopolymers in solution it was experimentally observed that relaxation domains are generally limited to 2 or 3. For instance, recent experiments |2| concerning the hydration of amino-acids with different chain length reveal the existence of a few water molecules which are strongly bound and the other water molecules which are practically free with ωr near 20 GHz. For chain length corresponding to amino caproic acids (CH_2 number equal to 5), a third relaxation domain appears associated with what is called "perturbed" water. In any case, water molecules are never spread in a disordered state but correspond to an integer number of relaxation domains. These general water properties developped in other chapters, are fundamental to describe the interaction of waves with living systems and are essential to understand a possible collective excitation of these water molecules which are bound to any biopolymer by means of waves with specific frequencies.

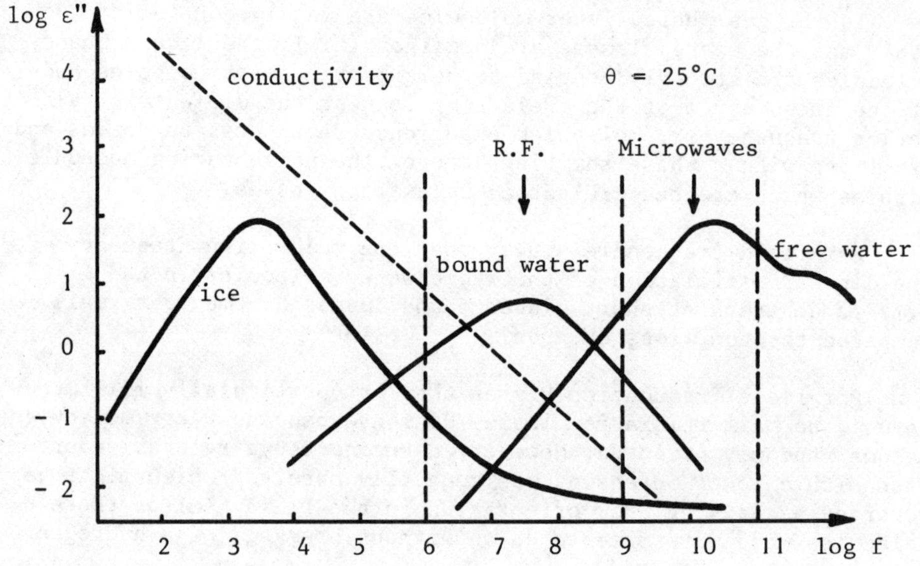

Fig. 2 - Dielectric losses of water (after J.B. HASTED)

Heating and thermalization mechanisms

In any case, the mechanism from which heating is produced in hydrated media such as living matter is basically different from other conventional heating processes which correspond to a thermal activation of mechanical vibrations (phonon excitation).

Another consequence of the existence of several excitation frequency bands for reorientation process of water molecules is the ability of hydration water bound to specific macromolecular substrates to absorb more energy from the incident e.m. fields than free water whether the field frequency is conveniently chosen (for instance r.f. frequency rather than microwaves) as it clearly appears from figure 2. From this consideration, the increase of the energy absorption by bound water compared to free water can produce a higher temperature increase near the macromolecular substrates which will experience hot spots compared to surrounding free water if thermalization processes correspond to relaxation times higher than that of reorientation processes. The exact pathway of thermalization for water molecules must therefore be considered at microscopic scale which is rather different from cooling pathway by heat conduction in fluids at macroscopic scale.

Equipartition of electric energy into vibrational modes is not immediate. The energy transfer between translationnal kinetic energy of a sonic wave direction and other degrees of freedom of molecules needs time which depends on sonic relaxation processes |3|. For a single relaxation process, the heat capacity at constant volume is expressed as a "reaction" heat capacity caused by the temperature variation of the molecule distribution among those energy levels which are responsible for the relaxation process. The rate of sonic energy transfer is proportional to the deviation from the equilibrium distribution with a macroscopic decay time associated to a relaxation equation similar to that of the dielectric relaxation of the Debye theory.

In general, the macroscopic decay time for sonic vibrations or dielectric relaxation has values of the same order particularly in the liquid phase such as free water. The result can be rather different with very condensed matter or when conformational equilibria of flexible molecules as biopolymers are considered. The application of ultrasonic absorption to the study of conformational equilibria in molecules such as n-butane reveals trans-gauche conversion which causes a relaxation at 15 to 20 MHz with an energy barrier near 3.5 kcal/mole which corresponds to a relaxation time of 10^{-9}s., at room temperature, a value which is considerably higher than dielectric relaxation times for group relaxation which are near 10^{-11} to 10^{-12} S.

Similarly, when considering hydration water molecules attached to biopolymer molecules for which the reorientation relaxation can be discerned at frequencies between that of biopolymer molecule and that of the free water, an ice-like structure can be associated to this bound water which contributes toward the structural stability of the biopolymer molecule. In this case, it is well known that the reorientation process by which the electric energy gained by bound water molecules from e.m. activation is transferred into the surrounding network takes place through various mechanisms related to the defect density |4|. It was observed that the activation enthalpy for thermal conductivity is equal to the activation energy for formation of a defect plus the activation energy for defect diffusion. In ice structure, this is considered as the rate determining step for the principal reorientation process.

One can presently conclude that further work will be necessary in order to arrive at a clear description by which microscopic heat loss takes place when bound water molecules responsible for structural stability of biomacromolecules are absorbing e.m. energy with certain frequencies corresponding to their dielectric relaxation. Thermalization processes which are clearly described in liquids and pure solids must also be precisely determined in concentrated biological macromolecule solutions with solid-liquid interfaces in order to clarify the possibility of a local temperature increase if the microscopic decay time of bound water molecules was higher than that of an e.m. dielectric excitation. It was indeed observed that the structural stability of macromolecules was very temperature dependent.

EXPERIMENTS AT CELLULAR LEVEL

Thermal equivalent of microwaves

An important factor generally considered is the specific absorption rate (SAR) for a living system which takes the nature and dimensions of the irradiated constituents into account for a given power density. The absorption capacity of a cell suspension was then interesting to consider in order to estimate the temperature increase inside the living cell when submitted to a specific irradiation wave.

Since it is known that the formation of zygotes in the yeast "*Saccharomyces Cerevisiae*" is very sensitive to changes in temperature, DARDALHON et al |5,6| used this property to determine the global temperature of the cellular system after various microwave irradiations. Two haploïds strains of different type were used which are able to undergo zygote formation giving rise to stable heterozygote diploïd cells. Irradiations were performed at the frequencies 9.4 GHz, 17 GHz and 73 GHz using power levels between 1 to 60 mW/cm^2. The estimations of equivalent temperatures were achieved by comparing the results to those obtained after conventional heating. Figure 3 indicates the main results at the three different irradiation frequencies and Figure 4 the results with a thermal bath to determine the temperature equivalent. From there, it can be concluded:

- a power density of 10 mW/cm^2 is equivalent to a global rise in temperature of the cells by 0.5 to 1 degree depending on the frequency used;
- for the same power density, the number of formed zygotes at 17 GHz is 2 to 3 timeshigher than that at 9.4 and 73 GHz. The result indicates that heating is essentially due to the dielectric absorption of microwaves by free or loosely bound water molecules inside the cytoplasm.

Several other experiments were recently described devoted to know whether the same biological response is to be expected from heat treatment produced either from waterbath heating or from microwave energy deposition. A strong controversy is always present even when authors used frequencies (1 to 2.45 GHz) and sometimes the same cellular system.

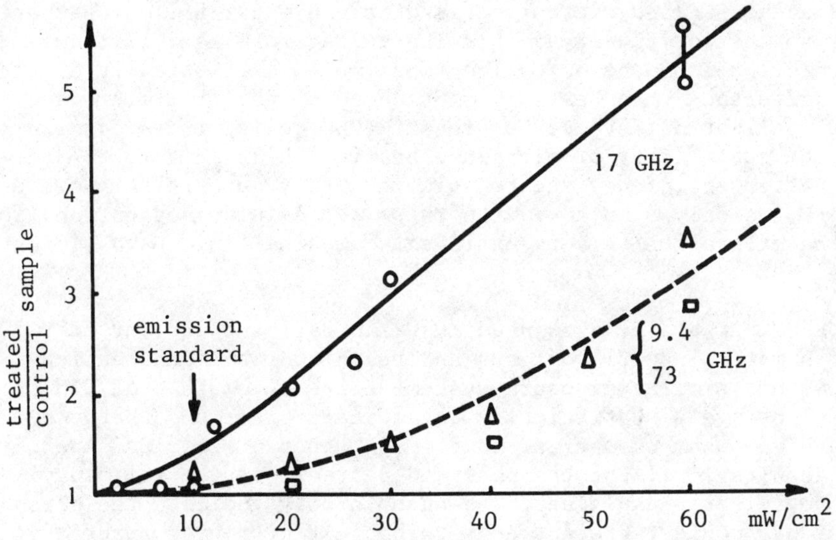

Fig. 3 - Zygote formation as a function of microwave power density at 3 frequencies.

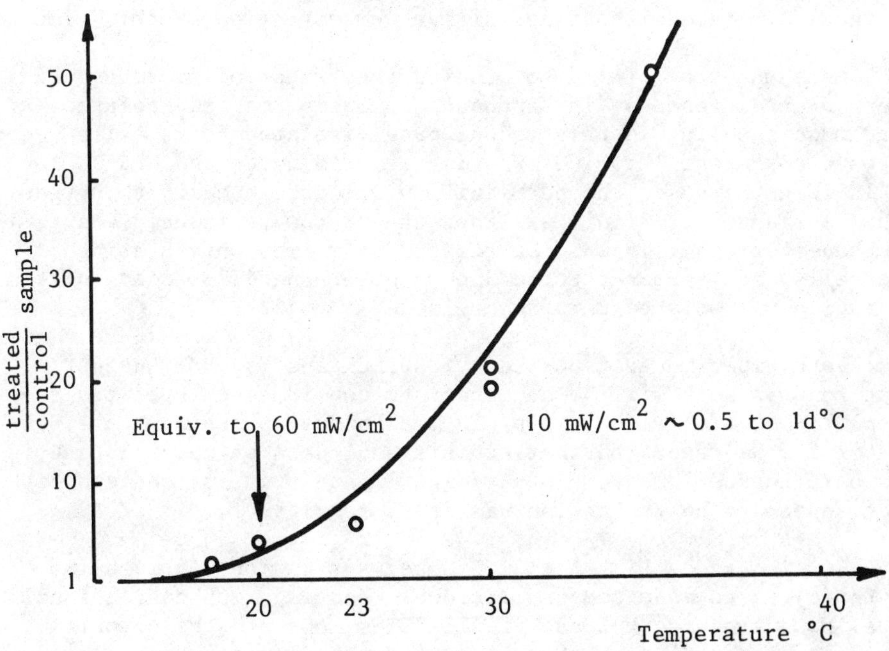

Fig. 4 - Zygote formation in water bath at various temperatures.

HARRISON et al |7| used mammalian cells (CHO) and bacterial cells heated in glass micropipettes within a water filled chamber similar to that of LIN et al |8|. The colony forming ability was measured between 43 and 50°C. They observe no statistically significant difference when heating is produced or not from microwave. When a slight difference is present (CHO cells) it is correlated to the specificity of microwave heating which is able to produce a better efficiency due to volumic energy deposition. However, this work has only been done with *in vitro* cellular suspensions for which thermalization is very efficient compared to *in vivo* living systems.

SUBJECK et al |9| also used *in vitro* cell suspensions of V 79 Chinese hamster lung fibroblasts and red blood cell enucleation heated with a similar exposure system derived from that of LIN et al. They observe a statistically significant difference between microwave and sham exposures, confirming other preceeding experimental results |10|. But the observed decrease of the cell survival is not clearly explained. The authors only indicate the plasma membranes could represent a hydrophobic region with absorption characteristics different from adjacent cellular regions. This indication is clearly based on the same concept of specific energy absorption by bound water which we previously indicated. The authors suggest membrane damage can be associated with the presence of the e.m. field without definitive demonstration at this time.

Mac REE et al |11| also studied the effect of microwave radiation on cardiogeneses in Japanese quail embryos and isolated cardiac muscle cells. In this second case, isolated heart cells were exposed to SAR of 1 to 100 mW/g during 90 minutes and SAR as low as 10 mW/g increased the permeability of cardiac cells to trypan blue. The author's finding is that the microwave induced change in membrane permeability was not related to macroscopic heating of the cells, but appeared to be due to other specific action of the radiation on isolated cardiac cells.

Both experiments reported by SUBJECK and Mac REE suggest that further work will be necessary to confirm such specific action of e.m. field and to explain mechanisms on the membrane permeability. We report further experimental data on the membrane in the next chapter but some other experimental results can exhibit what appear to be rather contradictory results.

For instance, LIU et al |12| used suspensions of mamalian erythrocytes to also compare microwave heating with conventional ones. Measuring the release of potassium ions and the osmotic fragility, they did not observe a difference, potassium release depending on the temperature elevation rather than the e.m. field intensity.

They observe that the membrane permeability of erythrocytes does not display a selective sensitivity to microwaves of 2 to 4 GHz with SAR of 80 to 200 mW/g.

Field effects on the cell cytoplasm

In spite of the fact that a number of experiments on living cells often show inconsistent results (the same contradiction could be demonstrated in considering the microwave experiments on colicin induction reported by several authors), a scientific evidence accumulated during the last few years leads a number of scientists to the hypothesis that rather low intensity microwave or r.f. fields can, in some cases, induce alterations to biological systems in the living cells such as cytoplasm or biomembranes. This is the case for DARDALHON and co-workers who made experiments on bacteria cells and yeast cells (wild strains or muted strains) at 2.45, 9.4, 17 GHz and at millimeter waves studying growth, letality, mutagenicity (mitochondrial and nuclear). No significant effects were observed on cell survival, on the induction of cytoplasmic "*petite*" mutations or of mitotic recombination. There was also no effect on sporulation, i.e. meiosis |13|. This excludes that microwaves induce genetic effect in nuclear and mitochondrial DNA and confirms results already obtained with millimeter waves |14,15|. In order to investigate whether microwaves could interfere with the repair of lesions induced in cellular DNA by UV radiation, the effects of combined treatments were studied. An exposure for one hour to 17 GHz at 50 mW/cm^2 before UV radiation compared with UV exposures alone, produced biological effects of small amplitude but statistically significant: decrease of survival and increase in mitotic recombination. The results are similar to those obtained by the same authors in interaction experiments with Xrays |16|.

These results suggesting that the action on cells could exert on the cytoplasmic or membraneous level, a new kind of experiments was performed to directly study the microviscosity inside the cell cytoplasm and try to correlate its variation with microwave irradiations. It is indeed well known that in fluid structures where cooperative forces such as hydrogen bonds dominate, parameters such as permittivity and viscosity have a very high and similar sensitivity to temperature or structure variations. A microwave irradiation stress can be detected by measurements of complex permittivity or viscosity.

Amongst several methods which can be used to measure the cell viscosity, a method of fluorescence depolarization was already proposed for other biological studies |17| and this method was recently studied to detect the variation of microviscosity of the cell after the cells in solution were exposed to microwave irradiations |18,19|. Fluorescein diacetate enters into the cell cytoplasm through the cellular membrane; fluorescein is produced by enzymatic hydrolysis in the cytoplasm and the polarization degree is measured using a fully automatized system (see ref 19 for details). The precision and reproducibility seem sufficiently high to allow a sensitive measurement of the cytoplasm viscosity to be attained when other parameters (such as temperature variations) are stabilized.

Previous experiments were made to detect the temperature stress which results from heating of the cells in suspension. After heating during 30 minutes either by microwaves of various power densities or by a water bath at different temperatures, the cell cytoplasm exhibits an increase of the microviscosity and a decrease of the enzymatic activity even several hours after heating, whereas the cytoplasm temperature decreases shortly after the end of heating (figures 5 and 6). The specificity of microwave power deposition inside the cell suspension is also clearly apparent. Fluorescence depolarization reveals good abilities to detect any effect on the cell cytoplasm in particular the stress which can result from microwave irradiations.

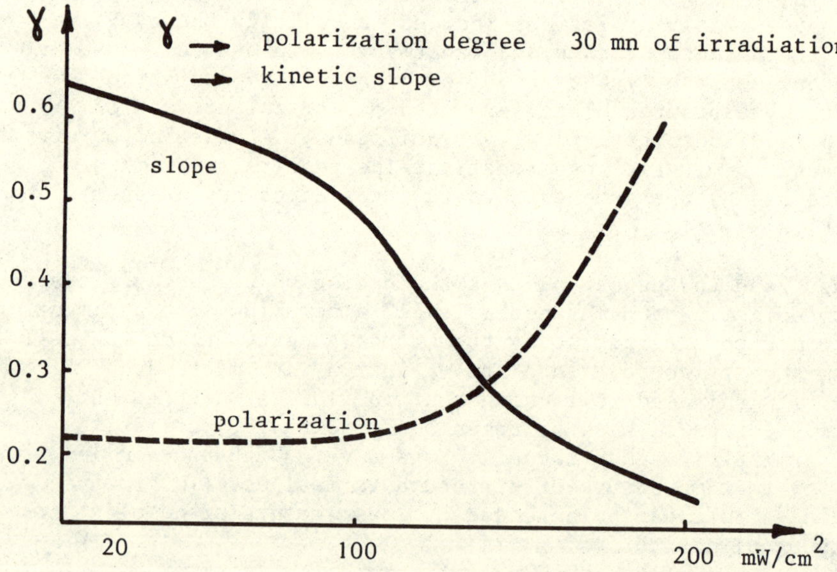

Fig. 5 - Variations of polarization degree and kinetic slope. The temperature increase is proportional to the power density.

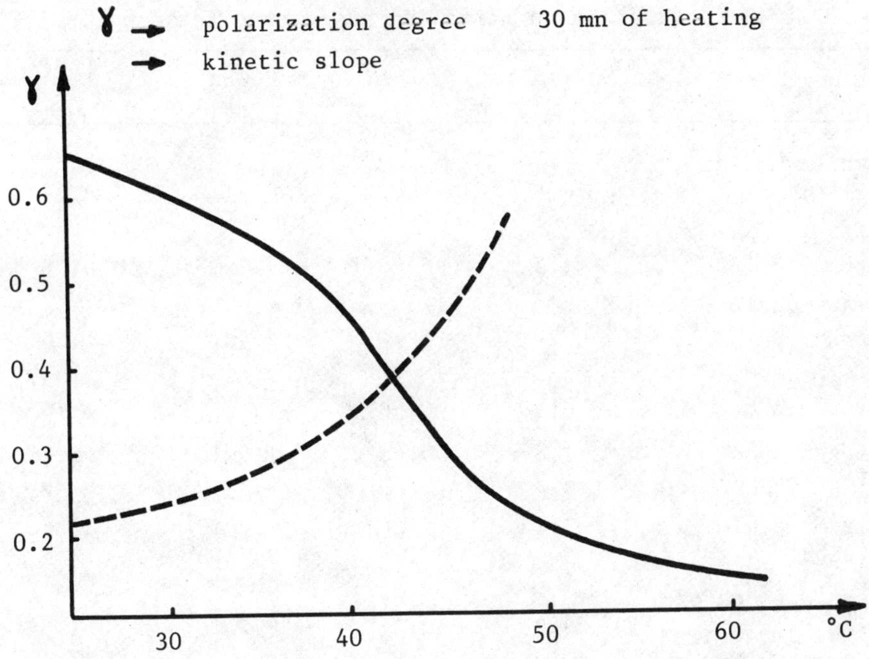

Fig. 6 - Variation of polarization degree and kinetic slope due to water bath heating at various temperature.

EXPERIMENTS AT MOLECULAR LEVEL

Activation energy associated to microwaves

Possible molecular effects of exposure to low intensity e.m. fields have been proposed to ultimately understand the basis mechanisms of interaction and it is interesting to estimate the exact conditions for the existence of molecular interactions. R.f. and microwave radiations are associated to photons with a quantized energy which is too small to directly modify any chemical bonds, even an hydrogen bond. Table I gives the activation energies and the corresponding frequencies and wavelengths of a few characteristic chemical bonds.

Table 1 - Activation energies and associated frequencies.

	kcal/mole	eV	F GHz)	λ(μ)
Brownian motion (27°C)	0.6	0.026	6.3×10^3	47.6
Covalent bond disruption	115	5	1.2×10^6	0.25
Van der Waals interactions	23	1	2.4×10^5	1.25
Bound water disruption	13	0.56	1.4×10^5	2.14
Hydrogen bond disruption	1.8 to 4.6	0.08 to 0.2	1.9×10^4 4.8×10^4	16 to 6.25
Polar molecule rotation	1 to 9	0.04 to 0.4	9.7×10^3 9.7×10^4	30 to 3
Reversible conformation change	9.2	0.4	9.7×10^4	3
Ionizing potential	230	10	2.4×10^6	0.12

Besides the activation energy hν associated to any specific e.m. radiation with a frequency ν, Brownian motion must be considered as a permanent excitation source of metastable states without specific frequencies and is represented by kT (T is the absolute temperature, k the Boltzmann's constant). The excitation conditions corresponding to a room temperature of 300°K (near 27°C) for any molecular system submitted to low level e.m. fields is summarized at figure 7. The absolute temperature of 300°K corresponds to an activation energy of 0.026 e.V. (0.6 kcal/mole), a wavelength of 47 μm and a frequency near 6.10^3 GHz. For lower frequencies (i.e. microwaves and r.f.), a permanent excitation of metastable states due to thermal noise is present. It results that microwave and r.f. fields with low intensity are unable to produce any effect which is already naturally occuring from thermal energy except for specific conditions. Two conditions are particularly known:

a) the amplification of metastable states by e.m. fields frequencies which correspond to specific states of living matter. The situation is then very similar to a phase lock coherent detector which can give a selective amplification of signal 10^4 times lower than thermal noise.

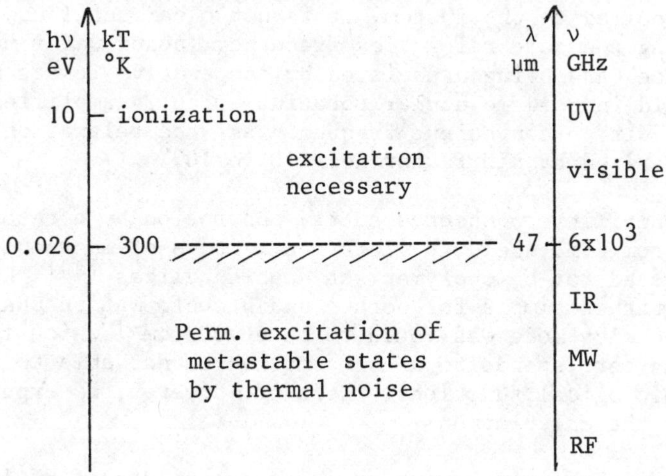

Fig. 7 - Compared data for Boltzmann's motion and energy activation, at room temperature.

b) The action upon cooperatively bonded systems which exist with periodic structures such as cellular membranes. Weak secondary forces are then responsible for the stabilization of the tertiary structure of biomolecules. These weak cooperative bondings hold together lipids and proteins of biomembranes but long range interactions with e.m. fields can actually modify the system equilibrium. This is rather similar to the magnetization process of ferromagnetic substances in which magnetization comes from a displacement of the magnetic domain walls whereas the external d.c. field applied to magnetize the substance is much lower than the molecular field between magnetic moment units.

Coherent excitation

Coming to the first condition, i.e. coherent amplification of metastable states, the basis of thermodynamics is the recognition that energy can exist in two forms: coherent energy freely convertible to mechanical work (such as dipole orientation in an applied field) and incoherent energy or heat. Then the distinction between heat and work is a matter of the coherence of the applied field. Whether any resonant system is present in living matter, one can wait for energy absorption when a coherent excitation by an e.m.

field is applied to the system. It is not clear until now if molecules having the same relaxation frequency (bound water molecules, for instance) and being associated by cooperative forces can also have a field induced molecular rotation which is amplified by an e.m. field with a convenient frequency as the relaxation process is characterized by a Q factor near 10 to 100.

A possibility to observe energy absorption by a resonant transfer from e.m. field to vibrational modes of macromolecules was calculated for homopolymer DNA double helices |20|. Calculations are rather simple for both A and B conformation DNA. The lowest frequency mode was found to be at 0.3 cm^{-1} which is rougly 100 GHz and corresponds to a conformation change able to alter specific biological functions. There is, however, no experiment to confirm the calculations.

Another theoretical work suggests the existence of long range collective molecular interactions, within membranes, with coherent e.m. fields resulting in coupled enzyme-substrate reactions |21,22| Experimental works on the millimeter wave spectra were made to verify this theory and have received a particular consideration in other chapters.

Effects on membranes

Very few experiments were made to study the effects of microwaves upon synthetic or natural phospholipid membranes.

TYAZHELOV et al |23,24| have studied the change in the conductivity of phospholipid membranes (lecithin) modified by various antibiotics. When microwave fields with a frequency near 0.9 GHz are applied normally to the bilayers, conductance can increase or decrease according to the nature of antibiotics. A particular attention was given to gramicidin A modified bilayers |24| for which a monophasic conductance increase was induced by microwaves with an intensity which depends linearly on the specific absorption rate of the system. Apparently, the microwave effect is independant from the type of ions which pass over the channels. The authors propose an interpretation based on a local overheating of membrane channels due to the fact that the electric field intensity is higher inside the channels than in the electrolyte.

Studies, reported by SHERIDAN |25,26| drew attention to the possibility that the membrane may be the best model system to explain the sensitivity of biological systems to e.m. fields. It was demonstrated, using Raman spectroscopy, that phase transitions in lipid bilayer occur over a narrow temperature range during low e.m. field irradiation than in its absence. This effect was then attributed to differential thermal gradients induced by the e.m. field.

A model involving absorption of microwave energy by bonded water and two different mechanisms of thermalization was discussed.

CONCLUSION

Many different mechanisms can be responsible for the absorption of e.m. radiation by biological molecular systems and living cells and a more detailed knowledge is still necessary to correctly describe these absorption mechanisms. Moreover, the dissipation of e.m. energy poses unresolved questions concerning microscopic thermalization of the absorbed radiation. As it was indicated, many experimental data reveal contradictory results when authors try to estimate the specificity of microwave heating at the cellular level. Thus there is an obvious need for additional research on the interaction mechanisms of e.m. radiation with living systems at cellular and molecular levels, though with the present experimental data the induced field effect seems always reversible and with a small intensity. It may also be suggested that cell cytoplasm and biomembranes may be the primary site for e.m. field alterations.

REFERENCES

1 J.B. HASTED, Aqueous Dielectrics, 1973.

2 J.L. SALEFRAN, Thesis work, Université de Bordeaux, 1978.

3 F. KOELHER, The Liquid State, 1972.

4 N. BJERRUM, Klg. Danske Videnskab. Selskab Mat. Fys. Medd., 27, 32, 41, 1951.

5 M. DARDALHON, D. AVERBECK and A.J. BERTEAUD, J. of Microwave Power, 14(4), 307, 1979.

6 M. DARDALHON, A.J. BERTEAUD and D. AVERBECK, Proc. of URSI Symposium, Jouy-en-Josas, 225, July 1980.

7 G. HARRISON, J. ROBINSON, D. MAC CULLOCH and A. CHEUNG, Proc. of URSI Symposium, Jouy-en-Josas, 41, July 1980.

8 J.C. LIN, W.D. PETERSON, J. Bioengineering, 1, 471, 1977.

9 J. SUBJECK, J. SCIANDRA, E. REPASKY and R. JOHNSON, Proc. of URSI Symposium, Jouy-en-Josas, 321, July 1980.

10 J. SUBJECK, MOREAU and R. JOHNSON, Eur. J. Radiother. (in press).

11 D. MAC REE, M. GALVIN, C. HALL, M. LIEBERMANN, Proc. of URSI Symposium, Jouy-en-Josas, July 1980.

12 L.M. LIU, F.G. NICKLESS and S.F. CLEARY, Radio Science, 14, 6S, Nov-Dec. 1979.

13 D. AVERBECK, M. DARDALHON and A.J. BERTEAUD, J. of Microwave Power, 11(2), 143, 1976.

14 A.J. BERTEAUD, M. DARDALHON, N. REBEYROTTE and D. AVERBECK, C.R. Acad. Sci., 281, 843, 1975.

15 M. DARDALHON, D. AVERBECK, Proc. IXe Congrès SFRP, 279, 1978.

16 M. DARDALHON, D. AVERBECK and A.J. BERTEAUD, Proc. of URSI Symposium, Jouy-en-Josas, 17, 1980.

17 L. CERCEK and B. CERCEK, Biophysik, 9, 109, 1973.

18 C. MORE, M. DARDALHON, A.J. BERTEAUD and D. AVERBECK, Proc. of URSI Symposium, Jouy-en-Josas, 25, 1980.

19 C. MORE and A.J. BERTEAUD (to be published).

20 E.W. PROHOFSKY, Proc. of Workshop at Univ. Maryland, 133, June 1977.

21 H. FRÖLICH, Nature, 228, 1093, 1970.

22 H. FRÖLICH, Proc. Nat. Acad. Sci. 72, 4211, 1975.

23 V.V. TYAZHELOV, S.I. ALEKSEYEV and P.A. GRIGOREV, Biophysics, 23, 750, 1978.

24 V.V. TYAZHELOV, S.I. ALEKSEEV, L. KH. FAIZOVA and V.V. CHERTISHCHEV, Proc. of URSI Symposium, Jouy-en-Josas, 105, July 1980.

25 J.P. SHERIDAN, R. PRIEST, P. SCHOEN, Proc. of Workshop at Univ. Maryland, 145, July 1977.

26 B.P. GABER and J.P. SHERIDAN, Proc. Bioelectromagnetic Symp. URSI, Seattle, 469, June 18-20 1979.

BIOLOGICAL EFFECTS AND HEALTH HAZARDS OF RF AND MW ENERGY: FUNDAMENTALS AND OVERALL PHENOMENOLOGY

Sol M. Michaelson

Department of Radiation Biology and Biophysics
University of Rochester
School of Medicine and Dentistry
Rochester, New York 14642

INTRODUCTION

Extensive investigations into microwave bioeffects during the last quarter century have shown that for frequencies between 200 and 24,500 MHz, exposure to a power density of 100 mW/cm^2 for several minutes or hours can result in pathophysiologic manifestations of a thermal nature in laboratory animals. Such effects may or may not be characterized by a measurable temperature rise, which is a function of thermoregulatory processes and active adaptation of the animal. The end result is either reversible or irreversible change, depending on the irradiation conditions and the physiologic state of the animal. At lower power densities, clear evidence of pathologic changes or physiologic alteration is nonexistent or equivocal. A great deal of discussion, nevertheless, has taken place on the relative importance of thermal or nonthermal effects of radiofrequency (RF) and microwave (MW) radiation.

Elucidation of the biologic effects of microwave exposure requires a careful review and critical analysis of the available literature. This entails differentiating established effects and mechanisms from speculative and unsubstantiated reports. Although most of the experimental data support the concept that the effects of microwave exposure are primarily, if not only, a response to heating or altered thermal gradients in the body, there are large areas of confusion, uncertainty and misinformation.

Fundamental Aspects

Twenty-five years ago Schwan and his associates[1-5] elucidated and enunciated many of the biophysical principles of electromagnetic field/biologic tissue interactions. Other investigators[6,7] also measured the *in vitro* dielectric properties of biological tissues. These earlier studies reviewed by Johnson and Guy[8] and more recent measurements in the microwave frequency range[9,10] established a useful base of *in vitro* dielectric data for various normal tissues over the extremely wide frequency range from 10 kilohertz (kHz) to 10 Gigahertz (GHz).

The amount of electromagnetic energy absorbed by tissue is determined by interaction of the electromagnetic field with the tissue's biological constituents. This interaction is defined by the tissue's anatomy, geometry and electrical properties. On a physiologic basis these principles suggest that if biological perturbations from EM fields should occur, they would initially be manifested by subtle responses characterized by functional changes in regulatory systems of the body.

Physiologic Integration

The main integrator of mammalian regulatory systems is the brain which through the hypothalamus mediates the classical biological responses to factors that may impose a strain on the homeostatic mechanisms of the body. Physiological integration results from cooperating processes at work within an individual. For example, heart rate and other circulatory properties are modified in response to messages from specific muscles, viscera, or glands in which augmented blood flow increases the supplies of oxygen and other substances at active local sites. Messages are transmitted at various kinds of functions and chemical receptors.[11]

To maintain homeostasis, mammals possess control mechanisms that react to changes in internal and external environments (stimuli or stressors). Two of these control mechanisms are primarily the neural and endocrine systems. Separation of endocrine from neural control is extremely difficult as neural signals are integrated at the hypothalamus to react to deviations in internal or external environments. Hypothalamic-hypophysial-adrenocortical and medullary (HHA), hypothalamic-hypophysial-thyroidal (HHT), hypothalamic-hypophysial-somatotrophic (HHS) prolactin and opiocortin neuroendocrine/neurotransmitter systems participate in this homeostatic or homeokinetic activity. Generally, they operate through negative feedback mechanisms. As an example, adrenergic neurons in the hypothalamus stimulate thyrotropin (TSH), entering the general circulation to stimulate thyroid secretion of triiodothyronine (T_3) and thyroxine (T_4). The T_3 and T_4 then act by negative feedback control on hypophysial TSH secretion. Because of the importance of these hierarchical systems to the body's economy, perturbation at any link in the chain could have multiple pathophysiologic consequences.

Microwave Hyperthermia and Physiologic Regulation

The organs and organ systems affected by exposure to microwave/radiofrequency(MW/RF) energy are susceptible, in terms of functional disturbance and/or structural alterations. Some reactions to MW/RF exposure may lead to measurable biological effects which remain within the range of normal (physiological) compensation and are thus not necessarily hazardous; some effects may improve the efficiency of certain physiological processes and can thus be used for therapeutic purposes. Some reactions on the other hand, may lead to effects which may be potential or actual health hazards.

Most of the MW/RF responses are explained by thermal energy conversion, almost exclusively as enthalpic energy phenomena. The complicated mechanisms of heat regulation are integrated by hormonal and nervous control as well as by a direct temperature effect of the blood supplying the hypothalamus which can also be influenced experimentally by direct heating.

The non-uniform, largely unpredictable distribution of energy absorption may give rise to temperature increases and rates of heating that could result in unique biological effects. It is important to recognize nevertheless, that the mammalian body normally is not a uniform incubator at 37°C but does contain significant temperature gradients.[12] Furthermore, induced temperature gradients in deep body organs may act as a stimulus to alter normal function both in the heated organ and in other organs or organ systems. Thus indirect effects can be elicited in organs far removed from the site of the primary interaction.

The maintenance of a certain temperature is of vital importance to the organism because all biologic processes are conditioned by temperature. The temperature of the tissues is an important factor which determines the extent of the physiologic response to heat. Much is known of the mechanisms by which endotherms achieve and maintain a characteristic stable internal body temperature in the face of environmental and internal thermal stresses. Microwave/radiofrequency energies provide a unique thermal challenge to deep as well as peripheral tissues that must be dealt with by these same mechanisms.

Active thermoregulation makes use of passive heat transfer mechanisms by employing internal circulating fluids (such as blood) to transfer heat from internal regions to external regions where passive heat radiation and convection are more effective. In some fur-bearing animals, an efficient mechanism is the movement of internally-warmed blood to the lungs; heat in the lungs is then transferred to the inspired air by convection and is then expired into the environment. Another mechanism (especially in man) is cutaneous vasodilation, resulting in the transfer of internal heat to the skin, where it can be radiated and convected into the surrounding environment. Sweating from the skin of humans and the paws and snout of fur-bearing animals provides a means of heat transfer; evaporation of the fluid permits rapid heat loss to the environment.

A body temperature increase implies a breakdown of thermoregulatory mechanisms. On the other hand, low intensity exposures (previously considered "non-thermal") usually initiate immediate and efficient thermoregulatory processes that insure the constancy of the internal body temperature.

Temperature changes can act as stimuli to different organs, influencing their reaction. The rate at which the heat is dissipated will vary in different species depending on heat-regulating mechanisms or metabolic characteristics. The breakdown of protective mechanisms for heat control causes an uncontrolled rise in body temperature.

The maintenance of a certain temperature is of vital importance to the organism because all biologic processes are conditioned by temperature. The temperature of the tissues is an important factor which determines the extent of the physiologic response to heat.

For the body as a whole, each response to temperature sensations appears to recognize a threshold. This threshold can be conveniently imagined to contribute to a so-called set-point. The set-point, however, is not fixed under all conditions.[11] In addition to the physiological responses of heat production and vasoconstriction, other actions that the individual takes may be regarded as behavioral. Localized tissue heating is known to greatly increase local tissue blood flow and to alter the metabolic processes in the affected tissues. This has generated interest in the use of microwave diathermy (and other means to produce localized hyperthermia) as an adjunct to effective cancer treatment.

Specific organ or tissue systems may "function" at a significantly different rate if local thermal gradients are altered. Relatively large changes in circulation are provoked by quite small deviations from neutral temperature.[13] The mechanisms of heat regulation are activated in several ways: by thermal receptors in the skin, by direct stimulation of the hypothalamus and receptors in the spinal cord and viscera. Under certain conditions, the thermal stimuli to the skin can be of greater significance in causing cardiovascular reactions than the level of core temperature.

In order to extrapolate observations in animals to predict results that might be obtained during human exposures, both physiologic and physical scaling must be employed.[14-16] The best method available at present, albeit fraught with oversimplifications, is frequency scaling. This approach assumes the use of shorter wavelengths (higher frequencies) for smaller animals and longer wavelengths (lower frequencies) for larger animals. Approximating the bodies of animals and man as prolate spheroids, an attempt has been made to ascertain what (lower) frequency must be used with the larger animal if the total absorbed dose rate (at the same plane wave exposure field intensity) is to be the same as that obtained at a higher frequency for a smaller animal.

Exposure of biological systems to MW/RF energy of sufficient intensity may lead to temperature elevation when the rate of energy absorption exceeds the rate of energy dissipation. Whether the resultant temperature elevation is general or confined to specific anatomical sites, depends on:

a) the electromagnetic field characteristics and distributions within the body and

b) the passive and active thermoregulatory mechanisms available to the organism.

The passive thermoregulatory mechanisms consist of heat radiation, conduction, convection, and evaporative cooling. The efficacy of heat convection between a body and its immediate environment is a function of the environmental conditions.

Cellular Effects - Chromosomes - Genetic Effects

Some investigators have reported chromosome changes in various plant and animal cells and tissue cultures.[17,18] These studies have been criticized by those who feel that the systems were subjected to a thermal stress; the chosen parameters of the applied field caused biologically significant field induced force effects in *in vitro* experiments and many of these experiments have not yet been independently replicated. Generally in studies concerned with response of cells in culture, undetected temperature deviations between irradiated and control systems can lead to erroneous interpretations. In investigations concerning the effects of microwave and radiofrequency energies on biological systems, especially when some form of cellular response is involved, temperature control must be a major consideration.

There is no satisfactory evidence of microwave-induced genetic effects at low to modest power densities.[19] It is known that the rate of induction of mutations will increase with increasing temperature. It is possible, therefore, that artifacts or thermal stress could be factors in some of the reported studies. Work with primitive organisms and rodents indicate that microwave exposure at power densities below 10 mW/cm^2 are not mutagenic.[20-22]

Growth and Development

There are a few reports which suggest that particular combinations of exposure frequency, duration, and power density produce effects on embryological development and postnatal growth. Some of these reports suggest that observed prenatal effects are deleterious, or teratogenic. In almost all instances, however, the reported effects can be ascribed to excessive temperature elevation caused by the exposure.

The reports on effects of microwave exposure on early development have been reviewed by Baranski and Czerski[19] who conclude "no serious effects are to be expected at power densities below 10 mW/cm^2 under usual exposure conditions". They further note that defects, when observed, are the result of hyperthermia.

The Gonads

The effect of microwaves on the testes has been studied fairly extensively. Although reports indicate that high power density exposure can affect the testes,[23] these responses can be related to the heating of the organs. The sensitivity of the testes to heat is well known.

Neuroendocrine Effects

Some investigators believe that endocrine changes result from stimulation of the hypothalamic-hypophysial system due to thermal interactions at the hypothalamic or adjacent levels of organization, the hypophysis itself, or the particular endocrine gland or end-organ under study.[24-30] According to other investigators, the observed changes are interpreted as being the result of direct microwave interactions with the central nervous system.[31-33] In either case, one should not consider neuroendocrine perturbations as necessarily pathologic because the function of the neuroendocrine system is to maintain homeostasis and hormone levels will fluctuate to maintain such organismic stability.

Immunology

Microwaves have been reported to induce an increase in the frequency of complement receptor-bearing lymphoid spleen cells in mice.[34] MW/RF radiation-induced hyperthermia in mice has been associated with transient lymphopenia with a relative increase in splenic T and B lymphocytes,[35] and decreased *in vivo* local delayed hypersensitivity. The influence of increased temperature on immune responses is well known.[36] Neural function and immunologic reaction are related. The influence of microwave-induced hypothalamic-hypophysial adrenal stimulation[23] and microwave-induced immune suppression has been suggested by Liburdy.[35]

Effects on the Nervous System

Transient functional changes referrable to the central nervous system (CNS) have been reported following "low-level" (<10 mW/cm^2) microwave exposure. Although some reports describe the thermal nature of microwave energy absorption, others implicate nonthermal or "specific" microwave effects at the molecular and cellular level. It should be noted, however, that specific (i.e., nonthermal) microwave effects have not been experimentally nor clinically verified. The first report of the effect of microwave energy on conditional response activity in experimental animals was made by investigators in the USSR.[37] In subsequent years, the study of "nonthermal" effects of microwaves gradually occupied the central role in electrophysiological studies in the Soviet Union.

Many effects of microwaves on the central nervous system are attributable to heating.[15,38,39] Neurophysiological responses to raised local tissue temperature are basically twofold: (1) direct effects on nervous tissue functions, and (2) reflex effects operating through sensors or tranducers of these thermal changes, and thence through effector mechanisms in the central nervous system.[40] Skin thermal receptors can respond to temperature changes of a few thousandths of a degree in a second. Hypothalamic sensitivity to direct thermal stimulation exhibits thresholds for local temperature increases of 0.5-0.6°C. This central sensitivity is consistent with induction of altered circulating pituitary hormone levels.[26,41] Ismailov and Subkova,[42] however, have criticized thermal models of these endocrine responses, on the grounds of higher lethality resulting from exposure to microwaves over identical intensities of infrared radiation and have proposed that microwave fields produce "nonthermal" effects which progress against a background of tissue heating.[43,44] It should be emphasized, nevertheless, that any evaluation of apparent differences between microwave heating and other thermalizing factors must consider specific absorption rates of energy at the hypothesized locus of interaction, including possible resonant effects of various frequencies in different sized animals or body structures.[40]

The Blood-Brain Barrier

Considerable interest has been engendered by a report of transient alteration in the permeability of small inert polar molecules across the blood-brain barrier of rats exposed to microwaves.[45] Attempts to replicate these findings have yielded equivocal results unless the brain is subjected to a large increase in temperature.[46,47]

It should be noted the methods used to investigate blood-brain barrier permeability are controversial. Permeability changes in cerebral blood vessels occur under various conditions, i.e., cold, heat, pressure, ionizing radiation, drugs, osmotic imbalance, edema and anoxia. Most techniques used to measure blood-brain barrier permeability in fact measure the net influence of several variables in the vascular space, alterations of blood flow, and membrane permeability.

MW/RF energy absorption within the cranial cavity may be focused as "hot spots." A model of lossy spheres simulating brain tissue shows that these occur inside spheres with radii 8 cm $< R >$ 0.1 cm for frequencies between 300 MHz and 12.0 GHz.[48] At lower frequencies and at much higher frequencies, heating occurs primarily at the surface of the sphere facing the field source. Small animals may also exhibit high focal microwave energy absorption at the craniocervical junction where body size approaches a significant fraction of the exposure energy wavelength.[49,50] Kritikos and Schwan[51] have modeled conduction and convection from hot spots in central brain structures, with inclusion of a factor for blood flow. For a spherical "head" 10 cm in diameter exposed to a 1.0 GHz 10 mW/cm^2 field with a central hot spot 2 cm in diameter, the expected temperature rise would be 0.5°C with normal blood flow and heat conduction. In this model, heat conduction and normal blood flow appear to contribute equally to heat removal from the hot spot. For a given incident field flux, the heating potential in the hot spot decreases rapidly with increasing head radius and for humans expected temperature elevations in the center of the head would be much lower at this frequency (1.0 GHz).[48,52,53] The physiological significance of raising cerebral temperature by 1-2°C is not known.[40] General, as distinct from focal, increments in brain temperature up to 2°C occur in normal subjects during exercise and in moderate heat stress, without evidence of major alterations in higher nervous functions.[54]

Behavioral Effects

Studies have been conducted on the effects of MW/RF on performance of trained tasks by rats, rhesus and squirrel monkeys. Many of these studies indicate that exposure to MW/RF energies can suppress performance of a trained task, and that a power density/dose rate and duration threshold for achieving the suppression exists. Depending on duration and other parameters of exposure, the threshold power density for affecting trained behavior ranges from 5 to 50 mW/cm^2.

An interesting study was performed by de Lorge[55] who exposed rats, squirrel monkeys, and rhesus monkeys to 2450 MHz under far-field conditions. Stable performance on operant schedules was disrupted in all three species at power densities positively correlated with the body mass of the animals. The power densities associated with behavioral disruption approximated those power densities that produced an increase in colonic temperature of at least 1°C. These data support the concept of scaling factors for extrapolation among species of animals of different size.

In assessing the implications of behavioral reactions to MW/RF exposure, it is important to realize that behavior among animals reflects adaptive brain-behavior patterns and behavioral thermoregulation is seen as an attempt to maintain a nearly constant internal thermal environment. Changes in body temperature bring about not only autonomic drives but also behavioral drives.[56] That "low-level" microwaves can elicit behavioral thermoregulation has been shown by Stern et al[57] and Adair and Adams.[58] Behavioral responses are not necessarily manifestations of specific changes in the CNS and may be a function of direct or indirect action of microwaves on other body systems.

Thermoregulatory behavior provides one mechanism for altering the heat exchange between an animal and its environment, thereby ensuring a constancy of core, as well as more peripheral, temperatures. Thermoregulatory behavior is functionally defined as behavior that directly affects, and is often controlled by, the thermal environment of the subject. As part of a feedback process, such behavior helps to regulate, or maintain the body temperatures. Since behavior may be functionally related to varying regional or peripheral temperatures, while core temperature remains constant, the absence of a core temperature change during microwave exposure cannot be used as evidence that an observed change in behavior was due to some mechanism other than a reaction to heat produced by microwaves.

Cardiovascular Effects

Several investigators report that exposure to microwaves may result in direct or indirect effects on the cardiovascular system. Some authors suggest that exposure to microwaves at intensities which do not produce appreciable hyperthermal effects may lead to functional changes as a result of acute as well as chronic exposures. Such effects as hypotonus, bradycardia, delayed auricular and ventricular conduction, decreased blood pressure, ECG alterations in workers in radiofrequency or microwave fields have been reported.[59,60] These changes do not diminish work capacity, and are reversible.[61] No cardiovascular pathology has been noted in man or animals as a result of microwave exposure.[62]

Hematopoietic Effects

Reports of hematopoietic effects from exposure to MW/RF energies are inconsistent. Although a number of investigators state that the blood and blood forming system are not affected by acute or chronic microwave exposure,[63-65] effects on hematopoiesis have been reported.[66-70] The time of onset and degree of hematopoietic change are dependent on the field intensity, duration of exposure, and induced hyperthermia.

In evaluating reports of hematologic changes one must be cognizant of the relative distribution of blood cells in a population of animals or humans and the thermal influence on these alterations. Early and sustained leukocytosis in animals exposed to thermogenic levels of microwaves may be related to stimulation of the hematopoietic system, leukocyte mobilization, or recirculation of sequestered cells. Eosinopenia and transient lymphocytopenia with rebound or overcompensation, when accompanied by neutrophilia, may be indicative of increased hypothalamic-hypophysial-adrenal function as a result of thermal stress.

Ocular Effects

During the past 25 years, numerous investigations in animals and several surveys among human populations have been devoted to assessing the relationship of exposure to microwaves and subsequent development of cataracts. It is significant that of the many experiments on rabbits by several investigators using various techniques, power density above 100 mW/cm^2 for 1 hour or longer appears to be the time-power threshold for lens opacification in the tested frequency range of 200 MHz to 10,000 MHz. In other species of animals such as dogs and non-human primates, the threshold for experimental microwave-induced lens opacity appears to be higher. All of the reported effects of microwave radiation on the lens can be explained on the basis of thermal injury.

That lens opacity can be produced in rabbits by exposure to microwaves is well established. Extrapolating interpreted results from animal studies to humans is, however, difficult because the conditions, durations and intensities of exposure are usually quite different. Several cases of alleged cataract formation in humans exposed to microwaves have been reported in the literature but precise exposure parameters are generally impossible to determine. It is also difficult to relate cause and effect, because lens imperfections do occur in otherwise healthy individuals, especially with increasing age. Numerous drugs, industrial chemicals and certain metabolic diseases are associated with cataracts.

Cutaneous Perception

Perception of microwave energy is a function of cutaneous thermal sensation or pain. The physiology of thermal sensation and pain has been the subject of several studies which suggest that a threshold sensation is obtained when the temperature of the warmth receptors in the skin is increased by a certain amount (ΔT).[71-73]

Health Aspects

A number of retrospective studies have been done on human populations exposed or believed to have been exposed to MW/RF energies. In general, studies performed in the U.S. have not revealed any conditions that could be ascribed to radar exposure.[74] On the other hand, surveys of Eastern European workers have noted functional changes in the nervous and cardiovascular systems.[59,60]

There is considerable difficulty in establishing the presence of, and quantifying the frequency and severity of "subjective" complaints. Individuals suffering from a variety of chronic diseases may exhibit the same dysfunctions of the central nervous and cardiovascular systems as those reported to be a result of exposure to microwaves; thus, it is extremely difficult, if not impossible, to rule out other factors in attempting to relate microwave exposure to clinical conditions.[75] In this context an extensive 12 year study performed in Poland did not reveal instances of irreversible damage or disturbances caused by exposure to microwave energy.[76]

Cataract has been incriminated for many years, as one of the chief hazards of exposure to microwaves. Many cases of cataracts attributed to microwaves have been reported in the literature. It is not possible to accept these as proven. Documentation of exposure history (field intensity, wavelength, duration and geometry) have been inadequate, but in all cases in which field intensity was known it was well in excess of 100 mW/cm^2.[77] There is no clinical or experimental evidence that lens damage allegedly due to microwave energy is morphologically different from lens abnormalities from other causes including the aging process.

Review of human survey data that are available and information derived from human case reports adds little to our knowledge of microwave cataractogenesis. None of the case reports of cataracts can be conclusively attributed to microwave exposure although in some cases there may possibly be an association. The scoring methods used, both for degree of exposure and lenticular defects, has not been particularly sound and their validity has been questioned. It is difficult to extrapolate from studies in anesthetized (and often hypothermic) animals to findings in radar workers and others who may be occupationally exposed at low levels on a daily basis, with possible infrequent exposures to intense fields that would be frankly thermalizing.[40]

Reports of cataracts in man must be put in perspective. Most studies suffer from inadequate documentation of exposure history (field intensity, wavelength, duration and geometry). It is essential that evaluation be made of the multiple environmental factors which may interact among themselves and with personal characteristics of the individual. There is always the danger that real factors may be overlooked leading to false association with factors of initial interest.

Problems and Recommendations

Although there is considerable agreement among scientists concerning the biological effects and potential hazards of microwaves, there are areas of disagreement. There also is a serious philosophical question about the definition of hazard. One objective definition of injury is an irreversible change in biological function as observed at the organ or system level. With this definition it is possible to define a hazard as a probability of injury on a statistical basis. It is important to differentiate between the hazard levels at which injury may be sustained and effect or perception. All effects are not necessarily hazards. In fact, some effects may have beneficial applications under appropriately controlled conditions. Microwave induced changes must be understood sufficiently so that their clinical significance can be determined, their hazard potential assessed and the appropriate benefit/risk analyses applied. It is important to determine whether an observed effect is irreparable, transient or reversible, disappearing when the electromagnetic field is removed or after some interval of time. Of course, even reversible effects are unacceptable if they transiently impair the ability of the individual to function properly or to perform a required task.

A critical review of studies into the biological effects of microwaves indicates that many of the investigations suffer from inadequacies of either technical facilities and energy measurement skills or insufficient control of the biological specimens and the criteria for biological change. More sophisticated conceptual approaches and more rigorous experimental design must be developed. This will require increased and improved education and training in the biological effects of non-ionizing radiation (NIR). There is a need for systematic and quantitative comparative investigation of the biological effects of exposure to MW/RF energies using well-controlled experiments. This should be done by using sound biomedical and biophysical approaches at the various organizational levels from the whole animal to the subcellular level on an integrated basis, with full recognition of the multiple associated and interdependent variables.

Proper investigation of the biological effects of NIR requires an understanding and appreciation of biophysical principles and "comparative biomedicine". Such studies require interspecies "scaling", the selection of biomedical parameters which consider basic physiological functions and work capacity, identification of specific and nonspecific reactions, and differentiation of adaptational or compensatory changes from pathological manifestations.

Assessment of the predictive value of animal testing for human responses is needed. This should be specifically directed towards comparing responses in several species to determine whether there is anything unique about a particular test animal. A systematic examination of several species is needed so that answers may be provided as to whether several species are better than one in predicting human response.

It is important that research be conducted in such a way that all aspects of the study are quantified, the type and degree of the effect, whether the effect is harmful, harmless, or merely an artifact, and how it relates to the results obtained by other investigators. For microwave bioeffects, body size of the experimental animal must be taken into account. Since body-absorption cross-sections and internal heating patterns can differ widely, an investigator may think he is observing a low-level or a "nonthermal" effect in one animal because the incident power is low, while in actuality the animal may be exposed to as much absorbed power in a specific region of the body as another larger animal is with much higher incident power density. In the performance of experimental studies on animals, for extrapolation to man, interspecies scaling factors must be considered.

Although most investigators accept the fact that exposure to high power density microwaves can result in pathophysiological manifestations of a thermal nature, some reports have suggested that "low power density" microwave energy can affect neural function in animals and man. Most of these reports have emanated from the USSR and other Eastern European countries. Since most reported "low-level" effects relate to behavioral and central nervous system changes, studies are needed to determine the nature and mechanism(s) of the nervous system's reactions, if any, to electromagnetic fields and to investigate the degree to which the individual's performance capabilities may be affected. Because of their important integrative and regulatory functions, the neuroendocrine and central nervous system should receive attention as possible sensitive areas. Neurochemical assays and immunologic reactivity could indicate basic mechanisms of interaction. The question whether reported central nervous system changes in man, (if they are validated), would be important enough to affect his performance should be resolved. Better understanding of local, regional and whole-body thermal regulation is required. More precise and better controlled long-term, low-level laboratory studies have been suggested. But these have to be rigidly controlled to obviate circadian rhythm and biologic drift over time which will influence responses.

Particular attention should be paid to instrumentation problems, such as the development of more adequate probes for making measurements in the presence of electromagnetic fields. Field strength, electrophysiological, and thermal probes which will give artifact-free readings, will not distort the field in any way, and which will not give rise to inadvertent stimulation of the tissue due to induced currents, are essential.

Well-designed and appropriately controlled epidemiological and clinical investigations of groups of workers and others exposed to microwaves should be fostered. Studies of workers and individuals exposed to MW/RF energies along with appropriate control groups, should include a thorough analysis of the exposure environment, including co-factors as well as electromagnetic fields. Epidemiological study is applicable not only to disorders in which there may be a major, definable, etiologic agent, but is also useful in evaluating disorders in which multiple environmental factors may interact.

There is always the danger that real factors may be overlooked leading to false association with factors included in the study. Such interacting factors could be heat, cold, toxic agents, hypoxia, noise, other radiant energy such as X-rays, chronic disease state and medication.

Above all there is a need for scientific competence and integrity. It is important to maintain a proper perspective and assess realistically the biomedical effects of microwave exposure, so that the worker or general public will not be unduly exposed nor will research, development and beneficial utilization of these energies be hampered or unnecessarily restricted.

ACKNOWLEDGEMENT

This paper is based on work performed under Contract No. DE-AC02-76EV03490 with the U.S. Department of Energy at the University of Rochester Department of Radiation Biology and Biophysics and has been assigned Report No. UR-3490-1964.

REFERENCES

1. H. P. Schwan, Temperature dependence of the dielectric constant of blood at low frequencies, Z. Naturforschung 3b:361 (1948).
2. H. P. Schwan, Electrical properties of tissue and cell suspensions, Adv. Biol. Med. Phys. 5:147 (1954).

3. H. P. Schwan, Electrical properties of tissues and cell suspensions, in: "Advances in Biological and Medical Physics," J. H. Lawrence and C.A. Tobias, eds., Academic Press, New York (1957).
4. H. P. Schwan and G. M. Piersol, The absorption of electromagnetic energy in body tissues, a review and critical analysis: Part I: Biophysical aspects, Am. J. Phys. Med. 33:371 (1954).
5. H. P. Schwan and G. M. Piersol, The absorption of electromagnetic energy in body tissues, a review and critical analysis: Part II: Physiological and clinical aspects, Am. J. Phys. Med. 34:425 (1955).
6. H. F. Cook, The dielectric behavior of some types of human tissues at microwave frequencies, Brit. J. Appl. Phys. 12:295 (1951).
7. J. F. Herrick, B. G. Jelatis and G. M. Lee, Dielectric properties of tissues important in microwave diathermy, Fed. Proc. 9:60 (1950).
8. C. C. Johnson and A. W. Guy, Nonionizing electromagnetic wave effects in biological materials and systems, Proc. IEEE 60:692 (1972).
9. H. P. Schwan and K. R. Foster, RF-field interactions with biological systems: electrical properties and biophysical mechanisms, Proc. IEEE 68:104 (1980).
10. M. A. Stuchly and S. S. Stuchly, Dielectric properties of biological substances - tabulated, J. Microwave Power 15:19 (1980).
11. E. F. Adolph, Look at physiological integration, Amer. J. Physiol. 237:R255 (1979).
12. J. D. Hardy, Thermal comfort: skin temperature and physiological thermoregulation, in: "Physiological and Behavioral Temperature Regulation," J. D. Hardy, A. P. Gagge and J. A. J. Stolwijk, eds., C. C. Thomas, Springfield (1980).
13. R. Thauer, Circulatory adjustments to climatic requirements, in: "Handbook of Physiology," Section 2, Circulation III, W. F. Hamilton, ed., Am. Physiol. Society, Washington, DC (1965).
14. S. M. Michaelson, Comparative biology in assessment of electromagnetic bioeffects, in: "Biomedical Aspects of Nonionizing Radiation," W. C. Milroy, ed., U.S. Naval Weapons Lab Tech. Report TR-3110, Dahlgren, VA (1974).
15. S. M. Michaelson, Thermal effects of single and repeated exposures to microwaves - a review, in: "Biologic Effects and Health Hazards of Microwave Radiation," P.Czerski, et al., eds., Polish Medical Publishers, Warsaw (1974).
16. S. M. Michaelson and H. P. Schwan, Comparative aspects of radiofrequency and microwave biomedical research, in: "Digest of Tech Papers IEEE G-MTT," S. W. Maley, ed., Internat. Symp. (1973).

17. J. H. Heller, Cellular effects of microwave radiation, *in*: "Biological Effects and Health Implications of Microwave Radiation, Symposium Proceedings," S. F. Cleary, ed., U.S. Department of Health, Education and Welfare, Public Health Service BRH/DBE 70-2 (1970).
18. D. E. Janes, W. M. Leach, W. A. Mills, R. T. Moore and M. L. Shore, Effects of 2450 MHz microwaves on protein synthesis and on chromosomes in Chinese hamsters, *Nonioniz. Radiat.* 1:125 (1969).
19. S. Baranski and P. Czerski, "Biological Effects of Microwaves," Dowden, Hutchinson and Ross, Stroudsburg, PA (1976).
20. S. Baranski, H. Debiec, K. Kwarecki and T. Mezykowski, Influence of microwaves on genetical processes of Aspergillus nidulans, *J. Microwave Power* 11:146 (1976).
21. C. F. Blackman, M. C. Surles and S. G. Benane, The effects of microwave exposure on bacteria mutation reduction, *Symp. Biol. Eff. of E.M. Waves.* U.S. Department of Health, Education and Welfare Publ. (FDA) 77-8010, 1:406 (1976).
22. M. M. Varma and E. A. Traboulay, Jr., Evolution of dominant lethal test and DNA studies in measuring mutagenicity caused by non-ionizing radiation, *in*: "Biological Effects of Electromagnetic Waves," C. C. Johnson and M. L. Shore, eds., Vol I, U.S. Department of Health, Education and Welfare, Food and Drug Adminstration, Publication (FDA) 77-8010, Rockville, MD (1976).
23. T. S. Ely, D. Goldman, J. Z. Hearon, R. B. Williams and H. M. Carpenter, Heating characteristics of laboratory animals exposed to ten centimeter microwaves, Bethesda, MD, U.S. Nav. Med. Res. Inst. (Res. Rep. Proj. NM 001-056.13.092), *IEEE Trans. Biomed. Eng.* 11:123 (1964).
24. W. G. Lotz and S. M. Michaelson, Temperature and corticosterone relationships in microwave exposed rats, *J. Appl. Physiol. Respirat. Environ. Exercise Physiol.* 44:438 (1978).
25. W. G. Lotz and S. M. Michaelson, Effects of hypophysectomy and dexamethasone on rat adrenal response to microwaves, *J. Appl. Physiol. Respirat. Environ. Exercise Physiol.* 47:1284-1288 (1979).
26. S. T. Lu, N. Lebda, S. Pettit, D. Rivera and S. M. Michaelson, Thermal and endocrinological effects of protracted irradiation of rats by 2450 MHz microwaves, *Radio Science* 12(6S):147 (1977).
27. S. T. Lu, N. Lebda, S. Pettit and S. M. Michaelson, Delineating acute neuroendocrine responses in microwave exposed rats, *J. Appl. Physiol. Respirat. Environ. Exercise Physiol.* 48:927 (1980).
28. S. T. Lu, W. G. Lotz and S. M. Michaelson, Advances in microwave-induced neuroendocrine effects: the concept of stress, *Proc. IEEE* 68:73 (1980).

29. R. L. Magin, S. T. Lu and S. M. Michaelson, Microwave heating effect on the dog thyroid gland. IEEE Trans. BME 24:522 (1977).
30. R. L. Magin, S. T. Lu and S. M. Michaelson, Stimulation of dog thyroid by local application of high intensity microwaves, Am. J. Physiol. 233:E363 (1977).
31. H. Mikolajczyk, Microwave irradiation and endocrine functions, in: "Biologic Effects and Health Hazards of Microwave Radiation," P. Czerski, et al., eds., Polish Medical Publishers, Warsaw (1974).
32. A. A. Novitskii, B. F. Murashov, P. E. Krasnobaev and N. F. Markozova, The functional condition of the system hypothalamus-hypophysis-adrenal cortex as a criterium in establishing the permissible levels of superhigh frequency elecromagnetic emissions, Voen. Med. Zh. 8:53 (1977).
33. I. R. Petrov and V. A. Syngayevskaya, Endocrine glands, in: "Influence of Microwave Radiation on the Organism of Man and Animals," I. R. Petrov, ed., Meditsina Press, Leningrad (1970).
34. W. Wiktor-Jedrezejczak, A. Ahmed, K. W. Sell, P. Czerski and W. M. Leach, Microwaves induce an increase in the frequency of complement receptor-bearing lymphoid spleen cells in mice, J. Immunol. 118:1499 (1977).
35. R. P. Liburdy, Radiofrequency radiation alters the immune system: modulation of T- and B-lymphocyte levels and cell-mediated immunocompetence by hyperthermic radiation, Radiat. Res. 77:34 (1979).
36. N. J. Roberts, Jr. and R. T. Steigbigel, Hyperthermia and human leukocyte functions: effects on responses of lymphocytes to mitogen, antigen and bactericidal capacity of monocytes and neutrophils, Infection and Immunity 18:673 (1977).
37. Z. V. Gordon, Y. A. Lobanova and M. S. Tolgskaya, Some data on the effect of centimeter waves (experimental studies), Gig. Sanit. (USSR) 12:16 (1955).
38. J. Bligh, Physiological response to heat, in: "Fundamental and Applied Aspects of Non-ionizing Radiation," S. M. Michaelson, et al., eds., Plenum, New York (1975).
39. S. M. Michaelson, Central nervous system responses to microwave-induced heating. Neurosci. Res. Program Bull. 15:98-100 (1977).
40. W. R. Adey, Tissue interactions with nonionizing electromagnetic fields. Physiol Rev. 61:435 (1981).
41. S. M. Michaelson, R. Guillet, W. G. Lotz, S. T. Lu and R. L. Magin, Neuroendocrine responses in the rat and dog exposed to 2450 MHz (CW) microwaves, in: "Biological Effects and Measurement of Radiofrequency/Microwaves," D. G. Hazzard, ed., Bureau of Radiological Health, HEW Publication (FDA) 77-8026, Rockville, MD p. 263 (1977).

42. E. S. Ismailov and S. M. Zubkova, Physicochemical mechanisms of the biological activity of microwaves (Russian), Biologicheskiye Nauki, 6:5 (Translation, JPRS 70101, Arlington) (1977).

43. A. S. Presman, "Elektromagnitzye Polya i Zhivaya Prioda" (Electomagnetic Fields and Animate Nature), Science Publishers, Moscow (1968).

44. A. S. Presman, "Elektromagnitzye Polya v Biosfere" (Electomagnetic Fields in the Biosphere), Znaniye, Moscow (1971).

45. K. J. Oscar and T. D. Hawkins, Microwave alterations of the blood-brain barrier system of rats, Brain Res. 126:281 (1977).

46. J. H. Merritt, A. F. Chamness and S. J. Allen, Studies on blood-brain barrier permeability after microwave irradiation, Radiat. Environ. Biophys. 15:367 (1978).

47. E. Preston, E. J. Vavasour and H. M. Assenheim, Permeability of the blood brain barrier to mannitol in the rat following 2450 MHz microwave irradiation, Brain Res. 174:109 (1979).

48. H. N. Kritikos and H. P. Schwan, The distribution of heating potential inside lossy spheres, Inst. Electrical Electronics Eng., Trans. Biomed. Eng. 22:457 (1975).

49. C. K. Chou and A. W. Guy, Quantitation of microwave biological effects, in: "Biological Effects and Measurements of Radio Frequency/Microwaves," D. G. Hazzard, ed., Bureau of Radiological Health, HEW Publication (FDA), Rockville, MD (1977).

50. A. W. Guy, Biophysical characteristics of electromagnetic fields, problems of dosimetry and dosimetric techniques, Neurosci. Res. Program Bull. 15:81-98 (1977).

51. H. N. Kritikos and H. P. Schwan, Potential temperature rise induced by electromagnetic fields in brain tissue, Inst. Electrical Electronics Eng. Trans. Biomed. Eng. 26:29 (1972).

52. H. N. Kritikos and H. P. Schwan, Hot spots generated in conducting spheres by electromagnetic waves and biological implications, Inst. Electrical Electronics Eng. Trans. Biomed. Eng. 19:53 (1972).

53. H. N. Kritikos and H. P. Schwan, Formation of hot spots in multilayer spheres, Inst. Electrical Electronics Eng., Trans. Biomed. Eng. 23:168 (1976).

54. M. A. Baker and L. W. Chapman, Rapid brain cooling in exercising dogs, Science 195:781 (1977).

55. J. de Lorge, Disruption of behavior in mammals of three different sizes exposed to microwaves: extrapolation to larger mammals, in: "1978 Symposium on Electromagnetic Fields in Biological Systems," S. S. Stuchly, ed., Ottawa (1978).

56. J. A. J. Stolwijk, Responses to the thermal environment, Fed. Proc. 36:1655 (1977).
57. S. Stern, L. Margolin, B. Weiss, S. T. Lu and S. M. Michaelson, Microwaves: effect on thermoregulatory behavior in rats, Science 206:1198 (1979).
58. E. R. Adair and B. W. Adams, Microwaves modify thermoregulatory behavior in squirrel monkeys, Bioelectromagnetics 1:1 (1980).
59. Z. V. Gordon, "Biological Effect of Microwaves in Occupational Hygiene," Izd. Med, Leningrad (1966).
60. M. N. Sadchikova and A. A. Orlova, Clinical picture of the chronic effects of electromagnetic microwaves, Ind. Hyg. Occupat. Dis. (USSR) 2:16 (1958).
61. Y. A. Osipov, "Occupational Hygiene and the Effect of Radio-frequency Electromagnetic Fields on Workers," Izd. Meditsina Press, Leningrad (1965).
62. Z. Edelweijn, R.L. Elder, E. Klimkova-Deutschova and B. Tengroth, Occupational exposure and public health aspects of microwave radiation, in: "Biological Effects and Health Hazards of Microwave Radiation," P. Czerski, et al., eds., Polish Medical Publishers, Warsaw (1974).
63. N. V. Tyagin, "Change in the blood of animals subjected to a SHF-UHF field," Voyenno-Medit. Akad. Kirov., 73:116, Leningrad (1957).
64. A. S. Hyde and J. J. Friedman, Some effects of acute and chronic microwave irradiation of mice, in: "Thermal Problems in Aerospace Medicine," J. D. Hardy, ed., Unwin Ltd., Surrey (1968).
65. J. F. Spalding, R. W. Freyman and L. M. Holland, Effects of 800 MHz electromagnetic radiation on body weight, activity, hematopoiesis and life span in mice, Health Physics 20:421 (1971).
66. S. M. Michaelson, R. A. E. Thomson and J. W. Howland, "Biologic Effects of Microwave Exposure." RADC: ASTIA Doc. No. AD 824-242, Griffis AFB, also United States Senate, Ninetieth Congress, second session on S 2067, S 3211 and HR 10790, 1968: Radiation Control for Health and Safety Act of 1967, (1967).
67. S. M. Michaelson, R. A. E. Thomson, M. Y. el Tamami, H. S. Seth and J. W. Howland, Hematologic effects of microwave exposure, Aerospace Med. 35:824 (1964).
68. S. Baranski, Effect of chronic microwave irradiation on the blood forming system of guinea pigs and rabbits, Aerospace Med. 42:1196 (1971).
69. P. Czerski, Microwave effects on the blood-forming system with particular references to the lymphocyte, in: "Biological Effects of Nonionizing Radiation," P. E. Tyler, ed., Ann. NY Acad Sci. 247:232 (1975).

70. P. Czerski, E. Paprocka-Slonka, M. Siekiersynzki and A. Stolarska, Influence of microwave radiation on the hematopoietic system, in: "Biologic Effects and Health Hazards of Microwave Radiation," P. Czerski, et al., eds., Polish Medical Publishers, Warsaw, (1974).
71. H. F. Cook, The pain threshold for microwave and infra-red radiations, J. Physiol. 118:1 (1952).
72. E. Hendler, J. D. Hardy and D. Murgatroyd, Skin heating and temperature sensation produced by infra-red and microwave irradiation," in: "Temperature Measurement and Control in Science and Industry," J. D. Hardy, ed., Reinhold, New York (1963).
73. E. Hendler, Cutaneous receptor response to microwave radiation, in: "Thermal Problems in Aerospace Medicine," J. D. Hardy, ed., Unwin Ltd., Surrey (1968).
74. C. D. Robinette, C. Silverman and S. Jablon, Effects upon health of occupational exposure to microwave radiation (Radar), Am. J. Epidemiol. 112:39 (1980).
75. A. K. Guskova and Y. H. Kochanova, Some aspects of etiological diagnostics of occupational disease as related to the effects of microwave radiation, Gig. Truda i Prob. Zabol 3:14 (1975).
76. P. Czerski and M. Piotrowski, Proposals for specification of allowable levels of microwave radiation, Medycyna Lotnicza (Polish) 39:127 (1972).
77. National Research Council, Effects of Microwave Radiation on the Lens of the Eye, National Academy of Sciences, Washington, DC (1981).

BIOLOGICAL EFFECTS OF LOW ENERGY ELECTROMAGNETIC FIELDS ON THE CENTRAL NERVOUS SYSTEM

W. Ross Adey

VETERANS ADMINISTRATION HOSPITAL, LOMA LINDA, CA 92357
AND DEPARTMENTS OF PHYSIOLOGY AND SURGERY, Loma Linda
University, School of Medicine, Loma Linda, CA 92357

INTRODUCTION

There has been extensive speculation about the possibility of enhanced sensitivities of central nervous tissue to environmental electromagnetic fields. Brain tissue possesses its own well known intrinsic oscillating field, the electroencephalogram (EEG). The functional significance of this internal field has been a matter of conjecture. Based on classical membrane electrophysiology, the majority of opinion has most frequently dismissed it as merely "the noise of the brain's motor." Evidence that this may not be an accurate evaluation has come from a variety of studies of effects of imposed oscillating electromagnetic fields which induce weak extracellular electrochemical oscillations in the fluid surrounding brain cells, and which mimic in varying degrees components of the natural electrochemical oscillations of the EEG in the same domain of brain tissue.

In addressing the problem of central nervous interactions with environmental electromagnetic fields, we may pose two key questions. Can the citadel of the neuron detect electrochemical oscillations in the perineuronal fluid that are many orders of magnitude weaker than the gradient of the membrane potential? If so, what are the anatomical substrates, and how do these substrates perform an amplification function for weak extracellular oscillations?

To the extent that these questions can be answered for brain tissue, they may provide a model for the search in other tissues for comparable effects. Our initial observations indicated that electromagnetic fields imposed on brain tissue at levels of the EEG and oscillating sinusoidally at frequencies in the EEG spectrum

(1-100 Hz), induced significant changes in ionic electrochemistry, in the electrophysiological rhythms of the EEG, and in certain learned patterns of EEG responses (Bawin and Adey, 1976; Bawin, Kaczmarek and Adey, 1975; Bawin, Gavalas-Medici and Adey, 1973; Blackman, Elder, Benane, Weil and Eichinger, 1979). These observations have now been extended in experiments to be described here to clonal lines of osteoblasts, pancreatic islet cells, cytotoxic T-lymphocytes and peritoneal macrophages. From these new data, it seems that a reasonable conclusion may be drawn that we are addressing a widespread phenomenon that may indeed be a general property of tissue; one that is vastly more exciting than classical models of cellular organization and excitatory processes based on equilibrium properties of membranes would have led us to expect. From these new studies of effects of weak electromagnetic fields that mimic various frequency and amplitude characteristics of intrinsic tissue electrochemical oscillations, it has become clear that the imposed fields can act as sensitive manipulanda in modifying a whole sequence of transductive steps that couple the initial cell surface triggering event to intracellular enzymatic and metabolic sequences. At this time, they include cell membrane receptor mechanisms for antibodies, hormones and neurotransmitters. Arising from field-modulated modification of these surface mechanisms, consequent effects have been noted on such important events as the sequence of adenyl cyclase activation, ensuing modifications in the conversion of adenosine triphosphate (ATP) to cyclic adenosine monophosphate (cAMP), and the ensuing activation of cAMP-dependent protein kinases.

Imposition of weak electromagnetic fields oscillating or modulated at low frequencies is becoming a valuable tool in studies of transductive coupling of pericellular electrochemical stimuli to cellular mechanisms. Observed sensitivities involve responses to stimuli far weaker than those initiating massive ionic perturbations that characterize excitation according to the Hodgkin-Huxley model. Some of these responses also show sharply lowered thresholds in certain narrow ranges of frequency and amplitude. Jointly, these data indicate that these sensitivities are based on nonequilibrium reactions. We will consider in more detail the possible nature of these nonequilibrium processes. In essence, the observed sensitivities to these weak electrochemical oscillations on cell membrane surfaces, conservatively measured or calculated to be many orders of magnitude less than the transmembrane potential gradient of 10^5 V/cm, support the view that cells in tissue "whisper together" (Young, 1951) by signals that pass from cell to cell as perturbations produced by each cell in the extracellular fluid which surrounds it. Obviously such a scheme in central nervous tissue would open the door to excitingly new concepts of neuronal and neuronal-neuroglial integration of information. Indeed, the anatomical structure and functional organization of cerebral neurons appear particularly suited to such a scheme; as discussed below, communication between cerebral neurons may occur by a variety of slow wave-like electrochemical oscillations as distinct from the transaction and transmission of information through trains of neuronal action potentials or impulses.

Use of electromagnetic fields having certain frequency and amplitude characteristics has thus become an important experimental tool in opening the door to a first understanding of the possible ways in which cells in tissue may communicate with each other. Our first perceptions indicate that this will prove to be a whole new world of scientific experience, and that we shall find the answers in mechanisms far removed from the classic biology of membrane excitation and modulation through chemical equilibrium processes.

Anatomical Substrates of Cerebral Organization

In seeking substrates at the cellular level for tissue interactions with intrinsic and imposed electromagnetic fields that induce electrochemical oscillations in the microenvironment surrounding each neuron, it is appropriate to focus on the unique organization of the profuse dendritic branches of these cells. These branches are beautifully displayed by the Golgi technique, which coats the entire surface (dendrites, cell body and axon) of a single neuron with silver chromate.

The striking feature of Golgi stained sections of cerebral cortex is the huge development of a tree of dendritic branches. These dendritic branches typically spread far from the small cell body, which has a diameter of 15 to 30 μm. Dendritic branches may extend many hundreds of micrometers from the cell body. Thus, the dendritic "tree" encloses a volume hundreds of times larger than the cell body from which it is derived. Also, by reason of the close proximity of neurons to one another in cerebral structures, the dendritic tree of one cell overlaps the space occupied by the trees of neighboring cells. Thus, there is very truly a "forest" of closely intertwined dendritic branches.

The elaboration of these dendritic trees is probably the most striking feature of the development of the cerebral cortex after birth. Golgi-stained histological sections of cerebral cortex in the newborn show only the main shafts of the future dendritic trees, resembling so many bare tree trunks stripped of branches after a forest fire. Gradually over the next 15 to 18 months, there is an enormous proliferation of finer dendritic branches which intertwine with those from other cells (Fig. 1).

This overlapping arrangement had long been known, but it was not until studies over the last 5 years have shown the extent to which actual dendrodendritic synapses are formed between dendritic branches of adjacent cells (Shepherd, 1979). Many of these synaptic contacts are designed to allow free movement of signals recip-

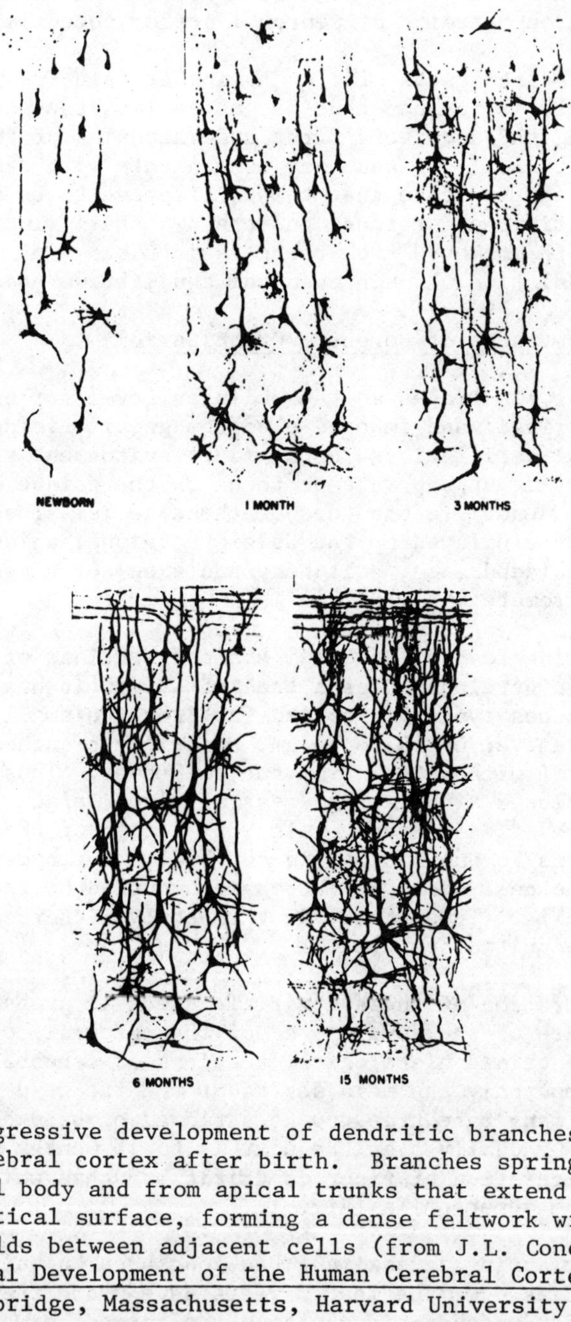

Fig. 1. Progressive development of dendritic branches in human cerebral cortex after birth. Branches spring from the cell body and from apical trunks that extend towards the cortical surface, forming a dense feltwork with overlapping fields between adjacent cells (from J.L. Conel, The Postnatal Development of the Human Cerebral Cortex, Vol. 1. Cambridge, Massachusetts, Harvard University Press, 1939).

rocally across a single junction. In this respect, they differ sharply from the typical unidirectional configuration of synapses between the fine axonal terminals of nerve fibers at the points where they make contact with the surface of the next neuron. Structurally, these dendrodendritic contacts display a variety of forms. Many of these arrangements are consistent with reciprocal conduction. For example, some gap junctions, in which the two dendritic elements make very close contact with each other for a short distance; others have the appearance of classical synapse , with a presynaptic vesicular concentration and a post synaptic bar in the adjoining membrane; and often a completely reciprocal arrangement is found in a closely adjacent synaptoid junction. These dual synaptic arrangements lying close together in a single domain of contacting membranes give a clear hint as to the capacity for reciprocal information flow across the region of contact.

Cerebral Neuronal Physiology

From elegant studies with liquid filled glass microelectrodes, fine enough to allow intracellular penetration of the tiny bodies of cerebral neurons, much has been learned about the electrophysiological integration occurring in cerebral neurons. Briefly, these intracellular records from many neurons are characterized by high amplitude intracellular electric waves. At the point of penetration of the electrode into the cell body (soma), the electrode records a membrane potential typically in the range 30 to 50 mV. This potential remains relatively steady when recorded in nerve cells outside the cerebral cortex, showing only transient modifications as the cell is excited or inhibited in the course of generating very brief action potentials (nerve impulses). By contrast, cerebral neurons frequently display a constantly shifting baseline in the membrane potentials. These wave-like perturbations are often of high amplitude, ranging from 5 to 20 mV. They are thus a sizable fraction of the membrane potential. In their frequency characteristics, they have a spectrum predominantly in the range from 1 to 20 Hz. The dominant energy bands are thus very similar to those in the EEG. The close relationship to the frequency spectrum of the EEG is further sustained if simultaneously recorded epochs of neuronal waves and EEG from the same domain of tissue are subjected to simultaneous spectral analysis. The EEG recorded in the fluid around nerve cells appears to be derived from the sum of portions of the intracellular neuronal waves that are "leaked" into the fluid around the generating neurons, and attenuated by reason of the high membrane resistance by a factor of approximately 200 from the amplitude recorded inside the cell. The amplitude of the intraneuronal waves expressed as a gradient across the thickness of the cell membrane is of the order of 10^4 V/cm, whereas the amplitude of the EEG expressed as a gradient across the dimensions of a single neuron is in the range 20 to 100 mV/cm. Thus, there is a disparity of approximately 5 orders of magnitude between the EEG recorded in the extracellular fluid and the magnitude of the cell membrane potential. It is not surprising that this disparity has long discouraged attempts to establish credibility for such weak pericellular electrochemical oscillations as playing some role in cellular communication in cerebral tissue. Parenthetically, it should be pointed out that despite the similarities in spectral content of the EEG and the contributing neuronal waves, they do not bear a direct relationship to one another in terms of exact synchronism; measurements of coherence have shown that the individual neuronal generator is only briefly and rarely synchronized with the field potential of the summed neuronal contributions, recorded as the EEG.

From this brief summary of the essential aspects of electrogenesis in cerebral tissue, we shall evaluate observed interactions of a variety of imposed electromagnetic fields on brain and other tissues.

Brain Tissue as a Tricompartmental Model

Cellular elements in brain tissue comprise both nervous and non-nervous elements. Nerve cells are surrounded by large cells of smaller non-nervous elements, the neuroglial cells, which substantially outnumber the neurons. Cerebral neuroglial cells respond sensitively to changing physiological states in the neurons which they enclose. Changes in enzyme content, protein synthesis and metabolic responses all exhibit correlated interactions as responses to sensory stimulation and as concomitants of learning procedures.

This communication between neurons and neuroglial cells occurs across the intervening space of the extracellular compartment. The space may occupy up to 20 per cent of the cerebral volume, but its size is highly variable and contingent upon the age of the cerebral tissue and on its metabolic status. It is very large in the newborn and rapidly decreases in response to trauma and asphyxiation.

As discussed below, the cerebral extracellular space has a significant macromolecular content. It constitutes a preferred pathway in the flow of current through cerebral tissue over alternate routes via cell membranes. Typical values for cell membrane resistance are of the order of 5,000 ohm/cm^2; by contrast, extracellular fluid has a typical specific resistance of 25 ohm.cm. Taking into account the contribution of the extracellular space to the tissue cross-section, the typical specific resistance for brain tissue is around 300 ohm.cm. Obviously, tissue currents associated with intrinsic and environmental electromagnetic fields will also find a preferred pathway through the extracellular medium. These narrow channels between cells possess a macromolecular structure meriting our detailed consideration. It should be pointed out that this region is not simply a saline bath. The ordered nature of certain of its macromolecular contents offers a structural and functional basis for observed interactions between tissues and imposed electromagnetic fields.

Organization of Macromolecules at Cell Membrane Surfaces

Almost 20 years ago, use of a phosphotungstic acid staining method for electron micrographs of brain tissue disclosed dark bands of cell surface material, characterized chemically as glycoproteins or glycosaminoglycans. Interest in these substances was fostered by development of a series of membrane models, all designed to account for specific properties of membranes that unfolded progressively from the beginning of the 1950s. The Davson-Danielli model proposed that the lipid bilayer (plasma membrane) is enclosed in a sandwich of protein coating the outer and inner surfaces of the bilayer. Benson (1965) proposed that the proteinaceous material disrupted the continuity of the lipid bilayer by lying within it, with protrusions on the external and internal surfaces of the membrane. This led in turn to the formulations by Singer and Nicolson (1972) of a fluid mosaic model, which now enjoys wide acceptance. In the fluid mosaic model, the protein group forms an intramembranous particle (IMP), with external and internal stranded protrusions. For the purposes of our discussion, the external strand is of major interest, since it offers a vehicle for the transductive coupling of a weak extracellular oscillating electromagnetic field to the interior of the cell. Structurally, this glycoprotein strand has terminal amino sugars (sialic acids) with numerous fixed negative charges. The net effect of these charged terminals is to produce a polyanionic surface sheet, which may be likened to a field of corn waving in the weak breeze of local electrochemical oscillations. These stranded protrusions establish a surface mosaic which thus determines the location and specificity of receptor sites for neurotransmitters, neurohumoral agents, hormonal binding sites and antibody receptor regions (Fig. 2).

The lipid bilayer itself has fluid properties, so that the intramembranous particles of protein float in the lipid bilayer and have considerable mobility within it. There is striking evidence on this mobility of the cell surface mosaic. Cell-mediated immunity in binding of antibodies to cell surface receptors on lymphocytes causes the aggregation of intramembranous particles into patches, followed by aggregation of the patches into a single cap. In embryonic muscle cells, actual movement of membrane surface receptors can be induced by electrophoretic currents, which displace acetylcholine receptors, and those sites binding lectin substances, such as concanavalin A. In essence, the distribution of these surface receptors specifies more precisely the biological subset of classes of T-lymphocytes than any other method so far available.

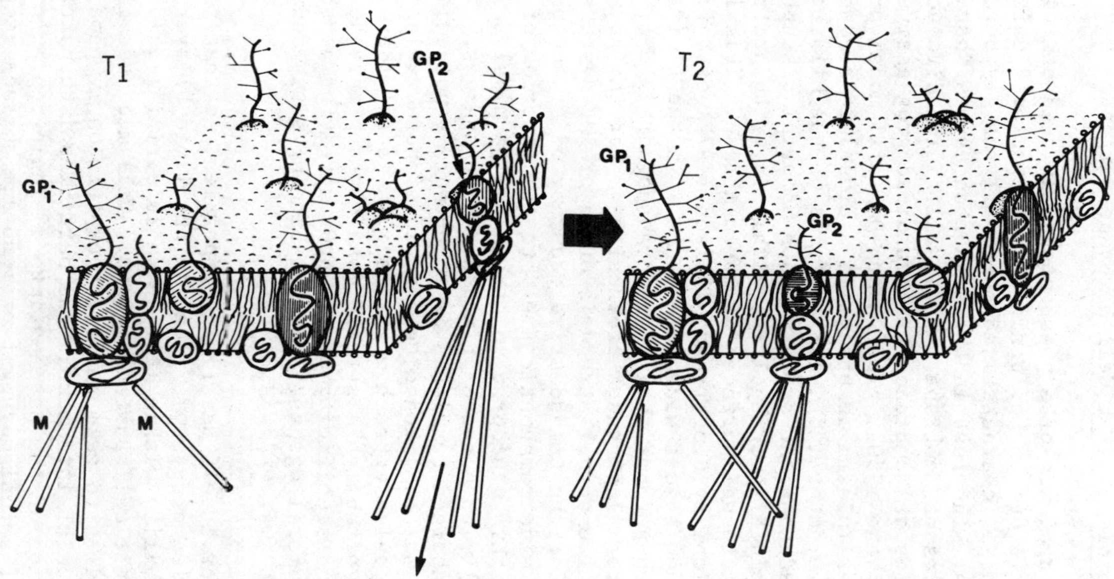

Fig. 2. Fluid mosaic model of cell membrane structure. T_1 and T_2 represent different moments in time. Some hypothetical glycoprotein particles are free to diffuse laterally in the lipid bilayer, whereas others (GP_1) may be constrained by microfilaments and microtubules (M). Some membrane macromolecules (GP_2) may be moved by microtubule contraction (From Nicolson, 1975, in: Functional Linkage in Biomolecular Systems. Raven Press, New York).

The polyanionic character of membrane surface glycoproteins attracts a counterion layer of cations. Of the constituent cations in extracellular fluid, calcium and hydrogen ions are the strongest competitors for the anionic binding sites, with strong competition between these two ionic species for available sites. In this respect, hydrogen ions compete far more powerfully than other monovalent cations, and Bass and Moore (1968) have modeled nervous excitation on the basis of local displacement of calcium ions by hydrogen ions at membrane surface sites. The ensuing depletion of hydrogen ions from the counterion layer would then produce a local alkalosis. As discussed below, the binding and release of calcium ions in cerebral tissue has proved a valuable tool in the detection of interactions of environmental electromagnetic fields with brain and other tissues.

Binding and Release of Calcium in Brain Tissue as Indices of Interactions with Environmental Electromagnetic Fields

The first indication that binding and release of calcium in cerebral cortex might be sensitive to electrical stimulation at intensities that mimicked the levels of the EEG in perineuronal fluid came from studies in the awake immobilized cat (Kaczmarek and Adey, 1974). Using large agar electrodes to deliver trains of 1.0 msec square wave pulses at 200/sec to the anterior and posterior poles of the cerebral hemisphere, relatively uniform fields at intensities of 50 to 100 mV/cm were produced in the major part of the cortical and subcortical zones of the stimulated hemisphere. Efflux of $^{45}Ca^{2+}$ and of ^{3}H-gamma-aminobutyric acid (GABA) were measured at the cortical surface. This electrical stimulation elicited increased efflux of calcium and GABA during and following the 10 min stimulus epoch. The magnitude of this increase approached 20 per cent for both calcium and GABA. In view of the role of GABA as an inhibitory transmitter substance, the findings raised questions about the functional capacity of natural and induced low frequency electrochemical oscillations at intensities no higher than the EEG in transaction and transmission of information in cerebral tissue. Findings in this study stimulated our search for evicence of modified calcium binding in cerebral tissue exposed to sinusoidal ELF fields in the frequency range of 1-100 Hz, and to radiofrequency and microwave fields sinusoidally amplitude modulated in the same ELF frequency range.

a. <u>$^{45}Ca^{2+}$ efflux from isolated brain tissue exposed to amplitude modulated 147 MHz fields.</u> Cerebral hemispheres of neonatal chicks were equilibrated with a physiological solution containing normal amounts of calcium (2.14 mM) and small amounts of $^{45}Ca^{2+}$. After equilibration, efflux of $^{45}Ca^{2+}$ from the surface of the hemisphere was compared between field exposed and control samples. Incident field intensity was 0.8 mW/cm^{2}, and the incident field was sinusoidally modulated to a depth of approximately 90 per cent at frequencies from 0.5 to 35 Hz.

Unmodulated fields produced no significant changes in $^{45}Ca^{2+}$ efflux. By contrast, efflux levels associated with exposure to modulated fields showed a striking "tuning curve" that at a modulation frequency in the vicinity of 16 Hz, exceeded 15 per cent over control levels. At higher and lower modulation frequencies, these induced alterations in efflux declined progressively from the peak at 16 Hz. Similar experiments were performed in the presence of 10^{-4} M sodium cyanide to preclude continued metabolic activity in the tissue. The increased $^{45}Ca^{2+}$ efflux persisted in the presence of the sodium cyanide. No responses were observed in samples of striated muscle comparable in volume to the cerebral hemispheres and tested concurrently with the brain tissue. There was thus a "window" of modulation frequencies effective in modifying the calcium efflux (Fig. 3).

A comparable window that was virtually the mirror image of that produced by these modulated RF fields was found with far weaker tissue components of ELF fields. In the latter case, ELF fields at 10 and 56 V/m in the same range of frequencies as those used to modulate the 147 MHz RF fields reduced the $^{45}Ca^{2+}$ efflux by about the same amount as it was increased by the RF fields. Again, the maximal interaction occurred at around 16 Hz. In this case, tissue components of these fields were calculated to be around 10^{-7} V/cm (Fig. 3).

We had also noted what appeared to be an amplitude "window" in these ELF experiments, with statistically significant responses at enviornmental field intensities of 10 and 56 V/m, but no significant responses at lower or higher field intensities. Separate studies by Blackman and in our own laboratories have confirmed occurrence of a number of frequency and amplitude windows in these calcium efflux responses in brain tissue exposed to ELF, RF and microwave fields. Blackman et al. (1979) noted that 147 MHz fields, sinusoidally modulated at 16 Hz, were only effective in increasing calcium efflux at incident intensities around 1.0 mW/cm^2. This was subsequently confirmed by Bawin, Sheppard and Adey (1978) using 450 MHz microwave fields sinusoidally modulated at 16 Hz; in the latter experiments, this amplitude window was found at intensities between 0.1 and 1.0 mW/cm^2. Blackman, Benane and Kinney(1981) have also observed frequency dependent field induced calcium ion efflux changes at incident field intensities between 1 and 70 V/m. These findings in freshly isolated cerebral hemispheres of the chick have prompted two further lines of study; we have examined the sensitivity of calcium efflux from synaptosome fractions and responses of intact cat cerebral cortex to sinusoidally modulated microwave fields.

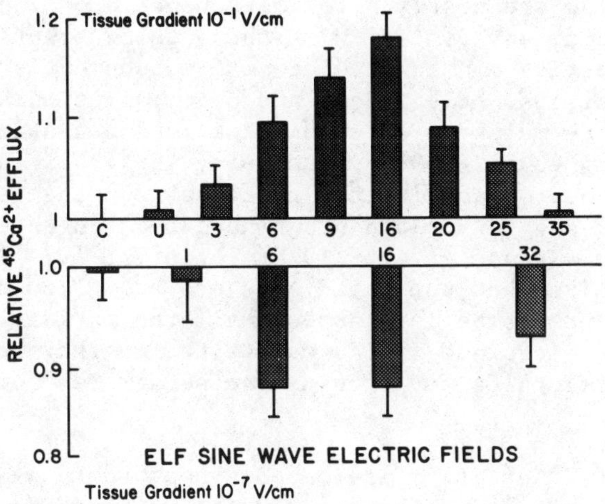

Fig. 3. A: $^{45}Ca^{2+}$ efflux from freshly isolated chick cerebral hemispheres exposed to weak radiofrequency fields (147 MHz, 0.8 mW/cm^2), amplitude-modulated at low frequencies (3-35 Hz). B: $^{45}Ca^{2+}$ efflux changes from exposure to far weaker electric fields (56 V/m) in the same frequency spectrum from 1 to 32 Hz. Peak magnitude of efflux change is similar for the 2 fields but opposite in direction. For radiofrequency field in A, the unmodulated carrier wave U had no effect when compared with controls C. Tissue field gradients differ by about 6 orders of magnitude between A and B. (Adapted from Bawin and Adey, 1976; and Bawin, Kaczmarek and Adey, 1975).

b. Calcium efflux rates from synaptosomes exposed to microwave fields amplitude modulated at low frequencies. Since evaluation of cell membrane properties is very difficult in whole hemisphere preparations, we have used synaptosomes, which are nerve terminals prepared from gently homogenized brain tissue. The membranes of these small terminal bodies reseal after their separation from the nerve fiber. When viewed with a transmission electron microscope, each individual synaptosome is an isolated entity resembling a synaptic terminal in its normal location. Its average diameter is about 0.7 μm, and its membrane enclosed numerous synaptic vesicles and frequently a few mitochondria. Since the synaptosomes are in direct contact with the bathing solution, their membrane properties can be studied more conveniently in whole brain or in tissue slices. Electrical and chemical stimulation depolarize the membrane, stimulating calcium uptake and neurotransmitter release (Redburn, et al., 1976; Blaustein, 1975). In addition to receptors for neurotransmitters, receptors for the lectin concanavalin A (con A) and for opioid drugs have been detected on synaptosomal membrane (Matus, et al., 1973; Terenius, 1973). These properties emphasize that the lipid bilayers and glycoconjugates are probably well preserved in synaptosomal preparations. Synaptosomal sensitivity to microwave fields was tested on the premise that these surface macromolecules may provide the substrates for field tissue interaction.

Efflux of $^{45}Ca^{2+}$ from preloaded synaptosomes was studied with a continuous perfusion technique and the rate constants of a 2-phase efflux process calculated. When a 450 MHz microwave field (incident intensity, 0.4 mW/cm^2), sinusoidally amplitude modulated at 16 Hz to a modulation depth of 75 per cent was applied during the second efflux phase, the rate constant increased by 38 per cent (Fig.4). Unmodulated or 60Hz modulated signals were not effective. These data suggest that the microwave field-induced change in calcium efflux probably did not involve intracellular calcium. Also, this change in the dynamic properties of synaptosomes did not require gross anatomical structure as a substrate for field-tissue interaction (Lin-Liu and Adey, 1981).

c. Effects of weak amplitude-modulated microwave fields on calcium efflux from awake cat cerebral cortex. Efflux of $^{45}Ca^{2+}$ was studied from preloaded cerebral cortex in cats immobilized under local anesthesia, and exposed to a 3 mW/cm^2 450 MHz field sinusoidally amplitude modulated at 16 Hz (modulation depth 85%). Tissue dosimetry showed a field of 33 V/m in the interhemispheric fissure (energy deposition 0.29 W/kg). Field exposure lasted 60 min. By comparison with controls efflux curves from field exposed brains were disrupted by waves of increased $^{45}Ca^{2+}$ efflux. These waves were irregular in amplitude and duration, but many exhibited periods of 20 to 30 min. They continued into the post exposure period (Fig.5).

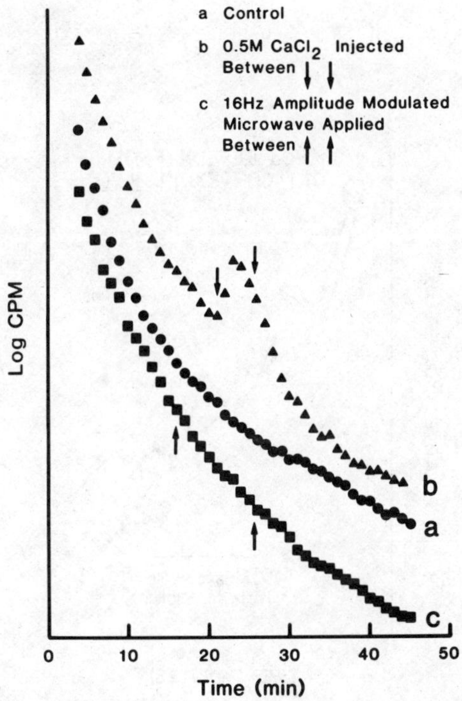

Fig. 4. Efflux of $^{45}Ca^{2+}$ from cerebral synaptosomes studied with a continuous perfusion technique. Curves were displaced vertically for clarity. Stimulation of calcium efflux by microwaves (450 MHz, 0.5 mW/cm^2, 16 Hz sinusoidal modulation, 75% depth) could be distinguished from that of a stimulated Ca-Ca exchange. Ca-stimulated efflux may be derived from the intracellular compartment. Microwave stimulation appeared to involve membrane surface binding sites, and increased the rate constant for $^{45}Ca^{2+}$ efflux in the second (slower) efflux phase by 38 ^{o}/o. (From Lin-Liu and Adey, 1981).

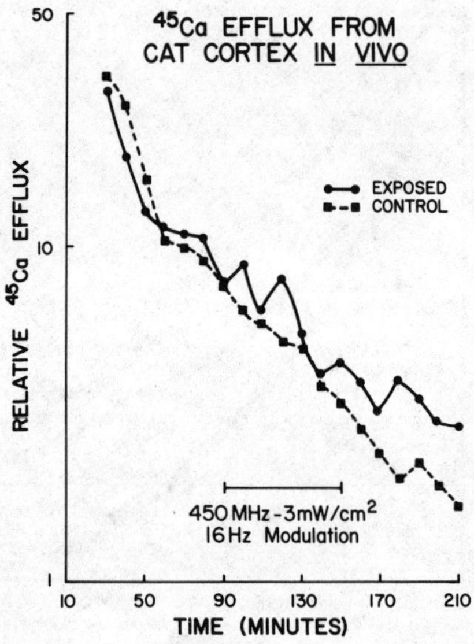

Fig. 5. Efflux of $^{45}Ca^{2+}$ from preloaded cerebral cortex in two experiments. Increased efflux in comparison with control occurred during and following exposure for 1 hour to a 450 MHz 3 mW/cm^2, sinusoidally modulated at 16 Hz. This curve of increased efflux shows slow oscillations sustained beyond the exposure epoch. (From Adey, Bawin and Lawrence, 1981)

Binomial probability analysis indicates that the field-exposed efflux curves constitute a different population from controls at a confidence level of 0.96 (Adey, Bawin and Lawrence, 1981).

In about 70 per cent of cases, initiation of field exposure was followed by increased end-tidal CO_2 excretion for about 5 min. However, hypercapnea induced by hypoventilation did not elicit increased $^{45}Ca^{2+}$ efflux. Thus, this increase with exposure did not appear to arise as a secondary effect of raised cerebral CO_2 levels. Radioactivity measurements in cortical samples after superfusion showed $^{45}Ca^{2+}$ penetration at about 1.7 mm/hr, a consistent with diffusion of the ion in free solution.

From the foregoing brief account of efflux studies from cerebral tissue under the influence of a variety of weak electromagnetic fields, it has become clear that fields raising tissue temperature orders of magnitude less than 0.1C may result in major physiological changes not attributable to raised temperature _per se_. These weak fields have been observed to produce chemical, physiological and behavioral changes only within "windows" in frequency and incident energy. For brain tissue, a maximum frequency sensitivity occurs between 6 and 20 Hz. Two different intensity windows have been seen, one for ELF tissue gradients around 10^{-7}V/cm, and one for amplitude modulated RF and microwave gradient around 10^{-1}V/cm. The former is at the level associated with navigation and prey detection in marine vertebrates and with control of human biological rhythms; the latter is at the level of the electroencephalogram (EEG) in brain tissue. Coupling of the field to living cells appears to require amplifying mechanisms that may be based on nonequilibrium processes, with long-range resonant molecular interactions.

Significance of Windowed Interactions as Indices of Nonequilibrium Processes

The low frequency and power windows so far defined for some field interactions with cerebral calcium binding strongly bespeak a cooperative interaction (Adey, 1975), based on long-range interactions in the length of a coherently organized charge system. From studies of the biopolymer poly-L-glutamic acid, Schwarz (1967, 1975) concluded that its fixed charge sites may behave coherently, with adjacent charge sites having the same energy level. It is implicit in the concept of a coherent domain that, for the duration of the coherent state, this patch of membrane would be thermally quiet, isolated from the randomization of energy levels characteristic of the noncoherent condition. A coherent domain of anionic, fixed-charge sites on membrane surface glycoproteins would require energy to raise them above the ground state. For some membrane-surface phenomena, energy is supplied by metabolic processes (Yahara and Edelman, 1972), but there is as yet no precise knowledge about sources of energy that might contribute to coherent surface charge states. Such a system can be restored to the ground state by an extremely weak trigger at the level of Boltzmann (kT) noise or below (Bawin and Adey, 1976).

The windowed character of these responses in frequency and amplitude domains unequivocally establishes a series of highly nonlinear mechanisms in the control of cerebral calcium ion binding. It also points to long-range interactions requiring ordered molecular states that persist for appreciable time over considerable atomic distances (Adey, 1979; Adey, 1981a, 1981b). It is also clear that the levels of cooperativity in these interactions must be high, since for the ELF field effects cited here, the effective stimuli may appear to be below the level of Boltzmann thermal noise. Though this is probably not the case (see discussion on models below), both the biological thresholds cited above and these chemical thresholds for ELF electric and magnetic fields are mutually consistent with sensitivities within an order of magnitude of thermal noise levels (Kalmijn, 1980). The search for a physical basis for this cooperativity may prove difficult. By comparison with tissue electric gradients induced by environmental EM fields, the requisite gradients for some known cooperative macromolecular transitions are very large. The helix-coil conformational change in poly(Y-benzyl L glutamate) can be induced as a cooperative transition by a gradient of 260 kV/cm (Schwarz and Seelig, 1968), based on nearest neighbor interactions. Long-lasting conformation changes occur in poly(A).2poly(U) and in ribosomal RNA with pulsed electric fields of 20 kV/cm and with a decay time 10 sec (Neumann and Katchalsky, 1972; Neumann, Nachmansohn and Katchalsky, 1973). They are viewed as a model for nerve excitability. It is clear that these phenomena and related models involve energy levels orders of magnitude greater than those associated with weak EM fields that elicit such a wide range of proven bioeffects. We may hypothesize that one or more transductive steps are necessary before the pericellular electric fields becomes an effective transmembrane signal. Models of these processes fall into two categories, one considering properties of polyanionic membrane surface macromolecules, and the other the behavior of the phospholipid bilayer (for more extensive review see Adey, 1981a).

Evidence for Location of Field-sensitive calcium binding sites at cell membrane surfaces

Calcium efflux changes from cerebral tissue induced by EM field exposure *in vitro* are typically 10-20 per cent. Changes of this magnitude are likely to arise from extracellular rather than intracellular pools. Cytosolic concentrations of calcium are so low (typically 10^{-7} M) that few of the molecules present within the cytosol or on the inner membrane surface facing the cytosol have any calcium bound in the resting cell (for review, see Kretsinger, 1981). With typical extracellular concentrations of 2 mM, there is thus an enormous differential between extracellular and intracellular levels. The primary function of calcium within the cytosol has been described as the transmission of information; therefore, even small increments of intracellular calcium levels by selective calcium influx allows selection of the appropriate intracellular physiological response.

The inflow of calcium into the interior of the cell in response to a broad range of stimuli increases cytosolic levels of free calcium to about 10^{-5} M (pCa about 5) for short periods between 1 and 100 sec, even though physiological results of this signal may last for hours. The effective free-ion concentration of calcium at the inner end of a membrane pore following its opening in excitation has never been measured, but probably never exceeds 2 X 10^{-5} M (pCa 4.7). This level would reflect significant resistance to calcium flow through the channel which would prevent attainment of levels around 5 X 10^{-4} M or more found at the outer end of the channel and on the membrane surface. From these observations and models a differential extracellular calcium concentration of at least an order of magnitude would be expected in both resting and excited cell states. Further evidence that it is the extracellular calcium pools that are associated with EM field interactions comes from use of lanthanum to block transmembrane movement in cerebral tissue; sinusoidally modulated 450 MHz fields continued to elicit modified $^{45}Ca^{2+}$ efflux after lanthanum blockade, but the response involved decreased efflux, in contrast to the increase occurring without lanthanum (Bawin, Adey and Sabbot, 1978).

In these *in vitro* experiments, calcium efflux was enhanced by addition of hydrogen ions, and inhibited in the absence of normal bicarbonate level. Omission of HCO_3^- from the medium resulted in a marked decrease (10 per cent) in efflux, by comparison with concurrent results for tissues in the standard physiological solution. This decrease was not due to an early rapid $^{45}Ca^{2+}$ efflux in the rinsing solution. These *in vitro* experiments indicate the importance of CO_2 in the homeostasis of the brain cell environment as a substrate in calcium binding mechanisms. The findings are consistent with transduction of weak, low-frequency oscillating electric fields in a specific class of extracellular negative binding sites normally occupied by Ca^{2+} and susceptible to competitive H^+ binding.

These nonequilibrium processes at the membrane surface constitute a hierarchy of interacting systems. Schwarz (1967) has described coherent states between nearest-neighbor anionic charge sites. In their interactions with cations in extracellular fluid, particularly calcium and hydrogen ions, these domains of coherent fixed charge sites offer a basis for cooperative processes in the length and area of the membrane surface. These coherent states persist for quite long times. In studies of interactions between acridine dyes and poly-L-glutamic acid, Schwarz observed coherent states lasting up to 0.8 msec. As discussed in Lecture 28, cooperative interactions induced by weak oscillating extracellular EM fields modify the interaction of hormone molecules with receptor coupling mechanisms, as for example, in the capacity of the peptide parathyroid hormone molecule to activate the enzyme adenyl cyclase on the inner aspect of the membrane. There appears to be a "ripple effect", also cooperative in character, that spreads away from the site of binding of the hormone molecule for considerable distances along the membrane surface. At a still more complex level, immunological events associated with the binding of antibodies at cell membrane surfaces are also highly coöperative in character. These interactions may involve actual movement of receptor sites to establish new patterns in the glycoprotein mosaic on the cell surface, as in the formation of patches which coalesce to a "cap" in the phenomena of patching and capping in lymphocytes. It should be emphasized that in all these cooperative membrane surface events, calcium ions play a required role. They are the mediators of the changed architecture of membrane structure by which weak electrochemical stimuli are first detected and then amplified at the membrane surface. They also mediate the coupling of these signals across the membrane to intracellular systems that initiate and mediate metabolic processes at energy levels many orders of magnitude higher than the energy levels associated with the initial membrane surface triggering events. Immunological responses that represent the more complex levels in this hierarchy are susceptible to impose low level EM fields.

Immunological Responses Modified by Amplitude Modulated Microwave Fields

There are two basic ways in which the immune system produces its effects in the tissues of an organism. One involves effects produced by antibodies circulating in the blood of the organism. In this humoral immunity, these antibodies combine with antigens on the surface of the target cell, producing effects that may include rupture of the cell membrane or lysis and consequent death of the cell. Cell killing may also occur by cytotoxic effects of T-lymphocytes in the process of cell-mediated immunity. In the latter, direct contact occurs between the cytotoxic lymphocyte and a target cell. The cytotoxic lymphocyte has already been stimulated to produce antibodies against the target cell, and these antibodies are located on the surface of the lymphocyte. Contact between the lymphocyte and the target cell again causes membrane rupture or lysis, releasing the intracellular contents of the target cell. Killing capacity of cytotoxic lymphocytes may therefore be measure by tagging the target cell with an isotope such as ^{51}Cr and measuring the release of ^{51}Cr associated with cell rupture and death.

We have measured the cytotoxic capacity of a mouse T-lymphocyte cultured cell line (CTLL-1) targeted against a human myeloma cell line (MPC-11) when the interacting cell systems were exposed to a 450 MHz field sinusoidally amplitude modulated at frequencies between 3 and 100 Hz (Lyle, Schechter, Adey and Lundak, 1981). Field intensity was 1.5 mW/cm^2. Modulation depth in these experiments was 75 to 85 per cent. When the 4 hour cytotoxicity assay was conducted in the presence of the microwave field modulated at 60 Hz, the cytotoxicity was reduced by about 20 per cent. This reduction in cytotoxicity related to effects of exposure on the lymphocytes, rather than on the target myeloma cells, since exposure of the lymphocytes to the field prior to adding them to the target cells in the cytolytic assay resulted in a similar inhibition. Most of this inhibitory effect was produced by the field in the early part of the 4 hour exposure period (early allogeneic recognition phase). Field- exposed cytolytic cells recovered their full cytolytic capacity in 12.5 hours.

When this suppression of cytolysis was tested over a spectrum of modulation frequencies from 3 to 100 Hz, a "tuning curve" was observed, similar to that observed for calcium efflux from brain tissue (Bawin, Kaczmarek and Adey, 1975) but centered around 60 Hz modulation instead of the peak in the vicinity of 16 Hz noted for brain tissue. Effects increased progressively for modulation frequencies of 3, 16 and 40 Hz, peaking at 60 Hz and declining for exposures at 80 and 100Hz. Unmodulated fields were without effect (Fig.6). Disclosure of this "window" for effects of low frequency modulation provides confirmatory evidence that the mode of field interaction is a non equilibrium process. Moreover, the site of interaction in these experiments is clearly at the membrane surface, and the effective field levels at the membrane surface (levels expected to be in the range of 10 to 100 mV/cm) would be expected to mediate their effects only if substantial "amplification" of their initial triggering effects occurred in the initial transductive steps at the membrane surface.

In continuing studies of these modulated microwave field effects on lymphocytes, we have examined their influence on mitogenic stimulation of human lymphocytes. We have used intracellular enzymatic activations as an index of the field influences on the mitogen acti-

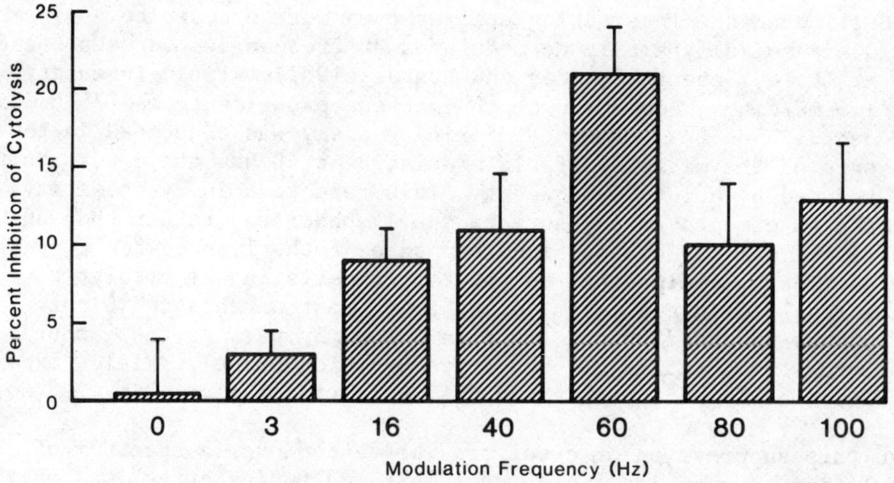

Fig. 6. Inhibition of cytoxicity of mouse T-lymphocytes targeted to destroy human bone tumor (myeloma) cells by a 450 MHz field, 1.5 mW/cm^2 peak envelope power, sinusidally modulated at frequencies from 3-100Hz. The "tuning curve" of inhibited cytotoxicity has a peak at 60 Hz. Unmodulated fields were without effect. (From Lyle, Schechter, Adey and Lundak, 1981 1981).

vation process. Pokeweed mitogen phythemagglutin activates the enzyme adenyl cyclase on the internal aspect of the membrane. In turn, the adenyl cyclase converts adenosine triphosphate to cyclic adenosine monophosphate (cAMP). The cAMP then activates a group of enzymes known as protein kinases. Normally, activation by the mitogen produces a sharp increase in cAMP-dependent protein kinase activity for about 60 min after initiation of the stimulus, with a peak at around 30 min. In preliminary observations, a 450 MHz microwave field (1.5 mW/cm^2) modulated at 16 Hz sharply reduced the magnitude of this initial peak, and enzyme activity returned to baseline levels in about 30 min. These initial findings suggest that the initial membrane surface events associated with the mitogen activity and coupled to intracellular enzymatic sequences essential in the initiation of cell division may be substantially modified by a weak modulated microwave field. The extent to which the _in vitro_ findings may reflect responses in the living organisms must await further research. Taken together with the evidence on field-sensitive sites for calcium binding and the data presented in Lecture 28 on sites of field-sensitive hormone binding mechanisms, these data collectively point strongly to the membrane surface as the prime site for cellular interaction with certain imposed electromagnetic fields.

Neurophysiological and Behavioral Effects of Modulated RF and Microwave Fields

In parallel with the foregoing studies in cellular biology, there have been investigations of the effects of modulated low-level environmental electromagnetic fields on EEG and behavior. These studies have involved ELF, RF and microwave fields. Findings with ELF fields will be discussed in Lecture 28.

In the first studies that specifically examined the possible signifigance of low frequency modulation of an RF field on brain electrical rhythms, cats were exposed to a 147 MHz, 0.8 mW/cm^2 field (Bawin, Gavalas-Medici and Adey, 1973). Because RF fields are more strongly coupled to tissues than ELF fields, RF fields at around 100 MHz can be expected to induce an EEG-level tissue gradient (10-100 mV/cm) with an incident energy around 1.0 mW/cm^2 (16 V/m), subject to variations attributable to body resonance effects. "Bursts" of EEG waves occurring in various brain nuclei of the awake cat as conditional responses to a flash of light (and thus constituting a learned response) were tested for interactions with the 147 MHz field, amplitude modulated at the dominant frequency of the selected transient EEG pattern. The irradiated animals were superior to a control group in the rate of performance, accuracy (in terms of bandwidth of EEG spectrum during the learned response), and resistance to extinction (minimun of 50 days vs. 10 days). The specificity of the frequency of the modulation was tested on another group of untrained animals where spontaneous transient patterns were used to trigger for short periods (20 sec after every burst) the RF fields amplitude modulated at various frequencies. The fields acted as reinforcers (increasing the rate of occurrence of the spontaneous rhythms) only when modulated at frequencies close to the biologically dominant frequency of the selected intrinsic EEG rhythmic episodes. Although this study used metal brain electrodes, spectral analysis of EEG records between wave "bursts" disclosed no artifactual rectification of imposed fields at brain-electrode interfaces.

Persistent EEG changes occurred for several days in rabbits after exposure for 2 hours daily for 4 to 8 weeks to a 5.0 MHz field amplitude modulated at 14-16 Hz (Takashima, Onoral and Schwan, 1979). Fields with amplitudes of 90 - 150 V/m in air enhance EEG activity at 10 - 15 Hz, and 500 V/m fields enhanced 4 to 5 Hz waves. No brain heating occurred during these exposures.

A persistent component in rat EEG spectral analyses at the pulse repetition frequency of a microwave field after irradiation has been reported (Servantie, Servantie and Etienne, 1975). With a 3.0 GHz field at 500 - 600 pulses/sec (1.0 μsec pulse duration, average power density 5.0 mW/cm^2), exposure for 10 days was followed by a distinct EEG peak at the pulse repetition frequency that waxed and waned in cycles lasting several minutes. The high frequency of the entrained spectral peak reported in this study may indicate a transductive mechanism distinct from that underlying EEG entrainment, where dendrites of cerebral neurons are the presumed locus of interaction for natural dominant frequencies typically below 50 Hz.

Soviet investigators have also developed a therapeutic device utilizing low frequency square wave modulation of a radiofrequency field. This instrument known as the LIDA, was developed by L. Y. Rabichev and his colleagues in Soviet Armenia, and is designed for "the treatment of neuropsychic and somatic disorders, such as neuroses, psychoses, insomnia, hypertension, stammering, bronchial asthma, and asthenic and reactive disturbances". It is covered by U.S. Patent #3,773,049. In addition to the pulsed RF field, the device also delivers pulsed light, pulsed sound, and pulsed heat. Each stimulus train can be independently adjusted in intensity and frequency. The radiofrequency field has a nominal carrier frequency of 40 MHz and a maximum output of approximately 40 Watts. The RF field is applied to the patient on the sides of the neck through two disc electrodes approximately 10 cm in diameter. The electrodes are located at a distance of 2 - 4 cm from the skin. Optimal repetition frequencies are said to lie in the range from 40 to 80 pulses per minute. Pulse duration is typically 0.2 sec. In an 8 year trial period, the instrument was tested on 740 patients, including adults and children. Positive therapeutic effects were claimed in more than 80 per cent of the cases treated (Rabichev et al., 1976).

Models of RF Interaction with Tissue; Possible Substrates for Low Frequency Modulation Effects

The molecular biology of interactions with EM fields described above points to phase partitions at membranes of cells and organelles as probable sites of transductive coupling. The evidence points to membrane surface glycoproteins with a polyanionic structure as possible sensing sites for weak fields. If we consider further the possible sequence of events in the coupling to cells of weak EM fields in the fluid surrounding them, and ways in which they may be effective as triggers to excitatory or metabolic processes, our speculative options narrow rapidly. The possibility that microwave fields may exert a direct transmembrane effect has been considered (Barnes and Hu, 1977; Pickard and Rosenbaum, 1978), in a model evaluating effects on equilibrium concentration of ions on opposite sides of the membrane, estimating by the use of the nonlinear Boltzmann equation shifts in ion concentration and magnitude of current flow resulting from membrane rectification. Numerical substitution in this model shows that an incident field of 10 mW/cm^2 produced a gradient of 4.4 V/cm across a membrane enclosed in an aqueous dielectric medium. This corresponds to an electric gradient of 9 μV across a 200 Å membrane, with a concentration shift of 1 part in 10^6 and a flow of 400 ions per sec for a cell with a surface area of 10^{-6} cm^2. The biological significance of such small currents is not known, but "these nonlinearities provide a mechanism for possible biological change," particularly where cumulative ion shifts may result from modulation of the microwave carrier at low frequency.

Intrinsic oscillating gradients of the order of 100 mV/cm in extracellular fluid, typical of slowly oscillating gradients in brain and other tissues, are clearly unlikely to be effective in directly influencing the normal transmembrane potential of 10^5 V/cm that exists over approximately 40 Å in the transverse dimension of a plasma membrane. Therefore, we may anticipate effective coupling of these weak fields only through one or more mechanisms capable of "amplifying" the initial triggering gradient. If these mechanisms exist, they must be sought in the heirarchical organization of membrane ultrastructure, probably beyond the level of individual macromolecules and certainly within the vista of the separate but interrelated structural entities that constitute phase boundaries on and within cell membranes. Membrane surface glycoproteins behave as a longitudinally organized (though imperfect) biopolymer sheet that encodes the membrane in length and in area (Edelman, 1976). This contrasts with ionic transport channels organized in a transmembrane axis

(Mueller and Rudin, 1967). Each has been assigned a unique role in models that purport to explain aspects of low-level field interactions at "athermal" energy levels. We have reviewed mechanisms at the molecular level known to be the basis of cooperative processes, including coherent states between macromolecular fixed-charge sites (Schwarz, 1967; Schwarz and Balthasar,1970). The dimensions of the coherent domains must be small, since synaptosome fractions showed changes in calcium efflux with modulated microwave fields, even though their mean dimensions are of the order of 0.3 μm (Lin-Liu and Adey, 1981).

In our search for some form of amplification of initial transductive steps at an extracellular location, we may presume that it involves systems capable of integrating the weak field over some distance, and would thus occur in the length and area of the membrane surface rather than in a transmembrane axis (Adey, 1977). Einolf and Carstensen (1971) have addressed this problem in a study of the behavior of micron-sized resin particles considered as porous particles with uniformly distributed fixed-charge sites. Porous charged particles characterized by a low frequency dielectric relaxation leading to large static dielectric constants. This results in polarization of the ionic atmosphere at the surface of the particle in the presence of an external electric field. As a result, there is an additional "apparent" dielectric constant of the particle, exceeding the dielectric constant by several orders of magnitude at low frequencies. It is proportional to the diameter of the particle and the square root of the fixed-charge concentration in the porous material, with values as high as 10^6 at frequencies below 1 kHz for micron-sized resin particles. Similar properties may be expected at the surface of tubular structures with diameters in the micron range, including dendrites with polyanionic glycoprotein surface layers.

The Einolf and Carstensen model offers a basis for those bioeffects in which thermal noise at normal tissue temperature appears substantially larger than the tissue components of imposed electric fields (Bawin and Adey, 1976; Adey 1981a). The Boltzmann equation may be written in terms that model the cell surface in the region of the counterion layer as a low-pass filter:

$$e^2 = 4\ kT\ BR$$

where the transfer function for the root mean square noise voltage $\underline{e}$ is a function of the frequency bandwidth $\underline{B}$ and the specific resistance of the noise pathway $\underline{R}$. With a specific resistance for brain tissue of the order of 300 $\Omega.cm^{-1}$ and an effective frequency bandwidth from 0 - 100 Hz, the equivalent noise voltage gradient would be of the order of 10^{-8} V/cm. This is in close agreement with observed sensitivities in marine vertebrates, birds and mammals for certain low frequency fields, and these thresholds are consistent with a thermal "floor" as the limiting factor.

We have shown that the Einolf and Carstensen model of dielectric dispersion at the surface of small charged spheres also applies to long, thin cell processes which typify the dendrites of neurons (Sheppard and Adey, 1979). The degree of polarization induced at the surface depends on the orientation of the incident field with respect to the length of the dendrite or axon, radius of the cylindrical surface, ion mobility, and temperature. It may be speculated that the extraordinary degree of polarization produced by counterions at the cells surface may bring about a dynamic distribution of weakly bound ions of reduced momenta. From the Heisenberg equation relating positional and momentum uncertainties, we find that ions of sufficiently low momentum would exhibit quantum behavior usually not associated with such massive bodies at biological temperatures. For example, the momentum of a thermal proton at $300^{\circ}K$ is ordinarily 4.5×10^{24} kg-m/sec. The resulting positional uncertainty, Δx, is about 10^{-11} m, so small that classical notions are entirely adequate for dynamic considerations. However, an ion with attenuated momentum $p\varepsilon^{\frac{1}{2}}$ has a positional uncertainty of $\varepsilon^{\frac{1}{2}}\Delta x$. If we take a value for ε in the region surrounding the ion of the same order of magnitude as for the macroscopic ε measured with a cell suspension of 10^4 to 10^6, we see that the ion would have a positional uncertainty of about 10^{-8} to 10^{-9} m. Tunneling would then be possible from one potential well to another, because the ionic wave function would extend through the region of a typical potential barrier and even over appreciable regions along the surface. If momenta are sufficiently reduced, smaller ions -- particularly protons -- would have significant probabilities of tunneling from one potential minimun to another. We hypothesize that proton tunneling may occur between charge sites that interact across the boundary between coherent and incoherent charge zones on cell membrane surface glycoproteins (Adey, 1977, 1979; Adey and Bawin, 1980; Sheppard and Adey, 1979). This process would be most effective in the access of the field electric gradient, along this surface biopolymer sheet. Development of long range order among surface macromolecules interacting by low-momentum ions may induce significant changes over the entire polarized region.

Sensitivity of some biological systems to weak EM fields suggests that these systems can store signal energy and thus overcome thermal noise. These systems show relatively small activation energies but protected from thermal fluctuations. Fröhlich has hypothesized that ELF electric oscillations in the brain may be connected with such a system. These oscillations cannot arise from a collective mode based on interactions of various molecular groups, since enormous volumes of tissue would necessarily be involved to overcome their thermal noise. Fröhlich has instead applied a general theory of coherent vibrations in biological systems (Bhaumik, Bhaumik and Dutta-Roy, 1976; Fröhlich, 1968) for which there is some experimental evidence (Fröhlich, 1975). Frölich envisages collective chemical oscillations in which globular proteins and the surrounding ions and structural water behave as an entity and oscillate between a strongly electrically polar excited state and a weakly polar ground state. A slow chemical oscillation is thus connected with a corresponding electrical vibration at a much higher frequency, typically in the frequency range of 10^{11} Hz. The strong electrical interaction between the highly polar states in conjunction with strong damping of electric currents then imposes limit-cycle conditions on these polar systems, making the oscillations highly sensitive to external electrical and chemical influences, as described by Kaczmarek (1976).

Effects of low frequency (ELF) and ELF-modulated radio and microwave fields at levels below those inducing significant thermal effect clearly involve highly nonlinear mechanisms. Taylor (1981) has prepared an excellent review on nonlinear wave phenomena in tissue-microwave interactions, and has drawn attention to the far-reaching theoretical work of A.S. Davydov. In a series of papers concerned with the interaction of phonons and excitons along linear molecules, Davydov and his co-workers have developed a theory of nonlinear molecular vibrations and their significance in biology. These vibrations take the form of soliton waves. Due to their existence in a minimal energy state, these solitons are extremely long-lived in comparison to linear oscillations, and could act to convey energy released by chemical reactions from one site to another in an enzyme, an actin molecule or other long-chain protein (Davydov, 1977, 1979). These solitons are characteristic of dispersive (reaction-diffusion) systems, as opposed to the dissipative or cooperative systems considered above as substrates in the first steps of membrane surface transduction of weak electrochemical oscillations. We have proposed a model for interaction between excitable tissue and electromagnetic fields, based on nonlinear waves in the cell membrane, with ionic interactions as an essential step (Lawrence and Adey, 1981)(Fig.7), in this model, calcium fluxes in the extracellular space of the central nervous system are considered as a nonlinear reaction-diffusion system. Membrane molecular solitons may exist in long-chain molecules (Davydov type) and play a significant role in charge transfer; or as nonlinear waves (Bullough, 1981), conveying energy along gel-lipid domains from one protein site to another (sine-Gordon soliton). These nonlinear waves, which move at subsonic velocities, may couple events in the extracellular domain with intracellular systems by reaction-diffusion processes along lipoprotein molecules that extend thru the lipid bilayer (Fig. 8). We suggest that the mechanism of membrane excitability rest upon three basic principles. First, the membrane proteins serve to conduct the ions across the membrane.

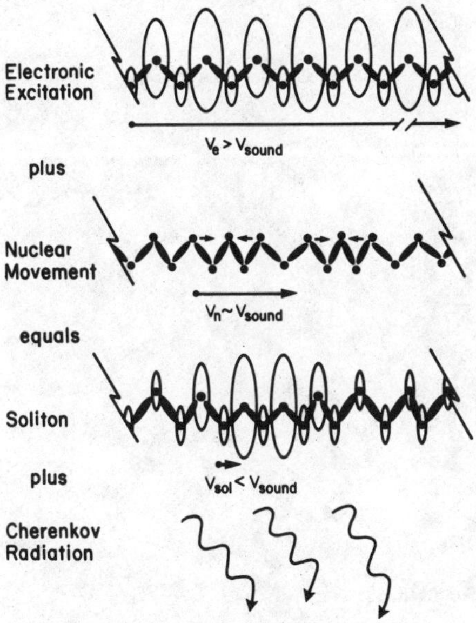

Fig. 7. The Davydov model for soliton formation. The "equation" along the left margin illustrates the energy balance in the formation of the soliton wave. The "Cherenkov radiation" in this figure consists of phonons produced by the interaction between the exciton mode and the chain deformation mode. The production of phonons associated with the formation of solitons accounts for the lower energy state of the soliton, and thus its stability (From Lawrence and Adey, 1981).

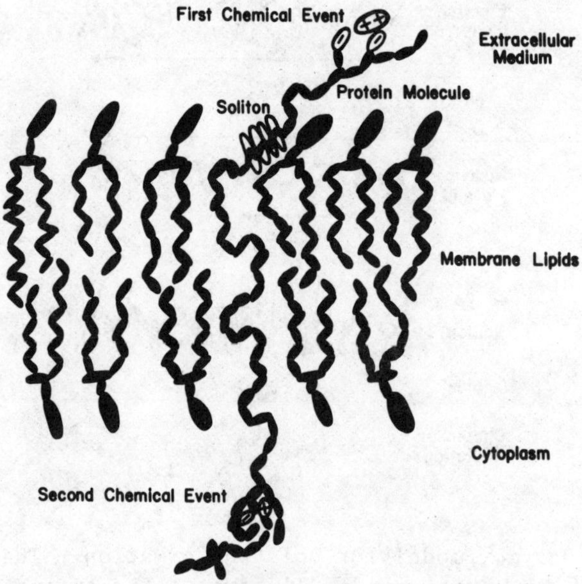

Fig. 8. The biological role of solitons. A hypothetical chemical event produces energy at one end of a long chain molecule. The energy is transferred in the form of a soliton along the molecule and induces a secondary chemical event at the other end. (From Lawrence and Adey, 1981).

Second, the presence of lipids and calcium in a particular thermodynamic phase specifically associated with the conducting proteins is essential to the propagation of the excitation. Third, nonlinearities in the physical properties of the system, rather than higher-order chemical kinetics, are the key to the process.

SUMMARY

1) The anatomical and physiological substrates of weak electromagnetic field interactions with the central nervous system have been reviewed, with emphasis on the role of the widely spreading "tree" of dendrites that are characteristic of cerebral neurons. 2) These dendrites generate large electrochemical waves at low frequencies (1-100 Hz) that "leak" into the surrounding extracellular fluid, where these small components of dendritic waves contribute to the electroencephalogram (EEG). 3) The amplitude of extracellular EEG waves (10-100 mV/cm) is far smaller than either the membrane potential (10^5 V/cm) or the intracellular neuronal wave (10^4 V/cm). Nevertheless, imposed radio frequency and microwave fields with the tissue amplitude of the EEG and sinusoidally modulated at EEG frequencies entrain the natural brain electrical rhythms at the field modulation frequency. 5) Similar "windowing" in relation to modulation frequency occurs in other tissues and cell systems, including the cytotoxicity of T-lymphocytes in cell-mediated immune responses. With low frequency (ELF) fields, cultured osteoblasts exhibit a field sensitivity in their responses to the peptide parathyroid hormone (see Lecture 28). Responses in calcium efflux, cell mediated immunity and endocrine effects all point to the cell membrane surface as the site of these initial nonequilibrium processes in cellular transduction of weak electrochemical stimuli. 6) Cell membrane transduction involves major "amplification" of the initial weak triggering events. A basis for nonlinear amplification is found in strands of polyanionic membrane surface glycoproteins and the transmembrane lipoprotein molecules to which they attach. Two classes of long range chemical interactions may be involved in the transductive signaling; cooperative (dissipative) events and reaction-diffusion (dispersive, soliton) mechanisms. Cooperative binding and release of calcium at cell membrane surfaces may occur at fixed charge anionic sites on sialic acid terminals of stranded glycoproteins. Transient coherent states between nearest-neighbor fixed charge sites over small surface domains would provide substrates for cooperative responses to weak electrochemical stimuli. Membrane molecular solitons may exist in long chain molecules and play a significant role in charge transfer; or as nonlinear waves conveying energy at subsonic velocities along gel-lipid domains from one protein site to another, as in transfer of signals from extra- to intracellular sites. 7) There is good experimental evidence from a variety of tissues that a form of cell-

to-cell communication can occur through weak electrochemical stimuli that are sensed by highly cooperative processes at cell membrane surfaces. In varying degrees, this may be a general property of tissue organization.

REFERENCES

Adey, W.R., 1975, Evidence for cooperative mechanisms in the susceptibility of cerebral tissue to environmental and intrinsic electric fields, in: "Functional Linkage in Biomolecular Systems", F.O. Schmitt, D.M. Schneider and D.M. Crothers, eds. Raven, New York. p. 325-342.

Adey, W.R., 1979, Models of membranes of cerebral cells as substrates for information storage, BioSystems, 8:163-178.

Adey, W.R., 1979, Experiment and theory in long-range interactions of electromagnetic fields at brain cell surfaces, in: "Magnetic Field Effects on Biological Systems", T. Tenforde, ed. Plenum, New York. p. 57-78.

Adey, W.R., 1981a, Tissue interactions with nonionizing electromagnetic fields, Physiol. Rev. 61:435-514.

Adey, W.R. 1981b, Ionic nonequilibrium phenomena in tissue interactions with electromagnetic fields, in: "Biological Effects of Nonionizing Radiation", K.H. Illinger, ed. American Chemical Society Symposium Series, No. 157. American Chemical Society, Washington, D.C. p. 271-297.

Adey, W.R., and Bawin, S.M., 1980, Nonequilibrium processes in binding and release of brain calcium by low-level electromagnetic fields, in: "Bioelectrochemistry: Ions, Surfaces, Membranes", M. Blank, ed. American Chemical Society, Advances in Chemistry Series, No. 188. American Chemical Society, Washington, D.C. p. 361-378.

Adey, W.R., Bawin, S.M., and Lawrence, A.F., 1981, Nonlinear wave mechanismss in tissue-electromagnetic field interactions. Bioelectromagnetics, in press.

Barnes, F.S., and Hu, C.L.J., 1977, Model for some nonthermal effects of radio and microwave fields on biological membranes, IEEE Trans. Microwave Theory Tech. 25:742-746.

Bass, L., and Moore, W.J., 1968, A model of nervous excitation based on the Wien Dissociation effect, in: "Structural Chemistry and Molecular Biology," A. Rich and C.M. Davidson, eds. Freeman, San Francisco. p. 356-368.

Bawin, S.M., and Adey, W.R., 1976, Sensitivity of calcium binding in cerebral tissue to weak environmental electric fields oscillating at low frequency, Proc. Natl. Acad. Sci., USA, 73:1999-2003.

Bawin, S.M., Adey, W.R., and Sabbot, I.M., 1978, Ionic factors in release of $^{45}Ca^{2+}$ from chick cerebral tissue by electromagnetic fields, Proc. Natl. Acad. Sci., USA, 75:6314-6318

Bawin, S.M., Gavalas-Medici, R., and Adey, W.R., 1973, Effects of modulated very high frequency fields on specific brain rhythms in cats, Brain Res., 58:365-384.

Bawin, S.M., Kaczmarek, L.K., and Adey, W.R., 1975, Effects of modulated VHF fields on the central nervous system, Ann. NY Acad. Sci., 247:74-81.

Bawin, S.M., Sheppard, A.R., and Adey, W.R., 1978, Possible mechanisms of weak electromagnetic field coupling in brain tissue, Bioelectrochem. Bioenergetics, 5:67-76.

Benson, A.A., 1966, On the orientation of lipids in chloroplast and cell membranes, J. Amer. Oil Chem. Soc., 43:265-270.

Bhaumik, D., Bhaumik, K., and Dutta-Roy, B., 1976, On the possibility of Bose condensation in the excitation of coherent modes in biological systems, Phys. Lett., 56A:145-148.

Bullough, R.K., 1981, Bose-Fermi equivalence and soliton theory in solid-state physics, Nature, 292:411-412.

Davydov, A.S., 1977, Solitons as energy carriers in biological systems, Studia Biophysica, 62:1-8.

Davydov, A.S., 1979, Solitons in molecular systems, Physica Scripta, 20:387-394.

Edelman, G.M., 1976, Surface modulation in cell recognition and cell growth, Science, 192:218-226.

Einolf, C.W., and Carstensen, E.L., 1971, Low-frequency dielectric dispersion in suspensions of ion-exchange resins. J. Phys. Chem., 75:1091-1099.

Fröhlich, H., 1968, Long-range coherence and energy storage in biological systems, Int. J. Quant. Chem., 2:641-649.

Fröhlich, H., 1975, The extraordinary dielectric properties of biological materials and the action of enzymes. Proc. Nat. Acad. Sci., USA, 72:4211-4215.

Kaczmarek, L.K, 1976, Frequency sensitive biochemical reactions, Biophys. Chem., 4:249-252.

Kaczmarek, L.K., and Adey, W.R., 1974, Weak electric gradients change ionic and transmitter fluxes in cortex. Brain Res., 66:537-540.

Kalmijn, A.J., 1980, Electromagnetic guidance systems in fishes, in: "Magnetic Field Effects on Biological Systems", T. Tenforde, ed. Plenum, New York.

Kretsinger, R., ed., 1981, Mechanisms of selective signaling by calcium, Neurosci. Res. Program Bull., 19:213-332.

Lawrence, A.F., and Adey, W.R., 1981, Nonlinear wave mechanisms in tissue-electromagnetic field interactions. Neurol. Res.,in press.

Lin-Liu, S., and Adey, W.R., 1981, Low-frequency amplitude-modulated microwave fields change calcium efflux rates from synaptosomes. Bioelectromagnetics, in press.

Matus, A., de Petris, S., and Raff, M.C., 1973, Mobility of concanavalin A receptors in myelin and synaptic membranes, Nature New Biology 244:278-279.

Neumann, E., and Katchalsky, A., 1972, Long-lived conformation changes induced by electric impulses in biopolymers, Proc. Natl. Acad. Sci., USA, 69:993-997.

Neumann, E., Nachmansohn, D., and Datchalsky, A., 1973, An attempt at an integral interpretation of nerve excitability, Proc. Natl. Acad. Sci.,USA, 70:727-731.

Pickard, W.F., and Rosenbaum, J.F., 1978, Biological effects of microwaves at the membrane level: two possible athermal electrophysiological mechanisms and a proposed experimental test, Math. Biosci., 39:239-253.

Rabichev, L.Y., Ilynna, T.G., Ilynk, V.A., and Raku, P.V., 1976, Elektroson y ritmoteflperticheskii son, Korsakov J. Neuropath. Psychiat., 3:443-446 (Russian).

Redburn, D.A., Shelton, D., Cotman, C.W., 1976, Calcium-dependent release of exogenously loaded γ-amino-[U-^{14}C]butyrate from synaptosomes; time course of stimulation by potassium, veratridine, and the calcium ionophore, A23187, J. Neurochem., 26: 297-303.

Schwarz, G., 1967, A basic approach to a general theory for cooperative intramolecular conformation changes of linear biopolymers, Biopolymers, 5:321-324.

Schwarz, G., 1975, Sharpness and kinetics of cooperative transitions, in: "Functional Linkage in Biomolecular Systems", F.O. Schmitt, D.M. Schneider, and D.M. Crothers, eds. Raven Press, New York. p. 32-35.

Schwarz, G., and Balthasar, W., 1970, Cooperative binding of linear biopolymers. 3. Thermodynamic and Kinetic analysis of the acridine orange-poly-L-glutamic acid system, Eur. J. Biochem., 12:461-467.

Servantie, B., Servantie, A.M., and Etienne, J., 1975, Synchronization of cortical neurons by a pulsed microwave field as evidenced by spectral analysis of electrocorticograms from the white rat, Ann. NY Acad. Sci., 247:82-86.

Shepherd, G.M., 1979, "The Synaptic Organization of the Brain", 2nd ed. Oxford University Press, New York, 436 pp.

Sheppard, A.R., and Adey, W.R., 1979, The role of cell surface polarization in biological effects of extremely low frequency fields, U.S. Department of Energy Symposium Series, No. 50, "Biological Effects of Extremely Low Frequency Electromagnetic Fields", Washington, D.C. pp. 147-158.

Singer, S.J., and Nicolson, G.L., 1972, The fluid mosaic model of the sturcture of the cell membrane, Science, 175:720-731.

Takashima, S., Onoral, B., and Schwan, H.P., 1979, Effects of modulated RF energy on the EEG of mammalian brains, Radiat. Environ. Biophys., 16:15-27.

Taylor, L.S., 1981, Athermal millimeter/microwave effects, Science, in press.

Terenius, L., 1973, Stereospecific interaction between narcotic analgesics and a synaptic plasma membrane fraction of rat cerebral cortex, Acta Pharmacol. Toxicol., 32:317-320.

Yahara, I., and Edelman, G.M., 1972, Restriction of the mobility of lymphocyte immunoglobulin receptors by concanavalin A, Proc. Natl. Acad. Sci., USA, 69:608-612.

Young, J.Z., 1951, "Doubt and Certainty in Science", Oxford University Press, New York.

BEHAVIOURAL EFFECTS OF RADIOFREQUENCY ENERGY

B.M. Servantie*
J. Gillard**

*Médecin en Chef, Maître de Recherches du Service de Santé des Armées
**Médecin Principal, Spécialiste de Recherches du Service de Santé des Armées
EASSM-CERB
B.P. 610
83800 - TOULON-NAVAL (France)

PRESENTATION

The studies about behaviour of living beeings, animal or human, are complex, and extrapolations are hazardous. Using such studies as a tool to study another factor may be very useful, but is also risky, specially when the factor is non ionizing electromagnetic radiation (N.I.R). We will not consider here the problems of human behaviour, and we will limit ourselves to various animal species which are object of such studies. We will present the following steps :

a - Behaviour and techniques;
b - Attempt of classification of experimental studies;
c - Technological problems raised by N.I.R;
d - Experimental results;
e - Mechanisms involved.

BEHAVIOURS AND TECHNIQUES

A behaviour can be defined as a spatio-temporal sequence of motor responses, caused and oriented by information of external or internal origin, present or remembered. It is not only the expression of automatic links between stimulus and answers : the information presented to a living beeing is processed and receive a meaning by reference to previous data.

Belonging to the field of biological sciences, behaviours can be considered from a double point of view. Either they are object of studies performed to elucidate their mechanisms, or, as codified tests, they can be used to study biological effects of environmental factors or of pharmacological agents.

To illustrate the first aspect, we will describe, as an example, the feeding behaviour. The progress of pharmacological and neurophysiological knowledges has allowed, here as for other behaviours, to use models more scientifically gratifying than the old explanations which invoked the ideas of instinct or impulse.

The first step was to identify the modifications of "internal environment" which cause the search for food. The study of effects of insuline and of 2-deoxy-6-glucose (2DG), which trigger this behaviour, has allowed to identify the lack of glucose as inducing factor.

The use of neurophysiological techniques such as selective destruction or electrical stimulation of brain structures has put in light the outstanding importance of hypothalamus in control of feeding. Destructions of area in lateral hypothalamus cause a complete aphagia and suppress the 2DG action. Electrical stimulation of this area induces feeding. Then chemoreceptors for hunger were localized at this point.

Remained to solve two problems : one for satiety, the other for hyperphagia induced by destruction of the ventro-medial area of the hypothalamus. The mechanism invoked for satiety was connected, at least partly, to a sensory activity of food on olfactory and gustatory receptors. And the ventro-medial area of the hypothalamus appears to rule the management of lipidic storage which regulates the frequency of feeding along the day.

In fact, the neurophysiological reality is more complex. Many facts compel to forsake the too simple idea of a limited hypothalamus center. The limbic system seems to play, here as for many other behaviours, an essential role : particularly, it would be responsible for competition for food and for choice of food.

Along this neurophysiological way, a neurochemical approach has occured during the last years, following progress in knowledge of central monoamine pathways. Thus was evidenced the triggering of feeding by application of noradrenaline on lateral hypothalamus, this triggering being suppressed by alpha blocking agents ; likewise, beta receptors would be responsible for satiety.

This fast survey of various constituants of a behaviour however simple shows the complexity of mechanisms implied in animals. We have left behind the problems of choice of foods and of their palatability. They are complex in animals, where interfere genetic factors and acquired datas. What about the complexity of such problems in man (and woman) where intervene cultural and social components.

As we have said, behaviours can be used as tools to evaluate the changes in relations between an animal and its environment, under the action of pharmacologic drugs or ambient factors. So numerous behavioral tests were designed to study psychotropic drugs effects. Such tests allow the study, in carefully controlled conditions, of behaviours obeying to naturally existing causes.

Some tests are devised to look at spontaneous motor activity : the animal is then put into an actographic cage. This kind of activity is very sensitive to catecholamine-like drugs. Spontaneous exploratory behaviour can be evaluated by other tests such as hole test, stair case test or open field test. For the last one, the animal is placed, as a rule only one time, on a grid floor with some objects ; an observer counts the number of squares crossed by the animal, the number of rearings, the number of contacts with objects and the number of defecations, the last parameter being linked to emotionality. Such tests are used to evaluate anxiolytic drugs.

The intra-specific aggressive behaviour can be analysed inducing it by electric shocks in pairs of animals.

Lastly, it is possible to use more sophisticated techniques using learning, memory and reminiscence. Frequently, they call upon operant conditioning. Then the reinforcement may be positive, generally by food, the subject being able to obtain a pellet by pressing upon a lever. The complexity of the task may be increased either by increasing the number of lever pressings (fixed ratio), or by introducing a temporal component (fixed interval or differential reinforcement of low-rate). The reinforcement may be negative, the animal evading an electric shock by pressing on a lever (Sidman-type avoidance) ; anologous is the shuttle-box test where the subject jumps in an other compartment of the cage to evade the electric shock, or the pole climbing test where the avoidance is achieved by climbing a pole.

Conflictual situations are also used. For conditioned emotional response (CER), an aversive event marked by a warning signal is randomly superimposed to a positive reinforcement. Generally, the result is a suppression of the behaviour in presence of the signal ; tranquillizing drugs cancel this inhibition.

The number of tests must not mask the difficulties to understand results. The methods described allow the study of pharmacological factors such as dose-effect relationship or synergistic actions, but understanding remains difficult : thus a minor tranquillizing drug can reduce spontaneous activity while stimulating conditioned activity. Amphetamine decrease response rate for fixed ratio and increase it for fixed interval.

More promising seems the explanation of behavioral changes by modifications of central monoamine systems. We have already pointed out their role in the feeding behaviour, but their action is encountered in all behaviours. For example, dopamine seems determinant to start behavioural sequences and particularly locomotor activity ; in fact, this phenomenon would be the result of a balance between dopaminergic and cholinergic systems. Likewise, noradrenergic systems would intervene in operant conditioning, in feeding and drinking, in self stimulation behaviour. Cholinergic system would be implied, as dopamine, in sham rage and aggressiveness. Serotonin and norepinephrine are implied in sleep mechanisms. Such examples demonstrate the interest to correlate behavioral tests with neurochemical assays.

ATTEMPT OF CLASSIFICATION OF EXPERIMENTAL STUDIES

All things previously said can be applied to researches about biological effects of N.I.R. They are environmental factors, able to interfere with function of living beeings. Then, we can presume they will be able to modify some behaviours in animals, the difficulties being perhaps to find the test (or the tests) which will show at the best these perturbations and will allow the analysis, and the animal species which will be the best experimental subject.

For this review, we have restricted ourselves to papers of the last period of researches about bioeffects of RF/MW, period which may be taken as beginning with the Symposium "Biological Effects and Health Implications of Microwave Radiation", held at Richmond (Virginia) in 1969.

Investigation of experimental papers published since this symposium shows that some species are more estimated than others : 54% of works are performed using rats, 20% using monkeys, 13% using mice and 9% using birds ; the remaining 4% are sparse among other species as cats, dogs, rabbits and even hornet.

Fields are also various : 6% are frequencies upper than 3 GHz ; 52%, a crushing majority, are between 1 and 3 GHz, essentially 2.45 GHz ; 11% are at 918 MHz ; 7% between 100 and 900 MHz ; 4% are between 5 and 40 MHz ; 19% are at very low frequencies (VLF) mainly at power frequency or at submarine communication system frequency.

The distribution of incident power densities or of absorbed powers is also large. We have sorted them according to the proposals of the Warsaw Symposium in three classes : "high level" for values upper than 10 mW/cm2 ; "low level" for values lower than 1 mW/cm2 ; "medium range level" for values between 1 and 10 mW/cm2. We find 25% of papers at low level, 25% at medium range level and 50% at high level.

It is now generally accepted that the average incident power density is not a very good criterion, at least for mechanisms relevant to thermal degradation of radiofrequency energy. We have then attempted to evaluate the absorbed dose (in W/kg) and the absorbed energy (in W) according to Durney (36) : the values range from 0.01 W/kg to 420 W/kg and from 0.001 W to 134 W ; no difference appears in the distribution of these values, according to the positiveness of the conclusions of the papers. In fact, such values are not very useful, because the SAR is often difficult to ascertain and it is impossible to take in account the local variations of energy deposition.

50% of studies are performed using CW fields, and 50% using pulsed or modulated fields. It is conceivable that a relation exists between field frequency and modulation : frequencies used for radar are generally pulse modulated, while I.S.M. frequencies are mainly CW.

Exposure durations are also variable, from few seconds (BERMANT et al - 10, JUSTESEN et al - 59) until many months (D'ANDREA et al - 26, SHANDALA et al - 107). Irradiation is performed continuously or, at the contrary, in multiple sessions, of which numbers and durations are almost as numerous as authors themselves.

The experimentations are also various and difficult to classify : 48% of papers use a complex technique such as reinforcement or fixed ratio ; 21% use tests evaluating exploratory or motor activity, as open field test ; other techniques are spread from self stimulation to audiogenic seizure.

Lastly, nature of fields is generally electromagnetic but, and specially at V.L.F., magnetic and electric fields, alone or associated, are also studied.

TECHNOLOGICAL PROBLEMS RAISED BY N.I.R.

To study behavioural effects of radiofrequencies necessitates to solve some technological problems and to avoid others, all due to the electromagnetic nature of these fields. KING (63) has stressed, as far back as 1969, that the field to study is modified by the animal used for a subject.

Physical laws ruling propagation of radiowaves and interactions with matter compel to do not use high conductivity materials inside N.I.R. to reduce artifacts and field distorsions. Sometimes, this is not convenient for some experiences and the searcher (FREY - 41) may be obliged to build devices specially designed for this kind of situation. Materials mainly used are low conductivity plastic, and polyfoam is a good one, but their use must be careful : LIN et al (72) have studied perturbations of fields provoked by plastic cages and by plastic restrainers used to maintain animals inside the fields ; the theoretical study is completed by an experimental one with a 2.45 GHz field.

Exposure conditions may be altered by such perturbations, due to the presence of animals and materials. Sometimes, and for example in multimodal cavities (JUSTESEN - 60), differences can be important, one or two order of magnitude between two points of the exposure area ; with anechoic chambers, analogous phenomenon can be produced by reflexions on ancillary materials.

It is then difficult to determine and to control exposure conditions, and the relation between field frequency, target dimensions and energy absorption, evidenced by C.C. JOHNSON and coworkers, does not simplify the problem : D'ANDREA (24,25) has confirmed that some behavioural effects were linked to incident radiation frequency.

EXPERIMENTAL RESULTS

Investigation of published papers shows the same variety than for other biological effects of radiofrequency energy.

For upper frequencies, THOMAS et al (117) show a difference in answer rate of rats with fixed ratio and D.R.L. experiments ; GILLARD et al (49) see a deterioration of performances with open field test ; NELSON (97) notes a decrease of performance of squirrel monkeys if central temperature increases. McAFFEE et al (79,80) does not find changes with rhesus monkeys, as KLEIN et al (66) with macaques.

In the low level 1 - 3 GHz range, BILOKRINICKIJ (13) observes modifications in conditionnal reflexes for low level fields with dogs ; FREY et al (38, 39, 40, 41) see a decrease of agressiveness and a loss of equilibrium with rats which besides look to be able to detect the electromagnetic field ; square wave modulated fields seem more active than CW fields of identical frequency ; SHANDALA et al (107, 108) find a decrease of performances of rats after long duration exposures, this phenomenon being diphasic ; THOMAS et al (117) note same results on rats with 2.45 GHz CW et 2.86 GHz PW, more than with 9.6 GHz ; moreover, there is potentiation of the action of dextroamphetamine.

For medium range field levels, HJERESEN et al (53) show an increase of motor activity in rats, eventually linked to an hearing phenomenon ; LOBANOVA (75) sees a difference in conditionnal reflexes in rats and rabbits after 4 months with 1 hour per day irradiation ; MITCHELL et al (88), with rats irradiated 5 hours per day for 22 weeks, find a deterioration of performance with operant conditioning and an increase of motor activity, but Sidman avoidance is not modified ; YAKOVLEVA et al (124) note differences in cardiac conditional reflexes associated to cortical cells oedema, in rats ; ADAIR (1) observes a change in thermoregulatory behaviour in monkeys (Saimiri sciureus) which regulated the temperature of the exposure room.

Researches performed with high level fields are more numerous : essentially, they indicate a deterioration of performances often linked to an increase of central temperature. CRIBORN (23) finds a decrease of learning ability in mice, if they survive after 3 to 6 minutes to 100 mW/cm2, GUSAROV (51), HUNT et al (54), MATRENINA et al (83), MONAHAN et al (91, 92, 93) and OLSSON (98) see a decrease in motor activity, sometimes with detection of field by mice. With rats, results are analogous : JUSTESEN et al (59, 60), KING (63), SANZA et al (104) observe a deterioration of performances, of activity, etc... DIACHENKO et al (34), GAGE (43), HUNT et al (55), DE LORGE (31), McREE et al (81), MATRENINA et al (83), MITCHELL et al (89) obtain similar findings and correlate them with a thermal factor, generally an increase of internal temperature of 1° C or more ; GALLOWAY (45) has the same decrease of performance with macaque monkeys and DE LORGE (30, 31, 32) with squirrel monkeys, linking it to an increase of rectal temperature of 1° C. HAWKINS et al (52), HUNT et al (54) note a decrease of sensitivity to audiogenic seizure in rats ; STERN et al (114) show that rats in cooled exposure chamber use less an infrared heating when they are irradiated, but without increasing internal temperature. On the contrary, FARRER et al (37), KLEIN et al (66), SCHOLL et al (105) with macaque monkeys, and LAMBERT et al (70) with dogs, do not find any effect of irradiation.

Using a medium level 918 MHz field, JOHNSON et al (56, 57) see a detection of the field, probably due to an hearing effect, and a speeding up of development after irradiation "in utero" ; LOVELY et al (77) obtain similar results, as MOE et al (90) ; they use the same irradiation device (cylindrical wave guide). LIN et al (73) and LOVELY et al (76) observe a decrease of performances with increased incident power densities ; but rats of CARROLL et al (19) do not avoid an analogous field and MONAHAN et al (94) are unable to produce aversion for sugar solutions with a 915 MHz field.

Works with fields in the range between 900 MHz and very low frequencies are not numerous. However, ANTIMONII et al (3) using a 39 MHz field, see a diphasic response in rats subjected to self stimulation ; BAWIN et al (7) with a 147 MHz field, note a facilitation of electroencephalographic conditioning in cats ; KORBEL et al (67, 68) show a decrease of motor activity in rats, caused by fields between 300 and 900 MHz ; MEDICI et al (86) at 450 MHz observe a reduction of latencies in new born chicken, reduction which is not found by SAGAN (103) ; SUDAKOV et al (115) obtain perturbations in conditional reflexes of rats with 40 MHz field. With higher levels, D'ANDREA et al (24, 25), using fields between 20 and 700 MHz, provoke a decrease of performance in rats with increase of central temperature, the resonance frequency beeing more efficient.

The problem of very low frequencies is not easier. CLARKE et al (21) show that chicken can detect a constant magnetic field, probably modulating it by moves of the head ; OSSENKOP (99) and PERSINGER et al (100) see an increase of activity in rats exposed to a low frequency modulated magnetic field ; YAKOVLEVA et al (124) provoke an increase of heart frequency by exposing pigeons to a constant magnetic field. But GRISSETT et al (50) in squirrel monkeys and DE LORGE (29) in macaque monkeys do not observe any effect of 60 Hz magnetic fields.

FREY et al (42) modify the conditioned emotional response of rats by a 60 Hz electric field ; GAVALAS et al (47) obtain, with an analogous field, a difference in fixed interval responses in macaque monkeys ; MEDICI et al (85), always in macaque monkeys, cause an increase in response frequency. But SMITH et al (104) do not find any effect.

Birds are a problem by themselves. They are often (pigeons, chickens) used as laboratory animals ; and the orientation of migratory birds is not still explained. Some works, as those from TANNER et al (116), show that birds are particularly sensitive to electromagnetic fields. Many authors, as BURKS et al (16), LARKIN et al (71), SOUTHERN (112), assert that the so numerous radio waves used for radar, TV and telecommunications are able to perturb the orientation sense of birds ; KRUPP (69) denies this effect, at least for radar frequencies.

BIGU DEL BIANCO et al (11, 12) show that bird feathers are a sensor specifically adapted to microwave fields ; CLARKE et al (21) evidence the sensitivity of domestic hen to very low frequency fields ; WALCOTT et al (121) find in the pigeon head a magnetic material, able to constitute an organ sensitive to magnetic fields ; BLISS et al (14) observe that circadian rhythms of a sparrow are changed when earth magnetic field is suppressed.

MECHANISMS INVOLVED

A physical factor is able to modify a behaviour of a living beeing if the organism can perceive this factor, then if the organism has one or more organs sensitive to this factor.

We have seen that WALCOTT et al (121) have found a material which, in pigeon, can constitute such an organ ; BIGU DEL BIANCO et al (11, 12) have shown that bird feathers are sensitive to microwaves. Then it seems to be logical that behaviours of birds may be modified by some fields.

For mammalians, such organs have never been described. But skin contains sensors sensitive to heat, and MICHAELSON (87) reminds that man can react to an increase of cutaneous temperature of 0.001° C/s, which can be caused by average power densities incident upon the skin of few tens of mW/cm2. Heat produced inside the organism by the field may be the perceptible factor in many experiments performed using high level fields, particularly with rodents exposed to field close to their resonance frequency. Radiofrequency fields are also able to penetrate inside organisms and to increase the central temperature which, perhaps more than the peripheral temperature, can constitute a major factor : this is evidenced by papers previously quoted, which correlate behavioural disturbances with temperature increase.

There is a discrepancy between results obtained with rodents and those obtained with monkeys, and particularly the negative results reported by McAFFEE (79) ; instead of a difference in sensitivity, this discrepancy may be ascribed to differences in dimensions and morphology between these species, perhaps also to different experimental techniques, and also to differences in energy deposition either in the whole body or in parts such as the head.

For lower levels, we must not neglect the hearing effect of modulated microwaves. It was studied by many workers, as for example CAIN et al (17) or JOHNSON et al (57), and may explain some results obtained at medium or low levels with PW fields in a range of frequencies between 0.9 and 3 GHz.

But some results remain, which call for different mechanisms. Presenting his "dopamine hypothesis", FREY (41, 42) meets present behavioural researches which attempt to explain animal behaviours by interactions between various cerebral monoamine systems. Perhaps also intervene results reported by ADEY (2), BAWIN et al (6), SERVANTIE et al (106), which find that pulsed fields can modify rhythms of brain electrogenesis ; and that strengthens the hypothesis that the more a field is complex, the more it is efficient from a bioeffects point of view.

We must also keep in mind another possibility : the field itself can be not perceived by the animal, but it can modify the ability of this animal to react to other environmental factors. Some of our works, recent or older (49), evidence this phenomenon.

CONCLUSION

Non ionizing electromagnetic fields of frequency lower than infra red are able to modify some behaviours in different animal species. The involved mechanisms are not completely understood, and if we can explain some experimental findings with a good chance to be right, for other we can only offer hypothesis, of which certain are classical and other (ARKAD'YEV - 4) are more venturesome. And things are still more complicated about human behaviours !

REFERENCES

-1- ADAIR E.R., "Microwave modification of thermoregulatory behavior : effects of exposure duration ",in" Ondes Electromagnétiques et Biologie - Proc. Symp. internat. URSI/CNFRS, Jouy en Josas, 30 juin-4 juillet 1980", 1 vol. édit. J. Berteaud, B. Servantie, 332 p, pp 183-187, 1980.

-2- ADEY W.R. "Neurophysiologic effects of radiofrequency and microwave irradiation", Bull. NY Acad. Med. 55 : 1079-1093, 1979.

-3- ANTIMONII G.D., BADIKOV V.I., KEL A.A., KRASNOV E.A., & SUDAKOV S.K., ("Changes in the selfstimulation reaction in rats under the action of modulated electromagnetic field" (Rus.)), Biull. Eksper. Biol. Med., 82 : 1163-1165, 1976.

-4- ARKAD'YEV V., "Electromagnetic hypothesis on the transmission of mental suggestion", AD A.048995, 1977.

-5- BARANIUK G.V. ("Orientation of the catfish in homogeneous and inhomogeneous electric fields" (Rus.)), Fiziol. Zh. SSSR, 65 : 673-677, 1979.

-6- BAWIN S.M., GAVALAS-MEDICI R.J. & ADEY W.R., "Reinforcement of transient brain rhythms by amplitude-modulated V.H.F. fields ",in" Biologic and clinical effects of lowfrequency magnetic and electric fields", Ed. J.G. Llaurado, A. Sances & J.H. Battocletti, 1 vol. C.C. Thomas (Springfield), pp 172-186, 1974.

-7- BAWIN S.M. & ADEY W.R., "Amplitude-modulated very high frequency (V.H.F.) electric fields", Neurosci. Res. Prog. Bull., 15 : 36-38, 1977.

-8- BERMANT R.I. & JUSTESEN D.R., "Pavlovian conditioning of microwave-induced hyperthermia", Proc. Annual Meeting USNC/URSI, Amherst 11-15 Oct. 1976.

-9- BERMANT R.I., "Pavlovian conditioning of microwave-induced hyperthermia in the rat", Ph. D. dissertation, Univ. of Kansas, 159 p, 1977.

-10- BERMANT R.I., REEVES D.L., LEVINSON D.M. & JUSTESEN D.R., "Classical conditioning of microwave-induced hyperthermia in rats", Radio Sci., 14 (65) : 201-207, 1979.

-11- BIGU DEL BIANCO J. & ROMERO-SIERRA C., "The properties of bird feathers as converse piezoelectric transducers and as receptors of microwave radiation - I - Bird feathers as converse piezoelectric transducers.", Biotelemetry, 2 : 341-353, 1975.

-12- BIGU DEL BIANCO J. & ROMERO-SIERRA C, "The properties of bird feathers as converse piezoelectric transducers and as receptors of microwave radiation. II - Bird feathers as dielectric receptors of microwave radiation", Biotelemetry, 2 : 354-364, 1975.

-13- BILOKRINICKIJ V.S., ("Influence of high doses of S.H.F. electromagnetic field on nervous system of conditioned animals" (Rus.)), Zh. vyssh. nerv. Dejateln. I.P. Pavlov, 21 : 325-334, 1971.

-14- BLISS V.L. & HEPPNER F.H., "Effects of a field free space on the circadian activity rhythm of the house sparrow, Passer domesticus", in" Biological effects of electromagnetic waves - Selected papers of the USNC/URSI annual meeting, Boulder 20-23 oct. 1975", vol. 1, pp 225-237, 1976.

-15- BOHILLS S.T., LEONARD S.P. & MEEHAN A.P., "Attempts to influence the feeding behaviour of brown rats using electromagnetism", Int. Pest Control, 21 : 114-116, 1979.

-16- BURKS D.G. & GRAF E.R., "Investigation of electromagnetic effects of a 1000 ft. T.V. Tower on migratory birds", Proc. Annual Meeting USNC/URSI, Boulder, 20-23 Oct, 1975.

-17- CAIN C.A. & RISSMANN W.J., "Mammalian auditory responses to 3 GHz microwave pulses", IEEE Trans B.M.E, 25 : 288-293, 1978.

-18- CARPENTER R.L., FERRI E.S. & HAGAN G.J., "Perturbations of the microwave field by experimental animal and apparatus in biological research", Proc. 1972 IMPI Symp., pp 196-197, 1972.

-19- CARROLL D. & LEVINSON D.H., "Failure of rats to escape from an intense 918 MHz microwave field", Proc. 1978 IMPI Symp., Ottawa, 27-30 June 1978.

-20- CHERNOVETZ M.E., "Behaviorial and physiological reactions to intense R.F. fields", Proc. 146th Nat. Meeting AAAS, San Francisco, 3-8 Jan, p 64, 1980.

-21- CLARKE R.L. & JUSTESEN D.R., "Behavioral sensitivity of a domestic bird to 60 Hz AC and to DC magnetic fields", Radio Sci., 14 (65) : 209-216, 1979.

-22- CLEARY S.F., "Physiological and behavioral response to microwave radiation in mammals", Radiat. Res., 74 : 492, 1978.

-23- CRIBORN C.O., "(Effect of microwaves in the thermal intensity range on mice : body weight, rectal temperature, respiration, activity in running wheel, perception reactions and training" (SWE)), NTIS, N78-29730/6GA, 1978.

-24- D'ANDREA J.A. & GANDHI O.P., "Behavioral effects of resonant electromagnetic power absorption in rats", Proc. Annual Meeting USNC/URSI, Boulder, 20-23 Oct., 1975.

-25- D'ANDREA J.A., GANDHI O.P. & LORDS J.L., "Behavioral and thermal effects of microwave radiation at resonant and non resonant wavelengths.", Radio Sci., 12 (65) : 251-256, 1977.

-26- D'ANDREA J.A., GANDHI O.P., ASTIE L. et al., "Behavioral and physiological effects of chronic low level 2450 MHz microwave radiation in rats", Proc. 1978 IMPI Symp., Ottawa, 27-30 Juin 1978.

-27- DARDANO J.F., "Research and development of fundamental performance relevant to the behavioral effects of low level microwave exposure", DDC 697161, 1969.

-28- DE LORGE J.O., "Operant behavior of rhesus monkeys in the presence of extremely low frequency low intensity magnetic and electric fields", Rep. N° NAMRL-1155, 18 p, 1972.

-29- DE LORGE J.O., "A psychobiological study of rhesus monkeys exposed to extremely low frequency low intensity magnetic fields", Techn. Rep. N° NAMRL-1203, 25 p, 1974.

-30- DE LORGE J.O., "Operant behavior and colonic temperature of squirrel monkeys (Saimiri sciureus) during microwave irradiation", 33 p, AD A043706, 1977.

-31- DE LORGE J.O., "Disruption of behavior in mammals of three differents sizes exposed to microwaves : extrapolation to larger mammals", Proc. 1978 IMPI Symp., 1978.

-32- DE LORGE J.O., "Operant behavior and rectal temperature of squirrel monkeys during 2.45 GHz microwave irradiation", Radio Sci, 14 (6S) : 127-225, 1979.

-33- DE LORGE J., "The effects of microwaves on animal behavior", in "Ondes Electromagnêtiques et Biologie. Proc. Symp. internat. URSI/CNFRS, Jouy en Josas, 30 juin-4 Juillet 1980", 1 vol. édit. J. Berteaud, B. Servantie, 332 p, pp 171-176, 1980.

-34- DIACHENKO J.A. & MILROY W.C., "The effects of high power pulsed and low level CW microwave radiation on an operant behavior in rats", NSWC/DL Rep N° TR-3230, 16 p, 1975.

-35- DURFEE W.K., POLK C., SMITH L. et al., "Influence of extremely low frequency electric and magnetic fields upon growth development and behavior in domestic birds", AD A034526, 47 p, 1976.

-36- DURNEY C.H., JOHNSON C.C., BARBER P.W. et al., "Radiofrequency radiation dosimetry handbook (2d ed.)", Rep. SAM-TR-78-22, 1978.

-37- FARRER D.N., YOCHMOWITZ M.G., JAEGER R.J. et al., "Primate performance assessment following 3.2 GHz exposures", AD A023495, 14 p, 1976.

-38- FREY A.H. & FELD S.R., "Perception and avoidance of illumination with low power pulsed U.H.F. electromagnetic energy", Proc. 1972 IMPI Symp., 1972.

-39- FREY A.H. & FELD S.R., "Avoidance by rats of illumination with low power non inonizing electromagnetic energy", J. Comp. Physiol. Psychol. 89 : 183-188, 1975.

-40- FREY A.H., FELD S.R. & FREY B., "Neural function and behavior : defining the relationship", Ann. NY Acad. Sci, 247 : 433-439, 1975.

-41- FREY A.H., "Behavioral effects of electromagnetic energy", in "Symposium on Biological Effects and Measurement of Radiofrequency/Microwaves. Proceedings Conf. Rockville, 16-18 Feb., 1977", pp 11-22, 1977.

-42- FREY A.H. & WESLER L.S., "Conditioned emotional response modification associated with exposure to 60 Hz electrical field", to be published, 1980.

-43- GAGE M.I., "Effects of single exposures to 2450 MHz microwave irradiation on rat behavior", Proc. Annual Meeting USNC/URSI, Amherst, 11-15 Oct, 1976.

-44- GAGE M.I., BERMAN E. & KINN J.B., "Videotape observation of rats and mice during an exposure to 2450 MHz microwave irradiation", Radio Sci., 14 (65) : 227-232, 1979.

-45- GALLOWAY W.D., "Microwave dose-response relationships on two behavioral tasks", Ann. NY. Acad. Sci., 247 : 410-416, 1975.

-46- GALLOWAY W.D., BAWIN S.M., FRAZER J. et al., "A summary of the ERMAC work session on nervous system and behavioral effects of nonionizing electromagnetic radiations", J. Microwave Power, 10 : 127-140, 1975.

-47- GAVALAS R.J., WALTER D.O., HAMER J. et al., "Effect of low level - low intensity electric fields on E.E.G. and behavior in Macaca nemestrina", Brain Research, 18 : 491-501, 1970.

-48- GAVALAS-MEDICI R., "Effects of weak electric fields on behavior and E.E.G. of laboratory animals", Neurosci. Res. Prog. Bull., 15 : 27-36, 1977.

-49- GILLARD J., SERVANTIE B., BERTHARION G. et al., "Study of the microwave-induced perturbations of the behavior by the open-field test into the white rat" in "Biological Effects of Electromagnetic Waves. Selected Papers USNC/URSI Ann. Meet. Boulder, 20-23 Oct 1975", 2 vol., vol. 1, 494 p, USDHEW, pp 175-186, 1976.

-50- GRISSETT J.O. & DE LORGE J., "Central nervous system effects as measured by reaction time in squirrel monkeys exposed for short periods to extremely low frequency magnetic fields", Rep. N° NAMRL-1137, 13 p, 1971.

-51- GUSAROV D.V., ("Effect of a S.H.F. field on the physical training ability of laboratory animals" (Rus.)), Voennomed Zh., (3) : 61-66, 1971.
-52- HAWKINS T.D. & HUNT E.L., "Reduction in sensitivity to audiogenic seizure following a single 2450 MHz CW irradiation of rats", Proc. Annual Meet. USNC/URSI, Boulder, 20-23 Oct. 1975.
-53- HJERESEN D.L., DOCTOR S.R., SHELDON R.L. et al. "Shuttlebox side preference as mediated by pulsed microwave and conventional auditory cues", Proc. 1978 IMPI Symp., 1978.
-54- HUNT E.L., PHILLIPS R.D. & KING N.W., "Effects of exposure to pulsed microwaves (radar) on central nervous system excitability in laboratory animals", 62 p, AD 786753, 1974.
-55- HUNT E.L., KING N.W. & PHILLIPS R.D., "Behavioral effects of pulsed microwave radiation", Ann. N.Y. Acad. Sci., 247 : 440-453, 1975.
-56- JOHNSON R.B., MYERS D., GUY A.W. et al., "Discriminative control of appetitive behavior by pulsed microwave radiation in rats", in "Biological Effects of Electromagnetic Waves. Selected Papers of the USNC/URSI Annual Meeting, Boulder, 20-23 20-23 Oct 1975", 2 vol., vol 1, 494 p, USDHEW, pp 238-247, 1976.
-57- JOHNSON R.B., LOVELY R.H., GUY A.W. et al., "Microwave control of behavior : an auditory phenomenon", Proc. Annual Meeting USNC/URSI, Amherst, 11-15 Oct 1976.
-58- JOHNSON R.B., MIZUMORI S., MYERS D.E. et al., "Effects of pre- and post-natal exposures to 918 MHz microwave radiation on development and behavior in rats", Proc. Annual Meeting USNC/URSI, Airlie, 1977.
-59- JUSTESEN D.R., PENDLETON R.B. & PORTER P.B., "Effects of hyperthermia on activity and learning", Psychological Reports, 9 : 99-102, 1961.
-60- JUSTESEN D.R. & KING N.W., "Behavioral effects of low level microwave irradiation in the closed space situation", in "Biological Effects and Health Implications of Microwave Radiation. Symposium Proceedings", 1 vol, 265 p, USDHEW, pp 154-179, 1970.
-61- JUSTESEN D.R., "Behavioral and psychological effects of microwave radiation", Bull. NY Acad. Sci., 55 : 1058-1078, 1979.
-62- KINDT C.W., BOWDEN D.M., SPELMAN F.A. et al., "Some developmental and behavioral factors of low intensity X band radiation", Proc. Annual Meeting USNC/URSI, Boulder, 20-23 oct. 1975.
-63- KING N.W. "The effects of low level microwave irradiation upon reflexive, operant and discriminant behaviors of the rat", Thesis, Univ. Kansas, 114 p, 1969.
-64- KING N.W., JUSTESEN D.R. & CLARKE R.L., "Behavioral sensitivity to microwave irradiation", Science, 172 : 398-401, 1971.

-65- KISLIUK M. & ISHAY J.S., "Influence of the earth's magnetic field on the comb building orientation of hornets", Experientia, 35 : 1041-1042, 1979.

-66- KLEIN M.J. & MILHAUD C.L., "(Preliminary results of the study of effects of microwaves on the central nervous system of a primate (Macaca mulatta)" (Fr.)), in "Effects biologiques des rayonnements non ionisants. Utilisation et risques associés". Proc. 9 th Internat. Congress SFRP, Nainville les Roches, pp 315-336, 1978.

-67- KORBEL S.F. & FINE A.L., "Effects of low intensity U.H.F. radio fields as a function of frequency", Psychonomic Sci., 9 : 527-528, 1967.

-68- KORBEL S.F., "Behavioral effects of low intensity U.H.F. Radiation" in " Biological Effects and Health Implications of Microwave Radiation - Symposium Proceedings", 1 vol, 265 p, USDHEW, pp 180-184, 1970.

-69- KRUPP J.H., "Radar and migrating birds", 11 p, AD A030346, 1976.

-70- LAMBERT P.D., NEALEIGH R.C. & WILSON M., "Effects of microwave exposures on the central nervous system of beagles", J. Microwave Power, 7 : 367-380, 1972.

-71- LARKIN R.P. & SUTHERLAND P.J., "Migrating birds respond to project Seafarer's electromagnetic field", Science, 195 : 777-779, 1977.

-72- LIN J.C., BASSEN H.I. & WU C.L., "Perturbation effect of animal restraining materials on microwave exposure", IEEE Trans. B.M.E., 24 : 80-83, 1977.

-73- LIN J.C., GUY A.W. & CALDWELL L.R., "Thermographic and behavioral studies of rats in the near field of 918 MHz radiations", IEEE Trans. MTT, 25 : 833-836, 1977.

-74- LOBANOVA E.A. & GONCHAROVA A.V., ("Study of conditioned reflexes in white rats irradiated by short and ultra short waves" (Rus.)) Gig. Truda Prof. Zabol, 15 : 29-33, 1971.

-75- LOBANOVA E.A., "The use of conditioned reflexes to study microwave effects on the central nervous system", in "Biological Effects and Health Hazards of Microwave Radiation", 1 vol., 350 p, Polish Med. Publ., pp 109-118, 1974.

-76- LOVELY R.H. & GUY A.W., "Conditioned taste aversions in the rat induced by a single exposure to microwaves", Proc. 1975 IMPI Symp, 1975.

-77- LOVELY R.H., MYERS D.E., JOHNSON R.B., et al., "Behavioral and physiological effects of chronic pulse-modulated microwave radiation in rats", Proc. Annual Meeting USNC/URSI, Amherst, 11-15 oct. 1976.

-78- McAFEE R.D., "Low power density behavior effects of microwave irradiation of experimental animals : real or artifact?", J. Microwave Power, 7 : 83-85, 1972.

-79- McAFEE R.D., ELDER S.T., LIPSCOMB R.J. et al., "Microwave and infrared radiation effects on an operant response in rhesus monkeys", Proc. Annual Meeting USNC/URSI, Boulder 20-23 oct. 1975.

-80- McAFEE R.D., CAZENAVETTE L., SHUBERT H., et al., "Microwave irradiation and ocular effects on rhesus monkeys", Biophys. J., 17 : 145a, 1977.

-81- McREE D.I., ELDER J.A., GAGE .M.I., et al., "Effects of nonionizing radiation on the central nervous system, behavior and blood : a progress report"., Environ. Health Perspect., 30 : 123-131, 1979.

-82- MANTHEI R.C. & GLASER Z.R., "The sleep process of rabbits exposed to low intensity nonionizing electromagnetic radiation. I. Development of methodology". in "Biological Effects of Electromagnetic Waves. Selected Papers of the USNC/URSI. Annual Meeting, Boulder, 20-23 oct. 1975", 2 vol., vol 1, 494 p, USDHEW, pp 341-351, 1976.

-83- MATRENINA V.L., POSADSKAIA V.M. & RUDAKOV I.A., ("Temperature changes and survival of laboratory animals after exposure to various intensities of microwaves" (Rus.)), Biull. Eksper. Biol. Med., 86 : 282-285, 1978.

-84- MATSSON J.L. & OLIVA S.A., "Effect of electromagnetic pulse on avoidance behavior and electroencephalogram of a rhesus monkey", Aviat. Space Environ. Med., 47 : 644-648, 1976.

-85- MEDICI R.G. & DAY S.R., "Effects of weak ELF electric fields on schedule-controlled behavior of monkeys", in "Biological Effects of Electromagnetic Waves. Selected Papers of the USNC/URSI Annual Meeting, Boulder, 20-23 oct 1975", 2 vol., vol. 1, 494 p, USDHEW, pp 215-224, 1976.

-86- MEDICI R.G. & SAGAN P.M., "Behavioral protocols and preliminary observations of chicks exposed to weak amplitude modulated 450 MHz fields", in "Symposium on Biological Effects and Measurement of Radio Frequency/Microwaves", Proceedings Conf. Rockville, 16-18 Feb., 1977, pp 34-40, 1977.

-87- MICHAELSON S.M. "Cutaneous perception of microwaves", J. Microwave Power, 7 : 67-73, 1972.

-88- MITCHELL D.S., SWITZER W.G. & BRONAUGH E.L., "Effects of chronic athermal microwave radiation on innate and learned behaviors in rats", Proc. Annual Meeting USNC/URSI, Amherst, 11-15 oct., 1976.

-89- MITCHELL D.S., SWITZER W.G. & BRONAUGH E.L., "Hyperactivity and disruption of operant behavior in rats after multiple exposures to microwave radiation", Radio Sci, 12 (6S) : 263-271, 1977.

-90- MOE K.E., LOVELY R.H. & MYERS D.E., "Physiological and behavioral effects of chronic low level microwave radiation in rats" in "Biological Effects of Electromagnetic Waves. Selected Papers of the USNC/URSI Annual Meeting, Boulder, 20-23 Oct. 1975", 2 vol., vol. 1, 494 p, USDHEW, pp 248-256, 1976.

-91- MONAHAN J.C. & HO H.S., "Microwave induced avoidance behavior in the mouse", in "Biological Effects of Electromagnetic Waves. Selected Papers of the USNC/URSI Annual Meeting, Boulder, 20-23 oct 1975", 2 vol., vol. 1, 494 p, USDHEW, pp 274-283, 1976.
-92- MONAHAN J.C & HO H.S., "Temperature dependance of microwave avoidance", Proc. Annual Meeting USNC/URSI, Amherst, 11-15 oct 1976.
-93- MONAHAN J.C. & HENTON W.W., "Free-operant avoidance and escape from microwave radiation", in "Symposium on Biological Effects and Measurement of Radiofrequency/Microwaves", Proc. Conference Rockville, 16-18 Feb 1977, pp 23-32, 1977.
-94- MONAHAN J.C. & HENTON W.W., "Microwave absorption and taste aversion as a function of 915 MHz radiation", in "Symposium on Biological Effects and Measurement of Radiofrequency/ Microwaves", Proc. Conference Rockville, 16-18 Feb 1977, pp 23-32, 1977.
-95- MONAHAN J.C. & HENTON W.W., "The effect of psychoactive drugs on operant behavior induced by microwave radiation", Radio Sci, 14 (6S) : 233-238, 1979.
-96- NEALEIGH R.C., GARNER R.J., MORGAN R.J., et al., "The effect of microwave on Y maze learning in the white rat", J. Microwave Power, 6 : 49-54, 1971.
-97- NELSON T.D., "Behavioral effects of microwave irradiation on squirrel monkey (Saimiri sciureus) performance of a repeated acquisition task", AD A055953/4GA, 18 p, 1978.
-98- OLSSON P.U., "FOA animals experiments show the physical and psychic effects of microwaves", FOA Tidningen, 16 : 7-9, 1978.
-99- OSSENKOPP K.P., "Maturation and open-field behavior in rats exposed prenatally to an ELF low-intensity rotating magnetic field", Psychol. Rep., 30 : 371-374, 1972.
-100- PERSINGER M.A. & OSSENKOPP K.P., "Behavioral changes in adult rats exposed to ELF magnetic fields", Int. J. Biometeor., 16 : 155-162, 1972.
-101- PERSINGER M.A., LUDWIG H.W. & OSSENKOPP K.P., "Psychophysiological effects of extremely low frequency electromagnetic fields : a review", Perceptual Motor Skills, 36 : 1131-1159, 1973.
-102- ROBERTI B., HEEBELS G.H., HENDRICX J.C.M., et al., "Preliminary investigations of the effects of low level microwave irradiation on spontaneous motor activity in rats", Ann. NY Acad. Sci., 247 : 417-424, 1975.
-103- SAGAN P.M. & MEDICI R.G., "Behavior of chicks exposed to low-power 450 MHz fields sinusoidally modulated at E.E.G. frequencies", Radio Sci., 14 (6S) : 239-245, 1979.
-104- SANZA J.N. & DE LORGE J.O., "Fixed interval behavior of rats exposed to microwaves at low power densities", Radio Sci., 12 (6S) : 273-277, 1977.

-105- SCHOLL D.M. & ALLEN S.O., "Skilled visual motor performance by monkeys in a 1.2 GHz microwave field", Radio Sci., 14 (6S) : 247-252, 1979.

-106- SERVANTIE B., SERVANTIE A.M. & ETIENNE J., "Synchronization of cortical neurons by a pulsed microwave field as evidenced by spectral analysis of electrocorticograms from the white rat", Ann. NY Acad. Sci., 247 : 82-86, 1975.

-107- SHANDALA M.G., RUDNEV M.I. & NAVAKATIAN M.A., "Patterns of change in behavioral reactions to low power densities of microwaves", Proc. Annual Meeting USNC/URSI, Airlie, 30 oct-4 Nov. 1977.

-108- SHANDALA M.G., DUMANSKII U.D., RUDNEV M.I., et al., "Study of nonionizing microwave radiation effects upon the central nervous system and behavior reactions". Environ. Health Perspect., 30 : 115-121, 1979.

-109- SHANDALA M., "The biological effects of microwave exposure at different non thermal levels", in "Ondes Electromagnétiques et Biologie- Proc. Symp. internat. URSI/CNFRS, Jouy en Josas, 30 Juin-4 Juillet 1980", 1 vol., édit. J. Berteaud, B. Servantie, 332 p, pp 57-65, 1980.

-110- SMITH M.T., D'ANDREA J.A. & GANDHI O.P., "Behavioral effects of strong 60 Hz electric fields in rats", J. Microwave Power, 14 : 223-228, 1979.

-111- SMITH R.F. & JUSTESEN D.R., "Effects of a 60 Hz electromagnetic field on locomotive et aggressive behavior of mice," Proc. Annual Meeting USNC/URSI, Amherst, 11-15 oct. 1976.

-112- SOUTHERN W.E., "Orientation of gull chicks exposed to project Sanguine's electromagnetic field", Science, 189 : 143-145, 1975.

-113- SPALDING J.F., FREYMAN R.W. & HOLLAND L.M., "Effects of 800 MHz electromagnetic radiation on body weight, activity, hematopoesis and life span in mice", Health Phys., 20 : 421-424, 1971.

-114- STERN S., MARGOLIN L., WEISS B. et al, "Microwaves effect on thermoregulatory behavior in rats", Science, 206 : 1198-1201, 1979.

-115- SUDAKOV K.V. & ANTIMONII G.D. ("The hypnogenic effect of modulated electromagnetic field" (Rus.)), Biull. Eksper. Biol. Med., 34 : 146-149, 1977.

-116- TANNER J.A., ROMERO-SIERRA C. & DAVIE S.J., "The effects of microwaves upon birds : preliminary experiments.", J. Microwave Power, 4 : 122-128, 1969.

-117- THOMAS J., FINCH E.D., FULK D.W. et al., "Effects of low-level microwave radiation on behavioral baselines", Ann. NY Acad. Sci., 247 : 425-432, 1975.

-118- THOMAS J., YEANDLE S.S. & BURCH L.S., "Modification of internal discriminative stimulus control of behavior by low levels of pulsed microwave radiation", in "Biological Effects of Electromagnetic Waves. Selected Papers of the USNC/URSI Annual

Meeting, Boulder, 20-23 oct 1975", 2 vol., vol. 1, 494 p., USDHEW, pp 201-214, 1976.

-119- THOMAS J.C., BURCH L.S. & YEANDLE S.S., "Microwave radiation and chlordiazepoxide : synergistic effects on fixed interval behavior", Science, 203 : 1357-1358, 1979.

-120- THOMAS J.C. & MAITLAND G., "Microwave radiation and dextro-amphetamine : evidence of combined effects on behavior of rats", Radio Sci., 14 (6S) : 253-258, 1979.

-121- WALCOTT C., GOULD J.L. & KIRSCHVINK J.L., "Pigeons have magnets", Science, 205 : 1027-1029, 1979.

-122- WANGEMANN R.T. & CLEARY S.F., "The in vivo effects of 2.45 GHz microwave radiation on rabbit serum components and sleeping time", Rad. Environ. Biophys., 13 : 89-103, 1976.

-123- WILLIAMS W., "Conditioned taste aversion in rats exposed to 2450 MHz CW microwaves", Proc. 1978 IMPI Symp., Ottawa, 27-30 Juin 1978.

-124- YAKOVLEVA M.I., SHLJAFER T.P. & SVETKOVA I.P., ("About problem of conditioned heart reflexes. Functional and morphological status of cortical neurones under the action of U.H.F. electromagnetic fields" (Rus.)), Zh. vyssh. nerv. Dejateln I.P. Pavlov., 18 : 973-978, 1968.

-125- YAKOVLEVA M.I. & MEDVEDEVA M.V., ("Conditioned regulation of heart activity and of respiration, and morphological changes in brain of pigeons under the action of a uniform magnetic field" (Rus.)), Zh. vyssh. nerv. Dejateln I.P. Pavlov, 22 : 288-293, 1972.

NEUROENDOCRINE RESPONSE TO MICROWAVE/RADIOFREQUENCY ENERGIES

Sol M. Michaelson

Department of Radiation Biology and Biophysics
University of Rochester
School of Medicine and Dentistry
Rochester, New York 14642

INTRODUCTION

To maintain homeostasis, a mammal possesses two control mechanisms that react to changes in internal and external environments (stimuli or stress). These two control mechanisms are the neural and endocrine systems. Separation of endocrine from neural control is not always possible as neural signals are integrated at the hypothalamus to react to deviations in the internal or external environments. Hypothalamic-hypophysial-adrenocortical (HHA), hypothalamic-hypophysial-thyroidal (HHT), and hypothalamic-hypophysial-somatotrophic (HHS) are three endocrine systems that participate in the "stress" response. Generally, they operate through a negative feed-back mechanism.

The neuroendocrine system (NES) is an exquisitely sensitive organ and chemical system intimately involved with, and under the influence of the central nervous system (CNS). This system exhibits a profound influence on the body, often through the effects it has on the metabolism of various tissues. The NES in coordination with higher nervous centers is a major regulatory system in the body. The functional relationships of the neuroendocrine system follow a cybernetic pattern, with feedback mechanisms playing an essential role. These relationships are distinguished by a hierarchy of activities, which consist of three levels of organization (hypothalamus, hypophysis, endocrine gland) in which overall output function, the secretion of hormones by the endocrine gland, is controlled by the balance of signals.

This balance is further modified by direct neural inputs from higher brain centers and peripheral nerves. As an example, adrenergic neurons in the hypothalamus stimulate thyrotropin-releasing hormone (TRH) acting on the anterior pituitary to increase thyrotropin (TSH), which enters the general circulation to stimulate thyroid secretion of triiodothyronine (T_3) and thyroxine (T_4). The T_3 and T_4 then act by negative feedback control on hypophysial TSH secretion.

The sensitivity of the neuroendocrine system to perturbation is greatest at its highest level, the hypothalamus, where small chemical or electrical stimuli can produce significant alterations in the amount of hormones secreted by the endocrine gland. Thus, the neuroendocrine system forms a sensitive mode of analyzing responses of the endocrine system itself and of higher CNS centers under the influence of environmental changes and organismic readjustments.

Acting alone or in concert, the various components of the neuroendocrine system play a central role in the integrative activities known as homeokinesis. Normal integrative function of the body or those activities that result from stimuli within the individual or due to alterations in the physical environment are integrated or "linked" together by the reciprocal relationships of the CNS and the endocrine system.

The classic triad of the Alarm Reaction (adrenocortical stimulation, thymicolymphatic hypotrophy and gastrointestinal ulcer) denotes the stereotyped response of the body to any demand that severely taxes the regulatory processes. The pathophysiologic picture of "stress" has been characterized as the General Adaptation Syndrome, which develops in three stages, the alarm reaction, the stage of resistance and the stage of exhaustion.[1] The triad of the alarm reaction also points out the involvement of the hypothalamic-hypophysial-adrenocortical system and autonomic control. It is now well established that in rats acute stress inhibits growth hormone (GH) secretion and stimulates adrenocorticotropic hormone (ACTH)[2] and prolactin release.[3] In general, stress-induced hormonal changes are not related to the nature, but rather to the intensity and duration of the stressing agent.

Hypothalamic-adrenocortical interaction displays a diurnal rhythmicity. The interaction is intensified during "stress" to the point of changing or obliterating the diurnal pattern of secretion. Among the strongest of the stressful stimuli are surgery, anesthesia, cold, narcosis, burning, high environmental temperature, and rough handling or restraint. A new environment or new manipulation technique alters animals' behavior patterns to induce anxiety, avoidance behavior, and weight loss and thus could be interpreted as being "stressful."

Standard laboratory stressors can easily be found in the experimental procedures that are used in biomedical studies. Such commonplace procedures as handling, novelty of experimental environment and procedures, extreme environmental temperatures, forced muscular exercise, immobilization, transportation, noise, electrical shock, ether anesthesia ...etc. can act as stressors under certain conditions. Great care must thus be exercised to ensure that the changes in hormone levels are the response to a specific stressor in question, (i.e., electromagnetic field) rather than to some extraneous factor. Therefore, investigation of the reactions of the endocrine axes to microwaves must be carefully designed and controlled, and investigations should be conducted in animals properly adapated to environmental conditions. For rats, the adaptation period should be at least 14 days.[4] Unless these factors are taken into consideration, it is not possible to eliminate stress reactions due to extraneous factors in experiments intended to investigate adrenal cortex function in relation to microwave exposure.[5] This is of paramount importance if one is interested in studying subtle indicators of microwave exposure, especially at lower intensities applied for long periods of time.

Functional alterations in the neuroendocrine system of both animals and humans exposed to microwave radiofrequency (MW/RF) energies have been reported by several investigators. The findings include changes in the secretions of the pituitary gland, adrenal cortex, thyroid gland, and the gonads. It is reasonable to expect that alterations in the levels of the secretory products of these organs will occur in response to microwave exposure at some time/intensity relationship. Shifts of a few millidegrees may alter firing rates in hypothalamic cells.[6] On the other hand, brain temperature changes in the range of 0.1-2.0°C are possible with exercise and a consequence of certain environmental stressors.[7]

Neuroendocrine and Endocrine Effects

Several reviews have considered neuroendocrine responses in relation to microwave exposure.[8-12] Response of the endocrine system of rats to whole-body exposure to microwaves has been studied in recent years, but most of the reports are based on relatively short exposures at modest to high power densities.[5,11,13-34]

Some investigators believe that endocrine changes result from stimulation of the hypothalamic-hypophysial system due to thermal interactions at the hypothalamic or adjacent levels of organization, the hypophysis itself, or the particular endocrine gland or end-organ under study. According to other investigators, the observed changes have been interpreted as being the result of direct microwave interactions with the central nervous system. In either case, one should not consider neuroendocrine alterations as necessarily pathologic because the function of the neuroendocrine system is to maintain homeostasis and hormone levels will fluctuate to maintain such organismic stability.

Hypothalamic-hypophysial-adrenal Response

Several investigators have reported biochemical and physiological changes as a result of microwave exposure which suggest an adrenal effect. According to Petrov and Syngayevskaya,[35] 3 and 24 hours after dogs were irradiated with 3000 MHz, 10 mW/cm^2, the corticosteroid content of their blood had increased by 100-150 percent above the original level. Serum potassium was decreased by 5-10 percent and sodium was increased by the same amount. Kirchev[36] reported that under the influence of an unspecified RF field (3-300 MHz) the weight of the adrenals increased as a result of hyperplasia, indicating adrenal stimulation.

Dumansky et al.[37] have reported that chronic exposure of animals to microwaves (CW or pulsed) is accompanied by reduced activity of blood cholinesterase and an increased amount of 17-ketosteroids in the urine, a reduced amount of ascorbic acid in the adrenal glands, and reduced weight of the adrenal glands. Blood cholinesterase activity is mostly "pseudocholinesterase" which has no correlation with acetylcholine activity which the authors imply.

Schliephake[38] observed an increase in 17-ketosteroids in the urine of humans "intentionally" exposed to "centimetric" microwaves (50 mW/cm^2, 10 min); in rats, a marked increase in the ascorbic acid content of the adrenal cortex was observed. The results of Leytes and Skurikhina[39] also indicated increased adrenocortical hormone production 1-2 hours after the beginning of exposure to microwaves. It has been suggested that these results are an indirect indication of increased pituitary adrenocorticotropic function.

According to Bereznitskaya,[40] the pituitary gland in female mice, when exposed to 3000 MHz (10 mW/cm^2) twice daily for five months, retained its gonadotropic function, although its activity was reduced in comparison with that of nonexposed animals. Tolgskaya and Gordon,[41] in discussing the dynamics of changes in the neurosecretory function of the hypothalamus, noted the reversibility of the process when exposure was terminated.

Rabbits exposed to 3000 MHz (50-60 mW/cm^2) 4 hours daily for 20 days tended to show a decline in the amount of urinary 17-hydroxycorticosteroids (17-OHCS) at the beginning of exposure, followed by a gradual return to normal.[42] During the control period, a mean output of 4.0 mg of 17-OHCS per 24 hr was observed, while exposure to microwaves was found to result in 2.8 mg/24 hr. No change was evident in the excretion of 17-ketosteroids in the urine.

In rats exposed to microwaves of varying intensity, no quantitative changes in corticosterone were found in the adrenals and blood plasma.[29] Prepubescent hypophysectomized rats displayed no differences in adrenal growth rate when treated with pituitary homogenates collected either from rats exposed to microwaves, or from control rats.

Rats exposed to 2450 MHz (CW), 10 mW/cm^2 for 4 hours, showed no change in adrenal weight, phenylethanolamine-N-methyl transferase (PNMT) activity or epinephrine levels.[32] After 16 hours of exposure (0.4°C increase in rectal temperature compared to controls), however, decrease in adrenal epinephrine (32 percent) was significant and PNMT activity was elevated (25 percent). There were no statistically significant differences ($P > 0.1$) in adrenal or plasma corticosterone levels between exposed and sham-exposed animals.

Michaelson et al.[43] reported that exposure of dogs to 2880 MHz pulsed microwaves at power densities above 100 mW/cm^2 resulted in physiologic responses indicative of adrenocortical stimulation which was consonant with the concept of non-specific "stress". It was suggested that microwaves of high power density can act as a "stressor" affecting regulatory and integrative homeokinetic activity resulting in an alteration in homeostasis.

Dumansky and Shandala[44] reported adrenocortical changes in rats and rabbits chronically exposed (10-12 hr/day, 180 days) to 2 and 5 mW/cm^2 respectively. Petrov and Syngayevskaya[35] suggest that the enhancement of corticosteroid activity during and after irradiation could be an adaptive reaction. Some animals develop inhibition of adrenocortical function (corticosteroid activity), attended by a decline in resistance to microwaves reflecting insufficient adrenocorticotrophic hormone (ACTH). Increased resistance may be related to an increase in the secretion of ACTH, which would also be an adaptive reaction of the organism. This is supported by the finding that the resistance of some animals to microwaves is slightly increased when ACTH is administered.

Lotz and Michaelson[20] and Lu et al.[10] reported plasma corticosterone (CS) levels in rats exhibited a variable power density/threshold pattern of response, with a different threshold for 120 minute exposure than for 30 or 60 minute exposure to 2450 MHz, CW. For all these durations of exposure, a strong correlation was evident between mean colonic temperature and mean plasma corticosterone levels. The threshold power density was 50 mW/cm^2 for a 30- or 60-min, and 20 mW/cm^2 for 120 min exposure. These thresholds occurred with whole-body specific absorption rates of 8.0 and 3.2 W/kg, respectively. Plasma CS increases within 15-30 minutes of the start of exposure to 2450 MHz and falls sharply within 15-30 minutes after termination of exposure.[13] Thus the adrenocortical response is transient.

In contrast to the pronounced adrenocortical response observed in intact rats, plasma CS levels in acutely hypophysectomized rats exposed to 60 mW/cm^2 for 60 minutes were below control levels. The CS response to microwaves at 50 mW/cm^2 for 60 minutes was suppressed by 3.2 μg dexamethasone/100 g body weight.[21] These results are consistent with the hypothesis that the stimulation of the adrenal axis in the microwave exposed rat is a systemic, integrative process due to a general hyperthermia. The results indicate that the microwave-induced CS response observed in rats is dependent upon adrenocorticotropin secretion by the pituitary, i.e., the adrenal gland is not directly stimulated by microwave exposure. Adrenocortical function may be a sensitive, quantifiable indicator of the physiological compensation required of an animal exposed to microwaves.

Novitskii et al.[45] studied the corticotropin releasing factor (CRF) of the median eminence, ACTH of the hypophysis and 11-oxycorticosteroid (11-OCS) of the plasma in 180 - 230 gram Wistar rats whole-body exposed to 0, 0.01, 0.1, 10 and 75 mW/cm^2 of 12.6 cm (2.6 GHz) microwaves with horizontal polarization for 30 min. Results indicated that the threshold intensity was 0.1 mW/cm^2 for increases in CRF, ACTH and 11-OCS; peaking at 1 mW/cm^2. The finding suggested that the adrenocortical stimulation was a process mediated by the central nervous system.

In a study by Lu et al.[23] to assess the neuroendocrine responses to protracted exposure, adult rats were exposed to 2450 MHz CW at 0, 1, 5, 10 or 20 mW/cm^2 for 1, 2, 4, or 8 hours. Exposure below 10 mW/cm^2 pushed the appearance of the peak colonic temperature to an earlier time of the day. In rats exposed to 20 mW/cm^2 for 8 hours, serum CS increase was significantly inhibited from the expected circadian elevation. This inhibition of CS circadian elevation was also noted in rats exposed to 0.1 and 1 mW/cm^2 for 4 hours.[25] A significant correlation between colonic temperature and CS level was found in sham-exposed rats sacrificed between 1230 and 1930 hours. Similar correlation was noted in rats exposed to 1 to 70 mW/cm^2 for 1 hour and sacrificed at 1230 hours, and rats exposed to 0.1 to 40 mW/cm^2 for 4 hours and sacrificed at 1530 hours. The temperature coefficient decreased sequentially among sham-exposed, one-hour exposed and 4-hour exposed rats, respectively. Thus, a dual action on the hypothalamic-hypophysial-adrenocortical axis was demonstrated in which "low intensity" exposure of the rat (<10

mW/cm^2) inhibited CS levels during the peak period of the CS circadian oscillation while "higher" intensity exposure (>20 mW/cm^2) stimulated CS secretion during any portion of the circadian periodicity.[23]

In their study, Novitskii et al.[45] suggested that increased hypothalamic-hypophysial-adrenocortical (HHA) stimulation with increasing intensities from 0.01 to 1 mW/cm^2 (2.6 GHz) could be an indicator of an adaptive reaction of the organism to a harmful agent. The findings in repeated 30 min exposures to 2.6 GHz at 1 mW/cm^2 was considered to be evidence of "cumulative effect" and "exhaustion" by microwave exposure. However, the pattern of this HHA reaction could very well fit into the picture of the general adaptation syndrome.[46]

Adrenocortical stimulation has been generally accepted to be a result of a stressor stimulus, i.e. a level of stimulation that requires bodily adjustment to counteract the insult. There is consistent evidence that microwave exposure of rats above 25 mW/cm^2 (~4 mW/g) stimulates the HHA axis, and is modulated by the central nervous system. The responses from exposures below 25 mW/cm^2, are variable suggesting stimulation or inhibition in some cases, or no change in others. Alterations in adrenocortical function at "low" intensities are smaller than the magnitude of the daily oscillation of this system and are modified by their timing with respect to the normal biological periodicities.[25]

Hypothalamic-hypophysial-thyroid Response

The thyroid gland plays an essential role in regulating basal metabolism in the organism as well as in the metabolic generation of heat in the tissues. The functional and structural integrity of the thyroid gland is essential for normal homeokinesis of the organism. Not only do the thyroid hormones act at the fundamental level of cellular metabolism by regulating cellular processes to maintain homeostasis, but the thyroid is also an integral member of the neuroendocrine system whose activity is dependent upon and responsive to functional disturbance in other members of the system.

The release of thyrotropin (TSH) by the anterior pituitary gland is regulated by an interaction between hypothalamic thyrotropin-releasing hormone (TRH) which stimulates TSH release and calorigenic ("metabolically active") thyroid hormones, thyroxine (T4) and triiodothyronine (T3) which suppress it. Of interest also is the indication that somatostatin (GH-RIH) the growth hormone-release inhibiting hormone, may regulate TSH secretion by its inhibitory action on TSH release. Interest in this endocrine axis is, therefore, appropriate when considering the possible physiologic perturbations of the thyroid as a consequence of microwave exposure.

The literature offers comparatively few experimental studies of the effect of RF or microwaves on the thyroid. In a study by Milroy and Michaelson,[31] rats exposed to microwaves in various regimens (2450 MHz, CW, 1 mW/cm^2 continuously for 8 weeks or 10 mW/cm^2, 8 hr/day for 8 weeks) showed no alterations in thyroid structure or function. Michaelson et al.[43] reported transiently increased radioactive iodide uptake (RAIU) in dogs exposed to 1280 or 2880 MHz pulsed microwaves, 100-165 mW/cm^2. Baranski[47] showed a stimulatory influence of 5 mW/cm^2 on the trapping and secretory function of the thyroid gland of rabbits.

In rats exposed for 16 hours to 2450 MHz (CW) at 10 to 25 mW/cm^2, tests of thyroid function in general showed no statistically significant deviations from the norm except that in animals with a 1.0 to 1.7°C increase in colonic temperature there was a reduction in the ability of the thyroid to concentrate iodide.[32]

Indirect evidence has been obtained of some protective influence of lowered general and tissue metabolic rate following hypophysectomy on the time-related lethal exposure of rats to microwaves. Mikolajczyk[30] found that the survival time of normal rats exposed to microwaves was largely a function of body mass; survival time per unit of body weight was significantly longer in hypophysectomized rats than in normal ones.

Lu et al.[22] reported that serum thyroxine levels were transiently elevated in rats after exposure to 2.45 GHz at 1 mW/cm^2 for 4 hours. This transient increase was not accompanied by changes in serum TSH.[23] Magin et al.[27,28] demonstrated that localized thyroid exposure (2.45 GHz) which resulted in thyroid temperature elevation can stimulate thyroid secretion in the absence of pituitary influence.

Levels of thyroid hormone were found by Vetter[34] to decrease as power density of 2.45 GHz microwaves increased from 5 to 25 mW/cm^2. Lu et al.[22] also noted decreased thyroxine levels in rats exposed to 2.45 GHz at 20 mW/cm^2 for 4 to 8 hours.

The thyroid depression apparently reflects inhibition of hypophysial TSH secretion as evidenced by decreased TSH prior to and accompanied by the decreases in serum thyroxine in rats exposed to 2.45 GHz microwaves (CW) at 10 mW/cm^2 for 1 and 2 hours and 20 mW/cm^2 for 2 hours and 8 hours.[23] Lotz et al. (unpublished observations) investigated TSH levels in rats exposed to 2.45 GHz at 13 to 60 mW/cm^2 for 30, 60 and 120 minutes. Their results indicated that a 30 minute exposure did not affect the TSH levels. Depressed TSH levels were noted in rats exposed at 30 mW/cm^2 (SAR = 4.8 W/kg) or higher for 60 min and 13 mW/cm^2 (SAR = 2.1 W/kg) or higher for 120 min. A high correlation between decreases in serum thyroxine and TSH was also reported in rats exposed to 2.45 GHz, 8 mW/cm^2, 8 hr daily up to 20 days.[33]

To counteract the influence of decreased TSH, stimulation of thyroid function could be revealed in rats exposed to a relatively high power density (2.45 GHz, 70 mW/cm^2) for 1 hr[25] or in rats with TSH obliterated by triiodothyronine at the time of exposure to 2.45 GHz at 40 mW/cm^2 for 2 hr.[24]

Perturbation of the thyroid gland may be the result of an indirect effect, the thermal stress on the body producing an hypothalamic-hypophysial response. This is consistent with microwave-induced thermal stimulation of hypothalamic-hypophysial-thyroid (HHT) activity.[48] These changes in thyroid activity could be the result of increased TSH and/or increased metabolic activity of the thyroid gland due to heating. Temperature elevation and heat stress have been associated with alterations in radioactive iodine (RAI) turnover rate. The HHT axis is sensitive to environmental temperature.[49] Differences in rate of temperature change or alteration in thermal gradients in the body would also result in qualitative differences in endocrine response.

Thus, there appear to be two types of action of microwave exposure on the hypothalamic-hypophysial-thyroid axis, i.e. local thyroid stimulation and axial inhibition. The local thyroid stimulation is, in contrast to the ACTH dependent adrenocortical stimulation, caused by high intensity microwave exposure. The inhibition of the HHT axis by thermogenic microwave exposure is a homeostatic reaction to the increased heat load. The lower level of metabolism can be viewed as a specific stress response.

It has been reported that microwave-exposed workers have developed enlargement of the thyroid gland as well as increased radioactive iodine uptake (RAIU), but in some cases without clinical symptoms of hyperfunction.[50] None of the reported alterations in thyroid function was irreversible or resulted in morbidity. D'Yachenko[51] described the results of a study of thyroid function in 38 men who operated microwave equipment (centimeter band) for 3 to 15 years. Enhanced ^{131}I uptake by the thyroid was found which was attributed to secondary effects resulting from radiation-induced disturbances of the sympathetic nervous system in the vicinity of the hypothalamus. Denisiewicz et al.,[52] did not find significant disturbances in thyroid function among 142 men exposed to power densities of 10 μW-1 mW/cm^2 while servicing microwave equipment.

Growth Hormone

The polypeptide, growth hormone (GH) or somatotropin (STH) is a secretory product of the pituitary gland. It has been shown that fasting, various forms of physical and psychologic stress, onset of sleep, alterations of protein intake, changes in plasma glucose levels, and administration of L-dopa, glucagon, or vasopressin affect pituitary production and plasma GH levels.[53]

GH circulates in the plasma in an unbound form and has ubiquitous sites of action, unlike its adenohypophysial counterparts, thyroid-stimulating hormone (TSH) and ACTH, which rely on their target gland secretory products for effect. Among its actions GH antagonizes the effects of insulin, in that it inhibits cellular uptake of glucose (glucose-sparing or diabetogenic effect), and it causes the release of free fatty acids from tissue storage depots.

In man and certain nonhuman primates, a variety of stresses, both physical and psychologic, may produce an acute GH release. The concomitant stresses in the rat are known to effect reduction in plasma GH levels.[54] Pulsatile bursts of GH secretion occur for apparently inexplicable reasons that are not associated with any changes in plasma metabolites that affect or are affected by GH secretion (glucose, free fatty acids, or circulating amino acids).

It appears that GH is regulated by a specific releasing factor (GRF) and a specific inhibiting factor (GIF) that originate in the hypothalamus, whereas ACTH and TSH have only releasing factors. The absence of inhibiting factors for TSH and ACTH can probably be best explained by the fact that these hormones have specific target tissues, which, in turn, produce hormones that act via a negative feedback to the hypothalamus.

GH, which possesses no specific target tissue, requires some mechanism to control its production. This control is achieved via the concentration of circulating metabolites, integrated with higher center inputs which affect hypothalamic GIF or GRF release when appropriate. This area of the hypothalamus, located in the medial basal area, together with the lateral hypothalamus, also functions as a final integrative center for energy balance and food intake. Also, these areas are intimately associated with the region of the hypothalamus involved in temperature regulation.[53,55]

In the rat exposed to 2.45 GHz microwaves, at 13 mW/cm^2 there is an increase in GH whereas at 36 mW/cm^2 rat serum GH drops after 60 min of exposure, to significantly low levels.[11] Lotz et al.[19] noted the threshold intensity for GH inhibition is 50 mW/cm^2 (SAR = 8.0 W/kg) for rats exposed to 2.45 GHz, CW for 30-

and 60-min. For 2 hr exposure, at 13 mW/cm^2 (SAR = 2.1 W/kg) or higher, GH levels were lower than among sham-exposed with progressively lower GH at each successively higher power density. Part of this sensitivity may be attributed to the higher GH levels in 2-hr sham-exposed rats than among 30- or 60-min shams suggesting the possible stress effect of routine confinement of small experimental animals.

Neuroendocrine/Metabolic Correlations

While hypothalamic-hypophysial-adrenocortical activation and hypothalamic-hypophysial-growth hormone inhibition can be viewed as non-specific stress reactions, hypothalamic-hypophysial-thyroid (HHT) depression may be considered as a specific reaction. The acute reaction of the HHT to thermogenic levels of microwaves is to lower the hormone affecting resting metabolic rate. It has been shown that decreases in the resting metabolic rate of male rats is dependent upon the quantity of absorbed energy.[56] The threshold at 6.5 W/kg was approximately double the resting metabolic rate. Ho and Edwards[57] reported a similar observation on the "specific metabolic rate" in the mouse. However, the "specific metabolic rate" was much higher than the resting metabolic rate of the given species. The decreased resting metabolic rate is considered to reflect physiologic adjustment.

Investigators have to be aware of the effects of body temperature on pituitary hormones so that precise biological effects can be allocated specifically to microwave exposure; threshold intensities can vary in relation to what is considered to be the normal range in sham-exposed or unexposed populations of animals. As an example, pituitary non-specific stereotyped reactions could occur in rats exposed to 50 mW/cm^2 of 2.45 GHz (specific absorption rate, SAR = 8.0 W/kg) for 1 hr. TSH adjustments of rats to an increased thermal load could occur at 10 mW/cm^2 (SAR = 1.6 W/kg).

Gandhi[58] reported that radiofrequency energy near the scaled half wave resonant frequency for man of 68 MHz can produce hot spots in the lower neck of human figurines with a specific absorption rate (SAR) of approximately 31 W/kg for a vertically polarized 10 mW/cm^2 incident power density. The model presented by Magin et al.[27,28] can serve to predict the biologic effects of microwaves when hot spots occur in the neck region.

de Lorge[59] plotted a relationship between body weight and power densities at which disruption of ongoing operant behavior occurred with rats, squirrel monkeys and rhesus monkeys as a basis for interspecies comparison. Although comparable comparisons for neuroendocrine parameters have not been made, Lotz[17] found that rats responded to 1.29 GHz microwave (2 μsec pulse, 0.001 duty cycle) by increased corticosterone levels at 15 mW/cm^2 for 30 minutes or longer. The same pulsed microwave exposure (1.29 GHz) was without effect on adrenocortical and GH secretion in the male adult rhesus monkey exposed at 20, 28 and 38 mW/cm^2 for 8 hours.[16,18] The increases in rectal temperature were 0.6, 1.0 and 1.5°C, respectively. These differences may suggest that neuroendocrine function of the rhesus monkey is more stable during thermogenic microwave exposure. This illustrates the difference in the response of a given species of animal to various frequencies and the resulting difference in energy deposition and distribution.

CONCLUSION

The acute effects of microwaves on hypothalamic-hypophysial function are: generally increased adrenocorticotropic secretion, decreased thyrotropic secretion and decreased GH secretion. These stereotyped changes can be observed simultaneously in rats acutely exposed to 2.45 GHz microwaves at 50, 60 or 70 mW/cm^2 for 1 hr.[25] The characteristics of these changes in hypothalamic hormones constitute the pattern of stress reactions of animals. Because of their physiologic significance, these biological end-points of microwave effects can serve as meaningful criteria for hazard evaluation if sufficient care has been incorporated into the design of chronic or repeated exposure experiments.

In the present state of the art, endocrine activity cannot be separated from the functional state of the neural network. Non-specific stress reactions to microwave exposure have to be isolated from extraneous factors that are usually associated with experimental procedures. Furthermore, evaluation of neuroendocrine responses involves not only perturbation, but also its recovery or manifestation of delayed response if such should occur.

The neuroendocrine data are consistent with the hypothesis that the adenohypophysial responses are the integral results of CNS processing of multiple signals from many body locations, such that no single localization of absorbed energy is pivotal to the onset of a response. Factors such as circadian rhythmicity, stimulus intensity, and interspecies differences, are important in determining the pattern of these responses. Thus, in addition to further studies to characterize the basic neuroendocrine response to microwave exposure, studies are needed to determine the physiological mechanism or mechanisms by which this regulatory system is affected during microwave exposure.

The effects of MW/RF exposure on endocrine function are generally consistent with both immediate and long-term responses to thermal input and to non-specific stress, which can also arise from thermal loading. The long-term response of animals to whole-body exposure at thermally significant levels is a decrease in the level of pituitary thyrotropic hormone in the blood plasma, followed by a decrease in the level of thyroxine.

Changes found in plasma levels of corticosterone and growth hormone are typical reactions of animals to non-specific stress. Such results emphasize the great care that is required in performing experiments to ensure that the changes in hormone level do not result from stress caused by handling of the animals or novelty of the experimental situation.

Although some studies indicate that microwave exposure can be manifested by endocrinopathy or hormonal changes, the nature of microwave interactions with endocrine organs is not known. Evidence suggests that microwave energy can act as a "stressor" in that it may affect the integrative and regulatory mechanisms of the body, which would result in altered homeokinesis. Studies indicate hypothalamic-hypophysial-adrenal and hypothalamic-hypophysial-thyroid effects can be induced at relatively high exposure levels for the particular animal species.

Some investigators believe such changes are caused by stimulation of the hypothalmic-hypophysial system due to thermal interactions at the hypothalamus, or the particular endocrine gland or end-organ under study. Other workers interpret the observed changes as effects of direct microwave interactions with the central nervous system.

The hypothalamus exerts a central influence on thermal regulatory processes, and when temperature is increased, this structure assumes control over and integration of food and water intake, metabolic rate, osmoregulation, growth, and reproduction. Because neuroendocrine function is an integration of numerous underlying chemical and biologic processes, caution is required in interpreting the significance of changes in the endocrine system induced by exposure to MW/RF energies.

Several components of the neuroendocrine system have been shown to be critically sensitive to environmental temperature.[49,60-62] Thus, reported "low power density" microwave-induced neuroendocrine perturbations could be a manifestation of sensitivity to small changes in peripheral temperature or selective stimulation of any component of the neuroendocrine system through alteration of thermal gradients in the body.

In regard to "stress" and adaptation, it should be emphasized that a new environment or new manipulation techniques can alter animals' behavioral patterns, namely, by inducing anxiety, avoidance behavior, and weight loss, and thus could be interpreted as being "stressful." Therefore, investigations of neuroendocrine response to microwave exposure must be carefully designed and controlled and should be conducted in animals properly adapted to environmental conditions.

ACKNOWLEDGEMENT

This paper is based on work performed under Contract no. DE-AC02-76-EV03490 with the U.S. Department of Energy at the University of Rochester, Department of Radiation Biology and Biophysics and has been assigned Report No. UR-3490-1966.

REFERENCES

1. H. Selye, "Stress", Acta, Inc., Montreal (1950).
2. H. Matsuyama, A. Ruhmann-Wemhold, and D. H. Nelson, Radio immunoassay of plasma ACTH in intact rats, Endocrinol. 88:692 (1971).
3. J. D. Neill, Effect of "Stress" on serum prolactin and luteinizing hormone levels during the estrus cycle of the rat, Endocrinol. 87:1192 (1970).
4. L. Grant, P. Hopkinson, G. Jennings, and F. A. Jennre, "Period of adjustment of rats used for experimental studies," Nature, (London) 232:135 (1971).
5. H. Mikolajczyk, Microwave-induced shifts of gonadotropic activity in anterior pituitary glands of rats, in: "Biologic Effects of Electromagnetic Waves," Vol. I, C.C. Johnson and M. L. Shore, eds., DHEW (FDA) 77-8010, Rockville (1977).
6. T. Nakayama, H. T. Hammel, J. D. Hardy, and J. S. Eisenman, Thermal stimulation of electrical activity of single units of the preoptic region, Am. J. Physiol. 204:1122 (1963).
7. M. A. Baker and L. W. Chapman, Rapid brain cooling in exercising dogs, Science, 195:781 (1977).
8. S. Baranski and P. Czerski, "Biological Effects of Microwaves," Dowden, Hutchinson and Ross, Stroudsberg (1967).
9. S. F. Cleary, Biological effects of microwaves and radiofrequency radiation, in: "CRC Critical Reviews in Environmental Control", C. Straub, ed., Chemical Rubber Company, New York (1977).
10. S. T. Lu, W. G. Lotz, and S. M. Michaelson, Advances in microwave-induced neuroendocrine effects": the concept of stress, Proc. IEEE 68:73 (1980).
11. S. M. Michaelson, W. M. Houk, N. J. Lebda, S. T. Lu, and R. Magin, Biochemical and neuroendocrine aspects of exposure to microwaves, Ann. NY Acad. Sci. 247:21 (1975).

12. S. M. Michaelson, Endocrine and biochemical effects, in: "Microwave and Radiofrequency Radiation", World Health Organization, Copenhagen, Regional Office for Europe, Section 7 (1977).
13. R. Guillet, W. G. Lotz, and S. M. Michaelson, Time-course of adrenal response in microwave-exposed rats, in: "Proceedings of the 1975 Annual Meeting of USNC/URSI", University of Colorado, Boulder, National Academy of Sciences, p. 316, Washington, D.C. (1975)
14. R. Guillet and S. M. Michaelson, The effect of repeated microwave exposure on neonatal rats, Radio Sci. 12 6(S):125 (1977).
15. W. M. Houk, S. M. Michaelson and D. E. Beischer, The effects of environmental temperature on thermoregulatory, serum lipid, carbohydrate, and growth hormone responses of rats exposed to microwaves, in: "Proceedings of the 1975 Annual Meeting of USNC/URSI", University of Colorado, Boulder, CO, National Academy of Sciences, p. 309, Washington, D.C. (1975)
16. W. G. Lotz, Neuroendocrine function in Rhesus monkeys exposed to pulsed microwave radiation, in: "Abstracts of Scientific Papers, 1978 Symposium on Electromagnetic Fields in Biological Systems," Ottawa, Canada (1978).
17. W. G. Lotz, Adrenocortical response in rats exposed to 1.29 GHz microwaves, presented at Bioelectromagnetics Symposium, Seattle, WA (1979).
18. W. G. Lotz, Thermal and endocrinological effects of microwave exposures on Rhesus monkeys, presented at Bioelectromagnetics Symposium, Seattle, WA (1979).
19. W. G. Lotz, S. M. Michaelson, and N. J. Lebda, Growth hormone levels of rats exposed to 2450-MHz (CW) microwaves, in: "Abstracts of Scientific Papers, 1977 International Symposium on the Biological Effects of Electromagnetic Waves," p. 39, Airlie, VA (1977).
20. W. G. Lotz and S. M. Michaelson, Temperature and corticosterone relationship in microwave exposed rats, J. Appl. Physiol. Respirat. Environ. Exercise Physiol. 44:438 (1978).
21. W. G. Lotz and S. M. Michaelson, Effects of hypophysectomy and dexamethasone on the rat's adrenal response to microwave irradiation, J. Appl. Physiol. Respirat. Environ. Exercise Physiol. 47:1284 (1979).
22. S. T. Lu, N. J. Lebda, and S. M. Michaelson, Effects of microwave radiation on the rat's pituitary-thyroid axis, in: "Abstracts of Scientific Papers, 1977 International Symposium on the Biological Effects of Electromagnetic Waves, p. 37, Airlie, VA (1977).
23. S. T. Lu, N. J. Lebda, S. M. Michaelson, S. Pettit, and D. Rivera, Thermal and endocrinological effects of protracted irradiation of rats by 2450 MHz microwaves, Radio Sci. 12 6(S):147 (1977).

24. S. T. Lu, N. J. Lebda, S. Pettit, and S. M. Michaelson, Modification of microwave biological end-points by increased resting metabolic heat load in rats, presented at Bioelectromagnetics Symposium, Seattle, WA (1979).
25. S. T. Lu, N. J. Lebda, S. Pettit, and S. M. Michaelson, Microwave-induced temperature, corticosterone and thyrotropin interrelationships. J. Appl. Physiol. Respirat. Environ. Exercise Physiol. 50:399 (1981).
26. S. T. Lu, S. Pettit, and S. M. Michaelson, Dual action of microwaves on serum corticosterone in rats, presented at Bioelectromagnetics Symposium, Seattle, WA (1979).
27. R. L. Magin, S. T. Lu, and S. M. Michaelson, Stimulation of dog thyroid by local application of high intensity microwaves, Am. J. Physiol. 233:E363 (1977).
28. R. L. Magin, S. T. Lu, and S. M. Michaelson, Microwave heating effect on the dog thyroid, IEEE Trans. Biomed. Eng. 24:522 (1977).
29. H. Mikolajczyk, Hormone reactions and changes in endocrine glands under influence of microwaves, Medycyna Lotnicza 39:39 (1972).
30. H. Mikolajczyk, Microwave irradiation and endocrine functions, in: "Biologic Effects and Health Hazards of Microwave Radiation," P. Czerski, et al., eds., Polish Medical Publishers, Warsaw (1974).
31. W. C. Milroy and S. M. Michaelson, Thyroid pathophysiology of microwave radiation, Aerospace Med. 43:1126 (1972).
32. L. N. Parker, Thyroid suppression and adrenomedullary activation by low-intensity microwave radiation, Amer. J. Physiol. 224:1388 (1973).
33. W. D. Travers and R. J. Vetter, Low intensity microwave effects on the synthesis of thyroid hormones and serum proteins, in: "Proc. of the 1976 Annual Meeting of USNC/URSI," p. 91, University of Massachusetts, Amherst (1976)
34. R. J. Vetter, Neuroendocrine response to microwave irradiation, Proc. Nat. Electron Conf. 30:237 (1975).
35. I. R. Petrov and V. A. Syngayevskaya, Endocrine glands, in: "Influence of Microwave Radiation on the Organism of Man and Animals," I. R. Petrov, ed., Meditsina Press, Leningrad, (1970).
36. K. Kirchev, Some experimental data on the effects of an UHF electric field on the adrenals, in: "Problems of Physiotherapy and Health Reports, Moscow (1959).
37. Yu. D. Dumansky, A.M. Serdyuk, C.I. Litvinova, L.A. Tomashevskaya, and V.M. Popovich, Experimental research on the biological effects of 12-centimeter low-intensity waves, in: "Health in Inhabited Localities," ed. II Kiev, (1972).
38. E. Schliephake, Endocrine influence on bleeding and coagulation time, Zbl. Chir. 85:1063 (1960).

39. F. L. Leytes and L. A. Skurikhina, The effect of microwaves on the hormonal activity of the adrenal cortex, Byull. Eksp. Biol. i Med. 52:47 (1961).
40. A. N. Bereznitskaya, The effect of 10-centimeter and ultrashort waves on the reproductive function of female mice, Gig. Tr. Prof. Zabol. No. 9:33 (1968).
41. M. S. Tolgskaya and Z. V. Gordon, Changes in the neurosecretory function of the hypothalamus and the neuro-pituitary body during chronic irradiation with centimeter waves of low intensity, in: "The Biological Effects of Radio-Frequency Fields," Works of the Laboratory of Radio-frequency Electromagnetic Fields, Institute of Work Hygiene and Occupational Diseases, AMN SSSR, No. 3, 87 (1964).
42. J. Lenko, A. Dolatowski, L. Gruszecki, S. Klajman, and L. Januszkiewicz, Effect of 10-cm radar waves on the level of 17-ketosteroids and 17-hydroxycorticosteroids in the urine of rabbits, Przeglad Lekarski 22:296 (1966).
43. S. M. Michaelson, R. A. E. Thomson, and J. W. Howland, "Biologic Effects of Microwave Exposure," Griffiss Air Force Base, Rome Air Development Ctr., Rome, New York (1967).
44. Yu. D Dumansky and M. G. Shandala, The biological action and hygienic significance of electromagnetic fields of superhigh and ultrahigh frequencies in densely populated areas, in: "Biologic Effects and Health Hazards of Microwave Radiation," P. Czerski, et al., eds., Polish Medical Publishers, Warsaw (1974)
45. A. A. Novitskii, B. F. Murashov, P. E. Krasnobaev, and N. F. Markozova, The functional condition of the system hypothalamus-hypophysis-adrenal cortex as a criterium in establishing the permissible levels of superhigh frequency electromagnetic emissions, Voen. Med. Zh. 8:53 (1977).
46. H. Selye, The general adaptation syndrome and the diseases of adaptation, J. Clin. Endocrinol. 6:117 (1946).
47. S. Baranski, Histological and histochemical effect of microwave irradiation on the central nervous system of rabbits and guinea pigs, Amer. J. Phys. Med. 51:182 (1972).
48. S. M. Michaelson, R. A. E. Thomson, and J. W. Howland, Physiologic aspects of microwave irradiation of mammals, Amer. J. Physiol. 201:351 (1961).
49. K. J. Collins and J. W. Weiner, Endocrinological aspects of exposure to high environmental temperatures, Physiol. Rev. 48:785 (1968).
50. M. I. Smirnova and M. N. Sadchikova, Determination of the functional activity of the thyroid gland by means of radioactive iodine in workers with UHF generators, in: "The Biological Action of Ultrahigh Frequencies," A. A. Letavet and Z. V. Gordon, eds., Moscow (1960).

51. N. A. D'Yachenko, Changes in thyroid function with chronic exposure to microwave radiation, Gig. Tr. Prof. Zabol. 14:51 (1970).
52. R. Denisiewicz, E. Dziuk, and M. Siekierzynski, Evaluation of thyroid function in persons occupationally exposed to microwave radiation, Pol. Arch. Med. Wewnetrznej 45:19 (1970).
53. J. B. Martin, Neural regulation of growth hormone secretion, N. Engl. J. Med. 288:1384 (1973).
54. G. M. Brown and S. Reichlin, Psychologic and neural regulation of growth hormone secretion, Psychosom. Med. 34:45 (1972).
55. A. V. Schally, A. Akimura, and A. J. Kastin, Hypothalamic regulatory hormones, Science 179:341 (1973).
56. R. D. Phillips, E. L. Hunt, R. D. Castro, and N. W. King, Thermoregulatory metabolic and cardiovascular response of rats to microwaves. J. Appl. Physiol. 38:630 (1975).
57. H. S. Ho and W. P. Edwards, Oxygen-consumption rate of mice under differing dose rates of microwave radiation, Radio Sci. 126(S):131 (1977).
58. O. P. Gandhi, Conditions of strongest electromagnetic power deposition in man and animals, IEEE Trans. MTT-23:1021 (1975).
59. J. deLorge, Disruption of behavior in mammals of three different sizes exposed to microwaves: extrapolation to larger mammals, in: "Symposium on Electromagnetic Fields in Biological Systems," S.S. Stuchly, ed., Int. Microwave, Power Institute, Alberta, Canada (1979).
60. K. Brown-Grant, C. Von Euler, G. W. Harris, and S. Reichlin, The measurement and experimental modification of thyroid activity in the rabbit, J. Physiol. 126:1 (1954).
61. E. W. Dempsy and E. B. Astwood, Determination of the rate of thyroid hormone secretion at various environmental temperatures, Endocrinol. 32:509 (1943).
62. H. D. Johnson, M. W. Ward, and H. H. Kibler, Heat and aging effects on thyroid function of male rats, J. Appl. Physiol. 21:689 (1966).

RADIOFREQUENCY AND MICROWAVE EFFECTS ON IMMUNOLOGICAL AND HEMATOPOIETIC SYSTEMS

Norbert J. Roberts, Jr.

Infectious Diseases Unit, Department of Medicine
University of Rochester School of Medicine
Rochester, New York 14642

INTRODUCTION

In technologically advanced countries, radiofrequency and microwave radiation (RF/MWR) is interwoven with daily life, affecting all to some degree, many to a greater degree. Studies by numerous investigators have raised the possibility that the immunological and hematological systems of humans and experimental animals are particularly susceptible to RF/MWR. Several recent and extensive reviews are available (1-4). The major goal of this paper is to indicate the complex nature of the hematological and particularly the immunological systems, the impact of thermoregulation and temperature changes on immune function, and the general nature of available (published) data on RF/MWR effects. The possible effects of microwaves on one cell type of particular interest, namely the lymphocyte, will be examined in greater depth, to illustrate both the known and the missing data, as well as confounding parameters. Thus, it is hoped that this review will not only indicate our current limited knowledge, but will provide some guidelines for design and evaluation of future reports.

HEMATOLOGICAL AND IMMUNOLOGICAL SYSTEMS

Fundamental aspects of these systems can only be covered in a general fashion in this paper. For more detailed review see references 5-12. Our pluripotent hematopoietic stem cells produce progeny that develop along three major lines. Red blood cells, or erythrocytes, are eventually produced by one lineage and support tissue respiration by virtue of the oxygen-carrying capacity of their hemoglobin, as the cells circulate alternately between the lungs and other tissues. Megakaryocytes evolve in the bone marrow and produce platelets, which have as a major function the preservation of our vascular channels, the sealing of leaks. The third major division is composed of cells that, when developed, will constitute our immunological defense system. These are the phagocytic and lymphoid white blood cells, or leukocytes. While the lifespan of the different blood cells vary considerably, the populations overall are constantly recirculating and regenerating. Thus, the system may be altered by affecting one or several aspects: hematopoiesis or production (stem cell function); mobilization, circulation and margination; and viability, longevity and destruction.

The immune system is our defense against a large spectrum of pathogens, including pyogenic bacteria, facultative intracellular bacteria, viruses, fungi, parasites, tumors, toxins from organisms, and miscellaneous chemical substances. Even in an era of antimicrobial and antineoplastic agents, the immune system is a primary determinant of survival. There is tremendous adaptability and redundancy in the immune system. Thus, we can and do survive many perturbations of the immune response. For example, a perturbation may not have clinical significance if the challenge or insult, against which that immune function is our defense, is not encountered. The immune system can learn or adapt, both in the individual host and in the species over generations. That our genetic composition affects the immune response is illustrated by the association of certain genetic (histocompatibility) backgrounds with certain specific types of infections or inflammatory diseases, or with certain potentially harmful sequelae of infection or response to infection.

The immune response is initiated by the introduction of a foreign molecule or determinant, called an antigen. Thus, the host must be able to distinguish self from non-self. The immune system can respond specifically and nonspecifically to challenge. It can recognize a specific offender whose character it has learned previously, or recognize nonspecifically (as non-self) an offender that the host has not encountered previously. The responsive cells can produce antigen-specific or nonspecific mediators that recruit other immunocompetant cells. In fact, recruitment of cells and so-called "arming" or activation of cells are major features of the immune response.

The true immune system consists of cells that are specialized for defense, broadly classified into phagocytic cells and lymphoid cells, and cell-derived humoral substances such as antibodies and complement. The latter factors can attach to challenging organisms and lyse them directly, or serve as handles

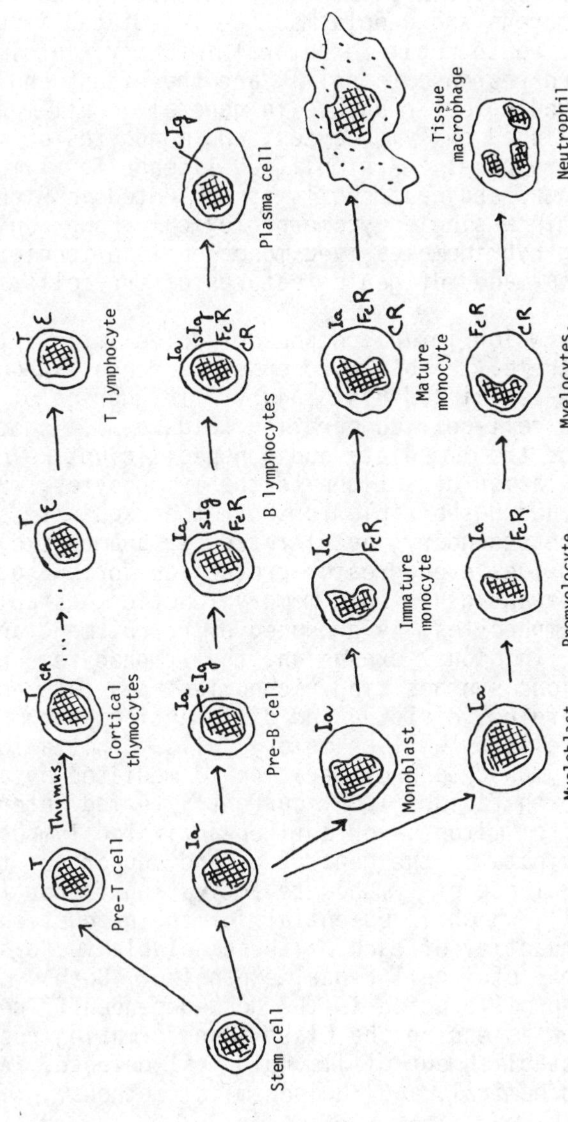

Figure 1. Lineage of T and B lymphocytes, monocytes-macrophages, and neutrophils.

to enhance the ability of phagocytic leukocytes to attach via receptors, and phagocytose (ingest) and kill the organisms. Humoral immunity and phagocytic cells (especially neutrophils) are of paramount importance in defense against the pyogenic microorganisms, which include most bacterial species. Cell-mediated immune mechanisms are the major defenses raised against intracellular pathogens and neoplasms. Cell-mediated immune mechanisms also serve to regulate humoral immunity, autoimmunity (recognition of and response to self), and the extent and magnitude of the immunological response in general. Cell-mediated immunity is established by lymphocytes, and monocytes or monocyte-derived tissue macrophages. A simplified lineage for lymphocytes, monocytes-macrophages and neutrophils is presented in Figure 1. Heterogeneity within a single cytomorphological group can be demonstrated using hybridoma-derived monoclonal antibodies directed against surface antigenic features of the cells.

The manner in which immune responses evolve after antigen stimulation is extremely complex, to ensure defense without unwarranted immune-associated host injury. Triggering of responses requires extensive cell-cell cooperation (Figure 2). Monocytes-macrophages provide the immediate and nonspecific uptake of antigen and presentation of antigen to the lymphocytes, which are antigen-specific, and responsible for both the exquisite specificity of response and the secondary, accelerated (or anamnestic) response, which provides even greater protection for subsequent encounters with the antigen. This memory function, established by both T and B lymphocytes, is produced by recruitment and clonal expansion. In clonal expansion, the lymphocytes undergo blast transformation: synthesizing ribonucleotides (RNA and DNA) and proteins, enlarging, dividing and differentiating to produce various effector cells as well as memory cells. Initiation and maintenance of T lymphocyte proliferation is mediated by a soluble T cell growth factor (TCGF, currently termed interleukin 2, IL2) released from mitogen- or antigen-activated lymphocytes. Macrophages participate in the generation and support of this response via the release of lymphocyte activating factor (LAF, or interleukin 1, IL1), which is essential for the production of IL2 by T cells. The quantity of each of these soluble factors dictates the extent of T cell clonal expansion. Both cytotoxic and helper T cell proliferation is IL2 dose-dependent. There are several methods for assessing the blast transformation response, integral to the establishment of immunological defense, including morphological, biochemical, and radiochemical methods.

Distinct lymphocyte subclasses carry out various functions. B cells produce antibody. Subsets of T cells express helper or suppressor functions, affecting the responses of other immunocompetent cells including B cells, as well as cytolytic func-

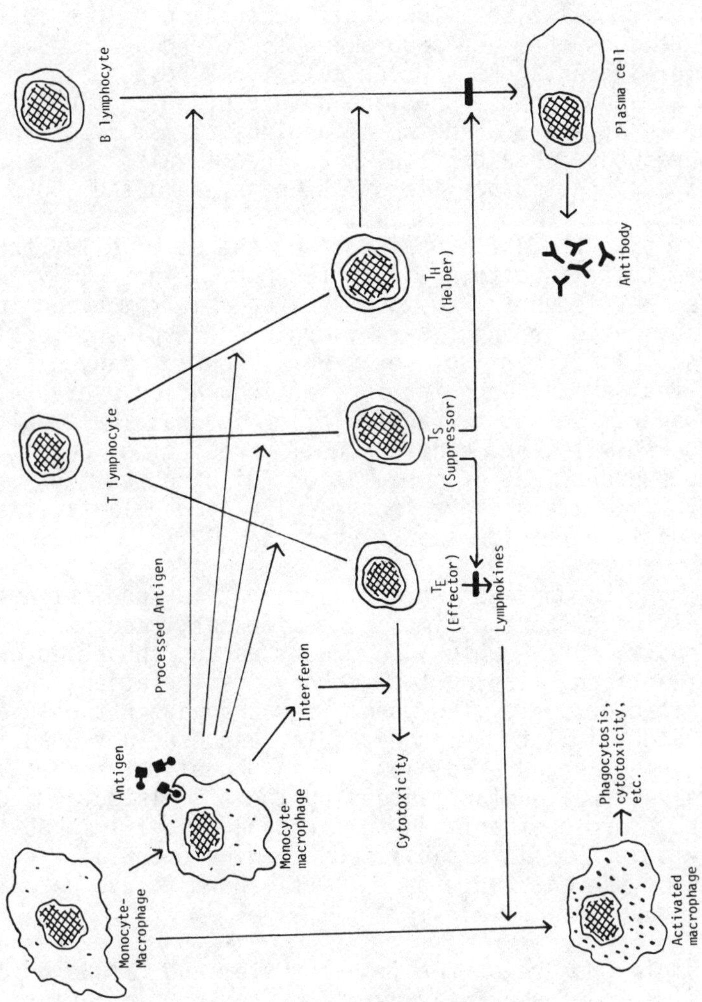

Figure 2. Cell-cell cooperation in immune responses.

tions. The balance of helper and suppressor activity is critical to immune homeostasis and health of the host. In fact, it is likely that we do not respond to self and develop autoimmune diseases because of the fine regulation of cell response. Autoimmune disease may thus result from an imbalance of suppressor and helper activity, allowing clonal expansion of those cells that are able to respond to self-antigens. While such regulation is critical, it must also allow rapid generation of the multiple effector functions that are programmed to defend against many different foreign antigens. Which cell types respond to a particular antigen depends upon the nature of the antigen, its dose and route of entry, and the immunological memory of the host. The response to a particular antigen is also influenced by the species and genetic profile of the host, as noted above.

Once lymphocytes differentiate from the stem cells, they partake in a traffic pattern within the host. Thus, T lymphocytes, once they leave the thymus, recirculate from blood into peripheral lymphoid organs (i.e., lymph nodes, spleen, tonsils) and back into blood, cycling over several hours. Many billions of lymphocytes may pass a point in the circulation every 24 hours. However, lymphocyte recirculation is drastically altered by antigenic stimulation, causing local arrest of circulation, followed by enchancement of circulation (with recruitment), followed by a proliferative response, with lymphoblastic transformation, differentiation and maturation.

The immune response is a continuum, but for understanding, it can be divided into two limbs: the afferent, recognition or induction phase, during which the monocytes-macrophages process and present antigen, leading to lymphocyte stimulation; and the efferent, effector phase. The monocyte-macrophage not only acts to recruit and stimulate lymphocytes in response to the antigen, it acts to ingest and degrade antigen in the effector phase when appropriately signalled (activated) by the stimulated lymphocytes. Thus, a cycle of antigen-to-macrophage-to-T-lymphocyte-to-macrophage-to-antigen is established, leading eventually to elimination of the antigen with as little harm to the host as possible (Figure 2).

The complex nature of the immune system and immunological homeostasis may confound interpretation (and particularly determination of mechanisms) of any potential RF/MWR effect.

TEMPERATURE AND IMMUNE FUNCTION

Many investigations of RF/MWR bioeffects properly call attention to the resultant thermal changes. In regard to potential effects on the hematological and immunological systems, it is particularly important to note that humans and animals have a sophisticated physiological system designed to raise body temperature upon encountering a challenge (13). Such a system may serve to amplify immunological responses. Many aspects of the afferent (recognition) and efferent (effector) mechanisms of the immune response are modified by relatively small temperature changes. In many animal species, febrile temperatures developing during lethal infections have been demonstrated to enhance survival (13,14). Preservation of the febrile response by natural selection (over time and across species) suggests that moderate temperature elevations (within the physiological range for the species) could be beneficial rather than detrimental in many instances. Many metabolic changes accompany the febrile response to challenge (15) and certain of these changes have been demonstrated to benefit host defense (14,16).

Studies of specific immune functions with _in vivo_ or _in vitro_ temperature elevation have provided evidence for temperature-dependent changes in immune response. Differences in cell function are often minimal or absent at rest, but accentuated by challenge (such as antigenic or mitogenic stimulation). For example, human leukocytes cultured at 38.5°C ambient temperature show enhanced recognition (lymphoblastoid transformation), recruitment (production of soluble mediators), and responder function (response to mediators) compared to leukocytes kept at 37°C (17,18).

The fact that minor temperature changes can significantly affect immune function confounds demonstration of potential temperature-independent RF/MWR effects.

THERMAL HOMEOSTASIS

The term nonthermal is generally used to describe those potential effects of RF/MWR that are ostensibly not related to measurable thermal stress or load. High level nonthermal effects (those occurring at power densities which do produce thermal stress) have not been clearly established or defined. Low level nonthermal effects have been the subject of many RF/MWR investigations, but their existence remains controversial.

A persistent problem to be addressed in RF/MWR studies is that of accurately measuring the amount of energy absorbed within the biological system. Great care must be taken in extrapolating results from one species to another, if this is to be done at all. For the exposed animal, there is no simple relationship between the applied RF/MWR energy and the given physiologic effect, such as a change in core (rectal) temperature (19). Such a temperature change is a complex function of the animal's physiological effector mechanisms, the power density, frequency and duration of exposure to RF/MWR, the familiarity of the animal with the procedure, the ambient conditions (such as temperature, humidity, and air flow), and other factors. Furthermore, different organs can sustain markedly different temperature changes when a thermal load is applied to different animal species (4). Hematological and immunological cells or organs may be situated within areas of localized heating ("hot spots").

The "set point" temperature for a species is maintained by physiological and behavioral processes that appropriately balance heat production or gain, and heat loss (20,21). A thermal load applied to the animal from an external source (such as exposure to RF/MWR) will precipitate maneuvers to increase heat loss, unless that stimulus has produced (as a primary or secondary effect) alteration of the set point. Thermal stress (or effects) may or may not be accompanied by detectable changes in core (rectal) temperature. If the thermal load can be dissipated by the host's physiological and behavioral responses, an increase in core body temperature may not be detectable. Alternatively, if the host cannot completely compensate for heat gain, a temperature rise would ensue. In either case, a thermal (stress) basis for possible effects might exist (activation of thermoregulatory adjusting maneuvers), although a "temperature change-dependent effect" may only be measurable in the latter situation. Although the rectal or colonic temperature reasonably reflects deep body (core) temperature in steady state conditions, it is slow to indicate changes in body temperature and does not indicate the magnitude of effective thermoregulatory responses (21).

In addition to the nature of the RF/MWR exposure and the species of animal, other experimental conditions (notably ambient temperature, humidity, and air circulation) would affect thermal-stress compensatory achievements during _in vivo_ exposure. If the ambient conditions already tax thermoregulation, even low RF/MWR absorption rates could lead to detectable temperature changes. Efficiency of heat dissipation for fur-bearing animals may be quite different from that for man under particular exposure and environmental conditions. Varying ambient conditions could lead to either accentuation or diminution of temperature changes. _In vitro_ systems with substantial environmental air or water flow can be similar to _in vivo_ situations in that a thermal load can be applied via RF/MWR, yet iatrogenic (instead of physiological) mechanisms dissipate the generated heat and prevent detection of a temperature change in the biological sample. (Such systems do not by their nature preclude a thermal basis for effects.) While _in vitro_ exposure of cells can limit or remove the contribution of many temperature-regulating physiological responses, the applicability of findings in such a setting to the _in vivo_ situation with RF/MWR exposure requires careful examination.

Both physiological (19,21) and behavioral (22) adjustments and adaptation by an animal can occur, including responses to levels of RF/MWR energy (thermal stress) that do not detectably change core (colonic) temperature. Subtle heating by RF/MWR at low power densities can be demonstrated by altering the thermoregulatory capacity, when no change in temperature would be detected in animals with intact thermal regulation (23). Endocrine and metabolic effects (which may in turn affect the immunological system) may ensue with or without detectable temperature changes (24,25). Such effects, as well as temperature changes with RF/MWR exposure, may in turn be modified by the circadian rhythm of the animal (26,27).

REPORTED RF/MWR EFFECTS ON THE HEMATOLOGICAL AND IMMUNOLOGICAL SYSTEMS

The literature pertaining to RF/MWR bioeffects is exceedingly difficult to interpret and apply, particularly in regard to exposure safety standards for humans. Many reports have not provided details of experimental design and research methodology (28), or have been anecdotal in nature. Alteration in one hematological parameter without concomitant change in dependent variables has been reported by several investigators. Where design and methods have been adequately described, they have varied so greatly that comparison remains elusive. Accurate measurement of the amount of energy absorbed by or dissipated within a particular biological system has been difficult, and exposure to RF/MWR causes inhomogeneous body heating (19), potentially affecting local immune function (which in turn can modify overall homeostasis). Many species of animals (and human cells *in vitro*) have been used, including dogs, rabbits, guinea pigs, rats, mice and others. Exposures to RF/MWR of 27 to 10,000 MHz, 0.5 to 800 mW/cm^2 or more, for durations from 5 minutes to several months, and under markedly variable environmental conditions have been reported. Comparison of studies using different species is difficult, not only due to differential absorption of RF/MWR, but also due to species-specific (and even strain-specific) physiological and immunological responses to any agent.

Only recently have studies regarding RF/MWR effects on cell markers been correlated with effects (or lack of effects) on functions or responses supported by cells identified by the markers. Complicating all of the literature is a rapidly evolving understanding of the nature of hematological and immunological homeostasis and response, leading to variation in interpretation of changes in cell markers by biomedical investigators. The often inadequate descriptions of methods and data can prevent reinterpretation of results in terms of our evolving knowledge of immunology. (We can know the significance of any change in leukocyte markers, for example, only if we know the significance or meaning of the markers themselves, or their relationship to leukocyte function or toxicity. Such understanding is rapidly evolving.)

Human System Investigations

Investigations of potential effects of RF/MWR on human immunocompetent cells have been limited in number and often inadequately described, excessively interpreted and inappropriately cited. For example, an initial and later (seven years) report of exposure of human mononuclear leukocytes to 2950 MHz RF/MWR in a 37°C chamber variably reported the absence or presence of a rise in culture temperature using the same protocols; several protocols were described in the methods but only limited data were presented resulting from approximately half of the study protocols; certain essential details of methodology were not included, and limited statistical analysis was provided (29,30). For example, changes in mitotic index were reported after 64 hours of culture, but were less after shorter (59 hours) or longer (70 hours) periods. Changes where cited were just beyond the lowest confidence levels, and did not consider the potential impact on probability that results from performing a large number of statistical analyses. (The chance that 1 in 20 comparisons could reach a probability value of 0.05 may make that value a less sound basis for conclusions.) The mitotic index and percent lymphoblastoid forms in the irradiated cultures were different "compared with controls", but values from control cultures were not reported, nor were the satistical methods or number of observations. Nonetheless, these studies were presented and are cited as evidence that RF/MWR exposure produces increased lymphoblastoid transformation of human leukocytes. Another investigator examined exposure of human leukocytes to 2950 MHz RF/MWR for "various periods, at several power densities" (31). Although he noted that results were poorly reproducible, non-quantitative (with regard to exposure *versus* effect) and only preliminary, he nonetheless stated that "in a few experiments, blastic transformation and inhibition of mouse macrophage migration by the incubation medium [MIF production, an immune mediator] occurred". The statement is often cited, without reference to the inadequate basis for acceptance according to scientific criteria.

Other investigators have exposed human mononuclear leukocytes to 27 MHz RF/MWR for 1 to 84 hours in a 37°C chamber (1°C difference between control and exposed cultures) in the presence of the mitogen PHA (32). They reported no substantial differences in DNA synthetic index, growth, or mitotic index (data not shown), but an increase in chromosome breaks in RF/MWR-exposed cells after 72 hours of continuous exposure.

Human mononuclear leukocytes were exposed to 10,000 MHz RF/MWR at varying power densities and for varying periods (Czerski P., cited in 19). Prolonged exposure to low levels ($<3mW/cm^2$) of RF/MWR eventually caused heating and thermal death of the cells, since culture vessels were not cooled. However no blastoid transformation was induced at levels below 5 mW/cm^2. In contrast, exposure at power densities between 5 and 15 mW/cm^2 (continued until the culture medium reached 38°C) was reported to induce lymphoblastoid transformation. The initial culture temperatures, durations of RF/MWR exposure, rates of temperature increase, and degrees of lymphocyte change were not reported.

Investigations of effects of RF/MWR on other human hematological cells have largely been confined to erythrocyte studies. Fresh erythrocytes have been exposed to 1000 MHz RF/MWR ($45mW/cm^2$, 30 min), and reported to show decreased active cation (potassium, sodium) transport and increased passive cation diffusion (33). Fresh erythrocytes have also been warmed from room temperature to 37°C by exposure to 2450 MHz RF/MWR ($90mW/cm^2$ initially, $30mW/cm^2$ maintenance); such cells showed no difference in loss of hemoglobin or potassium from erythrocytes kept at room temperature, or erythrocytes warmed conventionally in a hot air incubator (34).

Animal System Investigations

While studies of RF/MWR effects on human cells are limited, studies using exposure of animals or animal cells *in vitro* are extensive. However, the animal studies are so variable (species, exposure conditions, assays, etc.) that general conclusions are elusive, confounding eventual application to human exposure guidelines. (One exception is the conclusion that intense exposure and heating of the animal or animal tissue, to nonphysiologic temperatures, can damage the hematological and immunological systems, if the heating is not in fact lethal to the animal or tissues!) The breadth of different animal model investigations cannot be adequately described within the limits of this paper; an excellent recent review is available (1). Many animal studies have used small rodents, such as mice. A review of the complex data on potential RF/MWR effects in one such species will indicate many of the factors to be considered with regard to the hematological and immunological systems.

There are characteristics of the mouse that make it a difficult animal model for study of RF/MWR bioeffects relevant to humans. The mouse is a small rodent, with a very different resonance frequency (and hence RF/MWR absorption) from that of humans. The mouse has a very different mass-to-surface area relationship, fur, and a substantially less efficient thermoregulatory system compared to humans (19,21,35). The mouse has been shown to remain afebrile or become hypothermic in response to infectious or inflammatory challenges that evoke febrile responses in humans (36-38), even though the mouse has a similar system for endogenous pyrogen production and response (35). However, the mouse also has several important advantages for study of potential RF/MWR effects on hematological and immunological systems. As a small rodent, many animals can be used within most experimental protocols, allowing properly controlled studies. Furthermore, the immunological system has been most extensively described for the mouse, and inbred strains are available and have been characterized in terms of immunological responsiveness. Some of the most important and best performed and described investigations of RF/MWR effects on the hematological and immunological systems have used mice.

Even within a single species, such as the mouse, conditions of RF/MWR exposure have been exceedingly varied: 148 to 10,000 MHz RF/MWR, 0.5 to 450 mW/cm^2, 5 minutes to more than a year exposure period, and varying ambient exposure conditions (31,39-50). The latter have usually been least well detailed, along with temperature changes in the exposed animals or tissues. Statistical analyses have been limited, and often not presented at all. A number of these reports are summarized in Table I. They do not allow firm conclusions regarding RF/MWR effects in the absence of thermal insult. There have been suggestions that: (a) pulse-modulated (PM) RF/MWR exposure may produce changes not seen at equivalent constant wave (CW) power densities; (b) the animals can adapt to RF/MWR exposure; and (c) the greater the power density of exposure (and observed thermal stress), the greater the observed effect beyond a minimum level of exposure. It is difficult to be confident regarding reported differences in some of the most extensive studies. For example, one investigator reported studies using 100 control (not sham-exposed) mice, 100 mice exposed to RF/MWR for 6 weeks, and 100 mice exposed to RF/MWR for 12 weeks at low power densities (31;see Table). Statistical analyses were not presented for observed effects. Figures plotting absolute values for parameters such as antibody-producing cells did not indicate standard deviations or standard errors. Such results were described thus: "From these Figures, it _may seem that significant differences from controls_ were obtained in mice irradiated for 6 weeks. Exposure for 12 weeks did not, however, induce changes in the immune response. This finding may indicate that after a period of response, the animals became adapted to the microwaves "[emphasis added].

Table 3

Effects of RF/MWR Exposure on Hematopoietic and Immunocompetent Cells of Mice[a]

EXPOSURE[b] & Reference	OBSERVATIONS
148 MHz, 0.5 mW.cm^2; 1h/day, 5 days/wk, 10 wks. Neonates exposed starting at 4-7 days postpartum. (Ref 39)	Good growth, body weights in sham and exposed. Hemoglobin, hematocrit, erythrocyte count, leukocyte count differential not affected by exposure to RF/MWR. (Lymphocytes and neutrophils plotted; all others stated to show "virtual equivalence".)
800 MHz, 43 mW/cm^2; 2h/day, 5 days/wk, 35 wks. (ref 40)	No change in erythrocytes or leukocytes despite thermal burden.
In vitro exposure, 2450 MHz(CW) 30-1000 mW/cm^2 (SAR 60-2000 mW/g); 15 min., 37°C chamber. (Subset at 1000 mW/cm^2 in 7,22 and 37°C chambers) (Ref 41)	No obvious RF/MWR-induced ultrastructural damage by electron microscopy at 1000 mW/cm^2 (SAR=2000mW/g.) Viability (dye exclusion) unchanged at 500 mW/cm^2 (SAR=1000 mW/g) Decreased bone marrow colony forming units after RF/MWR exposure at 1000, 500, 250, 125 and 62 mW/cm^2, not at 31 mW/cm^2 when assayed 6 days after exposure; not at 62 and 31 mW/cm^2 when assayed 12 days after exposure. No late recovery after exposure at 1000 mW/cm^2 (SAR=2000 mW/g).
2450 MHz, 100 mW/cm^2; 5min. (Ref 42)	Increase (not significant), followed by decrease, followed by gradual increase in ^{59}Fe uptake (eventually greater than normal in spleen); all changes more marked in spleen than bone marrow. Splenic colony forming units initially unchanged, decreased at 24 hours, then increased.

[a]See text for detailed review of certain of these studies as well as additional reports.
[b]*In vivo* exposure to RF/MWR unless otherwise indicated. CW=constant wave; PM=pulse-modulated.

(Continued)

Table 3 (Continued)

2450 MHz, 100 mW/cm^2; 5 min. (2.3°C increase in rectal temperature; approximately same final temperature as animals heated in 43°C chamber). (Ref 43)	^{59}Fe uptake by spleen increased (to greater extent than with conventional heating); no change in bone marrow. Increased number of stem cells (colony forming units) in spleens and bone marrow. No change in peripheral blood erythrocyte count. Decrease, then increase in nucleated cells in spleen (similar with conventional heating); bone marrow not significantly changed. Increased peripheral blood leukocyte counts in two phases within 7 days after RF/MWR exposure. (Increased in single phase by conventional heating).
In vitro exposure, 2450 MHz; 50 mW/cm^2; 30 min., perfusion chamber (controls, 37°C; perfused, 31.8°C; perfused, RF/MWR-exposed, 34.3°C). (Ref 44)	Macrophage monolayer (non-induced peritoneal exudate cells). Phagocytosis of perfused human erythrocytes assayed. (RF/MWR exposure did not affect erythrocyte susceptibility to phagocytosis.) No changes in cells due to RF/MWR exposure, by light microscopy. Decreased phagocytic index (number of macrophages containing erythrocytes/total number of macrophages) with RF/MWR exposure during perfusion. No change if exposed to RF/MWR for 30 minutes, then perfused with erythrocytes for 30 minutes.
3000 MHz, 20 mW/cm^2; up to 15 min. (Ref 45)	No significant change in total or differential leukocyte counts or hemoglobin concentration immediately, 3, 7 and 20 days after exposure. Femoral bone marrow showed no changes except for an inconstant slight increase in eosinophils. (Not associated with peripheral blood eosinophilia.)

3105 MHz, 2 mW/cm^2 (PM); 145-160 hours. (Ref 46)	Increased ^{35}S-methionine incorporation (protein synthesis) by splenic, liver, and thymus cells. Increased lymphoblastic cells in spleen. Increased reticular and histiocystic cells in liver. Abundant lymphoblasts and reticular cells in thymus.
2950 MHz, 0.5 mW/cm^2 (PM); 2 h/day, 6 days/wk, 6 or 12 weeks. (Ref 31,47)	After last exposure, immunized with sheep erythrocytes; measured antibody-producing cells in lymph nodes. Increased antibody-producing cells after 6 weeks, not after 12 weeks exposure by direct PFC technique; fluctuation of control, 6-week-exposed, 12-week-exposed antibody-producing cells by indirect PFC technique. Increased lymphoblastoid transformation in lymph nodes, greater after 12 than after 6 weeks exposure.
2950 MHz, 1mW/cm^2 (PM; different hours of day. ("No change in colonic temperature".) (Ref 48)	Changes in normal circadian rhythm of bone marrow cell mitoses, dependent upon time of day when exposed and cell series.
9270 MHz, 100 mW/cm^2; 4.5 min/day, 5 days/wk, 59 wks. Exposure equivalent to one-half the LD_{50}. (3.3°C average increase in colonic temperature; range 2.0-5.0°C) (Ref 49)	"Neoplasia" of leukocyte lineage in exposed mice. (Monocytic-myeloid or lymphocytic). Intercurrent infection in colony.
10,000 MHz; 17.40 or 60 mW/cm^2; up to 15 minutes. (Ref 45)	Results as noted above for exposure at 3000 MHz.
10,000 MHz, 450 mW/cm^2 (PM); 5 min. (Ref 50)	Decrease in erythrocytes and leukocytes immediately and at one and five days after exposure. Recovery by 10 days. (Conventional heating produced less change, more rapid recovery.)

Another report, by Prausnitz and Süsskind (49; see Table for exposure details), on the effects of chronic exposure to RF/MWR stated that "neoplasms of the white blood cells" were more prevalent in the irradiated group than in control mice, but "longevity of the mice did not appear to be affected under the prevailing conditions". The data were presented in several sections, without statistical analyses. "Leucosis", defined as a non-circulating neoplasm of the white cells, or leukemia (a circulating "leucosis") was found in 35% of 60 irradiated mice and 10% of 40 control mice who died and had adequate postmortem examinations during the course of the longevity experiment. Other mice died without adequate postmortum data, or were sacrificed in three series during the study. By the third and last sacrifice series, 19 months after the first exposure and 4 months after the last exposure to RF/MWR, the findings of "leucosis" were equivalent in the two groups: 12 of 67 (18%) irradiated and 4 of 19 (21%) control mice.

Two major factors prevent citation of this report as an established indication of the link between RF/MWR and neoplasms. (In fact, further analysis of the primary data can lead to substantially different conclusions; see below.) First, no histological or biological criteria were provided to characterize or define a "leucosis", which was apparently the predominant neoplasm rather than leukemia. No pathological material was illustrated. Second, an antibiotic had to be administered to the mice "to fight secondary infection accompanying a small epidemic of pneumonitis". (Perhaps 66 deaths in 85 control mice, not sacrificed in the first two sacrifice series, indicates more than a "small epidemic".) Such pneumonitis could be expected to be of viral etiology, especially if leading to secondary bacterial infections. Such intercurrent infections in the study mice confound attempts to associate RF/MWR with differences in experimental observations. Even if there were an association between neoplasms and RF/MWR-plus-virus (a "two-hit" phenomenon, in contrast to control-plus-virus), the first factor cited above compromises acceptance of the authors' conclusions.

Further analysis of the primary data from the study by Prausnitz and Süsskind suggests alternate conclusions regarding the effects of exposure to RF/MWR. In fact, exposure to RF/MWR, resulting in intermittent increases in body temperature (see Table), may have enhanced host defense and survival of the mice under the experimental conditions. Equivalent percentages of the total number of mice in each experimental group were sacrificed in the first two sacrifice series. Nineteen of 100 (19%) control and 67 of 200 (34%) irradiated mice were alive when the study ended and all remaining mice were sacrificed. Thus, the RF/MWR-exposed group of mice showed enhanced survival ($p<0.01$ by χ^2

analysis) in the setting of intercurrent infection. Although the authors stated that "leucosis" was present in 30% (6 of 20) irradiated and only 10% (1 of 10) control mice sacrificed in the second sacrifice series, this increased incidence ($p>0.05$ by χ^2 analysis) was not associated with greater overall mortality. The presence of "leucosis" at any time during the longevity study could only be analyzed for 147 of the irradiated and 69 of the control mice: it was present in 39 (27%) and 9 (13%), respectively ($p<0.05$ by χ^2 analysis). The number of mice with "leucosis" (if any) was not stated for the mice in the first sacrifice series, but there was reportedly no correlation between the condition and irradiation in the 5 control and 10 RF/MWR-exposed mice. Unfortunately, "68 dead mice had undergone extensive postmortem changes that prohibited a meaningful histological assessment".

It is possible that the "leucosis" reported in these mice represented inflammatory localization of immunocompetent cells in response to the intercurrent infections, and this host defense mechanism was enhanced by the intermittent RF/MWR exposure-induced elevations of body temperature. The RF/MWR-exposed mice had average increases of 3.3°C in body temperature. Other studies have demonstrated enhanced resistance of mice to many different viral infections when elevated body temperatures are produced (13); one investigation specifically demonstrated reduced mortality of virus-infected mice who had been treated with RF/MWR-induced hyperthermia (51). Fever was shown to reduce morality from bacterial infection in another animal (lizard) model (52). Furthermore, the enhanced survival of the febrile lizards was correlated with inflammatory infiltration at the site of bacterial inoculation, resulting in prevention of spread of the microorganisms (53). The elevation in body temperature did not have to be continuous to have significant beneficial effect (54). In sum, a case could be made for the concept that the study by Prausnitz and Süsskind (49) demonstrated RF/MWR-induced beneficial rather than detrimental effects: protection from infection or, if histological and biological criteria were given and appropriate, neoplasms.

Recent studies of potential RF/MWR effects on mouse hematological and immunological systems have been more carefully described (especially methods and conditions), better controlled, with more extensive presentation of primary data. Such reports allow other investigators to reach their own conclusions, in agreement or disagreement with the interpretations of the original investigators. Ultimately, by the more complete presentation of methods and data, such studies advance the understanding of RF/MWR interactions with hematological and immunological systems.

Smialowicz and colleagues examined the effects of RF/MWR on spontaneous and stimulated blast transformation of mouse spleen cells (55). Splenic cells were exposed *in vitro* to 2450 MHz RF/MWR, for 1, 2 or 4 hours at 37°C, at an absorbed dose rate of approximately 19 mW/g. Culture temperatures and cell viability (determined by trypan blue dye exclusion) were assayed immediately after irradiation and showed no significant differences between exposed and control cultures. There were no significant differences in spontaneous (unstimulated) blast transformation between exposed and control cultures, nor in ability of the cultures to respond after stimulation with different mitogens at varying concentrations. There were no differences between the optimal responses (peak of the dose-response curve) of exposed and control cultures after stimulation with T lymphocyte mitogens or B lymphocyte mitogens.

Microwave exposure has been reported to affect expression of a marker associated with a stage in maturation of cells of the B lymphocyte lineage. Wiktor-Jedrezejczak and colleagues (56-58) have reported extensively on data generated from two sets of experiments, with a limited number of animals in each exposed and control group. However, the reports described results from assays of several immunological functions, the experiments were well described, and the data illustrate the potentially complex interaction of microwaves with the immunological system.

Wiktor-Jedrzejczak, et al (56) studied effects of RF/MWR on the quantitative relationships between different splenic lymphoid cell populations of inbred (CBA/J) mice. Mice were exposed for 30 minutes once or three times, in an environmentally controlled waveguide facility, to 2450 MHz RF/MWR (SAR= 12-15 mW/g) and compared to sham-exposed (control) animals. A constant and substantial airflow inside the chamber maintained an ambient 25°C temperature. Rectal temperature differences (after exposure relative to before exposure) ranged from -0.1°C to -0.5°C. The spleens were examined for cell populations 3, 6 and 9 days after the (last) exposure. Cells bearing surface immunoglobulin (Ig+), surface theta antigen (θ+), and surface complement receptors (CR+) were quantitated. Cells of the B lymphocyte lineage would be identified as Ig+, with more mature cells being CR+ as well (see Figure 1). T lymphocytes would be θ+. At all of the times after a single exposure to RF/MWR, there were no differences between control and exposed animals in total cell numbers, percent Ig+, or θ+ cells in the spleen. In contrast, a significant increase in percent of CR+ cells on day 6 (but not on day 3 or 9) after exposure was observed in spleens of the exposed mice. After three exposures (separated by 3 day intervals), there were again no significant changes in total cell numbers or percent θ+ cells. Percentages of Ig+ cells were increased (significantly 6 days after the last exposure), and significantly increased percentages of CR+ cells were noted on all days tested. These data were also reported elsewhere (57,58). Since the increase in CR+ cells was not accompanied by an increase in the total absolute cell number, it was unlikely that nonspecific cell proliferation was responsible for the effect (also see below). Other cell subpopulations were unchanged in percent contribution to total cell number. Among the other mechanisms considered (but not established or excluded by the reported data) were (1) stimulation of conversion of CR- precursor cells into CR+ cells; (2) inhibition of further maturation of CR+ cells into CR- plasma cells (with accumulation of CR+ cells); and (3) local effects of microwaves on the B lymphocyte membrane, altering expression of the CR without inducing maturation of the cell. Such potential mechanisms could be direct or indirect (via microwave effects on other systems or cells).

In another report (59) based upon the same experiments, Wiktor-Jedrzejczak, et al assayed spleen, bone marrow and peripheral blood leukocytes for DNA, RNA and protein synthesis, in order to determine whether the increased frequency of CR+ splenocytes after microwave exposure was associated with increased cell proliferation. (Such proliferation could occur in the spleen, or elsewhere with subsequent migration to the spleen). Cells were obtained by the same protocols noted above, and uptake of tritiated precursor substrates (without specific antigenic or mitogenic stimulation) was determined 4 hours, 3, 5 and 7 days after placing cells in culture. There were no significant differences (between exposed and control samples) in uptake of the precursors by spleen, bone marrow or peripheral blood leukocytes after single or multiple microwave exposure, at any of the time periods after cells were placed in culture.

Transformation responses of the RF/MWR-exposed splenic cells were normal after stimulation with B cell or T cell mitogens (57). Since protein synthesis was not increased after exposure to RF/MWR, it appeared that an increase in CR+ B lymphocytes was due to increased expression of (pre-formed) CR on the cell surface rather than new synthesis. A population of B lymphocytes with cytoplasmic CR exists, and induction of surface expression by these cells is one possible mechanism for the RF/MWR-induced increase in CR+ cells.

In a preliminary report (60), these investigators noted that a soluble factor produced by microwave-exposed spleen cells could mediate the increase in CR+ cells. Cells from RF/MWR-exposed (inbred) mice were placed within a diffusion chamber (allowing passage of cell-produced soluble mediators, but not passage of cells), and the chambers were placed in the peritoneal cavity of non-exposed mice. Several days later, the non-exposed recipient's spleen cells showed an increased percentage of CR+ cells. When non-exposed cells were placed in a diffusion chamber within the peritoneal cavity of RF/MWR-exposed recipients, again cells within and outside the chamber showed an increased percentage of CR+ cells. These studies provided both partial evidence against mediation of increased CR+ cells by an effect of RF/MWR on lymphocyte circulation, and evidence for mediation by a soluble factor.

To examine effects of microwaves on antigen-dependent maturation of B lymphocytes into immunoglobulin-secreting plasma cells, the mice were immunized with a T-dependent antigen, a T-independent antigen, and saline (control), and exposed to the RF/MWR for 30 minutes on days 1, 2 and 3 after immunization (57). Spleen cells were obtained on the 4th day and assayed (by plaque formation) for antibody formation. Results were variable, and differences between exposed and control cells were not statistically significant, or were of questionable significance. The data suggested that microwaves might cause polyclonal stimulation (without adding specific antigen) of B lymphocytes; there was a small increase in cells secreting antibodies to both antigens in spleens of saline-immunized RF/MWR-exposed mice. However, the RF/MWR exposure may have produced a diminished response to both the T-dependent and the T-independent antigens in the mice specifically immunized with the antigens.

Smialowicz, et al, (61) noting the results of Wiktor-Jedrzejczak et al, undertook more extensive investigations of the effects on lymphocyte function that might result from exposure of mice to 2450 MHz RF/MWR. Cell numbers and functions were extensively characterized for RF/MWR-exposed and sham-exposed animals (BALB/c mice). Mice were exposed daily (15 or 30 minutes) for up to 22 consecutive days to power densities ranging from 5 to 35 mW/cm^2 (SAR=4 to 25 mW/g), in 22°C exposure chambers (50% humidity and 25 m^3 air flow per minute), with all exposures performed in the morning. Colonic temperatures, taken prior to and immediately following exposure, showed no statistically or physiologically significant increase in exposed relative to sham-exposed animals on a given day or at a given power density. There were no differences between exposed and control animals in peripheral blood cell parameters (erythrocyte count, hemoglobin, hematocrit, leukocyte count and differential, or absolute count of lymphocytes and polymorphonuclear leukocytes), or in frequencies of T (θ antigen-positive) or B (complement receptor-positive) lymphocytes in the spleen. There were no differences in B and T lymphocyte transformation responses to several mitogens, nor were there differences in DNA synthesis, between cells from exposed and control animals, in the absence of mitogen stimulation. The antibody response (plaque-forming cell assay after immunization with sheep erythrocytes) did not differ between cells from exposed and control animals, nor did exposure to RF/MWR cause a difference in spontaneous antibody production. Such results (antibody production) were observed with immunization either preceding or following exposure to RF/MWR. Thus, these investigators did not find changes in hematological parameters such as described by Wiktor-Jedrzejczak, et al. The parameters of exposure were chosen to approximate those of the latter investigators. The differences in results were initially suspected to be due to differences in exposure systems: a waveguide system in the studies by Wiktor-Jedrzejczak, et al., and exposure under far field conditions in an anechoic chamber by Smialowicz, et al. Subsequent observations showed that the RF/MWR-induced effect (increased CR+ spleen cells) observed by Wiktor-Jedrzejczak, et al. was mouse strain specific: the effect could be induced (by those investigators) in CBA/J mice but not in BALB/c mice (1). (Circadian rhythm may also have affected results, since 9 mice per day, one at a time, were exposed for 30 minutes each in the studies by Wiktor-Jedrzejczak, et al).

Smialowicz, et al, remarked on the absence of colonic temperature changes in RF/MWR-exposed mice relative to sham-exposed animals. Mice exposed to 30 mW/cm^2 (SAR approximately 22 mW/g) would have accepted RF/MWR energy equivalent to more than three times their basal metabolic rate (approximately 6.4 mW/g). It is likely that the combination of temperature (22°C), humidity (50%) and air velocity (25 m^3/min) in the exposure chamber maintained the mice at their physiological temperature. Further evidence of a thermal burden, with temperature rise abroggated by the applied environment, was provided by results when mice were exposed, as above, without any change of air; such mice had significantly higher colonic temperatures following exposure.

The relationship between RF/MWR exposure and steroid release, associated with thermal stress, has been investigated by Liburdy (62,63), to further characterize the nature of potential RF/MWR effects on cell-mediated immunity. Liburdy exposed mice (C57Bl/6, CD/1, and B6D2F1) to 26 MHz RF/MWR (CW) at a power density of 8.62 W/cm^2 (12.9 mW/g) for 4 to 7 minutes, or to warm air (79°C oven) for 8 to 12 minutes, to induce equivalent increases (2 to 4°C) in rectal temperature (64). Sham-exposed mice were also used. Peripheral blood total white blood cell counts were unchanged after exposure to RF/MWR. In contrast, warm air-exposed and sham-exposed mice showed peripheral leukocytosis. The constant total leukocyte count in the RF/MWR-exposed mice was accompanied, however, by marked shifts in the proportion of leukocyte types, with maximum changes evident three hours after exposure. Circulating lymphocytes decreased and circulating neutrophils increased, with pre-exposure levels gradually reestablished over 55-96 hours. Warm air-exposed and sham-exposed mice showed an increase in both lymphocytes and neutrophils (approximately twofold for each), contributing to the overall leukocytosis observed in those groups. Liburdy noted that induction of a transient neutrophilia and lymphopenia by RF/MWR exposure was similar (in kinetics also) to the changes induced by endogenous release or exogenous administered adrenocorticotrophic hormones. Release of adrenocorticotrophic hormones can be triggered by physical, chemical or physiological stress. The difference between RF/MWR heating and warm air heating might be due to the fact that rapid RF/MWR heating may be a stress factor for a greater proportion of the exposure time than the more slowly acting (by convective transfer) warm air treatment.

In subsequent studies (62), Liburdy used two strains of mice (C57Bl/6 and BALB/c) to investigate the role of steroids; no differences between the two strains were observed in the studies. Mice were exposed to 26 MHz RF/MWR (800 mW/cm^2, 5.6 mW/g, 2-3°C increase in core temperature) once for 15 minutes, or 20 times (morning and afternoon) over a period of 10 days. Exposure of mice to two alternate hot environments were made using a vented dry-air oven (63°C) or a heated water bath (41°C), with all exposures matched to induce a net increase in core body temperature of 2-3°C over a similar period of time. Such detectably thermogenic (single) RF/MWR exposures induced a peripheral blood lymphopenia and neutrophilia that persisted for 12 hours. Exposure to RF/MWR that was not detectably thermogenic (26 MHz, 50 mW/cm^2; or 5 MHz, 800 mW/cm^2; each with a reduction in absorbed power to 0.36 mW/g) did not induce lymphopenia. Similarly, exposure to warm air did not lead to lymphopenia, although it closely approximated RF/MWR heating. Maximum lymphopenia was sustained by mice exposed three times (at 3-hour intervals) to the thermogenic RF/MWR, and return to normal levels in these mice was prolonged.

Steroid administration (4 mg/kg methyl prednisolone) led to lymphopenia and neutrophilia that was qualitatively similar to that induced by obviously thermogenic RF/MWR exposure. Thermogenic RF/ MWR exposure was associated with a stress-induced increase in measured plasma corticoid levels, after single or multiple exposures. Levels were three-fold greater than those found in sham-exposed or warm air-treated animals. Furthermore, thymic weight and cell density and splenic cell density in chronically (20 times) but not in singly RF/MWR-exposed animals were reduced relative to warm air-exposed or sham-exposed animals. Similar changes were induced by administration of exogenous steroids to the mice.

Splenic lymphocytes expressing Thy 1 surface antigen (T cells) and lymphocytes having complement-binding receptors (B cells) were enumerated at the time of maximum peripheral blood lymphopenia, three hours after the single or the last of multiple (20) exposures to the thermogenic RF/MWR. Single and, to a greater extent, multiple RF/MWR exposures resulted in marked increases in the percentage of both T and B lymphocytes in the spleen. Percentages of both cell types were also increased after administration of exogenous steroids. Multiple (but not single) exposures to warm air led to a relative increase in B lymphocytes only. Since the mice exposed (multiple times) to RF/MWR showed peripheral lymphopenia, a relative enrichment of T and B lymphocytes in the spleen, and no significant change in the absolute size of either subpopulation, it appeared that Thy 1-negative and complement receptor-negative cells were displaced from the spleen. This suggested that interpretation of experiments using splenic cells from RF/MWR-exposed mice should consider effects of induced changes in spleen cell populations.

Liburdy went on to characterize the effects of RF/MWR exposure on *in vivo* lymphocyte circulation, and the relationship of changes in circulation to steroid release associated with thermal stress and the process of thermoregulation (63). Mice (C57Bl/6 and BALB/c strains; no differences noted between strains) were exposed to 2600 MHz RF/MWR (CW) at 25 or 5 mW/cm^2 (19 or 3.8 mW/g) for one hour. Immediately before exposure, mice were injected with ^{51}Cr-labelled splenic lymphocytes. One, 6 and 24 hours after cell injection, the lung, liver, spleen, and lower extremity long bones (bone marrow) were removed and assayed for proportions of labelled cells. Sham-exposed, warm air-exposed (63°C oven) and steroid-treated groups (4 mg/kg methyl prednisolone) were also assayed. Both exposure to 25 mW/cm^2 RF/MWR and exposure to warm air led to an increase in core (colonic) temperature (2°C) within 15 minutes, followed by stable hyperthermia due to adjusted thermoregulation. Liburdy called attention to the fact that, although the absolute increases in temperature for the 25 mW/cm^2 RF/MWR and warm air exposures were identical, the rates of core temperature increase for the treatments were significantly different, with a more rapid increase noted in the RF/MWR-exposed animals. As noted above, steroid output in the RF/MWR-heated mice was threefold greater than that in warm air-heated mice, despite identical final core temperatures (62).

Normally, administered splenic lymphocyte traffic consists of a rapid influx of injected cells into the lungs, followed by migration of most cells ("homing") to the spleen with limited migration to the liver and little, if any, migration to the bone marrow. In Liburdy's studies, the hyperthermic (25 mW/cm^2)

RF/MWR exposure led to a 37% decrease in lymphocyte migration from the lung to the spleen, and a threefold increase in lymphocyte migration to the bone marrow. Similar changes were noted with administration of exogenous steroids, in concurrence with other reports of steroid effects on lymphocyte traffic. Lymphocyte traffic to the liver was unchanged by the RF/MWR exposure or other treatments. Neither exposure to RF/MWR (5 mW/cm^2) without a detectable increase in core temperature nor thermogenic warm air exposure resulted in altered lymphocyte traffic.

Ability of the mice to develop a delayed hypersensitivity (cell-mediated) reaction was assayed with a standard technique, namely, swelling of a footpad injected with sheep erythrocytes, to which the mice had previously been sensitized (62). Neither sham exposures nor multiple warm air exposures (twice daily from 5 days before sensitization and until the day of footpad challenge) changed the delayed hypersensitivity response. In contrast, multiple thermogenic RF/MWR exposures markedly suppressed the response of either strain (C57Bl/6 or BALB/c) of mice. Qualitatively similar immunosuppression followed administration of steroids before sensitization of the mice to the antigen.

Liburdy suggested that such *in vivo* whole-body RF/MWR exposure could be perceived as a heat stress that stimulates the hypothalamic-hypophyseal-adrenal axis to trigger the release of adrenal steroids into the blood (65). While RF/MWR was felt to act indirectly on lymphocytes through steroid-associated actions, Liburdy noted that other stress-associated products or reactants might act in parallel with steroids to produce effects on the immunological system. RF/MWR exposure without a detectable increase in core temperature in these experiments may have constituted a thermal stress, but one with different effects on the hypothalamic-hypophyseal-adrenal axis.

When Liburdy's observations (62) are compared to those of Wiktor-Jedrzejczak et al (56), differences in protocols and experimental conditions are apparent. Wiktor-Jedrzejczak, et al did not measure peripheral blood leukocyte levels or plasma corticoid levels, and measured rectal temperatures before and after (but not during) exposure of the mice to 2450 MHz RF/MWR. Temperature changes in the mice were minimal, and temperature generally decreased after exposure because of the environmental conditions, namely, forced air convection cooling. Although the animals in the experiments of Wiktor-Jedrzejczak, et al were exposed to RF/MWR at twice the specific absorption (13 mW/g versus 5.6 mW/g) that could lead to an increase (2-3°C) in core temperature (58), the environment provided additional (iatrogenic) thermoregulation. The thermal stress was balanced by a hypothermic stress, with potentially complex effects on the animal's physiological regulatory system. It could be expected that, to maintain the near-normal core temperature, the peripheral temperature (and likely the vascular circulation) were significantly changed. The results of Wiktor-Jedrzejczak, et al (an increase in percentage of splenic CR+ B lymphocytes only) were most similar to those observed when Liburdy exposed mice to warm air. The thermal load from RF/MWR exposure was likely to have been equal or greater in the experiments of Wiktor-Jedrzejczak et al, but the environment may have modified the stress (and thus, perhaps, the plasma corticoid levels) to be the equivalent of the warm air-exposed animals in Liburdy's experiments. In fact, the animals in the studies of Wiktor-Jedrzejczak, et al, appeared to undergo significant cold stress, partially counteracted by RF/MWR absorption (i.e., heating) in the exposed animals. The RF/MWR-exposed animals were thus compared to sham-exposed animals whose physiological thermoregulatory systems were responding to a greater burden in order to maintain core set-point temperatures.

CONCLUDING COMMENTS

It should be readily apparent from the above discussion that interactions of RF/MWR with the hematological and immunological systems are complex and difficult to define. Many but not all of the conflicting observations can be ascribed to species specificity and/or varied exposure conditions. Extrapolation from species to species and eventually to humans, in order to formulate safety guidelines for RF/MWR exposure, entails delineation of multiple confounding factors. A comparative approach with appropriate "scaling", or use of proportionality or conversion factors, is necessary for establishing relevance of experimental animal data for humans.

If future studies are to advance our understanding, they must include a thorough description of methodology and results, adequate controls, and uniform (or readily translated) reporting of exposure factors, including frequency, intensity, rate and length of exposure, total dose absorbed and dose distribution. Environmental conditions, often not described in earlier studies, must be delineated. There is a great need for continuing judicious *in vivo* and *in vitro* investigation of RF/MWR bioeffects. *In vivo* experimental protocols are subject to animal to animal variability, and it is more difficult to determine and reproduce the amount of RF/MWR energy absorbed. While average absorbed energy may be determined, the energy absorbed at specific sites within the animal is more difficult to measure. "Hot spots" may exist in critical areas, such as locations rich in immunocompetent or hematopoietic cells, or other types of cells whose altered physiology would in turn affect hematological and immunological homeostasis.

Many other systems maintaining homeostasis affect the hematological and immunological systems, and may confound interpretation of *in vivo* RF/MWR effects. Exposure of an animal to RF/MWR may result in thermoregulatory responses that bring increased blood flow to the connective surfaces, such as the skin, resulting in elevation of cutaneous temperatures. Lymphocyte transformation responses by human and murine mononuclear leukocytes may be delayed or even diminished at a usual skin temperature (32°C) relative to core (37°C) temperature (66). As skin temperature is increased, it is likely that immunocompetent cells in such areas will show enhanced responses to the multitude of resident or transient antigenic stimuli contacted at the body surface at any point in time. This could initiate an immune response leading to localized and/or circulating lymphoblastoid cells. The effect might be further accentuated by an elevation of the animal's core temperature into the febrile range for the species (13,17).

It is easier to determine and reproduce the amount of RF/MWR energy absorbed in *in vitro* experimental protocols. Immunocompetent cells can more truly be examined in an unstimulated state, and studies can often be more tightly controlled. Perhaps two of the greatest advantages of *in vitro* investigation are: (1) studies may be performed with human cells and systems; and (2) the impact of multiple non-immunological and non-hematological systems and responses on the function of exposed leukocytes, erythrocytes and stem cells can be limited. While the latter aspect allows dissection of mechanisms for described effects, it also is a disadvantage with regard to eventual formulation of guidelines for *in vivo* human exposure limits. Those other physiological systems and interactions would have to be considered. Thus, both *in vivo* and *in vitro* investigations are required to attain a clear understanding of RF/MWR interactions with hematological and immunological systems.

It is not yet established that RF/MWR effects on the hematological and immunological systems exist independent of thermal effects (including the rate as well as the magnitude of thermal burden). RF/MWR effects due to heating, with or without temperature increases, have been repeatedly demonstrated. It is conceivable that such thermal effects, especially if not exceeding the limits of the subject's physiological regulatory systems, could be beneficial rather than detrimental (13). The complex nature of immunoregulation may predict that some immune functions will be enhanced and some depressed. The ubiquitous distribution of RF/MWR exposure suggests that further investigations are warranted, both to define and limit potential health hazards, and to define and expand potential health benefits, such as the use of RF/MWR-induced hyperthermia in the treatment of cancer (13), a return to the "fever therapy" of history.

ACKNOWLEDGEMENTS

The author's work is supported in part by a Young Investigator Research Award (AI 15547) from the National Institute of Allergy and Infectious Diseases and in part by funds from the U.S. Environmental Protection Agency (R806390 and CR 808039), the U.S. Air Force Office of Scientific Research (AFOSR-80-0111), and the U.S. Air Force Aeronautical Systems Division (F33615-81-K-0616).

REFERENCES

1. R.J. Smialowicz, Hematologic and immunologic effects of nonionizing electromagnetic radiation, Bull. N.Y. Acad. Med. 55:1094 (1979).
2. S.M. Michaelson, "Microwave and radiofrequency radiation", World Health Organization, Copenhagen (1977).
3. S.M. Michaelson, Microwave biological effects: An overview, Proc. IEEE 68:40 (1980).
4. B.D. McLees, and E.D. Finch, Analysis of reported physiologic effects of microwave radiation, Adv. Biol. Med. Physics 14:163 (1973).
5. C.F. Nathan, H.W. Murray, and Z.A. Cohn, The macrophage as an effector cell, N. Engl. J. Med. 303:622 (1980).
6. E.L. Reinherz, and S.F. Schlossman, Regulation of the immune response - Inducer and suppressor T-lymphocyte subsets in human beings, N. Engl. J. Med. 303:370 (1980).
7. A.S. Rosenthal, Regulation of the immune response - Role of the macrophage, N. Engl. J. Med. 303:1153 (1980).
8. E.R. Unanue, Cooperation between mononuclear phagocytes and lymphocytes in immunity, N. Engl. J. Med. 303:977 (1980).
9. F.W. Ruscetti, and R.C. Gallo, Human T-lymphocyte growth factor: Regulation of growth and function of T-lymphocytes, Blood 57:379 (1981).
10. E.R. Stiehm, and V.A. Fulginiti, "Immunologic Disorders in Infants and Children," Second Edition, W.B. Saunders Company, Philadelphia (1980).
11. K.A. Smith, L.B. Lachman, J.J. Oppenheim, and M.F. Favata, The functional relationship of the interleukins. J. Exp. Med. 151:1551 (1980).
12. T. Diamantstein, R.E. Handschumacher, J.J. Oppenheim, D.L. Rosenstreich, E.R. Unanue, B.H. Waksman, and D.D. Wood, Nonspecific "lymphocyte activating" factors produced by macrophages. J. Immunol. 122:2633 (1979).
13. N.J. Roberts, Jr., Temperature and host defense, Microbiol. Rev. 43:241 (1979).
14. M.J. Kluger, The evolution and adaptive value of fever ,

Amer. Scientist 66:38 (1978).
15. W.R. Beisel, Metabolic response to infection, Ann. Rev. Med. 26:9 (1975).
16. M.J. Kluger, Fever, Pediatrics 66:720 (1980).
17. N.J. Roberts, Jr., and R.T. Steigbigel, Hyperthermia and human leukocyte functions: Effects on response of lymphocytes to mitogen and antigen and bactericidal capacity of monocytes and neutrophils, Infect. Immun. 18:673 (1977).
18. N.J. Roberts, Jr., and K. Sandberg, Hyperthermia and human leukocyte functions. II. Enhanced production of and response to leukocyte migration inhibition factor (LIF), J. Immunol. 122:1990 (1979).
19. S. Barański, and P. Czerski, Biological effects of microwaves. Experimental data, in: "Biological Effects of Microwaves," Dowden, Hutchinson and Ross, Stroudsburg, Pennsylvania (1976).
20. M.J. Kluger, "Fever. Its Biology, Evolution, and Function," Princeton University Press, Princeton, New Jersey (1979).
21. S.M. Michaelson, Thermal effects of single and repeated exposures to microwaves- A review, in: "Biologic Effects and Health Hazards of Microwave Radiation,"P. Czerski, K. Ostrowski, M.L. Shore, Ch. Silverman, M.J. Suess, B. Waldeskog, eds., Polish Medical Publishers, Warsaw (1974).
22. S. Stern, L. Margolin, B. Weiss, S-T Lu, and S.M. Michaelson, Microwaves: Effects on thermoregulatory behavior in rats. Science 206:1198 (1979).
23. R.J. Smialowicz, M.M. Riddle, P.L. Brugnolotti, R.R. Rogers, and K.L. Compton, Detection of subtle microwave heating in 5-hydroxytryptamine-induced hypothermic mice, Bioelectromagnetics 1:210 (1980).
24. E.R. Adair, Metabolic adjustments during whole-body 2450 MHz CW microwave exposure. Bioelectromagnetics 1:209 (1980).
25. S. Barański, and P. Czerski, Interaction of microwaves with living systems, in: "Biological Effects of Microwaves," Dowden, Hutchinson and Ross, Stroudsburg, Pennsylvania (1976).
26. W.G. Lotz, Influence of the circadian rhythm on the adrenocortical response to microwave exposure, Bioelectromagnetics 1:244 (1980).
27. J.A.J. Stolwijk, Responses to the thermal environment, Fed. Proc. 36:1655 (1977).
28. D.I. McRee, Review of Soviet/Eastern European research on health aspects of microwave radiation, Bull. N.Y. Acad. Med. 55:1133 (1979).
29. W. Stodolnick-Barańska, Lymphoblastoid transformation of lymphocytes in vitro after microwave irradiation, Nature 214:102 (1967).

30. W. Stodolnik-Barańska, The effects of microwaves on human lymphocyte cultures, in: "Biologic Effects and Health Hazards of Microwave Radiation," P. Czerski, K. Ostrowski, M.L. Shore, Ch. Silverman, M.J. Suess, B. Waldeskog, eds., Polish Medical Publishers, Warsaw (1974).
31. P. Czerski, Microwave effects on the blood-forming system with particular reference to the lymphocyte, Ann. N.Y. Acad. Sci. 247:232 (1975).
32. D.A. Holm, and L.K. Schneider, The effects of non-thermal radio frequency radiation on human lymphocytes in vitro, Experentia 26:992 (1970).
33. E. Sh. Ismailov, The effect of microwaves on erythrocyte potassium and sodium ion permeability, Biol. Nauki 14:58 (1971).
34. D.J. Peterson, L.M. Partlow, and O.P. Gandi, An investigation of the thermal and athermal effects of microwave irradiation on erythrocytes, IEEE Trans. Biomed. Eng. 26:428 (1979).
35. P. Bodel, and H. Miller, Pyrogen from mouse macrophages causes fever in mice, Proc. Soc. Exp. Biol. Med. 151: 93 (1976).
36. I.L. Bennett, Jr., and L.E. Cluff, Bacterial pyrogens, Pharmacol. Rev. 9:427 (1957).
37. F. Halberg, W.W. Spink, and J.J. Bittnew, Protection by aldosterone and 11, 17-oxycorticoids against effects of brucella somatic antigen in adrenalectomized mice, Endocrinol. 59:380 (1956).
38. W.P. Larson, R.N. Bieter, M. Levine, and W.F. McLimans, Temperature reactions in mice infected with pneumococci, Proc. Sci. Exp. Biol. Med. 42:649 (1939).
39. J.C. Lin, J.C. Nelson, and M.E. Ekstrom, Effects of repeated exposure to 148-MHz radio waves on growth and hematology of mice, Radio Sci. 14(suppl.):173 (1979).
40. J.F. Spalding, R.W. Freyman, and L.M. Holland, Effects of 800-MHz electromagnetic radiation on body weight, activity, hematopoiesis and life span in mice, Health Phys. 20:421 (1971).
41. J.C. Lin, M.J. Ottenbreit, SL Wang, S. Inone, R.O. Bollinger, and M. Fracassa, Microwave effects on granulocyte and macrophage precursor cells of mice in vitro. Radiat. Res. 80:292 (1979).
42. D. Rotkovská, and A. Vacek, Effect of high-frequency electromagnetic field upon haemopoietic stem cells in mice, Folia Biol. (Praha) 18:292 (1972).
43. D. Rotkovská, and A. Vacek, The effect of electromagnetic radiation on the hematopoietic stem cells of mice, Ann. N.Y. Acad. Sci. 247:243 (1975).

44. C.P. Mayers, and J.A. Habeshaw, Depression of phagocytosis: A non-thermal effect of microwave radiation as a potential hazard to health, Int. J. Radiat. Biol. 24:449 (1973).
45. A.S. Hyde, and J.J. Freidman, Some effects of acute and chronic microwave irradiation of mice, in: "Thermal Problems in Aerospace Medicine," J.D. Hardy, ed., Urwin Limited, Surrey (1968).
46. L. Miro, R. Loubière, and A. Pfister, Effects of microwaves on the cell metabolism of the reticulo-histocytic system, in: "Biologic Effects and Health Hazards of Microwave Radiation," P. Czerski, K. Ostrowski, M.L. Shore, Ch. Silverman, M.J. Suess, and B. Waldeskog, eds., Polish Medical Publishers, Warsaw (1974).
47. P. Czerski, E. Paprocka-Slonka, M. Siekierzyński, and A. Stolarska, Influence of microwave radiation on the hematopoietic system, in: "Biologic Effects and Health Hazards of Microwave Radiation," P. Czerski, K. Ostrowski, M.L. Shore, Ch. Silverman, M.J. Suess, and B. Waldeskog, eds., Polish Medical Publishers, Warsaw (1974).
48. P. Czerski, E. Paprocka-Slonka, and A. Stolarska, Microwave irradiation and the circadian rhythm of bone marrow cell mitosis, J. Microwave Power 9:31 (1974).
49. S. Prausnitz, and C. Süsskind, Effects of chronic microwave irradiation on mice, IRE Trans. Biomed. Electron. 9:104 (1962).
50. S.F. Gorodetskaya, The influence of an SHF electromagnetic field on the reproduction, peripheral blood composition, conditioned-reflex activity, and the morphology of the internal organs of white mice, in: "Biological Action of Ultrasound and Super-High Frequency Electromagnetic Oscillations," A.A. Gorodetsky, ed., Academy of Sciences, Kiev (1964).
51. S. Szmigielski, M. Luczak, M. Janiak, M. Kobus, B. Laskowska, E. DeClercq, and P. DeSomer, In vitro and in vivo inhibition of virus multiplication by microwave hyperthermia, Arch. Virol. 53:71 (1977).
52. M.J. Kluger, D.H. Ringler, and M.R. Anver, Fever and survival, Science 188:166 (1975).
53. H.A. Bernheim, P.T. Bodel, P.W. Askenase, and E. Atkins, Effects of fever on host defense mechanisms after infection in the lizard Dipsosaurus dorsalis, Br. J. Exp. Path. 59:76 (1978).
54. H.A. Bernheim, and M.J. Kluger, Fever: Effect of drug-induced antipyresis on survival. Science 193:237 (1976).
55. R.J. Smialowicz, The effect of microwaves (2450 MHz) on lymphocyte blast transformation in vitro, in: "Biological Effects of Electromagnetic Waves," C.C. Johnson, M.L. Shore eds., Rockville, Maryland, HEW Publ. (FDA)77-8010 (1976).
56. W.Wiktor-Jedrzejczak, A. Ahmed, K.W. Sell, P. Czerski, and W.M. Leach, Microwaves induce an increase in the frequency

of complement receptor-bearing lymphoid spleen cells in mice, J. Immunol. 118:1499 (1977).
57. W. Wiktor-Jedrzejczak, A. Ahmed, P. Czerski, W.M. Leach, and K.W. Sell, Immune response of mice to 2450-MHz microwave radiation: Overview of immunology and empirical studies of lymphoid splenic cells, Radio Sci. 12(suppl):209 (1977).
58. W. Wiktor-Jedrzejczak, A. Ahmed, P. Czerski, W.M. Leach, and K.W. Sell, Increase in the frequency of Fc receptor (FcR) bearing cells in the mouse spleen following a single exposure of mice to 2450 MHz microwaves, Biomedicine 27:250 (1977).
59. W. Wiktor-Jedrzejczak, A. Ahmed, P. Czerski, W.M. Leach, and K.W. Sell, Effect of microwaves (2450-MHz) on the immune system in mice: Studies of nucleic acid and protein synthesis, Bioelectromagnetics 1:161 (1980).
60. C.J. Schlagel, and W. Wiktor-Jedrzejczak, Possible humoral mechanism of 2450 MHz microwave-induced increase in complement receptor positive cells as studied using a modified diffusion chamber culture technique, Bioelectromagnetics 1:247 (1980).
61. R.J. Smialowicz, M.M. Riddle, P.L. Brugnolotti, J.M. Sperrazza and J.B. Kinn, Evaluation of lymphocyte function in mice exposed to 2450 MHz (CW) microwaves, in: "Proc. 1978 Symp. Electromagnetic Fields in Biological Systems," S.S. Stuchly, ed., International Microwave Power Institute, Edmonton, Canada (1979).
62. R.P. Liburdy, Radiofrequency radiation alters the immune system: Modulation of T- and B-lymphocyte levels and cell-mediated immunocompetence by hyperthermic radiation, Radiat. Res. 77:34 (1979).
63. R.P. Liburdy, Radiofrequency radiation alters the immune system. II. Modulation of in vivo lymphocyte circulation, Radiat. Res. 83:66 (1980).
64. R.P. Liburdy, Effects of radio-frequency radiation on inflammation, Radio Sci. 12(suppl):179 (1977).
65. W.G. Lotz, and S.M. Michaelson, Temperature and corticosterone relationships in microwave-exposed rats, J. Appl. Physiol. Respirat. Environ. Exercise Physiol. 44:438 (1978).
66. M. Lauwasser, and J.W. Shands, Jr., Depressed mitogen responsiveness of lymphocytes at skin temperature, Infect. Immun. 24:454 (1979).

MUTAGENIC AND DEVELOPMENTAL EFFECTS OF MICROWAVE RADIOFREQUENCY (MW/RF) ENERGIES

Sol M. Michaelson

Department of Radiation Biology and Biophysics
University of Rochester
School of Medicine and Dentistry
Rochester, New York 14642

INTRODUCTION

Some investigators have reported chromosomal changes in various plant and animal cells and tissue cultures exposed to MW/RF energies. Other investigators have reported no changes. Reported chromosomal changes include structural aberrations, polyploidy and stickiness.

Both inhibitory and stimulatory effects on the expression of genetically regulated enzyme synthesis and on bacterial and mammalian cell growth have been reported; a frequency dependent periodicity of the effects has been described. On the other hand some reports indicate no effect on growth or mutagenesis in bacteria at various mm and microwave frequencies.

The mutagenic potential of microwave energy has been evaluated by various techniques including the dominant lethal test in mammalian systems, genetic transmission in Drosophila, and point mutations in bacterial assays with inconsistent results. Increased mutagenesis in Drosophila has been reported, but no effects on mutagenesis has been observed by other investigators.

There are a few reports which suggest that particular combinations of wavelength, power density and duration of exposure produce effects on embryonic development and postnatal growth. Alterations in development have been reported in insects, chick embryos and rodents.

The reports on effects of microwave exposure on early development indicate that no serious effects are to be expected at power densities below 10 mW/cm^2 under usual exposure conditions. They further note that defects, when observed, are the result of hyperthermia. There are numerous reports of abnormalities from the induction of systemic hyperthermia of 2.5 -5°C above the normal temperature for the species, by exposure of a pregnant animal to elevated temperatures at specific critical developmental stages of the fetus. It would thus appear that in the reports of microwave-induced developmental abnormalities, it is the temperature rise in the fetus, irrespective of the manner in which it was produced, that caused the damage.

Cellular-Chromosome-Genetic Effects

Some investigators have reported chromosomal changes in various plant and animal cells in tissue culture[1-6]. In vivo exposure of Chinese hamster bone marrow and testis cells to 30-35 MHz for 1 to 9 days induced significant increases of abnormal cells[7]. The peak-to-peak field strength used was 460 V/cm and the pulse width was 77 μ sec, (pulse repetition rate=1000). Other investigators have reported no changes[8]. Reported chromosomal changes include structural aberrations[1,6], polyploidy[5] and stickiness[1]. Exposures range from 7 mW/cm^2 to more than 200 mW/cm^2.

Some of these studies can be criticized because the systems were subjected to a thermal stress; the chosen parameters of the applied field caused biologically significant field induced force effects in *in vitro* experiments and many of these experiments have not yet been independently replicated. Generally, in studies concerned with response of cells in culture, undetected small temperature deviations between irradiated and control systems can lead to erroneous interpretations. In investigations concerning the effects of microwave and radiofrequency energies on biological systems, especially when some form of cellular response is involved, temperature control must be a major consideration.

Inferences of apparent genetic effects as a result of chromosome studies should be viewed with circumspection. Chromosome scoring techniques are tedious and require considerable skill.[9] Thus conclusions made from only fragmentary data should be suspect.

Although studies of chromosome aberrations are potential early indicators of microwave-induced biological changes, such effects in tissue culture may reflect total response of a specific tissue, but not of genetic injury to the germinal epithelium where it is especially important. Chromosome aberrations may also be referable to somatic mutations which has no relevance for transmissible genetic mutations.

There are several sources of error in estimating chromosome aberration frequencies and in using the estimates to evaluate microwave exposures. When cells are cultured in vitro, aberration frequencies may vary with post-exposure time in culture. There are also many variables in the tissue culture techniques used in various laboratories, which must be taken into consideration when comparing and evaluating results. The possible influence of other agents such as viruses, heat, chemicals, etc., that are known to produce chromosome anomalies, should not be ignored. It is possible to measure changes in cells when they are not a part of an integrated living system; it is not always correct, however to extrapolate these findings to the intact organism where the cell may be in a different relationship and cell cycle and surrounded by other cells with differing sensitivities or protective capacities.

There have been some questions concerning the exact magnitude of the fields and temperature within the receptacles containing cell cultures, blood samples and solutions during exposure. Often the samples are placed in fields of known strength and power density, but due to the complex shapes of the vessels holding the samples, the actual fields acting on the cells or organisms is unknown. Also, it is difficult in some cases to determine whether the effects are specifically due to the fields or simply due to a temperature rise. Attempts to measure the temperature of fields within the sample by conventional methods can produce perturbations that may significantly modify the results of the experiment[10].

Effects on mitochondria isolated from exposed animals have been reported[11], but there was no effect on rat liver mitochondria exposed in vitro to 2.4 GHz microwaves 1-41 W/Kg[12] or 1-12 GHz, at a maximum of 2 mW/cm^2.[13] No effect of microwave exposure has been found on a number of enzymes and proteins irradiated in vitro.[14-17] Albert et al.[18] exposed Chinese hamsters at 2450 MHz, 50 mW/cm^2, for 0.5 - 4.5 hours over a period of 1-21 days and found no change in liver ATP.

Miro et al.[19] exposed Swiss albino mice to pulsed 3105-MHz at 20 mW/cm^2 average power density (400 W/cm^2 peak) for 145 h. Stimulation of splenic lymphopoiesis and increased ^{35}S methionine incorporation in spleen, thymus, and liver were found. The authors interpret these results as a sign of stimulation of cells belonging to the reticulo-endothelial system.

Both inhibitory and stimulatory effects on the expression of genetically regulated enzyme synthesis and on bacterial and mammalian cell growth were reported by Webb[20] at 59-143 GHz, 10-50 mW/cm^2; a frequency dependent periodicity of the effects was described. Hill et al.[21] found no effect on growth of *E. coli* exposed to 10-70 mW/cm^2 of 65-75 GHz.

Miro et al.[19] reported a "radioprotective" effect in exposure of bacteria to 3105 MHz, pulsed at a peak power of 39 W/cm^2, temporal average 2 mW/cm^2. Other reports show interference with genetically controlled synthesis in bacteria.[22,23] Blackman et al.[24] reported no effect on bacterial growth at 68, 69, 70, 71, 72, 73, or 74 GHz at an incident power density estimated to be 0.3 mW/cm^2, or at 1.70 or 2.45 GHz between 0.005 and 50 mW/cm^2 (0.008 - 75 mW/g), nor was there any effect on mutagenesis in bacteria exposed to 2.45 GHz (10 and 50 mW/cm^2, 15 and 70 W/kg) or to 1.70 GHz (88 V/m; 3 W/kg).

Microwave irradiation for 30 minutes at frequencies between 70 and 75 GHz and power densities up to 60 mW/cm^2 did not induce any killing in mutant and wildtype strains of *E. coli* and *Saccharomyces cerevisiae*.[25] Such exposure did not produce any DNA damage which can be recognized by the known DNA repair systems. The authors suggest that the effect of microwaves may be reversible. Simultaneous exposure to microwaves and X-rays produced increased survival of X-irradiated *E. coli* which suggested enhanced repair due to increased metabolism.

Baranski et al.[26,27] were not able to attribute mutagenic effects or metabolic changes in *Physarum polycephalum* or *Aspergillus nidulans* to specific effects of 10 mW/cm^2, 2450 MHz CW or pulsed microwaves. Correlli et al.[28] also reported no mutagenesis after exposure to 2.6 - 4.0 GHz at 20 W/Kg. They investigated the effects of RF on colony-forming-ability (CFA) and molecular structure (determined by infrared spectroscopy) of *Escherichia coli B* bacterial cells in aqueous suspension. Cells were exposed for 10 hours at SARs of 20 W/kg (equivalent to 50 mW/cm^2). No RF-induced effects on either colony forming ability (CFA) or molecular structure were observed.

The mutagenic potential of MW/RF energy has been evaluated by various techniques including the dominant lethal test in mammalian systems[29-31], genetic transmission in Drosophila[32,33], or point mutations in bacterial assays[24] with inconsistent results.

Although Mickey[34] reported increased mutagenesis in Drosophila exposed in a 20 MHz field, no effects on mutagenesis were observed by Pay et al.[33] using 2450 MHz or by Mittler[32] with 3 MHz and 150 MHz RF energy.

Varma and co-workers[29,30] reported increased mutagenesis, using the dominant lethal test with male mice exposed to 10 and 50 mW/cm^2 1.7 GHz CW for 90 and 30 minutes respectively. Mice exposed to 2.45 GHz CW at 100 mW/cm^2 for 10 minutes and at 50 mW/cm^2 three times, 10 minutes each, within one day, also showed increased mutagenesis. Mice subjected to four exposures of 50 mW/cm2, 10 minutes each, over a period of two weeks, showed no increase of dominant lethality above control levels.

Berman and Carter[31] exposed male rats daily to 425 MHz CW (Day 12 of gestation to 90 days of age, 10 mW/cm^2 4 hours/day) or 2450 MHz CW at 5, 10 or 28 mW/cm^2 from day 6 of gestation to 90 days of age, 4 or 5 hours/day. No significant evidence of germ cell mutagenesis or alteration in reproductive efficiency was detected.

In essence, there is no satisfactory evidence of microwave-induced genetic effects at "low" to "modest power densities".[35] Experimental studies of microorganisms[24,26,27] and rodents[29,30,36] suggest that microwave exposure at power densities below 10 mW/cm^2 are not mutagenic in these organisms. It is known that the rate of induction of mutations will increase with increasing temperature. It is possible therefore that artifacts or thermal stress could be factors in some of the reported studies.

Changes in cell membrane permeability have also been attributed to RF energy.[37] Other studies[38] have failed to find membrane permeability effects from RF-heating. Janiak and Szmigielski[39] reported no significant differences in the sequence and time-course of cell membrane injury between cells treated in a water bath and those heated with 2450 MHz microwaves.

Overt thermal effects due to radiofrequency and microwave energy absorption have been demonstrated and documented. The reports of effects which appear to depend on specific frequencies and amplitudes or "windows" would imply biological responses may not always be due to a rise in temperature. Prohofsky[40] has suggested that low-lying longitudinal vibrational modes of DNA molecules could be induced or enhanced by electromagnetic fields at microwave frequencies of 3 GHz or higher. Such induced modes could theoretically produce conformational changes in the DNA molecule and result in biologically significant functional alterations. Frohlich[41] has similarly suggested microwave interactions with macromolecular biologically active complexes. Illinger[42,43] has treated the problem of molecular interaction from a quantum mechanical approach. He suggests the possibility of field-induced quasi-resonant transitions occurring at frequencies higher than 10 GHz from the excitation of coherent vibrational modes. Though some experiments seem to provide results that support such a theory it has been pointed out that great care must be exercised in differentiating between actual biological interactions and cyclic and multiple resonances in cavity, waveguide and other exposure systems which have the capability of creating multiple reflections.[44]

The principal technical problems in studying RF-induced effects on cells is that the studies are often conducted using conventional apparatus designed for cell studies -- flasks, dishes, holders, agitators, water baths, incubators etc. -- and various elements of the apparatus may distort the RF fields in such a way that the specific absorption rate of energy in the cell cultures may be considerably higher or lower than field measurements would indicate. Often the samples are placed in fields of known strength and power density, but due to the complex shapes of the vessels containing samples, the actual fields acting on the cells or organisms are unknown. Also, it is difficult in some cases to determine whether the effects are specifically due to the fields or simply due to a temperature rise. Attempts at measuring the temperature of fields within the sample by conventional methods can produce perturbations that may significantly modify the results of the experiment.

Because of the questionable techniques utilized, reports concerning the genetic implications of microwave exposure are highly suspect, especially since hyperthermia by itself has been shown to induce chromosome damage and gene mutations in a wide range of organisms.[45] Some progress has been made in designing cell culture apparatus that will provide accurate, calibrated exposure to RF fields, but results of much of the earlier work on cell and tissue cultures must be questioned with regard to the actual absorbed RF energy in the cell culture media.[10,46,47]

Microwave energy is considered too low to produce nonthermal effects on DNA structure. Takashima[48] using changes in optical density and viscosity as criteria for strand separation, and thus, structural change, failed to observe structural changes in DNA from exposure to pulsed energy (10 Hz-10 KHz and 100 KHz-10 MHz) at levels of 300 volts (peak-to-peak) across the radiation cell.

The present knowledge of biophysical mechanisms underlying cell membrane function, and functional and structural properties of subcellular components is limited. Interpretation of studies of such phenomena and their biological significance therefore requires considerable circumspection. The anomalous behavior of the 'bound water' of membranes as reported by Grant[49] may help in providing explanations for such effects.

The effects of MW/RF energies on cells and tissues should be investigated by reliable and carefully controlled techniques that are sufficiently sensitive to detect cellular damage in the absence of thermal influence. An essential element in the proof of mutagenicity is the establishment of a field-intensity/time-related effect. Such studies should be free of interacting variables and should permit valid extrapolation to the whole organism with its multiple interdependent, integrated functions. In addition, testing must not be confined to one organism or cell type, but investigations must include a wide range of both *in vivo* and *in vitro* systems. If possible, testing should be done comcomitantly with recognized genetic tests, since only in this way will it be possible to decide which methods constitute a meaningful way of assessing genetic hazards from chromosomal aberration studies.

Drosophila melanogaster, the fruit fly, has been used in several studies to investigate possible genetic effects of microwave exposure since it has a well-described genetic system with a short generation time, large broods, ease of exposure, and minimal space requirements. Heller and Mickey[3] and Mickey[34] claim that somatic and genetic changes are produced in *Drosophila melanogaster* by radiofrequency energy. In some experiments, flies were apparently exposed 5 minutes to 1 hour to 5-40 MHz (15-30 μsec, 500-1000 pulses/sec, 250-6000 V/m peak). According to the authors the number of lethal and externally-manifested mutations increased approximately 13-fold as compared with the mean number of such mutations in control populations of flies. The most effective frequency appeared to be 21 MHz. The genetic tests employed are not described nor are any data given with regard to the frequency or consistency of their observations. No temperature recordings were reported. From a careful analysis of these reports, it would appear that such responses would be due to the high E-field exposure under pulsed conditions. The authors did not determine thresholds, yet the lowest field value for damaging effects appears to correspond roughly to 53 W/cm^2.

The effects of chronic exposure of colonies of *Drosophila melanogaster* larvae to 2450 MHz CW microwaves have been investigated by Imig et al.[50] and Searle et al.[51] The larvae were exposed throughout their entire period of growth to power densities up to approximately 1.0 W/cm^2. To eliminate the thermal effects the temperature of the experimental and control groups were maintained at a constant 28°C. The results of these investigations seem to indicate the absence of specific or "non-thermal" effects upon *Drosophila melanogaster*.

Beyer et al.[52] also investigated the potential mutagenicity of 2450 MHz microwave in *Drosophila melanogaster*. Males were placed in an acrylic capsule 18 cm from the antenna and exposed to 2450 MHz CW energy generated at forward powers of 2.1, 2.75, and 3.0 kW. The 2.75 kW level was lethal. Sex-linked lethal mutations were not observed.

In contrast to the studies of Heller and Mickey[3] and Mickey[34] who reported a ten-fold rise in sex-linked recessive mutations after pulsed radiation in the frequency range 30-60 MHz generated by capacitor plates, Beyer et al.[52] did not find such increase in sex-linked recessive mutations after 2450 MHz CW radiation. Mittler[32] also failed to obtain mutagenesis with 3 and 150 MHz RF. Beyer et al.[52] note that the extent of coupling between *Drosophila* and 2450 MHz microwave energy is in question because of the small size of the fly. The number and clustering of flies could affect the observed lethality. It has been suggested that body dehydration during exposure could cause lethality. This was supported by microscopic examination which revealed physical deformation of the thorax after receiving lethal microwave exposure[53].

In order to explain some of the results obtained with *Drosophila*, Tell[53] exposed a group of 6 day old male, wild-type *Drosophila melanogaster* to 2450 MHz for 55 minutes at an "intense" field. A dramatic change in body weight (about 65 percent reduction) was caused by the exposure. To assess the absorption efficiency of the fruit flies, their absorption cross-section to plane electromagnetic waves was computed. The important result of these calculations is that a fly presents an effective area for electromagnetic absorption of approximately 1/1000 of its geometrical cross-section. Clearly then, the fruit fly is a very inefficient test system with respect to imparting absorbed microwave energy at this frequency. It is possible, nevertheless, that the fruit fly might be reasonably responsive to absorbed energy provided adequate energy can be delivered and accurately measured. A rough estimate of the thermal dose-effect dependence from microwave exposure was made, based on the assumption that the fly is, for practical purposes, a black body radiator. If the fly is to be heated above the ambient temperature, it would take a power density of about 1.044×10^5 W/m^2 to raise the fly's temperature 1°C above an ambient of 25°C. This corresponds to a thermal flux of 0.562×10^{-3} calories.[53]

Growth and Development

There are a few reports which suggest that particular combinations of wavelength, power density, and exposure duration can produce effects on embryonic development and postnatal growth. Alterations in development have been reported in insects[54]; chick embryos[55,56]; and rodents.[57-63]

Larvae of the mealworm beetle, *Tenebrio molitor*, were exposed to two different intensities of 39 MHz. An electrode voltage of 3.6 kV was used for one experiment, and 0.9 kV was used for another. Adults developing from larvae exposed at sublethal levels exhibited malformed and missing legs. It was concluded that the deformities most likely resulted from heat damage to the histoblasts that project into the legs of the sixth or last-instar larva[64-66].

Carpenter and Livstone[54] studied the effects of 10 GHz CW microwaves on pupae of *Tenebrio molitor*. Each pupa was inserted in a waveguide and irradiated at 80 mW/cm^2 for either 20 or 30 min or at 20 mW/cm^2 for 120 min, after which development was observed. In control groups 90 percent metamorphosed to become normal adult beetles. In the exposed groups only 24 percent developed normally; 25 percent died and 51 percent developed abnormally. When these thermal conditions within pupae were duplicated by convectional heating, subsequent development of pupae was normal in 80 percent of the experiments. The authors concluded that the abnormalities induced by microwave radiation were not thermally mediated.

Later studies by Lindauer et al.[67] suggested that pulsed microwaves produced comparable effects as did CW at equivalent "dosage", defined as energy level-exposure duration. Apparently total dose and not dose rate more nearly determines the extent of the morphologic alteration[68]. In experiments conducted by Olsen[69] with exposures at 4.0 and 5.95 GHz, calculated energy doses of 37.8 to 1526 J/g, 5 min to 6 hours duration, morphologic alteration was found both for E-field and H-field exposures and both for parallel and for perpendicular polarization. The probability of extremely high local fields created in this type of exposure, nutritional and health status of the organism, or the possibility of post-hatching cannibalism was apparently not considered by other investigators working with Tenebrio larvae[70]. Olsen[71] has provided a thermal basis to explain the microwave-induced teratogenic effects in the meal worm _Tenebrio molitor_. Olsen[69] and Pickard and Olsen[72] noted the threshold of teratogenesis in Tenebrio to be associated with a rise of pupal temperature in excess of 10° C.

Van Ummersen[55,56] reported inhibition of growth and development of chick embryos exposed to 2450 MHz (CW) 400-20 mW/cm^2, 4.5 minutes to 5 hours (ΔT up to 19°C). Since all embryos in which effects were produced reached a temperature of 55°C, the results of these studies suggest that the deleterious effects observed were due to heating. Protein denaturation takes place in the neighborhood of 45°C, thus any factor which elevates the temperature to this level could start degeneration of cell structures. The high power densities that were used in this study would be sufficient to cause protein denaturation on a thermal basis. Osborne[73,74] found that at no stage of development was the chick embryo affected by prolonged 200 MHz (CW) exposure when the temperature rise within the egg was never more than 1°C.

Giarola and Krueger[75] exposed chicks to 260, 915, and 2435 MHz for four weeks at several power densities and observed decreased egg production but no effect on fertility, hatching or sex ratios. Also no macroscopic abnormalities were noted in newly-hatched chicks or in dead embryos. These experiments, however, were fraught with difficulties, including death and infertility in controls, small sample size, inadequate temperature controls, as well as a loss and change of power. It is thus inappropriate to make meaningful conclusions from this work.

Quail embryos exposed to 30 mW/cm^2, 2450 MHz (CW) for 4 hours on each of the first 5 days of incubation, did not develop gross deformities or changes in hatchability that could be correlated with exposure.[76] Microwave-induced temperature within the eggs varied from 34-37°C which is the normal incubation temperature.

In another study[77] Japanese Quail embryos were exposed during the first 12 days of development to 2.45 GHz microwaves at an incident power density of 5 mW/cm^2 and specific aborption rate of 4.03 mW/g. No gross deformities were observed in the exposed quail when examined and sacrificed at 24-36 hr after hatch. No significant changes in the total body weight or weights of the heart, liver, gizzard, adrenals, and pancreas were found in the treated birds. Hematological parameters were also measured in the study. The results showed a statistically significant increase in hemoglobin and statistically significant decrease in monocytes in birds exposed to microwaves. No statistically significant changes in hematocrit, red blood cells, total white blood cells, lymphocytes, heterophils, basophils or eosinophils were detected.

Rugh et al.[59,60] reported abnormalities in mouse fetuses exposed in an environmentally controlled wave-guide at days 7-13 of gestation to absorbed 2450 MHz (CW) microwaves in the range of 12.6 to 33.5 J/Kg, equivalent to 123 mW/cm^2 incident power. Hemorrhages, resorptions, exencephaly, stunting, and fetal death were observed. Differential effects at different gestation days suggest thermal sensitivity of embryos. In a further study, Rugh and McManaway[61,62] demonstrated that lowering the dam's body temperature with pentobarbital anesthesia could prevent the teratogenic effects of thermal loading with microwaves.

Rugh and McManaway[62] reported studies on CF-1 mice exposed to 2450-MHz microwaves for four minutes at dose rates of 78.8 to 136.2 mW/g. The majority of the observed abnormalities resulted from exposures on day 8 or 10 of gestation. It is important to note that 100 mW/g for 4 min is the convulsive threshold for this strain of mouse. In a later study[63] in which the averaged dose rate was 107.4 mW/g, 68 percent of the animals exposed on day 8 were either resorbed, dead, or abnormal as compared with 28 percent of the animals exposed on day 10, and with 20 percent of the animals exposed on days 3 or 4. Thus two main peaks of teratogenic susceptibility are suggested: the first on day 4, which corresponds to the time of implantation of the embryo in the uterine horn, and the second at day 8, which corresponds to the beginning of organogenesis.

Laskey et al.[78] exposed gravid rats to 2450 MHz CW microwaves, 100 mW/cm^2, for 8-13 min. on Days 2, 5 (pre-implantation stage), 8 (organogenesis stage), or 15 (fetal stage). These exposures produced group mean rectal temperatures ranging from 41.4 to 42.8°C (sham = 38.0°C). No changes occurred in the pre-implanted embryos, but there was an increased number of resorbed fetuses in the Day 8 exposure and a decrease in weight of live fetuses exposed on Day 8 or Day 13. No obvious abnormalities were seen in any of the litters when examined on Day 19 of gestation.

Dietzel et al.[79-81] exposed pregnant rats once between days 1 and 16 of gestation with a 27.12 MHz diathermy unit at 55, 70 or 100 W which was sufficient to raise the animals colonic temperatures to 39, 40, or 42° C. The fetuses were examined near term. The peak incidence of anomalies, was found to occur on gestation days 13-14, when 16 percent of the fetuses were abnormal. This fetal wastage, as in the studies by Rugh et al.[59,60] are clearly associated with a general body temperature increase in the dam.

Lin et al.[82] studied the effect of repeated exposure of C3H mice to 48 MHz. The animals were exposed to 0.5 mW/cm^2 (63.25 V/m) in a TEM exposure chamber for one hour a day, five days a week, beginning on the 4th to 7th days postpartum, for 10 weeks. The formed elements in the blood were not affected by the exposure. The means of body mass of the irradiated and control animals were comparable. No significant differences in lesion onset, incidence, prevalence, extent, or type were observed when repeated RF-exposed animals were compared with control groups. During the period of the study no cataracts were noted. Fertility differences among irradiated and control animals were not detected. Body growth patterns did not differ among sham and RF exposed animals.

Employing a multimodal cavity at 2450 MHz, Chernovetz et al.[83] irradiated pregnant mice with a single "intense" dose of 38 mW/g for 10 min (22.8 J/g) on gestation day 11, 12, 13, or 14. This dose resulted in 10 percent maternal lethality. The exposure during late organogenesis or early fetal stage caused no change in fetal mortality or morbidity when compared to shams. In another study, Chernovetz et al.[84] noted an increased rate of resorptions in rats after an absorbed dose of 30 mW/g for 20 min on days 10-16.

In studies of effects of in utero exposure of Long-Evans rats to 2450 MHz CW, Michaelson et al.[85,86] found no adverse effects on the dam or offspring when gestation length or litter size were examined. The rats were exposed at 10 or 40 mW/cm^2 (1.6 - 6.4 W/kg equiv.) for one hour on Day 9 (organogenesis) or Day 16 (fetal stage) of gestation. Accelerated maturation was suggested by increased adrenal weight and earlier corticosterone stability.

Berman et al.[87] exposed mice to 2450 MHz at 3.4-28 mW/cm^2 100 minutes daily throughout pregnancy. Mean live fetal weight per litter decreased with exposure at the highest power density. There was an increased incidence of cranioschisis in exposed fetuses. Estimates of mean dose rate ranged from 2.0 to 22.2 mW/g.

Nelson et al.[88] exposed C3H mice at 148 MHz for one hour daily from day 2 through day 19 of gestation in a rectangular coaxial exposure system at 0.5 mW/cm^2 corresponding to an SAR of 0.013 mW/g. The experiment was conducted as three separate replications. In each of the experiments some of the dams were allowed to come to term and the fetuses were weighed at birth and again at 60 days of age while in others the uterus was extirpated on day 19 of gestation. No differences in percentage of resorbed, stillborn, or abnormal fetuses were observed in any of the experiments.

McRee and Nawrot[89] exposed pregnant CD-1 mice to 2.45 MHz CW microwaves at power densities of 5 mW/cm^2 (17.9 mW/g), 21 mW/cm^2 and 30 mW/cm^2 (25.5 mW/g), for 8 hours daily. The 5 mW/cm^2 group was exposed from day 1 through day 15 of gestation while the 21 mW/cm^2 and 30 mW/cm^2 groups were divided into two groups and exposed either from day 1 through 6 or day 6 through 15 of gestation. Both cage controls (non-handled) and sham-irradiated (handled) controls were employed as well as handled and non-handled control groups that were subjected to elevated ambient temperatures. The results of the study indicated a decrease in pregnancy rate due merely to handling during days 1 through 6 of gestation (86 percent non-handled, 72 percent handled).

Bereznitskaya[57,58] exposed mice to 3000 MHz, 10 mW/cm^2 which resulted in increased fetal wastage. No definite abnormalities or inborn genetic defects were found.

Jensh et al.[90] reported on the effects of protracted prenatal exposure of Wistar derived rats to 2450-MHz microwaves for 8 hours daily throughout gestation. The mean exposure time was 115 hours to 20 mW/cm^2 incident power density. No statistically significant differences were observed between control and exposed animals for maternal mass, embryonic and fetal resorption rate, abnormality rate, and term fetal and placental masses. These authors also reported similar experiments in which 915-MHz microwaves were employed.[91,92] They exposed Wistar rats at 10 mW/cm^2 for 8 hours daily throughout gestation for an average of 110 hours. Post-exposure colonic temperatures of dams showed no increase over baseline rectal temperatures. No differences were observed in embryonic or fetal death, abnormalities, fetal mass, litter size, placental mass, fetal sex ratio, or maternal mass.

In another study[93] gravid Wistar rats were exposed 8 hours daily throughout pregnancy to 915-MHz microwaves at 10 mW/cm^2. The average exposure time was 109 hours. Dams were allowed to deliver their offspring. Within three days after birth the pups were given three tests for reflexes. After the pups were weaned, a series of performance tests were given. The post-weaning tests began on post-partum day 60 and were completed by the 90th day. No detrimental post-natal effects were observed on performance in a water T-maze, avoidance behavior, open-field behavior, forelimb hanging, or on performance in a 24-hour activity wheel. No teratology was observable in rats exposed throughout gestation to 35 mW/cm^2 microwaves at 6000 MHz. The authors of the three studies state that the irradiaton was "non-thermal", but no doses or dose rates were given for any of their exposure conditions.

Chernovetz et al.[84] exposed Holtzman derived, Sprague-Dawley rats to 2450-MHz microwaves in a multi-mode cavity at dose rate of 31 $\pm$ 3 mW/g for 20 minutes. The microwave treatment was matched to infrared exposure on the basis of duration and averaged increment of colonic temperature ($\Delta t = 3.4°C$). The animals were acutely exposed once on day 10, 11, 12, 13, 14, 15, or 16 of gestation. An increased number of fetal resorptions but no specific fetal abnormalities occurred in dams exposed to microwaves. Fetal mass was smaller than that of controls among dams subjected to either microwaves or infrared. Fetal brains among microwave-exposed animals contained less norepinephrine. Dopamine content of the fetal brain, although reduced in microwave-exposed animals, was not significantly different from that in control and infrared-irradiated animals. Microwave-exposed dams differed from infrared-irradiated dams only in exhibiting a greater number of resorptions. Both the microwave- and infrared-exposed dams differed from controls in exhibiting more resorptions; their fetuses were also smaller. No specific anatomical abnormalities were observed, although the dose of microwave energy was at the LD_{23} level for the dam. The authors speculated "the probability of teratogenic insult from the microwave exposure of the rat is smaller than the dam's probability of mortality".

In another study on rats, Chernovetz et al.[94] employed dose rates of 28 mW/g and 14 mW/g for 20 minutes and reported no specific abnormalities or increase of resorptions from exposure of fetuses to 2450-MHz microwaves in a multimode cavity on day 8, 10, 13, or 14 of gestation. No lethality resulted from the treatment although the post-treatment temperature of the dams in the 28 mW/g conditions reached 42°C. In a third study[95] the dose rates were elevated to 31 mW/g or 17 mW/g for 20 minutes on gestation days 8, 10, 12, or 14 resulting in average post-treatment temperatures of 43°C or 41°C with a lethality rate of 21 percent for the dams exposed to the higher level of microwaves. Both resorptions and abnormalities were increased in the 31 mW/g condition. Exencephaly was the most frequently observed abnormality. Fetal body mass was smaller in the high microwave conditions and fetal brain mass was affected both by the treatment and the day of gestation on which exposure occurred. Regression analysis revealed that both peak temperature and dose rate were related positively to the occurrence of resorptions and abnormalities. The regression of fetal brain mass on fetal body mass revealed a tendency for animals exposed to 31 mW/g to be macrocephalic while the 17 mW/g exposed animals tended to be microcephalic. The three studies[84,94,95] taken together would appear to support the authors' earlier speculation that in the laboratory rat the teratogenic threshold for thermal levels of microwaves is near the mortality threshold for the exposed dam. In addition, the results of the three studies clearly parallel the heat stress literature that fetal damage in the rat results from thermal inputs.

Berman et al.[96] exposed Sprague-Dawley rats to 2.45 GHz at a power density of 0 or 28 mW/cm^2 for 100 minutes daily from days 6-15 after breeding. Additional animals were exposed to 40 mW/cm^2. They concluded that 2.45 GHz microwaves does not produce a strong teratogenic effect in the rat unless the dam is thermally stressed.

Conover et al.[97] reported on single, 20- and 30-minute exposures of fetal rats on the 10th, 12th, or 14th day of gestation to 27.12-MHz at specific absorption rates of 17 to 35 mW/g. Preliminary results suggested that fetal wastage occurred after exposure on the 10th or 14 days of gestation. Grossly observable malformations occurred in animals exposed during the 10th day for 30 minutes while visceral abnormalities occurred after exposure on the 10th and 14th days.

In a recent review, O'Connor[98] noted that with respect to basic design, procedure, and variables assessed, the teratogenic studies reported to date have been more diverse than decisive. Wide variation in exposure parameters makes it difficult to compare the results; additional difficulty is generated because many of the reports do not contain information on critical variables such as the manner in which the day of gestation was timed. The day on which the animal is "sperm-", or "sperm-plug" positive can be timed as day 0, although a more common procedure is to consider this day 1.

Many of the investigators who have reported defects have employed acute, intense, irradiation which obviously has placed a thermal burden on the exposed subject. Some studies attempt to control for heat by including controls heated by means of infrared. Of importance in this regard are the comparisons with the literature on heat stress.

Many of the teratogenic studies of MW/RF have been performed without a sufficient number of animals, and others lack sophisticated design and thus do not allow for observation of low probability events. One could argue that any increase in the incidence of fetal damage, regardless of how low, should be considered as a possible biologically significant event even if it is not statistically reliable. While few adequate and rigorous designs have been employed, more critical to the assessment of demonstrated teratogenic potential of microwaves is the fact that the statistical analyses are usually not given in enough detail to permit evaluation.[98]

If attention is focused not on procedural questions but only on similarities in the results of the studies, several trends are apparent. The most common result from fetal exposure to microwaves would appear to be a non-specific, general response, that of reduced or retarded gains of body mass. Without further study it is impossible to know if this decrease is maintained after birth and when, if ever, the exposed stunted fetuses catch up. It is important to note that this general suppression of body mass is the only effect that appears to be common across the range of species that have been studied.

Another more general deleterious response seen in the mammal is increased rate of fetal resorption. The increase may be indicative of malformed fetuses, but the resorbed nature of the fetal material precludes a more fine-grained analysis and thus identification of which, if any, specific structure was damaged. The increased rate of resorption and the range of exposures within which it occurs is remarkably similar to the effects of heat stress. Particularly in the rat, the resorption rate appears to increase within a rather narrow thermal window, the other side of which is febrile death. The majority of defects has been observed following high level, acute exposures with obvious thermal components.[98]

It does appear that abnormalities in small animal fetuses can be produced with microwaves in conjunction, however, with systemic hyperthermia of 2.5 - 5°C above the normal temperature for the species at some period during specific critical development. From a survey of the literature, it appears that it is the temperature rise in the fetus, irrespective of the manner in which it is produced, that causes damage. It is important to realize that in all species there is a constantly evolving pattern of maturation during gestation and in the rat this continues during the first 3 weeks of postnatal life. In interpreting teratological effects of microwaves as with any agent it is important to realize that many fetal defects such as hemorrhage, resorption, stillbirth and exencephaly occur spontaneously in mice.[83]

In women, infections such as rubella, influenza, and smallpox, occurring during early pregnancy, are known to cause abortions and fetal malformations[99,100]. In general, it appears that any infection giving rise to fever in early stages of pregnancy in man or animals, is capable of producing fetal malformation or abortion. It is well known that induction of fever can lead to the early termination of pregnancy[101]. There are numerous reports of abnormalities from the induction of systemic hyperthermia of 2.5 - 5°C above the normal temperature for the species for one hour or longer during specific critical developmental stages of the fetus by exposure of the pregnant animals to elevated temperatures and humidity. Fetal resorption, growth retardation, microphthalmia, and malformations affecting the central nervous system, musculoskeletal system, and other organs, have been observed in animals.[102-105] Hyperthermia of 4 - 4.5°C for 40 to 60 minutes during specific developmental stages produces increased fetal resorptions, retardation of growth, microphthalmia, anencephaly, and defects of tail, limbs, toes, palate, and body in rats depending upon the gestational stage at which hyperthermia occurred.[102] These results indicate that the occurrence of fetal malformations in mammals from fever in early pregnancy is probably related to the hyperthermia occurring at a particular critical stage of organogenesis. The threshold appears to be an elevation of 2.5 - 5.0°C above the normal temperature of the species sustained for an hour or more.

From the standpoint of public health, one must consider the difficulty of extrapolating data from experimental teratology to the human fetus. Such an extrapolation becomes feasible only after detailed analysis of the fine mechanisms of teratogenesis.[106] Also of great importance is the need for appropriate scaling factors to permit extrapolation of experimental data obtained on small animals, to the human. The reports on effects of microwave exposure on early development have been reviewed by Baranski and Czerski[35] who concluded that no serious effects are to be expected at power densities below 10 mW/cm^2 under usual exposure conditions.

ACKNOWLEDGEMENTS

This paper is based on work performed under Contract No. DE-AC02-76EV03490 with The U.S. Department of Energy at the University of Rochester Department of Radiation Biology and Biophysics and has been assigned Report No. UR-3490-1965.

REFERENCES

1. K.M. Chen, A. Samuel and R. Hoopingavner, Chromosomal abberrations of living cells induced by microwave radiation. Environmental Letters 6:37 (1974).
2. J.H. Heller, Cellular effects of microwave radiation, in: "Biological Effects and Health Implications of Microwave Radiation," S.F. Cleary, ed., U.S. Department of Health, Education, and Welfare, Public Health Service BRH/DBE (1970).
3. J.H. Heller, and G. H. Mickey, Non-thermal effects of radiofrequency in biological systems. Digest 1961 Internat. Conf. Med. Electron. (1961).

4. D.E. Janes, W. M. Leach, W. A. Mills, R.T. Moore, and M.L. Shore, Effects of 2450 MHz microwaves on protein synthesis and on chromosomes in Chinese hamsters, Non. Ioniz. Radiat. 1:125 (1969).
5. K.T.S. Yao, Cytogenetic consequences of microwave incubation of mammalian cells in culture, Genetics 83:584 (1976).
6. K.T.S. Yao, Microwave radiation-induced chromosomal aberrations in corneal epithelium of Chinese hamsters, J. Heredit., 69:409 (1978).
7. G.H. Mickey, J.H. Adler, and E. Snyder, Nonthermal hazards of exposure to radiofrequency fields, Final Report, The New England Instit. Ridgefield, CT, (1975).
8. A.T. Huang, M.E. Engle, J.A. Elder, J.B. Kinn and T.R. Ward, The effect of microwave radiation (2450 MHz) on the morphology and chromosomes of lymphocytes, Radio Sci. 12:173 (1977).
9. J.R.K. Savage, Use and abuse of chromosomal aberrations as an indicator of genetic damage. Int. J. Environ. Stud. vol. 1:233-240 (1971).
10. A.W. Guy, A method for exposing cell cultures to electromagnetic fields under controlled conditions of temperature and field strength, Radio Sci., 12:87 (1977).
11. Y.D. Dumansky and V. F. Rudichenko, Dependence of the functional activity of liver mitochondria on the super-high frequency radiation, Hyg. and Sanit., Moscow. (1976).
12. J.A. Elder, J. S. Ali, M. D. Long and G.E. Anderson, A coaxial air line microwave exposure system: Respiratory activity of mitochondria irradiated at 2-4 GHz, in: "Biological Effects of Electromagnetic Waves," Vol. 1, pp. 352-365. U.S. Dept. Health Educat, and Welfare, FDA, Rockville, MD. HEW Publication (FDA) 77-8010. (1976)
13. K.D. Straub and P. Carver, Effects of electromagnetic fields on microsomal ATPase and mitochondrial oxidative phosphorylation, in: "Biological Effects of Nonionizing Radiation," P. E. Tyler, ed., Ann. N.Y. Acad. Sci., 247:292 (1975).
14. J.W. Allis, Irradiation of bovine serum albumin with a crossed-beam exposure-detection system, in: "Biologic Effects of Nonionizing Radiation," P. E. Tyler, ed., Ann. N.Y. Acad. Sci. 247:312 (1975).
15. M.L. Belkhode, D.L. Johnson, and A.M. Muc, Thermal and athermal effects of microwave radiation on the activity of glucose-6-phosphate dehydrogenese in human blood, Health Physics 26:45 (1974).
16. M. Bini, A. Checcucci, A. Ignesti, L. Millanta, N. Rubino, S. Camici, G. Manao, and G. Ramponi, Analysis of the effects of microwave energy on enzymatic activity of lactate dehydrogenase (LDH), J. Microwave Power, 13:96 (1978).
17. T.R. Ward, J.W. Allis, and J.A. Elder, Measure of enzymatic activity coincident with 2450 MHz microwave exposure, J. Microwave Power 10:315 (1975).

18. E.N. Albert, G. McCullars, and M. Short, The effect of 2450 MHz microwave radiation on liver adenosine triphosphate (ATP). J. Microwave Power 9:205 (1974).
19. L. Miro, R. Loubiere and A. Pfister, Effects of microwaves on the cell metabolism of the reticulo-endothelial system, in: "Biologic Effects and Health Hazards of Microwave Radiation, P. Czerski et al. ed., Polish Medical Publishers, Warsaw (1974).
20. S.J. Webb, Genetic continuity and metabolic regulation as seen by the effects of various microwave and black light frequencies on these phenomena, in: "Biologic Effects of Nonionizing Radiation, P. E. Tyler, ed., Ann. N.Y. Acad. Sci., 247:327 (1975).
21. D.W. Hill, M.J. Hagmann, A. Riazi, O.P. Gandhi, L.M. Partlow, and L.J. Stensaas, Effect of millimeter waves on bacteria and viruses. Proc. Biol. Eff. EM Waves, Int. Union Radio. Sci., Helsinki, August (1978).
22. A.Z. Smolyanskaya and R.L. Vilenskaya, Effects of millimeter-band electromagnetic radiation on the functional activity of certain genetic elements of bacterial cells (Trans.), Usp Fiz. Nauk 110:571 (1973).
23. N.P. Zalubovskaya, Reactions of living organisms to exposure to millimeter-band electromagnetic waves, Trans. Usp. Fiz. Nauk. 110:574 (1973).
24. C.F. Blackman, S.G. Benane, C.M. Weil, and J.S. Ali, Effects of nonionizing electromagnetic radiation on single-cell biologic systems, in: "Biologic Effects of Nonionizing Radiation, P.E. Tyler, ed., Ann. N.Y. Acad. Sci., 247:352 (1975).
25. D. Averbeck, M. Dardalhon, and A. J. Berteaud, Microwave action in procaryotic and eucaryotic cells and a possible interaction with X-rays, J. Microwave Power 11:143 (1976).
26. S. Baranski, H. Debiec, K. Kwarecki, and T. Mezykowski, Influence of microwaves on genetical processes of Aspergillus nidulans, J. Microwave Power, 11:146 (1976).
27. S. Baranski, J. Bal, H. Debiec, K. Kwarecki, and T. Mezykowski, The influence of microwaves on genetic apparatus functions. Proc. Biol. Eff. E.M. Waves, XIX Gen. Assembly, Int. Union Radio Sci., Helsinki, August (1978).
28. J.C. Correlli, R. J. Gutmann, S. Kohazi, and J. Levy, Effects of 2.6-4.0 GHz microwave radiation on E.-coli B, J. Microwave Power 12:141 (1977).
29. M.M. Varma, E.L. Dage, and S.R. Joshi, Mutagenicity induced by nonionizing radiation in Swiss male mice, in: "Biological Effects of Electromagnetic Waves, C.C. Johnson and M.L. Shore, eds., U.S. Department of Health, Education, and Welfare, Food and Drug Administration, Rockville, MD, HEW Publication (FDA) 77-8010 (1976).

30. M.M. Varma and E.A. Traboulay, Jr., Evaluation of dominant lethal test and DNA studies in measuring mutagenicity caused by non-ionizing radiation, in: "Biological Effects of Electromagnetic Waves," C. C. Johnson and M. L. Shore, eds., Vol. 1, pp. 386-396. U.S. Department of Health, Education, and Welfare, Food and Drug Administration, Rockville, MD. HEW Publication (FDA) 77-8010 (1976).
31. E. Berman and H. Carter, Mutagenic and reproductive tests in male rats exposed to 425 or 2450 MHz (CW) microwaves, Proc. Biol. Eff. E. M. Waves, Int. Union Radio Sci., Helsinki, August (1978).
32. S. Mittler, Failure of 2 and 10 meter radio waves to induce genetic damage in Drosophila melanogaster, Environmental Res. 11:326 (1976).
33. T.L. Pay, E.C. Beyer and C.F. Reichelderfer, Microwave effects on reproductive capacity and genetic transmission in Drosophila melanogaster, J. Microwave Power 7:75 (1972).
34. G.H. Mickey, Electromagnetism and its effect on the organism. N.Y. State J. Med. 63:1935 (1963).
35. S. Barański and P. Czerski, "Biological Effects of Microwaves," Dowden, Hutchinson & Ross, Stroudsburg, PA (1976).
36. W. M. Leach, On the induction of chromosomal aberrations by 2450 MHz microwave radiation, J. Cell Biol. 70:387 (1976).
37. S. Baranski, S. Szmigielski, and J. Moneta, Effects of microwave irradiation in vitro on cell membrane permeability, in: "Biological Effects and Health Hazards of Microwave Radiation," P. Czerski et al., eds., Polish Medical Publishers, Warsaw (1974).
38. L. M. Liu and S.F. Cleary, Effects of microwave radiation on erythrocyte membranes, in: "Abstracts of 1977 International Symposium on the Biological Effects of Electromagnetic Waves, Airlie, Virginia (1977).
39. M. Janiak and S. Szmigielski, Injury of cell membranes in normal and SV40-virus transformed fibroblasts exposed in vitro to microwave (2,450 MHz) or water-bath hyperthermia (43 deg C), in: "Abstracts of 1977 International Symposium on the Biological Effects of Electromagnetic Waves," Airlie, Virginia (1977).
40. E. Prohofsky, Microwave frequencies and the structure of the double helix, in: "The Physical Basis of Electromagnetic Interactions with Biological Systems," pp. 133-140 USDHEW Publication (FDA) 78-8055, Rockville, MD. (1978)
41. H. Fröhlich, The extraordinary dielectric properties of biological materials and the action of enzymes, Proc. Nat. Acad. Sci., 72:4211 (1975).

42. K. Illinger, The attenuation function for biological fluids at millimeter and far-infrared wavelengths, in: "Biological Effects of Electromagnetic Waves," C. L. Johnson and M. L. Shore, eds., Vol II pp. 169-183. USDHEW Publication (FDA) 77-8011, December (1976.)
43. K. Illinger, Millimeter wave and far-infrared absorption in biological systems, in: "The Physical Basis of Electromagnetic Interaction with Biological Systems," L. S. Taylor and A. Y. Cheung eds. USDHEW Publication (FDA) 78-8055, Rockville, MD., pp. 43-64 (1978).
44. W. D. Hershberger, Microwave transmission through normal and tumor cells, IEEE Trans. MTT 26:618 (1978).
45. D. Lindegren, The temperature influence on the spontaneous mutation rate, Hereditas 70:165 (1972).
46. S. M. Michaelson, Discussion following the paper "Effects of 2,450 MHz microwave radiation on cultivated rat kangaroo cells", in: "Biological Effects and Health Implications of Microwave Radiation, S. F. Clearly, ed., HEW Publication Number BRH/DBE 70-2, p. 133. (1970).
47. S. M. Michaelson, Biologic and pathophysiologic effects of exposure to microwaves, in: "Microwave Bioeffects and Radiation Safety," M.A. Stuchly, ed., IMPI Vol. 8, The International Microwave Power Institute, Edmonton Alberta Can, pp. 55-94. (1978)
48. S. Takashima, Studies on the effect of radio-frequency waves on biological macromolecules, IEEE Trans. Bio-Med. Eng., 13:28 (1966).
49. E. Grant, Determination of bound water in biologic materials from dielectric measurements, in: "The Physical Basis of Electromagnetic Interactions with Biological Systems, L. S. Taylor, and A. Y. Cheung, A.Y., eds., Rockville, MD. Dept. HEW, pp. 113-119, Publ. No. (FDA 78-8055) Rockville, MD, (1978).
50. C.J. Imig and G.W. Searle, Review of Work Conducted at State University of Iowa on Organisms exposed to 2450 mc cw Microwave Irradiation. 188p., Griffiss AFB, N.Y., Rome Air Dev. Center (1962).
51. G.W. Searle, R.W. Dahlen, C.J. Imig, C.C. Wunder, J.D. Thomson, J.A. Thomas, and W.J. Moressi, Effect of 2450 mc microwaves in dogs, rats and larvae of the common fruit fly, in: "Biological Effects of Microwave Radiation," M. F. Peyton, ed., Plenum Press, New York (1961).
52. E. C. Beyer, T. L. Pay, and E.T. Irwin, Jr., Developmental and genetic testing of Drosophila with 2450 MHz microwave radiation, in: "Radiation Bio-Effects Summary Report, January-December, 1970, USDHEW, PHS, BRH Publication No. BRH/DBE 70-7 (December) (1970).
53. R.A. Tell, Microwave absorption characteristics of Drosophila melanogaster, in: "Twinbrook Research Laboratory Annual Report 1971, U.S. Environmental Protection Agency, Washington, D.C., p. 155 (1972).

54. R.L. Carpenter and E.M. Livstone, Evidence for nonthermal effects of microwave radiation: abnormal development of irradiated insect pupae, IEEE Trans. MTT 19:173 (1971).
55. C. A. Van Ummersen, The effect of 2450 mc radiation on the development of the chick embryo, in: "Biological Effects of Microwave Radiation, M. F. Peyton, ed., Plenum Press, New York, (1961).
56. C. A. Van Ummersen, "An Experimental Study of Development Abnormalities Induced in the Chick Embryo by Exposure to Radio Frequency Waves, Ph.D. Dissertation, Tufts University, Medford, Mass. (1963)
57. A. N. Bereznitskaya, The effect of 10-centimeter and ultrashort waves on the reproductive function of female mice, Gig. Tr. Prof. Zabol. 9:33 (1968).
58. A. N, Bereznitskaya, Research on the reproductive function in female mice under the impact of low-intensity radio waves of different ranges, in: "Industrial Health and Biological Effects of Radio Frequency Electromagnetic Waves," Material of the Fourth All-Union Symposium, October 1972, Moscow (1972.
59. Rugh, R., E.I. Ginns, H.S. Ho and W.M. Leach, Are microwaves teratogenic?, in: "Biologic Effects and Health Hazards of Microwave Radiation, P. Czerski, et al., eds., Polish Medical Publishers, Warsaw (1974).
60. Rugh, R., E.I. Ginns, H.S. Ho and W.M. Leach, Responses of the mouse to microwave radiation during estrous cycle and pregnancy, Radiation Res. 62: 225 (1975).
61. R. Rugh and M. McManaway, Can electromagnetic waves cause congenital anomalies?, International IEEE/AP-S USNC/URSI Symposium, Amherst, Mass (1976).
62. R. Rugh and M. McManaway, Anesthesia as an effective agent against the production of congenital anomalies in mouse fetuses exposed to electromagnetic radiation, J. Exp. Zool., 197:363 (1976).
63. R. Rugh and M. McManaway, Mouse fetal sensitivity to microwave radiation, Congenital Anomalies, 17:39 (1977).
64. A.M. Kadoum, H.J. Ball, and S.O. Nelson, Morphological abnormalities resulting from radiofrequency treatment of larvae of Tenebrio molitor, Ann. Entomol. Soc. Amer. 60:889 (1967).
65. A.M. Kadoum, H.J. Ball, and L.E. Stetson, Metabolism in the yellow mealworm, Tenebrio molitor (Coleoptera tenebrionidae), following exposures to radiofrequency electric fields, Ann. Entomol. Soc. Amer. 60:1195 (1967).
66. A.M. Kadoum, S.O. Nelson, and L.E. Stetson, Mortality and internal heating in radiofrequency-treated larvae of Tenebrio molitor, Ann. Entomol. Soc. Amer. 60:885 (1967c)

67. G.A. Lindauer, L.M. Liu, G.W. Skewes and F.J. Rosenbaum, Further experiments seeking evidence of nonthermal biological effects of microwave radiation, IEEE Trans. Microwave Theory Tech. 22:790 (1974).
68. L.M. Liu, F.J. Rosenbaum, and W.F. Pickard, The relation of teratogenesis in Tenebrio molitor to the incidence of low level microwaves, IEEE Trans. Microwave Theory Tech. 23:929 (1975).
69. R.G. Olsen, Insect teratogenesis in a standing-wave irradiation system, Radio Sci., 12:199 (1977).
70. D.R. Green, F.J. Rosenbaum, and W.F. Pickard, Biological effects of microwaves on pupae of Tenebrio molitor, in: "Symposium on Biological Effects and Measurement of Radiofrequency/Microwaves HEW Publ. (FDA) 77-8026, D.G. Hazzard, ed., Rockville, MD. (1977).
71. R.G. Olsen, Constant dose microwave irradiation of insect pupae, Proc. Biol. Eff. E.M. Waves, XIX Gen. Assembly, Int. Union Radio Sci., Helsinki, August (1978).
72. W.F. Pickard and R.G. Olsen, Developmental effects of microwaves in Tenebrio molitor: Experiments to detect possible influences of radiation frequency and of culturing protocols, p. 66. In: Abstracts of the 1977 USNC/URSI Symposium on Biological Effects of Electromagnetic Waves. National Academy of Sciences, Washington, D.C. (1977)
73. C. Osborne, Studies on the biological effects of 200 mc, in: Investigators' Conference on Biological Effects of Electronic Radiating Equipments, Rome Air Development Center, Air Research and Development Command, Rome, N.Y., ASTIA Document No. AD 214 693, p. 20. (1959)
74. C. Osborne, Studies on the biological effects of 200 mc, in: "Proceedings of the Second Annual Tri-Service Conference on Biological Effects of Microwave Energy, E.G. Pattishall and F. Banghart, eds., University of Virginia, Charlottesville, ASTIA Document No. AD 131 477, 1958, p. 196 (1958).
75. A.J. Giarola, and W.F. Krueger, Continuous exposure of chicks and rats to electromagnetic fields, IEEE, Trans MTT 22:432 (1974).
76. D.I. McRee, P.E. Hamrick, J.E. Zinkl, P. Thaxton, and C.R. Parkhurst, Some effects of exposure of the Japanese quail embryo to 2.45 GHz microwave radiation, in: "Biologic Effects of Nonionizing Radiation, P.E. Tyler, ed., Ann. N.Y. Acad. Sci. 247:377 (1975).
77. D.I. McRee and P.E. Hamrick, Exposure of Japanese Quail embryos to 2.45 GHz microwave radiation during development. Radiat. Res. 71:355 (1977).
78. J. Laskey, D. Dawes, and M. Howes, Progress report on 2450 MHz irradiation of pregnant rats and the effect on the fetus. in: "Radiation Bioeffects Summary Report PHS USDHEW, BRH IDBE-70, Rockville, MD, pp. 167-173 (1970).

79. F. Dietzel, Effects of non-ionizing electro-magnetic radiation on the development and intrauterine implantation of the rat, in: "Biologic Effects of Nonionizing Radiation," P.E. Tyler, ed., Ann. N.Y. Acad. Sci., 247:367 (1975).
80. F. Dietzel, and W. Kern, Abortion following ultra-shortwave hyperthermia animal experiments, Arch. Gynakol. 209:445 (1970).
81. F. Dietzel, W. Kern, and R. Steckenmesser, Deformity and intrauterine death after short-wave therapy in early pregnancy in experimental animals, Munch. Med. Wschr. 114:228 (1972).
82. J.C. Lin, J.C. Nelson, and M.E. Ekstrom, Effects of repeated exposure to 148 MHz radiowaves on growth and hematology of mice, Radio Science, 14: 173 (1979).
83. M.E. Chernovetz, D.R. Justesen, N.W. King, and J.E. Wagner, Teratology, survival, and reversal learning after fetal irradiation of mice by 2450 MHz microwave energy, J. Microwave Power 10:391 (1975).
84. M.E. Chernovetz, D.R. Justesen, and A.F. Oke, A teratologic study of the rat: microwave and infrared radiations compared, Radio Sci. 12:191 (1977).
85. S.M. Michaelson, R. Guillet, M.A. Catallo, J. Small, G. Inamine and F.W. Heggeness, Influence of 2450 MHz microwaves on rats exposed in utero, J. Microwave Power 11:165 (1976).
86. S.M. Michaelson, R. Guillet, and F.W. Heggeness, The influence of microwave exposure on functional maturation of the rat, Proc. 17th Hanford Biology Symposium "Developmental Toxicology of Energy - Related Pollutants, Department of Energy Symposium Series 47, D. Mahlum et al., eds., pp. 300-316, CONF 771017 TIC. USDOE NTIS Springfield, VA. (1978).
87. E. Berman, J.B. Kinn, and H.B. Carter, Observations of mouse fetuses after irradiation with 2.45 GHz microwaves, Health Physics 35:791 (1978).
88. J.C. Nelson, J.C. Lin, and M.E. Ekstrom (1979). "Teratogenic effects of RF radiation on mice, "Presented at Bioelectromagnetics Symposium, Seattle, Washington, June 18-22.
89. D.I. McRee and P. Nawrot, Exposure of pregnant mice to 2.45 GHz microwave radiation, Presented at Bioelectromagnetics Symposium, Seattle, Washington, June 18-22 (1979).
90. R.P. Jensh, J. Ludlow, L. Weinburg, W.H. Vogel, T. Rudder, and R. L. Brent, "Studies concerning the postnatal effects of protracted low dose prenatal 915 MHz microwave radiation," Teratology 17:21 (1978).
91. R.P. Jensh, J. Ludlow, I. Weinberg, W.H. Vogel, T. Rudder and R.L. Brent, Teratogenic effects on rat offspring of non-thermal chronic prenatal microwave irradiation. Teratology, 15:14A (1977).

92. R.P. Jensh, J. Ludlow, L. Weinberg, W.H. Vogel, T. Rudder, and R.L. Brent, "Studies concerning the protracted prenatal exposure to a non-thermal level of 2450 MHz microwave radiation in the pregnant rat," Teratology 17:48 (1978).
93. R.P. Jensh, and J. Ludlow, Behavioral teratology: application in low dose chronic microwave irradiation studies, in: "Neural and Behavioral Teratology, T. V. N. Persand, ed., MTP Press Ltd., Lancaster, England (1980).
94. M.E. Chernovetz, D.R. Justesen, and D.M. Levinson, Acceleration and deceleration of fetal growth of rats by 2450 MHz microwave radiation, in: S. Stuchly, ed., IMPI, Edmonton, Alberta, Canada (1979).
95. M.E. Chernovetz, D. Reeves, and D.R. Justesen, "Teratology in rats exposed to 2450 MHz microwaves at intense and intermediate dose rates," Presented at Bioelectromagnetics Symposium, Seattle, Washington, June 18-22, (1979).
96. E. Berman, H.B. Carter, and D. House, "Observations of rat fetuses after irradiation with 2.45 GHz (CW) microwaves," Presented at Bioelectromagnetics Symposium, Seattle, WA, June 18-22, (1979).
97. D. Conover, J. Lary, and E. Foley, "Induction of teratogenic effects in rats by 27.12 MHz RF radiation," Presented at the 1978 Symposium on Electromagnetic Fields in Biological Systems, Ottawa, Canada, June 27-30 (1978).
98. M.E. O'Connor, Mammalian teratogenesis and radiofrequency fields, Proc. IEEE 68: 56 (1980).
99. P. Gruenwald, Mechanisms of abnormal development, Arch. Path. 44:398 (1947).
100. G.J. Wilson, Experimental studies on congenital malformations. J. Chron. Dis. 10:111 (1959).
101. J.A. Cameron, Termination of early pregnancy by artificial fever, Proc. Soc. Exp. Biol. and Med., 52:76 (1943).
102. M.J. Edwards, Congenital malformations in the rat following induced hyperthermia during gestation, Teratology 1:173 (1968).
103. M.J. Edwards, Congenital defects in guinea pigs: fetal resorptions, abortions, and malformations following induced hyperthermia during early gestation, Teratology 2:313 (1969).
104. L.H. Garrison, The effect of fever on the development of the rat incisor, J. Dental Res. 19:215 (1940).
105. C. Hsu, Influence of temperature on development of rat embryos, Anat. Rec. 100:79 (1948).
106. L.V. Martson and V.M. Voronina, Experimental study of the effect of a series of phosphoroorganic pesticides (Dipterex and Imidan) on embryogenesis, Environ. Health Perspec. 13:121 (1976).

CATARACTOGENESIS INDUCED BY RF AND MW ENERGY

Björn M. Tengroth

Department of Ophthalmology
Karolinska Institute
S-104 01 Stockholm, Sweden

INTRODUCTION

Since the end of the 19th century intense nonionizing radiation has been considered a biological threat. The research work in those days were of a surprisingly good standard, and some of the results from this time are still relevant.

Solar eclipse burns of the eye and some of the hazards reported on from carbon arc sources were studied both epidemiologically and experimentally during the first decades of this century. The hazards reported from the radiation in the visible region of the spectrum were mainly concerned with retinal burns and the consequent impairment of vision. Reports on cataract formation from infrared radiation were not fully understood from a pathophysiological viewpoint until after the first world war, but the term glassblower's cataract was well established for more than a century prior to this time.

The technical development during and after the second world war not only produced powerful radiation sources but also new quality radiation. The radar technique and later the masers, both working in the MHz and GHz bands as well as in the optical region of the spectrum, are examples of this development.

The mechanisms for the ionizing radiation's interaction with the tissues are rather well penetrated and the legal regulations and rules for handling ionizing radiation are developed all over the world. The need for corresponding rules for nonionizing radiation has first been recognized during the last decades, and hundreds of reports from epidemiological and experimental studies have appeared with increasing frequency. However, the agreement between these reports is still lacking in many fields. In this paper we are only concerned with the cataractogenous effects of microwave exposure. No serious reports on cataract formation as a result of radiofrequency radiation exposure have up to now been published, and the physical background for such effects would be very doubtful.

Definition

Most of our knowledge on the formation of cataracts and other lens changes secondary to exposure for microwaves is concerned with four main frequencies, i.e. 0.9 GHz, 2.45 GHz, 3.2 GHz and 9 GHz, either continuous wave or pulsed.

The Eye

The eye has been of the greatest interest in the discussions on the hazardous effects of nonionizing radiation, as this organ has a number of unique features compared to other organs of the human body. Visual impairment has been reported as the result of retinal burns, cataract formation and corneal clouding, all secondary to the exposure for electromagnetic radiation.

Electromagnetic radiation of wavelengths reaching from 370 nm in the ultraviolet to the near infrared in the region of 1 μm can be focused by the cornea and the lens to the posterior portion of the eye, i.e. the retina and the choroid. Radiation with longer wavelengths, as microwaves, is influenced by the orbital anatomy. Only between 400 and 770 nm the radiation should be considered as the adequate stimulus of the eye, i.e. light. Even if the microwaves cannot be focused by the optics of the eye, one has to know something about the optical properties in order to understand the deleterious effects that appear in these medias as a result of microwave exposure.

In order to work as a focusing system, the medias of the eye have to be transparent. The cornea, that consists of a number of different layers mainly built up by collagen fibres, polysaccharides and water, is through a regular arrangement completely transparent in its normal stage. No blood vessels penetrate this tissue and the nutrition has to depend upon other transport mechanisms. Active ion pumps as well as passive transportation across the different membranes take care of this delicate task, and these complicated mechanisms are still far from understood.

The Lens

In order to understand the effects of microwaves, a description of the lens and its physiology as well as the mechanism of cataract formation is necessary.

The lens is a continuously growing tissue of normally excellent transparency. Furthermore, the lens can change its form during most of the human life. It is the focusing device of the eye. Not only the form but also the index of refraction can be altered as a result of the interrelationship of the lens fibres.

The lens epithelium, i.e. the cell layer that produces the lens fibres throughout life, is situated underneath the elastic lens capsule. In the embryonic lens this epithelium forms a lens vesicle and later an embryonic nucleus. The lens capsule is a true basement membrane produced by the epithelial cells. It is thicker in the anterior portion than in the posterior portion of the lens. The epithelial cells elongate so that they reach from pole to pole to form the lens fibres, and they lose their cell nuclei. Whereas the lens fibres in the embryonic stage go from pole to pole to give the lens a spherical form, the continuous development is characterized by the formation of unequally long fibres. This means that they do not reach from pole to pole but terminate to form a Y-shaped suture. This results in a precision in the lens fibre joint and creates an eliptical form. After birth the sutures will be less regular and the Y-shape is turned into a more dendritic shape. In the adult lens the epithelium can only be seen in the anterior and equatorial portions of the subcapsular region, and only in the equator the fibres are formed and concentrically layered around the lens. From an optical viewpoint different layers can be defined in the lens, as the older parts will be more sclerotic. An embryonic, fetal, infantile and adult nucleus can be differentiated, as well as the cortex, the epithelium and the capsule. These zones will have a slight difference in refractive index. The hexagonal lens fibres will lose their nuclei so that the central part of the lens will be transparent. The lens has no nerves or blood vessels. Its metabolism is arranged through active and passive transportation of different substances.

Active transportation into the lens is performed through pumps of potassium, inositol and amino acids. Passive transportation takes place through diffusion or leak of water, chloride, glucose, and synthesis of certain protein and glutathione is also of importance. The complex enzymatic systems and transportation routes are of the greatest importance to withhold transparency, and one can easily understand how temperature changes and eventually other agents will interfere with these systems, which all are in equilibrium.

The Cataract

Opacities in the lens can result in decreased visual acuity, and these opacities are generally referred to as cataract. However, the term cataract can have different meanings, and certainly cataract is a clinical diagnosis when it can be visualized in retro-illumination. The number of different lens changes discussed in respect to radiation effects cannot all be attributed to cataract formation. Vacuoles, cysts, exfoliations and discontinuation zones in different parts of the lens do not necessarily relate to cataract formation.

Cataract formation is not a part of aging but something abnormal, even if 60-70% of all humans above the age of 70 can show cataractous changes. The mechanisms behind cataract formation, however, are not at all fully understood. This is apparent from the development of the lens, where areas are formed at different times as well as in a different way. The different mechanisms for cataract formation will be briefly summarized.

The newly formed fibres might be formed opaque, which is the case in congenital or developmental cataract, and may affect only small parts of the continuously growing lens. This resembles the rings in a tree, where it is possible to see changes in climate during certain periods by the analyses of these rings.

The opacification of previously clear lens fibres is often a disturbance of the youngest and therefore most vulnerable fibres, i.e. in the clear subcapsular zone. Hypocalcemia or hyperglycemia are typical metabolic disturbances. Concussion can also affect the fibres. The senile cataract is often the result of opacification of older fibres. Generally disturbances in the ionic balance will cause breakdown of cell membranes and cause local oedema in the lens fibre cells.

Formation of granular material can be seen to replace the new fibres if the metabolism of the epithelial cells is disturbed. This is the case in some radiation cataracts after exposure to ionizing radiation. The same is seen in toxic, metabolic and complicated cataracts. The mitotic activity of the cells first decreases and later increases, and cellular debris or proliferation of cells takes place in the subcapsular zone and migrates and concentrates to the posterior pole. With careful examination this can be observed also in the anterior portion as the clear zone is obliterated.

Pigment may accumulate, as is the case in the senile nuclear cataract called cataracta brunescens or even nigra.

The deposition of foreign material is seen as a result of accumulation of certain drugs.

To explain the opacities from a purely physical basis one must remember that the transparency of the normal lens is based on small spatial fluctuations in the number of protein molecules over dimensions comparable to the wavelength of light. Owing to the high concentration of these molecules in the lens, none scatters light independently of another. Cataract is thus explained by large molecular aggregates or by separation of molecules due to entry of water.

Gross changes, such as separation of the lens fibres, cause local variations in the refractive index and a proportionately larger amount of light scatter. Ultrastructure studies (1-4) of cataract show granules in the cytoplasm and electron dense inclusions, which are compatible with molecular aggregation and vesical formation of the cytoplasm. If the light scatter is compensated for by holographic filters, the degradation of image formation is improved when studying cataractous lenses _in vitro_. This supports the scatter theory (4). The senile cortical cataract might be explained by the fluctuations in _the orientational order of the proteins_ (5).

Whereas the ionizing radiation primarily will affect the germinal epithelium in the lens equator, changing the mitotic rate and affecting fibre formation, the nonionizing radiation results in a temperature increase. This in itself will result in a coagulation of proteins as well as an alteration in epithelial cell metabolism and function. The acute temperature change caused by infrared radiation is attributed to heat transportation from the iris pigment, where the radiation is absorbed, to the part of the lens capsule covered by the iris, with a thickening of the capsule as well as true exfoliation as a result. A more chronic exposure will lead to changes in the germinal epithelium, with the same result as after exposure to ionizing radiation. (Fig. 1-5).

Microwaves

High power microwaves, which might be suspected of being health hazards, are mainly emitted by radar equipment and microwave ovens. One of the main effects on the eye is cataractogenic. In a number of papers and articles the problems and risks of this radiation have been discussed by Michaelson (6-10).

In general one can say that microwave irradiation at thermal levels causes a number of changes in the eye, and mainly in the lens. Intense heat will in the acute stage give rise to conjunctival hyperemia, edema in the cornea, inflammation in the iris, and cloudiness in the lens. However, at these levels the heat is so strong that it is not bearable for a human being. The more interesting levels of irradiation will therefore be when the heat sensation is negligible and where there is a risk for a temperature change in the lens that slowly will result in tissue damage.

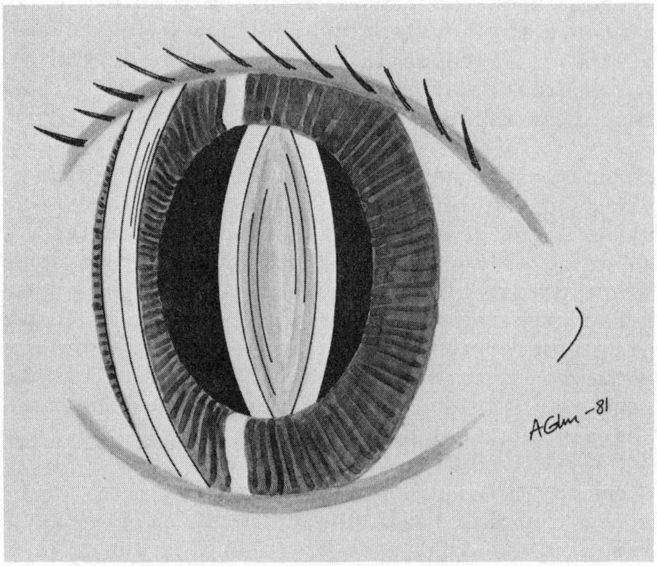

Fig. 1. Optical section of the anterior segment of the eye showing the cornea and the lens. Schematic drawing.

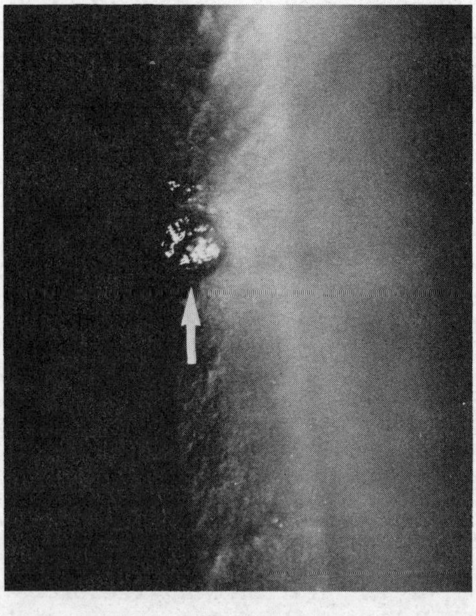

Fig. 2. Anterior subcapsular vacuoles (arrow). Slit lamp photo.

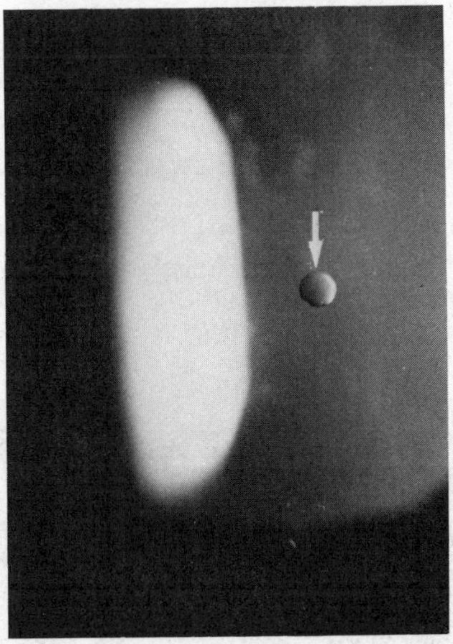

Fig. 3. Posterior subcapsular vacuole (arrow). Slit lamp photo.

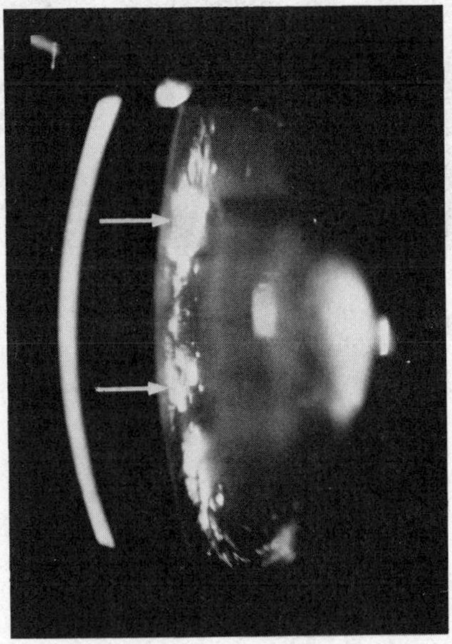

Fig. 4. Hydrated lens fibres forming wedge shaped opacities in the anterior cortex (arrows). Slit lamp photo.

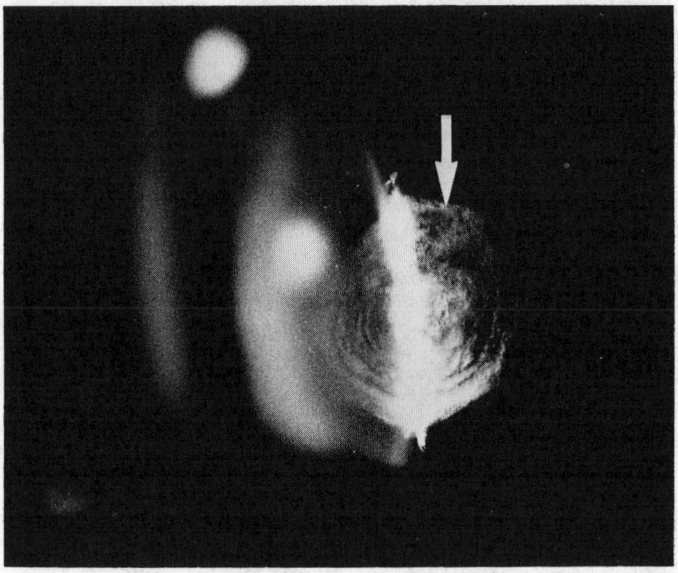

Fig. 5. Posterior subcapsular cataract. Slit lamp photo.

The more the frequency is increased, the more superficial is the thermal effect. One also knows that repeated exposure could result in damage, even if the level of irradiation in each exposure is below the threshold level (11-14). One also knows that pulsed microwave fields are stronger cataractogenic than the continuous field, at the same average power flux density.

From the detailed studies of the ultrastructural changes in the lens after exposure to microwaves, one can conclude that there is not only a pure thermal effect on the lens but also changes in cell metabolism and activity that will give secondary changes in the lens. To characterize these effects as non-thermal could be discussed, as the alteration that takes place in the cells might very well be the result of a temperature change.

A temperature rise secondary to the exposure for microwaves may result in the above mentioned changes. It is therefore impossible to talk about any specific microwave cataract with a characteristic morphology as has been proposed by some authors.

Epidemiological human studies in the modern sense of the term have never been performed. One of the reasons for this is that the population handling microwave equipment or exposed to significant amounts of microwave radiation is small and very often exposed to other types of radiation as well. Age matched studies of radar personnel have been presented (15-16) but one lacks information concerning exposure to other radiation sources or a thorough hereditary background story that rules out lens disease. It would be rather difficult to perform such studies, and I do not think that we will ever be able to organize them. However, one must not forget that the problem of the microwave cataract from a pure scientific viewpoint is more psychological than medical.

From a practical and clinical viewpoint a cataract that results in visual impairment is of interest. From the literature on microwaves it is difficult to show any such cases, as other cataractogenous agents might have intervened in the few cases presented. It is on the other hand apparent, from what has been said about the background for cataract formation, that it is not only possible but also probable that microwave exposure should be able to result in the acceleration of any pathological event in the lens or add to any other traumatic or metabolic disturbance. This is of the greatest importance and should be taken into account whenever safety measures and standards are discussed.

It is quite natural that a "new" radiation source, as the radar or the microwave oven, will rise the curiosity not only of the people exposed but also of my colleagues in the medical profession.

As a private practitioner, an eye-doctor will see a number of patients with unilateral or bilateral cataracts in age groups where he does not expect such changes to appear. This has always been the case. He now wants to satisfy his curiosity and will ask the patient about other diseases or exposure to external agents - traumatic, chemical, pharmacological or radiational - that could explain the cataract. The patient exposed to a new tool, as a radar equipment or a video display unit, will prabably mention this instead of discussing the family history of cataracts, which very few have any knowledge of. The problem is that the ophthalmologist, however trained in science, will soon have an impression of a connection between the radiation exposure and the cataract. This impression might be stronger as a number of patients have a similar story, and soon he presents the result of this "impression science" as an epidemiological study in a more public way. The result is apparent, and we would probably not be in this wonderful place if it had not been for these reports.

In humans the reports are of two different kinds. We have a few retrospective studies, as the ones presented by Appleton (15) et al., where no changes in exposed personnel could be shown as compared to controls. However, as can be seen from his first report, the conclusions might be an error.

Table I shows figures taken from Appleton et al. (15).

	Number		Opacities	
	Controls	Exposed	Controls	Exposed
20-29	37	15	0 (0%)	0 (0%)
30-39	32	21	6 (19%)	5 (24%)
40-49	38	31	10 (26%)	10 (32%)
50-59	20	18	6 (30%)	7 (39%)
60-69	8	6	1 (13%)	4 (67%)
	135	91		

In a later study with a total of 1.542 exposed and 801 controls no difference was seen (16).

In a study we performed (17) on microwave workers, the exposure levels were well above the safety level, some times 10 times that. Where a discomfort of heat sensation had been experienced an over-representation of opacities was demonstrated in the exposed group, but none showed a clinical cataract. The retinal changes that we reported on I will mention later.

In the number of reports presented by Zaret (18-19) no scientific evidence for a connection between the observed changes and exposure to microwave radiation can be demonstrated.

It is apparent that one cannot extrapolate the results from animal experiments to humans, for a number of reasons. There is a clear difference between species among the experimental animals, and this difference is probably more pronounced if one compares animals and man. As pointed out by Paulsson (20) in our group, there is a considerable difference between humans, only because of the anatomy of the face and orbit. The more proptosed the eyes are, the greater the risk for a high dose of microwave radiation in the S-band. This dependence upon eye position, that has been mentioned when the results of experiments on rabbits and monkeys have been explained, is well documented (21). As can be observed on the curves (fig. 9) taken from Paulsson (20) a considerable concentration of microwaves in the 2.45 MHz band takes place in the vitreous and the retina, and the dependence upon eye position is also demonstrated. Another difficulty is the time it takes for a cataract to develope. The cataracts reported on in humans might have developed during decades whereas in animals it would only have taken days or months.

Experimental Studies

One of the purposes of the experimental studies performed has been to estimate the power levels below which no cataracts or other lens changes can be induced.

Since 1948 a number of experimental studies on rabbits, monkeys, dogs and rats have been performed in order to estimate the level of microwave radiation which forms cataracts. However, not until the geometry of the near and far field of the microwave radiation was explained by Guy (22) and others in 1975 experimental studies have been of value.

The experimental studies are the basis for our understanding of microwave cataract. The studies of Guy (22) et al. as well as Ummersen and Cogan (23) not only show us the complexity of the radiation, but also one resembling the type of change one observes after feeding animals with galactose.

There is no doubt, as has been mentioned earlier, that there is a cummulative effect of microwave irradiation on the lens. Also we know that the pulsed radiation is more dangerous in this respect than the continuous field.

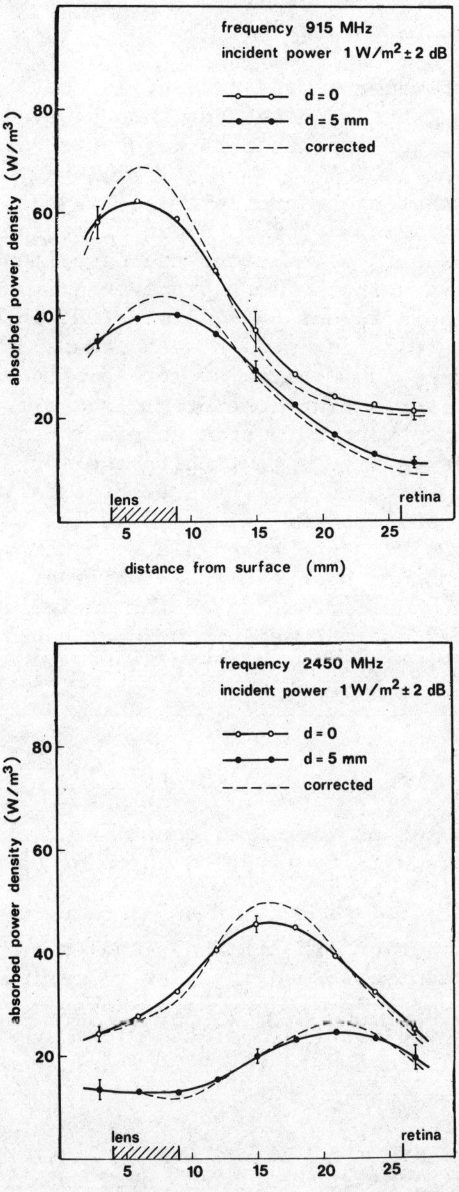

Fig. 6. Absorbed power pattern in the eye of a microwave irradiated model of a human head.

Above at 915 MHz and below at 2450 MHz.

The cataractogenic agents can also combine in the induction of cataracts. Experimental studies, where subthreshold irradiation of microwaves have been used in diabetic rabbit, have shown that the cataract development accelerates and that some cataractogenic agents can combine in the induction of cataract, even if each of them is given in a subcataractogenic dosage (24).

The combined effects of microwave radiation and galactose feeding in the rat lens, as reported from our group (25), is of interest in this context. Using 2.45 GHz CW or 3.2 GHz pulsed it was possible to show that a combination of microwave and glactose could result in cataract formation, whereas microwaves at this level of exposure as well as galactose diet separately did not produce any cataract, as can be seen in Table II. The techniques used for examing the eye was slip-lamp biomicroscopy, microradiography, light and electron microscopy. From this study it is concluded:

1. Rats irradiated with repeated sublethal microwave doses do not develop visible lens opacities. Electron microscopic examination shows extracellular vacuoles.

2. Rats given a diet contining 12% galactose do not develop visible lens opacities or microscopical changes.

3. Rats given a combination of galactose and repeated low microwave doses develop anterior subcapsular lens opacities, which biomicroscopically differ markedly from galactose cataract. Vacuoles appear similar to those seen in animals subjected to high microwave doses.

4. Microwave irradiation and galactose feeding seem to potentiate each other's damaging effect on the lens

When we reported (17) on retinal changes we did not know if there really could be any connection between the intense exposure to microwave and these changes. Experimental studies (26) using 550 W/cm^2 average power (3.1 GHz pulsed) revealed electron microscopic changes in che rabbit retina when exposed for 1 hour 53 times during 100 days. This can certainly not be taken as a proof of a connection in the human study mentioned, but I think one shall bear in mind that temperature changes in the delicate neuronal tissues of the retina might have to be taken into consideration when the hazardous effects of microwave exposure are discussed.

Table II

Experimental design and summary of results.

Treatment	Method: Slit-lamp biomicroscopy	Method: Micro-radiography	Method: Light and electron microscopy
A. Microwave irrad.			
1. 1.5 kW/m^2 2.45 GHz CW	neg.	pos.	not studied
2. 1.0 kW/m^2 3.2 GHz pulsed repeated exp.	neg.	not studied	pos.
B. Galactose feeding 12%	neg.	neg.	neg.
C. Galactose feeding 12% + Microwave irrad. 0.5 kW/m^2 3.2 GHz pulsed repeated exp.	pos.	pos.	pos.

SUMMARY

As can be concluded from this review, microwave cataract is not a common, nor a serious problem in the clinical ophthalmology. From what we know of how a cataract is formed, one cannot expect the microwave cataract to be of a certain type. It is of the greatest importance, however, to notice that the basis for microwave cataract formation, as well as the data from some of the experimental work, suggest that the combined effect of microwaves and any other cataractogeneous agent, or a genetic background for a senile or presenile cataract, might accelerate the cataract formation at exposure levels that are fairly low. How this should be handled from a legal or standard setting point of view I am certainly not prepared to comment on.

REFERENCES

1. T. Kuwabara, J. H. Kinoshita, and D. G. Cogan, Electron microscope study of galactose-induced cataract, Invest. Ophthal. 8:133 (1969).
2. B. T. Philipson, Changes in the lens related to reduction in transparency, Exp. Eye Res. 16:29 (1973).
3. A. Brini and J. Flamant, Cataracta glaucomatosa acuta, Exp. Eye Res. 16:19 (1973).
4. D. Miller, J. L. Zuckerman, and G. D. Reynolds, Holographic filter to negate the effect of cataract, Arch. Ophthal. 90:323 (1973).
5. R. A. Schachar and S. A. Solin, The microscopic protein structure of the lens with a theory for cataract formation as determined by Raman spectroscopy of intact bovine lenses, Invest. Ophthal. 14:380 (1975).
6. S. M. Michaelson, Cutaneous perception of microwaves, J. Microwave Power 7:67 (1972).
7. S. M. Michaelson, Human exposure to nonionizing radiant energy - potential hazards and safety standards, Proc. IEEE 60:389 (1972).
8. S. M. Michaelson, Thermal effects of single and repeated exposures to microwaves - a review, Proc. Intern. Symp. Warsaw, Oct. 1973, pp. 1-14.
9. S. M. Michaelson, Microwave and radiofrequency radiation, World Health Organization, Document ICP/CEP 803 (1977).
10. S. M. Michaleson, Effects of exposure to microwaves problems and perspectives, Environ, Health Perspectives 8:133 (1974).
11. R. L. Carpenter, D. K. Biddle, and C. A. Van Ummersen, Opacities in the lens of the eye experimentally induced by exposure to microwave radiation, IRE Trans. on Medical Electronics, ME-7:152 (1960).
12. R. L. Carpenter, D. K. Biddle, and C. A. Van Ummersen, Biological effect of microwave radiation with particular reference to the eye, Proc. 3rd Intern. Conf. on Medical Electronics, London, England, 1960, pp. 401-408.
13. R. L. Carpenter and C. A. Van Ummersen, The action of microwave radiation on the eye, J. Microwave Power 3:3 (1968).
14. R. L. Carpenter, Experimental microwave cataract: A review. Biological Effect and Health Implications of Microwave Radiation, ed. S. F. Cleary, Symp. Proc. Richmond, Virginia, 1969, pp. 76-81.
15. B. Appleton and G. C. McCrossan, Microwave lens effects in humans, Arch. Ophthal. 88 (1972).
16. B. Appleton, S. Hirsch, R. O. Kinion, M. Soles, G. C. McCrossan, and R. M. Neidlinger, Microwave lens effects in humans, Arch. Ophthal. 93 (1975).

17. E. Aurell and B. Tengroth, Lenticular and retinal changes secondary to microwave exposure, Acta Ophthal. 51:764 (1973).
18. M. M. Zaret, Cataract following use of microwave oven, 2032 N. Y. State Journal of Med., Oct. 1974.
19. M. M. Zaret, I. T. Kaplan, and A. M. Kay, Clinical microwave cataracts, in: "Biological Effects and Health Implications of Microwave Radiation" ed. S. F. Cleary, Symp. Proc., Richmond, Virginia, 1969, p. 82.
20. L. E. Paulsson, Measurements of 0.915, 2.45 and 9.0 GHz absorption in the human eye. Presented at 1976 European Microwave Conf.
21. P. Kramar, C. Harris, A. F. Emery, and A. W. Guy, Acute microwave irradiation and cataract formation in rabbits and monkeys. J. Microwave Power 13:3 (1978).
22. A. W. Guy, J. C. Lin, P. Kramar, and A. F. Emery, Effects of 2450 MHz radiation on the rabbit´s eye, IEEE Trans. Microwave Theory, vol. MTT-23, 6 June, 1975.
23. C. A. van Ummersen, D. G. Cogan, Effects of microwave radiation on the lens epithelium in the rabbit´s eye, Arch. Ophthal. 94 (1976).
24. O. Hockwin and H.-R. Kock, Combined noxious influences, in: "Cataract and Abnormalities of the Lens", ed. John G. Bellows, published by Gune and Stratton, Inc. pp. 243-254 (1975).
25. E. Lydahl, L. E. Paulsson, B. Philipson, and P. Fagerholm, Combined effects of microwave irradiation and galactose feeding on the rat lens. Technical Report 91, Chalmers, Gothenburg, Sweden (1979).
26. L. E. Paulsson, Y. Hamnerius, H. A. Hansson, and J. Sjöstrand, Retinal damage experimentally induced by microwave radiation at 55 mW/cm^2, Acta Ophthal. 57:183 (1979).

INTERACTION OF RF AND MW WITH THE LIVING SYSTEMS: RESEARCH AND EXPERIENCE IN CHINA

K.C. Yee

Microwave Institute of the
Chekiang Medical College
Hangchow, China

The uses of radio and microwave radiation extend into all areas of our life and into basic and applied research in engineering, medicine and science. Some examples include radio and television broadcasting, wood and paper drying, plastic curing, food processing, medical treatment, biochemical analysis, radar, long distance telephone, satellite communication, burglar alarms, microwave ovens and so on. It should be noted that the number of devices that emit radio and microwave radiation are rapidly increasing, as is their use in consumer, medical and industrial applications.

The effects of microwave radiation on animals and humans have been a subject of important investigation. It is known that at sufficiently high-power levels they can produce heating and many associated adverse effects (1).

During the last seven years, we had conducted animal research studying the effects of microwave exposure. The results are discussed as follows:

I. Acute Effects of Microwave Exposure in Rats

1. The Measurement of Lethal Dose in Rats

The exposed rats were subjected to a 100 mW/cm^2 power density. After 3-4 minutes of radiation, most animals displayed more and more activities varying from restlessness to extreme agitation. As exposure continued for about 7-8 minutes, the rats panted. Marked vasodilation of skin mucous membranes were observed. The rats desperately attempted to escape from the cages. Finally, they became prostrate and died after ten to twenty-three minutes of exposure. The animals were rigid and their rectal temperatures elevated to 43 ^oC, which was 4-6 ^oC higher than that before radiation. The lethal time of this group when half of the rats died was 18 minutes. The lethal dose was 0.03 W.h/cm2. The death time of the animals at 80 mW/cm^2 power density group was greatly increased. The lethal time was 40 minutes and its lethal dose was 0.05 W.h/cm2. The animals were necropsied, and blood was found in lungs. There was blood settled in liver and bloodshut in brain.

2. Acute Microwave Effects on Blood Pressure, Respiration, ECG, Rectal and subcutaneous Temperatures in Rabbits

a) Blood Pressure: In 80 mW/cm^2 power density group, the rabbit's blood pressure fell about 6 mmHg. At 10 minutes after the on set of 1 hour radiation, the fall in pressure was about 16 mmHg. After the exposure was stopped, the blood pressure fell 9 mmHg in half an hour. The comparisons were made between the changes in their blood pressures. Its probability was < 0.05. In 40 mW/cm^2 power density group, the blood pressure fell slowly. After 10 min. of exposure the kymograph records showed the fall in blood pressure at about 4 mmHg. After radiation, the blood pressure rose 2-3 mmHg in half an hour. The comparisons between the changes in blood pressure were made. Its probability was < 0.05. In 10 mW/cm^2 power density group the fall in blood pressure was 3 mmHg. The probability was > 0.05. (See Fig. 1) No changes in blood pressure of control group were observed in 1 to 1.5 hours.

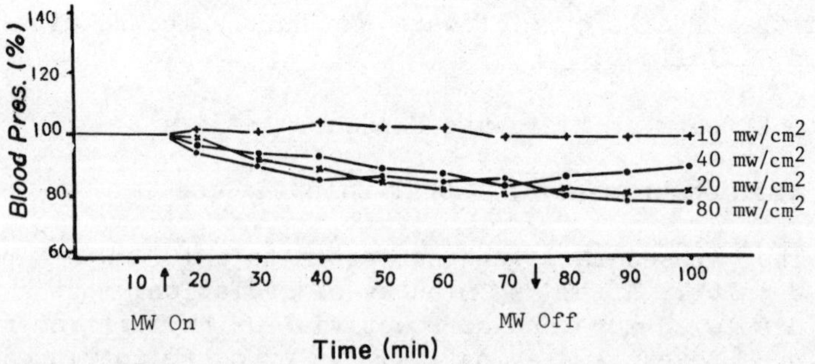

Fig. 1 The effects of microwave radiation on pressure.

Table 1. Relationship Between the Power Densities and Blood Pressure Drop

Pwr. Dens. / Avg. Blood Pressure Drop (mmHg)	80 mW/cm^2	40 mW/cm^2	20 mW/cm^2
After 10 min. Radiation	6	4	2
After 1 hr. Radiation	16	18	20
30 min. After Radiation End.	25	18	22

The acute microwave effect on the blood pressure at the first 10 minutes was almost a linear response. (See Table 1) The pressures drops were 6 mmHg for 80 mW/cm^2, 4 mmHg for 40 mW/cm^2, and 2 mmHg for 20 mW/cm^2.

For longer time, between the power densities and the pressure drops, there was a normal correlation function ($r = 0.9828$, $df = 4$, when 1% $r = 0.917$) excluding the 20 mW/cm^2 group. Because the probability of cardiac rhythmic disturbances of 20 mW/cm^2 group was more than 40 mW/cm^2, the pressure drop was also higher. This problem will be discussed in the sections on ECG and nonthermal effects.

b) Respiration: It is obvious that the effect of high power density on the respiratory rate is accelerative. In 80 mW/cm^2 group, the respiratory rate increased from 57 breaths/min. to 109 breaths/min. The change of respiratory rate in 40 mW/cm^2 was 55 breaths/min. Their probabilities were less than 0.05. The respiratory rate of 20 mW/cm^2 and 10 mW/cm^2 did not change very much. Their probabilities were greater than 0.05. The accelerative effect on the respiratory rate did not appear right after exposure. It usually occurred thirty minutes after the onset of exposure. (See Fig. 2) As the animal's temperature rose after radiation, the heat loss depended upon the acceleration of respiratory rate.

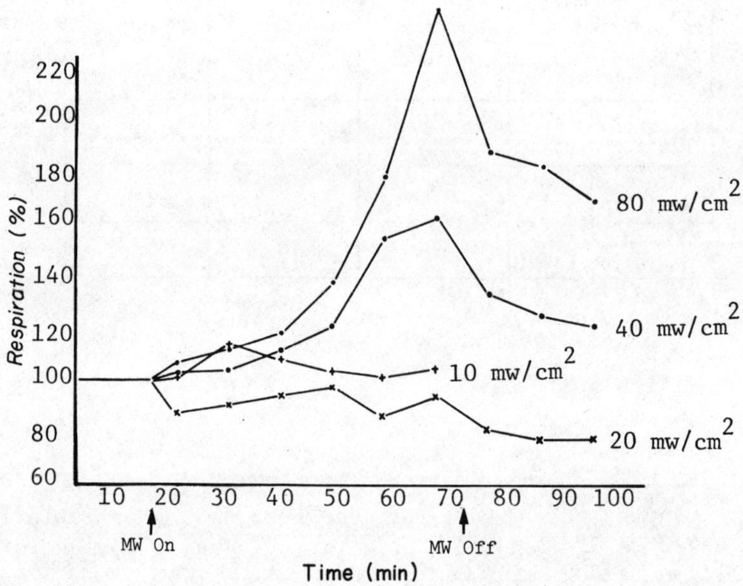

Fig. 2 The microwave effects on respiration.

c) Subcutaneous and Rectal Temperatures: The subcutaneous temperature of animals rose soon after radiation. The comparisons were made among the changes in subcutaneous temperature of 80 mW/cm^2, 40 mW/cm^2 and 20 mW/cm^2 groups. (See Fig. 3) Their probabilities were smaller than 0.05. At the end of 1 hour exposure, the temperature rose to the highest point, and it soon fell after radiation was turned off and returned to the pre-exposure level. Between the subcutaneous temperature and power densities there was a normal correlation function (r=0.9933, df=4, 1% r=0.917). (See Tab. 2)

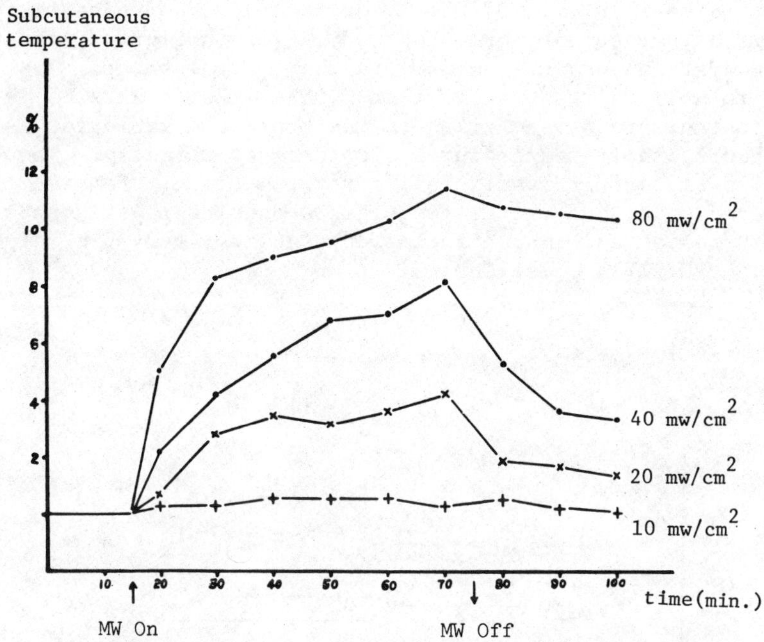

Fig. 3 Microwave effects on subcutaneous temperature.

Table 2. Relationship Between the Power Densities and the Rise of Subcutaneous Temperature.

Pwr. Dens. / Avg. Rise of Subcutaneous Temp. (°C)	80 mW/cm^2	40 mW/cm^2	20 mW/cm^2
After 1 hr. Radiation	5	3.1	1.6

The animal's rectal temperature slowly rose at the beginning of exposure, but it rose sharply after 20 minutes. The temperature reached the highest value at the end of the one hour exposure. The probabilities of 80 mW/cm^2 and 40 mW/cm^2 were smaller than 0.005. (See Fig. 4) The probability of 20 mW/cm^2 group was more than 0.05. For this group, the comparison was also made with the control group. Its probability was smaller than 0.001. The animals of the control group were fixed on the operation table for 1-1.5 hours, their temperatures also dropped slightly. The temperature gradually fell after radiation. Between the changes of the rectal temperature and the power densities there was a normal correlation function (r=0.9578, df=4, when 1% r=0.917). (See Tab. 3)

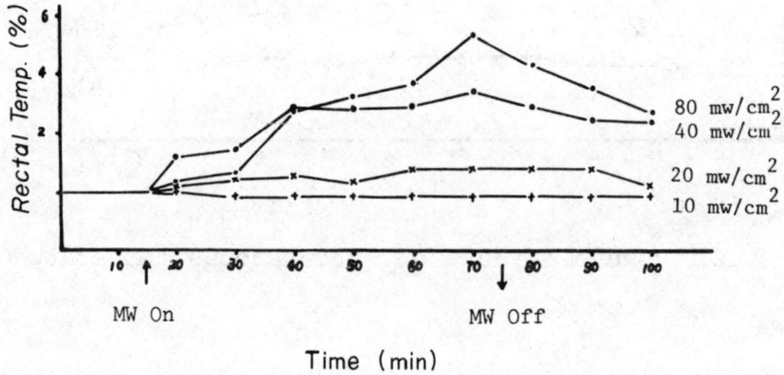

Fig. 4 Microwave effects on rectal temperature.

Table 3. Relationship Between the Power Densities and Rise of the Rectal Temperature.

Pwr. Dens. / Avg. Rise of Rectal Temp. (°C)	80 mW/cm^2	40 mW/cm^2	20 mW/cm^2
After 1 hr. Radiation	2	1.3	0.3

d) ECG: The value K of ECG decreased in most animals exposed to 80 mW/cm^2. The comparisons were made with the pre-exposure values of K. The change was obvious, and the probability is smaller than 0.01. The T/R&S increased after exposure. (See Tab 4.) The probability was smaller than 0.001. The K value returned to pre-exposure level soon after exposure. However, the T wave amplitude continued to increase for at least one hour and then recovered to pre-exposure level. In 40 mW/cm^2 power density group the of T/R&S wave increased slightly ($p < 0.05$), but there was no change in K and heart rate. (See Tab. 5)

Change in the K value of 20 mW/cm^2 group was smaller than that of 80 mW/cm^2 $p < 0.001$). The heart rates were faster than that of 40 mW/cm^2 group ($p < 0.01$), but there was no change in the T/R+S ($p > 0.05$). (See Tab. 6).

The specific effects of the microwave exposure of 20-80 mW/cm^2 on the ECG were the elevation of T wave, but after exposure its amplitude also recovered. (See Fig. 5)

Table 4. Effects of Microwave (80 mW/cm^2) on K, T/R&S of ECG and Heart Rate

Items / No. of Rabbits	K before	K after	T/R&S before	T/R&S after	Rate of Heart (beat/min.) before	Rate of Heart (beat/min.) after
1	0.37	0.28	0.33	0.56	250	316
2	0.35	0.30	0.10	0.60	230	261
3	0.31	0.29	0.27	0.45	230	261
4	0.32	0.29	0.27	0.36	273	300
5	0.33	0.31	0.82	0.85	300	333
6	0.31	0.27	0.41	0.71	333	428
7	0.38	0.28	0.70	0.55	400	400
8	0.35	0.33	0.30	0.41	286	300
9	0.37	0.28	0.17	0.39	250	461
10	0.36	0.31	0.39	0.53	240	300
11	0.34	0.29	0.39	0.64	273	316
12	0.30	0.38	0.56	0.44	273	261
P	< 0.01		< 0.001		< 0.01	

Table 5. Effects of Microwave (40mW/cm^2) on K, T/R&S of ECG and Heart Rate

No. of Rabbits \ Items	K before	K after	T/R&S before	T/R&S after	Rate of Heart (beat/min.) before	Rate of Heart (beat/min.) after
1	0.35	0.31	0.25	0.30	222	230
2	0.33	0.29	0.25	0.29	250	250
3	0.31	0.31	0.17	1.25	230	290
4	0.31	0.30	0.35	0.70	230	316
5	0.39	0.36	0.23	0.59	230	300
6	0.32	0.30	0.23	0.40	316	316
7	0.33	0.33	0.42	0.53	261	261
8	0.36	0.39	0.56	0.50	250	240
9	0.38	0.41	0.27	0.29	200	250
10	0.38	0.33	0.40	0.63	273	261
P	> 0.05		< 0.05		> 0.05	

Table 6. Effects of Microwave (20 mW/cm^2) on K, T/R&S of ECG and Heart Rate

No. of Rabbits \ Items	K before	K after	T/R&S before	T/R&S after	Rate of Heart (beat/min.) before	Rate of Heart (beat/min.) after
1	0.32	0.29	0.17	0.20	240	261
2	0.30	0.27	0.31	0.08	375	428
3	0.39	0.30	0.08	0.17	250	273
4	0.37	0.34	0.15	0.33	286	300
5	0.33	0.31	0.17	0.46	230	273
6	0.31	0.29	0.08	0.10	230	250
7	0.29	0.28	0.22	0.23	353	325
8	0.31	0.30	0.22	0.23	300	316
9	0.42	0.36	0.12	0.17	214	250
10	0.33	0.32	0.15	0.31	300	353
11	0.39	0.33	0.28	0.13	286	286
P	< 0.001		> 0.05		< 0.01	

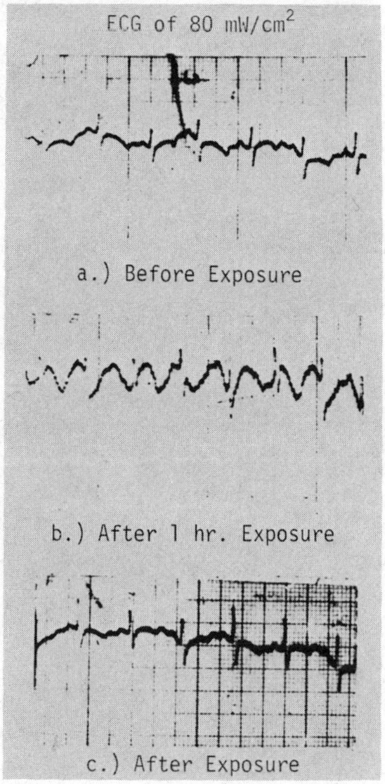

Fig. 5 The ECG of 80 mW/cm^2 group.

We had observed the ventricular tachycardia and bigeminus rhythm in the animals whose Q-T interval and K of ECG were decreased sharply. Their blood pressure fell greatly from 110 mmHg. to 50 mmHg during the rhythmic disturbances. After radiation, normal rhythm can recover in some animals. The depression of ST during the rhythmic disturbances means that the effective cardiac output decreases greatly which influence coronary blood supply. With the recovering of normal rhythm the blood pressure rose continuously in half an hour after taking off the radiation. The general condition of the animals completely improved. (See Fig 6). In only a few animals the rhythmic disturbance did not recover after stopping radiation, and their blood pressure continuously fell to 40 mmHg. Finally these animals died. (See Fig. 7 and 8).

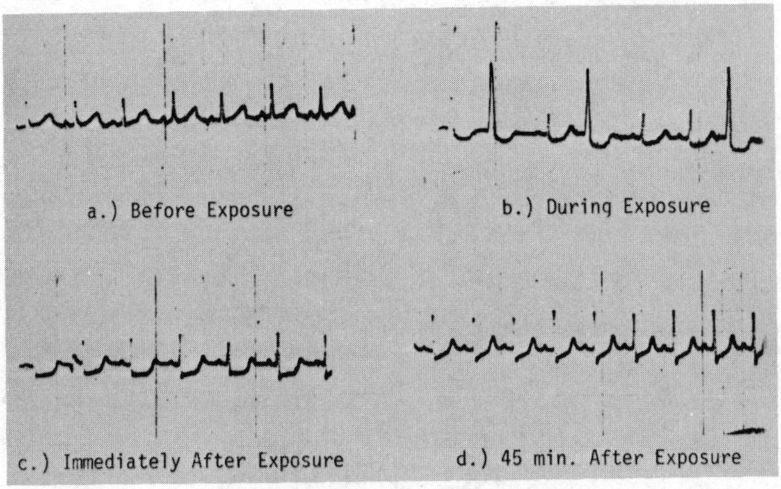

Fig. 6 ECG of 20 mW/cm^2 group. a. before microwave radiation, b. the multiventricular tachcardia during microwave radiation, c. after radiation the recovery of normal rhythm, but S-T still depressed, d. the S-T recovers forty-five min. after radiation.

General Discussion: When the animals were exposed to microwave radiation, some of the microwave energy was absorbed and converted into heat. The subcutaneous temperature rose as soon as animals were radiated by microwaves. The elevated subcutaneous temperature certainly caused the rise of rectal temperature, dilatation of artery walls, and fall of blood pressure. The animals could dissipate heat by accelerating respiration. There was a dose-response relationship between those changes and power densities. It is evident that thermal effects may play a significant role on acute effects of microwaves.

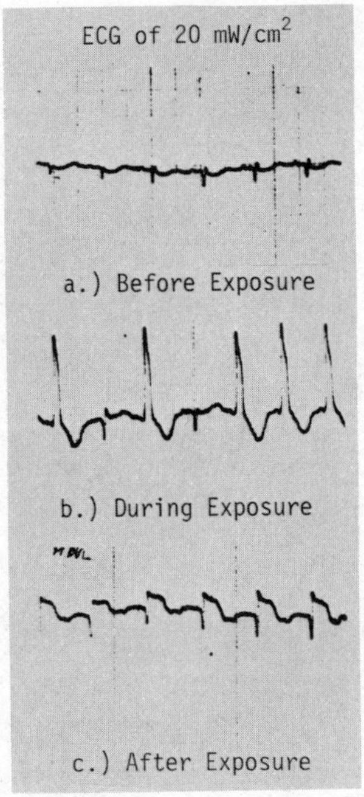

Fig. 7 Rhythmic disturbance (20 mW/cm^2) after microwave radiation, a. Normal ECG, b. Rhythmic disturbance (during radiation), and c. after exposure before death.

The large difference between the exposure standards of the United States and the USSR has been and continues to be a source of controversy (2.34). U.S. exposure standards are based principally on the understanding that the observed effects of radio and microwave radiation on animals are related to the heat generated from absorbed radio and microwave energy. Many of the earlier papers evaluating work in this field concluded that the only significant effect was the thermal one, and the insufficient evidence existed to substantiate the view that non-thermal effects were also of importance.

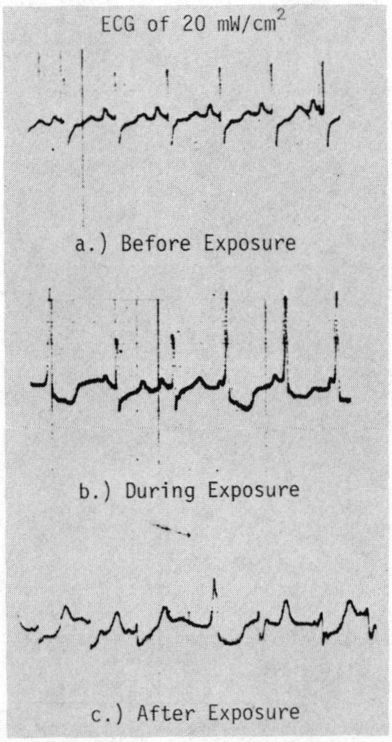

Fig. 8 The rhythmic disturbances of ECG (20 mW/cm^2), a. Normal ECG, b. the rhythmic disturbance during radiation, c. after exposure the normal rhythm didn't recover, the amplitude of T wave elevates and S-T depress. Finally the animal died.

In our experiment (5), the rectal temperature of animals (20 mW/cm^2) rose 0.3° C only, but there were changes of cardiac function including the decrease of K, Q-T interval of ECG, depression of S-T, and rhythmic disturbance. It is difficult to explain these changes in terms of thermal effects. The question remains whether the microwave radiation interferes with the excitability or conductivity of the heart. Further experiments on this subject will be needed.

II. Retinal Effects at Low-level Exposure

It is well known that the biological effects of high intensity microwave exposure are related to the local generation of heat. The organs most susceptible to microwave damage are the eyes and the testes, where heat dissipation is a problem. It is suspected that microwave can cause the formation of lens opacities. We have studied discrete populations of veterans who worked under several hundreds of uW/cm2 power density of microwave exposure. We didn't find visible changes of lens with conventional slit-lamp examinations, but many microwave workers complained about their fatigued eyes (4,6).

The nonthermal effects of microwave radiation are poorly understood. Some findings seem to point to the possible existence of a nonthermal factor as well. For instance, a delayed decrease in the ascorbic acid and glutathions have been demonstrated to occur in the irradiated lens.

The effects of low power density of microwave on the retinal potential in the rabbits were reported (7). The experiment is summarized as follows: Rabbits were first allowed to adapt to dark for 1 hour and then the anesthetic (urethane) was given by injection. The level of anesthesia was adjusted to a depth which would just prevent voluntary movement. Anesthetized rabbits were placed in a wooden bed.

The dark test-room was constructed of echosorb. Echosorb has a reflectivity of 1%. The metal electrode holder was replaced by plastic parts to eliminate any field interaction. Initial dark-adaptation was not disturbed by the manipulative procedures and records of retinal potential could be taken at once.

The retinal potential is an electrical potential developed between the inner and outer surfaces of the retina. The electrodes were a pair of cotton tufts sunken in 0.85% NaCl placed in the center of the cornea and the indifferent electrode was placed between the two eyes on a shaved area of the rabbit's forehead. The fluid surface tension kept the active electrode in position. This electrode system had less electrical disturbances due to movements of breathing (8). The active electrode and indifferent one were coupled to lowpass microwave filters (9) and then were connected to a double-sided cathode-follower unit and the input of the amplifiers (See Fig. 9). The output of the amplifiers was connected to a two-channel oscilloscope and a computer. The potentials were displayed on one beam of a double beam cathode ray tube; the other beam being used for the time tracing and recording of the marks of the light flashes, sometimes for the record of Visual Evoked Potential (VEP). Two channel of retinal potential and VEP are

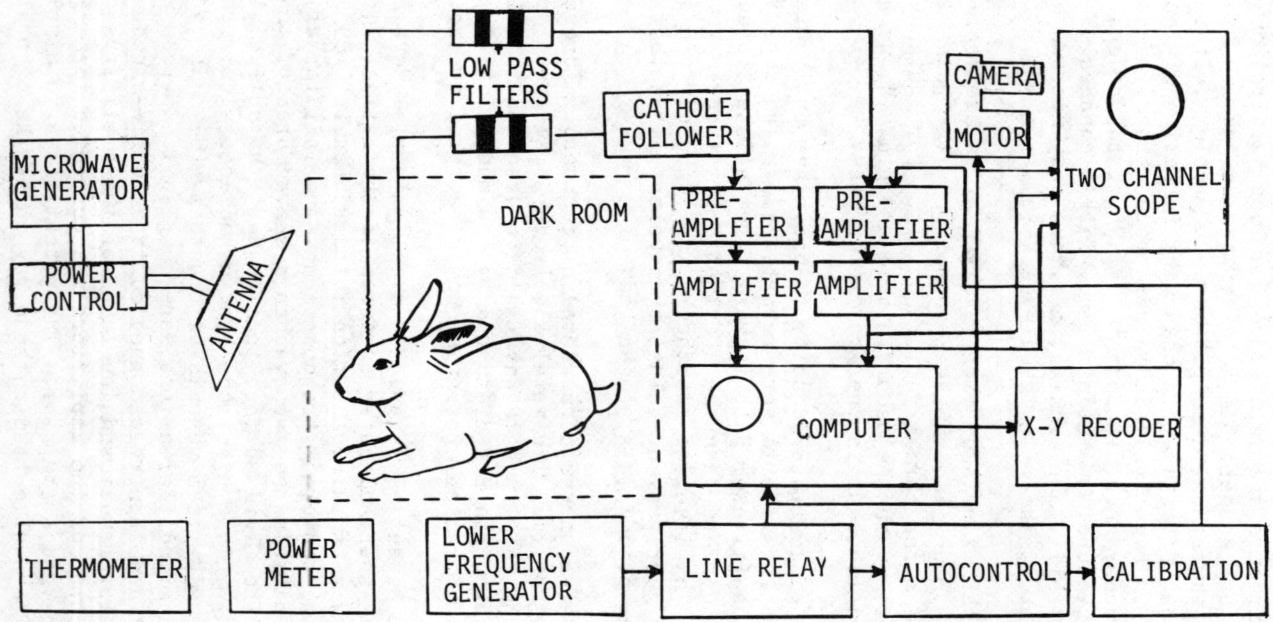

Fig. 9 Block diagram of instrumentation used to quantify retinal potential and visual evoked potential effects of microwave radiation in the rabbits.

amplified and displayed along with a master clock.

All channels were sampled by the computer's multi-channel analog- to-digital converter. The results of the analysis were displayed on a cathode ray tube and on X-Y instrument (10).

In the studies, a 6v. lamp white light source was used to provide a 1 s. flash once every 60 seconds. The light from the system passed through a plane of the pupil. The image of the light source lay fully within the pupil aperture. The size of the image in the pupil was approximately 3x2 mm.

We used pulsed microwave; 3 GHz. repeated frequency; 1875 pps. pulse width: 0.6us. We controlled the average power density at 700 uW/cm2.

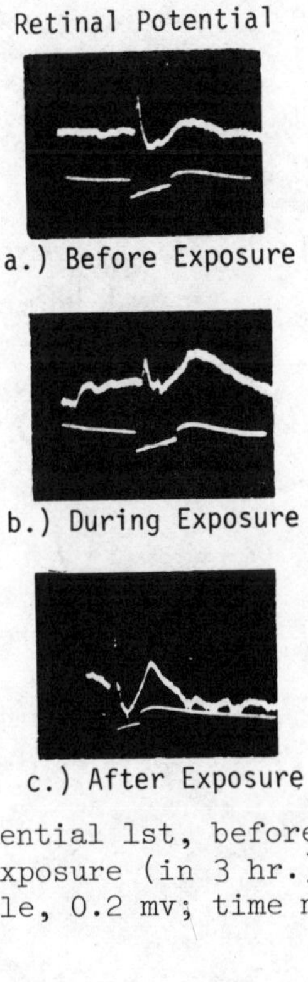

Fig. 10 Retinal potential 1st, before exposure. 2nd, during microwave exposure (in 3 hr.). 3rd, after exposure. Voltage scale, 0.2 mv; time marker, 1 second.

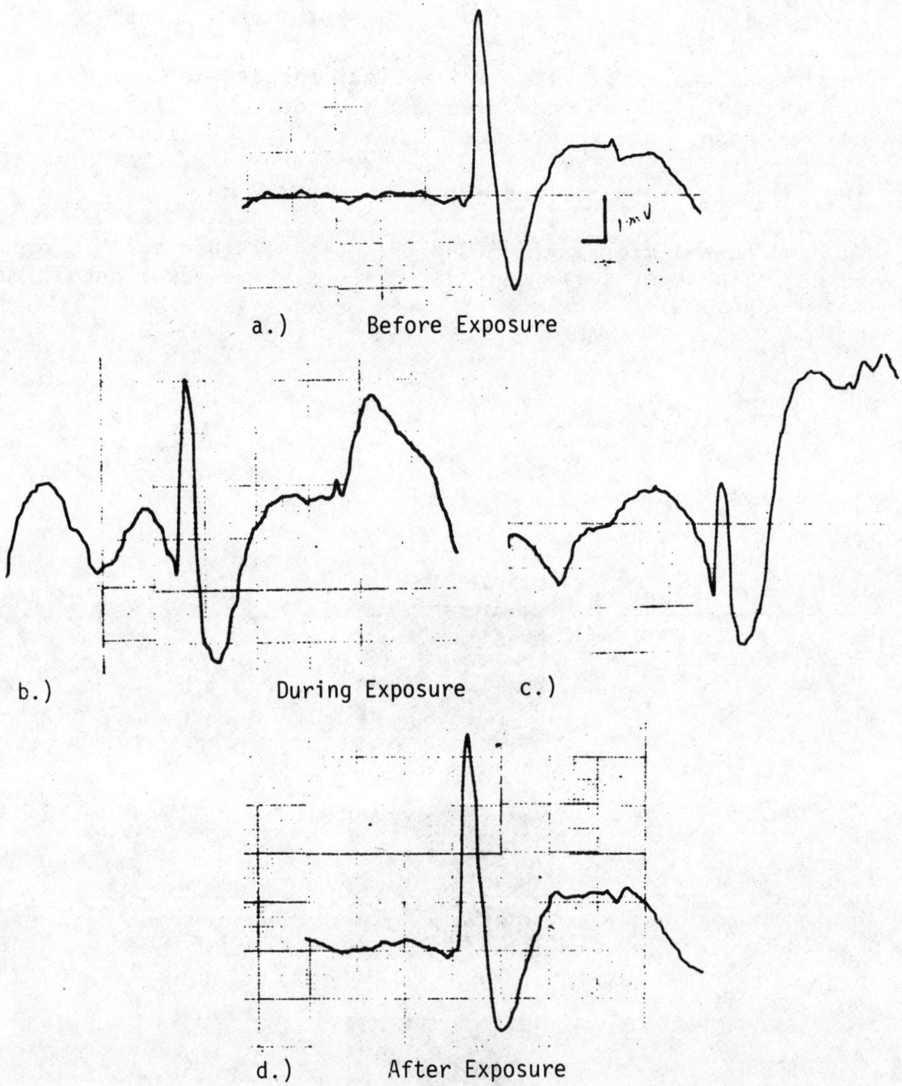

Fig. 11 Computer printout of superimposed curve of retinal potential data. Voltage scale; 1 mv time marker; 200 ms.

The rabbit was allowed to adapt to dark at least 1-2 hours in the morning and then the retinal potential was recorded (Fig. 10, 1st). A retinal potential showed a peculiar curve; its initial phase was characterized by a negative wave (a wave) rapidly followed by a positive wave (b wave), then came a low secondary rise of the curve--the positive phase (c wave). The cessation of the light stimulation was accompanied by a rise in the curve (d wave)--the so called "off-effect". The amplitude of b wave was 0.2 - 0.5 mv. in rabbits. A superimposed curve of evoked retinal potentials (ERP) responded to twenty photic stimulation and were recorded by X-Y instrument (Fig. 11, a).

The rabbit was usually radiated by microwave in the afternoon. The size of b wave was decreased in a lot of rabbits after 3-4 hours of exposure (Fig. 10, 2nd), diminishing gradually during continued exposure. In that time we usually observed c wave to rise. Naturally, the ERP was also decreased. (Fig. 11, b & c). We stopped radiation in the evening, the size of b wave, ERP as soon as recovered, sometimes on half an hour (Fig. 10, 3rd), (Fig 11, d). The time course of the development of these effects showed in Fig. 12.

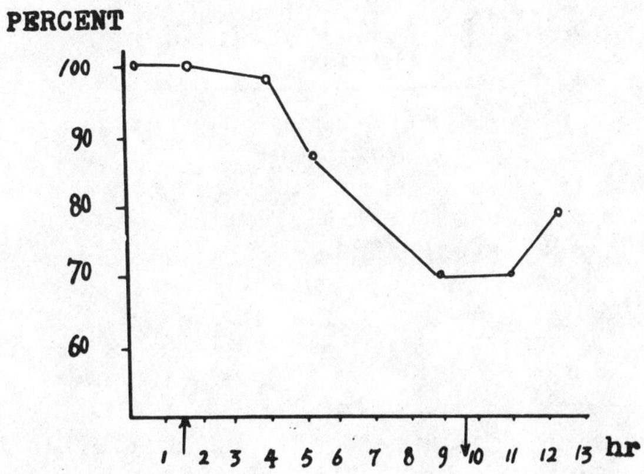

Fig. 12 The time course of the development of microwave effects on the ERP. Abscissae indicated experimental hours. Ordinates indicates the change of ERP in percentage. ↑ indicates radiation was turned on; ↓ indicates radiation was turned off.

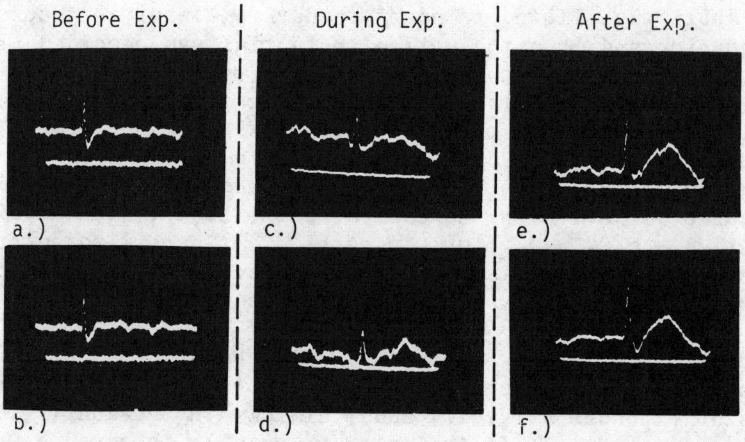

Fig. 13 Retinal potential. In every picture upper is retinal potential and lower is spontaneous potential recorded from the visual area of cortex in rabbit.

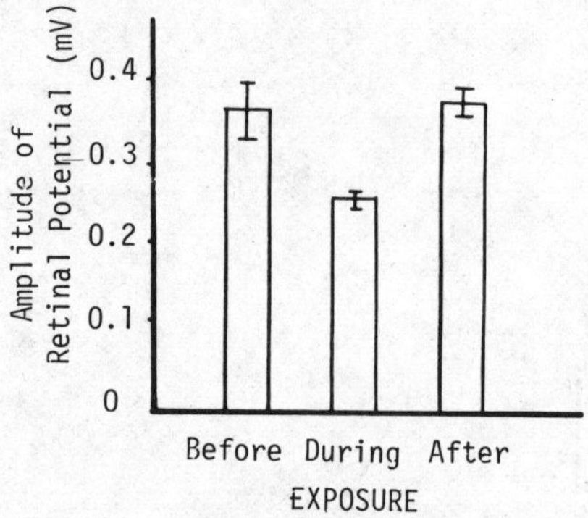

Fig. 14 The mean volume of retinal potential in twenty rabbits under microwave exposure.

Sometimes, the size of b wave decreased only slightly during exposure a in a few rabbits. The rebound phenomenon had been observed when the microwave generator was turned off in these rabbits (Fig. 13). The differences of size of b wave were statistically highly significant (Fig. 14).

Discussion: Many of the earlier papers evaluating work in this field concluded that the only significant effect was the thermal one, and the insufficient evidence existed to substantiate the view that non-thermal effects were also of importance.

The behavior of the human body in response to microwave radiation is very complicated. The conversion of microwave energy into heat is a principal mode of damage to living organisms, especially to the eyes, but much recent research supports the view that non-thermal effects are substantive (11). We are more concerned with the effect of microwave fields on information storage in living systems (12). For example, sensitivity of the eye and nose of some microwave workers (sight and smell) is decreased, but it is alleged that virtually these symptoms disappear when the subjects are assigned to other work or are given lengthy vacations (13,14).

There are general agreements about the existence of a slow cornea-positive component such as P I which is responsible for the secondary rise of c wave. There is much evidence to show that the cornea-negative a wave is the first sign of illumination and that it passes over a slower negative phase which is often submerged below a mainly cornea-positive response but is sometimes visible. Component PII in it's initial part forms wave b. The component P III appears to survive damage to the retina better than the other ones. It is assumed to be associated with the process of inhibition. As the microwave radiation diminishes the amplitude of b wave, it is reasonable to say that the microwave can decrease P II of the retina. The rebound phenomenon must take place immediately after exposure. One mechanism that fits these requirements is an inhibitory effect on the retina. When the radiation was turned off these effects disappeared and b wave rebounded. There was no change of temperature in vitreous body during exposure at 700 uW/cm^2. Naturally, thermal effect couldn't explain this phenomenon. We can't easily explain why the wave c was increased during exposure and didn't recover after exposure in 1-2 hours. This is an area that we hope to explore further in the near future with microelectrode techniques to record the firing of retinal element and cortical cells.

III. Subacute Experiments

Forty-eight rats were exposed to 2450 MHz cw microwaves. Before exper-iments, we had chosen the animals of which EEG and ECG were of normal value. We didn't observe any experiment animal; its ECG occurred bradycardia or tachychardia.

There were 10 mW/cm2, lmW/cm2, 100 uW/cm2, and control groups. The animals were exposed to microwaves five hours a day for one month. EEG and ECG were recorded before the radiation, the 7th day and 15th day of exposure, and during the 15 days after exposure.

The EEG frequency appeared a tendency to slow and the ECG occurred bradycardia, tachycardia and local ventricular block in 10 mW/cm^2 and 1 mW/cm2 exposed groups. The change of R-R interval in some animals were obvious from 210 ms. to 350 ms (Fig. 15). Comparison was made with the pre-exposed values of R-R interval. The probability was smaller than 0.05. There were no changes in 100 uw/cm^2 and control groups.

IV. Chronic Experiments

This experiment was conducted with sixteen rabbits and forty rats (15). The sixteen rabbits were divided into four groups at random from which three groups were irradiated with three levels (10 mW/cm^2, 1 mW/cm^2, 0.1 mW/cm^2) and one group served as control. The forty rats were divided into four groups, from which three groups were irradiated with the other three levels (5mW/cm^2, 0.2 mW/cm^2 and 0.01 mW/cm^2) and one was control. The exposed groups were irradiated six hours daily for four and half months. The observed items included rectal temperature, body weight, blood pressure, white blood count, whole blood cholinesterase, leukocytic alkali phosphatase (LAP), ECG, EEG (parietal and occipital region) ad Y-labyrinth test.

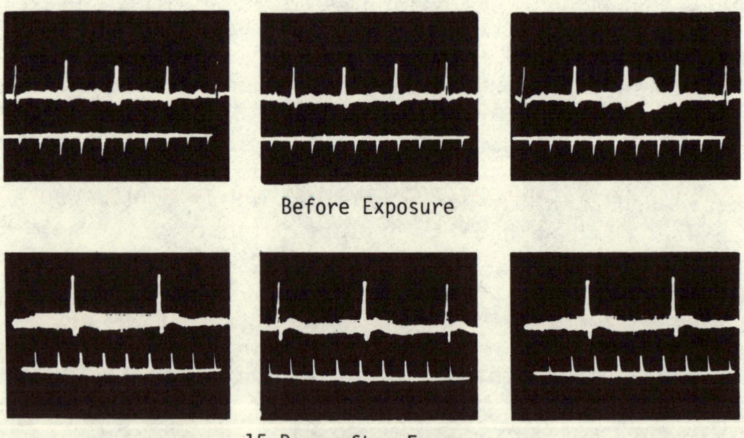

Fig. 15 ECG of rats recorded before and 15 days after microwave exposure.

There were certain power densities of microwave which induced EEG frequency slowing and amplitude increasing. The most pronounced changes of ECG were bradycardia, tachycardia and R wave widening. Leukocyte and LAP were increased in the first half of the month and then there were no changes. Blood pressure was fluctuated. Mistakes at y-labyrinth test appeared to increase. The relations between these variables of observed indexes and power densities are shown in Table 7.

V. Effects of Microwave Radiation on Bioelectric Activity of Cortex Quantity and Heart Rate in the Rabbits

The studies on the influence of microwave radiation on EEG of animals have been carried out by many authors. Most of them observed the effects of microwave radiation on EEG without quantitative method. There are near a thousandfold differences of the threshold power density levels of biological effect between the reports from Bertharion (16) and Asubaev (17). In this field, we tried to study encephalo-electro activity quantitatively with an instrument of spectral integral analysis. At the same time, the EEG and ECG of rabbit were also recorded.

Levitina et al (18) reported that several mW/cm2 of microwave radiation (CW and PW) decreased the heart rate of rabbits. Kaplan et al repeated this experiment (19) and found no effect, but they only used continuous wave. The effects of lower power density on heart rate still are obscure. In this experiment, we observed the changes of electroencephalo-integrated amplitude and heart rate in rabbits during pulsed microwave exposure at 2 mW/cm2 and 0.4 mW/cm2.

Our experiments were conducted with rabbits. Their body weights were about 2 Kg. Eighteen of them were implanted with a pair of recording electrodes into the skull on the occipital region, using stainless steel screws (1 mm diameter). The animals were divided into three groups. One week after operation, EEG of these rabbits returned to normal. Then, the experiment started. The first group was exposed to 2 mW/cm2, the second to 0.4 mW/cm2 and the third group was sham exposed. ECG and EEG were observed before and after exposure on the first, seventh and fourteenth day of irradiation. A total of 54 experiments were run. The microwave source was 2900 MHz pulsed wave with 1875 Hz modulated frequency; pulse width was 0.6 us. Groups of six rabbits were irradiated at a time in a small anechoic chamber, facing the horn antenna, 110 cm (far field) away from it. Rabbits were exposed 6 hours a day. The test-room was constructed of echosorb.

Table 7. Relation between the Variance of Observed Indexes & Power Densities.

Items	10 mW/cm^2	5 mW/cm^2	1 mW/cm^2	0.2 mW/cm^2	0.1 mW/cm^2	0.01 mW/cm^2	Control
EEG; Amplitude ↑	++	/	--	/	--	/	--
Frequency ↓	++	/	++	/	--	/	--
ECG; Heart Rate ↑↓	/	++	/	--	/	--	--
R Widen	/	++	/	++	/	--	--
Leukocyte ↑	/	++	/	--	/	--	--
LAP ↑	/	+	/	--	/	--	--
Blood Pressure Change	++	/	--	/	--	/	--
Rectal Temp. ↑	--	--	--	--	--	--	--
Weight ↓	/	+	/	--	/	--	--

++ Represents the variable with significant difference
\+ Represents the variable only with a tendency change
/ Represents no animal exposed at this power density level
-- Showed no significant changes

EEG was recorded with bipolar leads and was sampled by the quantitative instrument for 5 frequency ranges. The 5 frequency bands were: 2-3.5/s, 4-7/s, 8-13/s, 14.5-19/s and 22-30/s. the bipolar electrodes were coupled to lowpass filters to prevent microwave disturbance. ECG was recorded with thorax leads. The R-R intervals were recorded on a computer. EEG was recorded for 3-5 min. at the following periods: before exposure, 1.5 h. and 5 h. after the onset of microwave exposure, and 1 h. after radiation. ECG was recorded for 3-5 min. before and after 1.5 h. exposure.

1. Spectral Integrated Analysis of Encephalo-electric Activity

After exposure, the slow waves seemed to be dominant in rabbit EEG. However, there was no significant differences in integrated index for each spectrum between, before and after exposure (Tab. 8 and 9).

Since the differences in absolute EEG integrated amplitude values in rabbits for different individuals and dates were too great, the percentage of change in integrated amplitude during exposure was used as the quantitative index. The averaged change percents were indicated in Fig. 16 (the total integrated amplitude before exposure was 100%). After the microwave radiation was started, the amplitudes increased in both exposed groups. They were significantly different from the control ($p < 0.05$). The increase of total integrated amplitude appeared in about half of the experimental animals. Immediately after exposure, the amplitudes were decreased in both exposed groups. We call it an "off-effect".

Table 8. Averaged Integrated Index of α Wave (%).

Group / Time	1st. (2mW/cm^2)	2nd. (0.4mW/cm^2)	3rd. (Control)
Before Exposure	18	18	20
After 6 hrs. Exposure	19	18	21

Table 9. Averaged Integrated Index of Slow Wave (θ and δ) (%)

Time \ Group	1st. (2mW/cm^2)	2nd. (0.4mW/cm^2)	3rd. (Control)
Before Exposure	64	58	57
After 6 hrs. Exposure	63	59	53

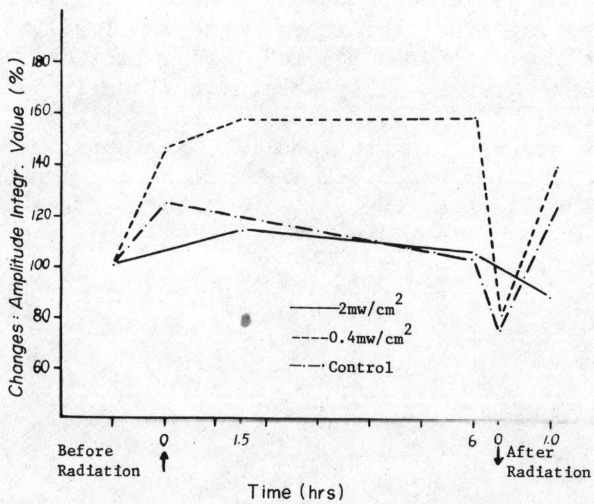

Fig. 16 Changes in amplitude integrated value.

2. Changes of Heart Rate

The averaged heart rate of rabbits was 209.5 beats/min. (2mw/cm^2), 223 beats/min. (0.4 mW/cm^2) and 216.7 beats/min. (control). There were no obvious changes at the time the microwave started. After 1.5 hours exposure, the decrease of heart rate happened in 18 experiments of total in the first group. The changes of every animal were more than 10%. Although there were no changes in some animals and even increase in a few, the use of t-test on the averaged change value indicated significant difference with before exposure. There was no significant difference in the control group after sham irradiation (Tab. 10). There was no effect in the second group exposed to 0.4 mW/cm2.

Arrhythmia accompanying with bradycardia was observed in only a few experiments of the first microwave group. (See Fig. 17) One hour after radiation, the heart rate was recuperated and arrhythmia disappeared.

Discussion: Differences in the microwave effects on EEG were published. Baranski et al (20) summarized the changes in EEG amplitude as follows: High amplitude slow waves of EEG appear during microwave irradiation. There is a certain response lantency. When in the long-term study, the average amplitudes decrease. In our experiments, the total integrated amplitude was increased at 0.4 mW/cm^2 and 2 mW/cm^2 for several and hundreds of minutes respectively. After termination of irradiation, desynchronization appeared, and there was no change of spectral integrated index in both exposed groups. Perhaps the microwave dose was not enough to influence the spectrum. Bertharion et al (17) reported that microwave exposure at 5 mW/cm2 for 24 hours caused no EEG change in rats, but induced high amplitude slow waves if exposed for 48 hours Asubaev (17) and Dumanskii (21) indicated the 10 uW/cm^2 and 5 uW/cm^2 respectively as the EEG threshold of microwave's effect. The former reported that high amplitude slow waves occured only after 40 to 50 seconds of radiation. However, the latter reported that rapid waves increased within half a month of radiation. The slow waves did not increase until after one month exposure. We suppose that the spectral integrated analysis might be used as an objective functional index of the nervous system for large groups of microwave workers. We consider the limitations of current data and underscore the need for further research.

Table 10. Effect on Heart Rate.

Group	No. of Rabbit	No. of Experi.	Avg. Drop (beat/min.)	P
Exposed	16	28	20.29	< 0.01
Control	16	27	6.90	> 0.05

Frequency = 3 GHz Repetition Rate 1875 pps
Inc. Pwr. Density = 2 mW/cm^2 Pulse Width = 0.6μs

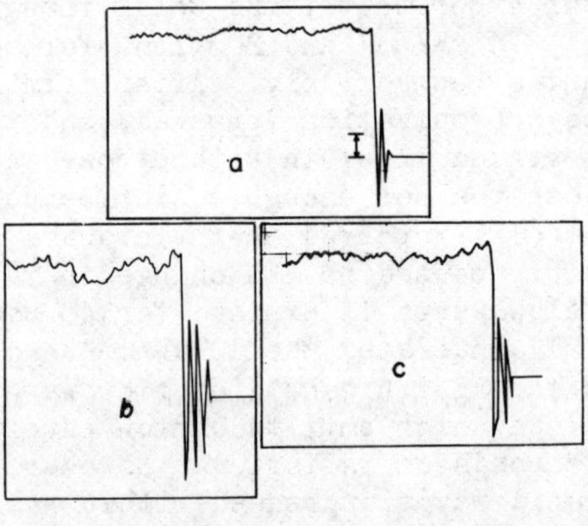

Fig. 17 Effect of 2 mW/cm^2 microwave radiation on the R-R interval of ECG in one rabbit (No. 29 rabbit of 1st group). a. Before exposure (interval,308 ms) b. After 1.5 h. exposure (392 ms) c. After exposure 1 h. (324 ms).

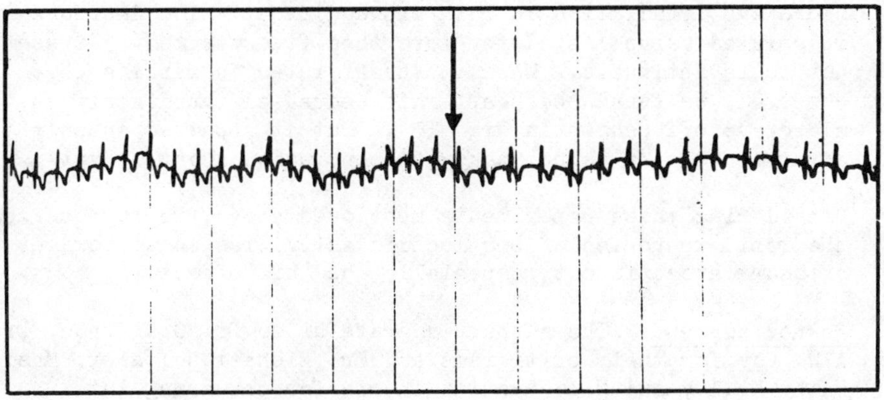

Fig. 18 Change in the heart rate at microwave off, distance between two black lines is 1 s.

Microwave effects on heart rate in our study are compatible with the reports of Presman (22). Pulsed microwave exposure at 2 mW/cm^2 may decrease heart rate in rabbits. The effects did not occur at 0.4 mW/cm^2. Nevertheless, Frey and Siefert (23) indicated that rate of change of beat may be influenced by microwaves, with the exposure pulses synchronized with the R wave at quite low average power densities.

Rapid responses of bioelectric activities to microwave exposure are interesting to us. Cholodev reported that in 31 percent of animals examined desynchronization of the bioelectric activity of the cortex was observed at the moment of switching the transmitter on or off, which he explains as a reaction to microwave stimulus (100-1000 uW/cm^2). Baranski (20) supposed it was an artifact. Goldstein (24) also found there was a possible indication of an "on-effect" and an "off-effect" in two experiments (2%) when the microwave (700 uW/cm^2) was turned on and off.

Seaman and Wachtel (25) reported that two types of responses to microwaves were observed in Aplysia pacemakers. The response developed slowly and was seen in all neurons. The other rapid responses were seen in a few neurons. An increase in firing rate within one interspike internal of the onset of irradiation. In two cells an immediate decrease in firing rate occurred at the termination of an irradiation. He pointed out that rapid changes cannot be attributed to a thermal mechanism. In the present experiment, the integrated amplitude value of bioelectric activities of cortex dropped at the termination of a microwave irradiation in both exposed group. The decrease in integrated value lasted for more than five minutes. It seems not to be artifacts. When the heart rates in rabbits were observed, we found the heart rate decreased immediately at the microwave off (shown in Fig. 18). But it appeared in only two experiments. We cannot make the conclusion about it yet.

Considering these experiments mentioned above, we suppose that the rapid responses of bioelectric activities on microwave exposure are existent, especially the "off-effect".

Acknowledgment: The authur is grateful to Dr. C.K. Chou, Dr. A.W. Guy for their criticisms and Mr. Michael Heltsley, Mrs. Kathy Kelley and Miss Rustina Thorpe for preparing this document.

REFERENCES

1. S.M. Michaelson, "Thermal effects of single and repeated exposures to microwaves." "Biologic Effects and Health Hazards of Microwave Radiation", Polish Medical Publish, Poland Warsaw, 1-14, 1974.
2. H.P. Schwan, Keynote Address and C.C. Johnson Memorial Lecture "Microwave Bioeffects Research; Historical Perspectives On Productive Approaches". J. of Microwave Power 14(1), 1979.
3. Karel Marha, "Microwave radiation safety standards in Eastern Europe" IEEE Transaction on Microwave Theory and Techniques, vol, MTT-19(2), 165-168, 1971.
4. Hua Chiang and K.C. Yee: "Study of Safety Standards of Microwave, Acta of Chekiang Medical College," 8(2), 57-62, 1979.
5. K.C. Yee and Hua Chiang: "Experimental Research of biological acute effects of microwave exposure," Acta Physiological Sinica 32(1), 10-17, 1980.
6. K.C. Yee: "Research and Development in Biological Effects of Microwave." Progress in Physiological Sciences. 11(4), 309-315, 1980.
7. K.C. Yee and Hua Chiang: "Effect of Microwave on Retinal Potential in Rabbits at Lower Density," Acta Physiologica Sinica, 32(4) 370-374, 1980.
8. H.B. Parry, K. Tansley, and L.C. Thomson, "The Electroretinogram of the dog.", J. Physiol., 120, 28-40 (1953).
9. A.W. Guy, "Quantitation of Induced Electromagnetic Field Patterns in Tissue and Associated Biologic Effects." "Biologic effects and health hazards of microwave radiation" Polish Medical Publishers. Poland Warsaw, 203-216 (1974).
10. J.W. Hartwell and C.W. Erwin. "Evoked Potential Analysis; On-line Signal Optimization Using a Mini-computer." EEG and Clin. Neur., 41, 416-421 (1976).

11. W. R. Adey, "Frequency and power windowing in tissue interactions with weak electromagnetic fields" proceeding of the IEEE, 68(1),119 - 125, 1980
12. K.C. Yee: "Effects of Microwave on Nervous System." Bioengineering Section of Foreign Medicine, 2, 7-11, 1979.
13. K.C. Yee: "Biological Effects of Microwave and its Prevention." Hygienical Section of Foreign Medicine. 2, 66-73, 1976.
14. K.C. Yee: "Microwave Radiation and its Prevention, Technology of Microwave Dry". 49-55, 1976.
15. K.C. Yee and Hua Chiang: "Experimental Research on Biological Effects of Microwave Chronic Exposure," Acta of Chekiang Medical College, 10(2) 1981.
16. Bertharion, G., Servantie, B. and Joly, R. "Electro-Cortico-Graphic Modifications after exposure to microwave fields on white rat". J. Microwave Power 6(1); 62, 1971.
17. Asubaev, C.H. "Evaluation of threshold sensitivity of the rabbit brain to pulsed electromagnetic fields of a superhigh frequency range". Byull Eksp Biol Med. 74, 56-59, 1972.
18. Levitina, N.A. "Investigation of non-thermal action of microwave on the rhythm of cardiac contractions in the frog". Byull Eksp Biol Med. 12, 64, 1966.
19. Kaplan, I. T., Metlay, W., Zaret, M., Birenbaum, L., and Rosenthal, S.W. "Absence of heart rate effects in rabbits during low level microwave irradiation" IEEE Trans. Microwave Theory and Techniques, MTT-19(2), pp. 168 - 173, 1971.
20. Baranski, S. and Czerski, P. "Biological Effect of Microwaves," Dowden, Hutchinson and Ross, Inc., U.S.A., 1976.
21. Dumanskii, Yu D. "Influence electromagnetic fields on human". Kieu, 1975.
22. Presman, A. S. and N. A. Levitina "Non-thermal action of microwaves on cardic contraction in animals Report II: Investigation of the action of impulse microwaves", translated from Bulleten Experimental noi Biologii medising, Vol. 53, pp. 39-43, 1962.
23. Frey, A. H. and Siefert, "Pulse modulated UHF energy illumination of the heart associated with change in heart rate." Life Sciences, 7(11) 505-512, 1968.
24. Goldstein L. and Sisko, Z. "A Quantitative electroencephalographic study of the Acute effects of X-band microwaves in Rabbits." "Biologic Effects and Hazards of Microwave Radiation" Warsaw, Poland, 128, 1973.
25. Seaman, R.L. and Wachtel, H. "Slow and Rapid responses to cw and pulsed microwave radiation by individual Aplysia pacemakers." J. Microwave Power. 13(1), 77-86, 1978.

ABSTRACT

Our Experimental Results Showed:

1) The threshold of acute effects of microwave radiation (C.W. 2450 MHz) is 20 mW/cm^2 in rabbit. The effects are fall of blood pressure, acceleration of respiration, the elevation of subcutananeus and rectal temperatures. There is a normal correlated function between the changes and power densities. All effects are thermal in nature.

2) The microwave radiation may effect the Q-T interval, K and amplitude of T wave of ECG in rabbits. We observed rhythmic disturbances of heart a in few animals.

3) At 0.7 mW/cm^2 power density, the size of the b wave of retinal potential was decreased during pulsed microwave radiation (3 GHz, 1875pps,0.6us) and the rebound phenomenon of b wave have been observed when the microwave was off.

4) Forty-eight rats were exposed to 2450 MHz cw microwave. There were 10 mW/cm^2, 1 mW/cm^2, 100 uW/cm^2 and control groups. The animals were exposed to microwaves five hours a day for one month. The EEG frequency appeared a tendency to slow and the ECG occurred bradycardia, tachycardia and local ventricular block in 10 mW/cm^2 and 1 mW/cm^2 exposed groups.

5) The 16 rabbits were divided into four groups: 10 mW/cm^2, 1 mW/cm^2, 0.1 mW/cm^2 and control. The 40 rats were divided into 4 groups: 5 mW/cm^2, 0.2 mW/cm^2, 0.01 mW/cm^2 and control. The exposed groups were irradiated 6 hours daily for 4 1/2 months. The microwave source was 2450 MHz, cw. There were certain power densities of microwave which induced EEG frequency slowing and amplitude increasing. The most pronounced changes of ECG were bradycardia, tachycardia and R wave widening. There was no significant difference in rectal temperature, body weight, white blood count, whole blood cholinesterase, or leukocytic alkali phosphatase.

6) We had studied encephalo-electro activity quantitatively with an instrument of spectral integral analysis. The total integrated amplitude was increased in both exposed groups (2 $mW/cm2$ and 0.4 mW/cm^2). There was significant difference from the control ($p < 0.05$). When the exposure stopped, the amplitude decreased immediately in both exposed groups. After exposure, the heart rate decreased in the groups exposed to 2 mW/cm^2. It was significantly different from before exposure.

DIFFERENTIATION BETWEEN BIOLOGICAL EFFECTS AND HEALTH HAZARDS: SCALING FROM ANIMALS

Michael H. Repacholi

Radiation Protection Bureau
Health and Welfare Canada
Ottawa, Ontario K1A 0L2

INTRODUCTION

Since its beginning the earth has been bombarded by both ionizing and non-ionizing radiations from terrestrial and extraterrestrial origin. Life as we know it today has evolved with this natural background radiation. Living organisms utilize various parts of the electromagnetic spectrum for day to day existence, especially the infrared, visible and ultraviolet components. Little is known of the use that living organisms make of the natural radiofrequency and microwave environment. With the recent increases in the power density levels from artificial sources to the general ambient microwave and radiofrequency radiation environment, there is a need to know whether changing this background to a significant degree will produce unacceptable changes to life. Unfortunately such a question may never fully be answered because as living organisms evolve, changes in the environment from factors other than radiofrequency and microwave radiation (e.g. chemicals) are likely to have a much greater impact. Evidence from the scientific literature would indicate that if changes occur from these non-ionizing radiations, they are likely to be very subtle in nature. Thus from the viewpoint of a health agency one has to place a greater priority with potential adverse health effects that are likely to occur within a few generations.

There are many thousands of reports in the scientific literature that describe "biological effects" from exposing living organisms to microwave/RF radiation. A continuing problem confronting health agencies is to differentiate between those biological effects that may be phenomenological in nature and tend to be transient or easily repaired, and those effects that are truly a hazard to human health. Perhaps before considering this problem one should understand what is meant by the term "good health". A healthy person can be defined as being of sound body, mind or spirit, or being free from physical disease or pain and in a state of mental well-being. An adverse health effect can be defined therefore as one which adversely affects this state of physical and mental well-being.

In this paper, examples of biological effects from exposure to microwave and radiofrequency fields are discussed with a view to providing some insight into the complex evaluation that must be made of effects, to determine if they constitute a health hazard. Some disturbed people believe that they are being exposed to microwave fields that in fact do not exist, and their behavioral patterns can be changed by this imagined microwave exposure. The value of in-vitro experiments is also discussed in terms of assessment of risk to health. Finally the value of scaling of effects in animals to effects that may occur in man will be discussed.

Biological Effect or Health Hazard?

Radiant energy can produce an effect only when it is absorbed by matter. This does not necessarily mean that the significance of the effect produced bears a direct relationship to the amount of energy absorbed. The primary modes of action of these radiations are either photochemical or thermal[1]. The Grotthus and Draper Law states that no photochemical reaction can occur unless radiant energy is absorbed. This absorption requires an energy transfer from the incident photons to the absorbing molecules[2]. When microwave or radiofrequency energy is absorbed, at the molecular level, either the electronic energy levels of its atoms are affected, or changes occur in the rotational, vibrational or transitional energies of the molecule. In biological systems, microwave or radiofrequency energy absorption causes polar molecules to rotate and increases the kinetic energy of the molecule (producing heat).

An analysis of biological effects from exposure to microwave and radiofrequency energy requires the consideration of a sequence of events: the physical interaction of radiant energy with matter followed by physiological reactions - either local or generalized, and immediate or delayed biological effects. The possibility of adaptive mechanisms leading to exhaustion via the classical sequence of events of stress - adaption - fatigue, has to be considered. Consequently the effects of single or repeated exposures have to be analysed separately, even when exposures take place under identical conditions[3].

Czerski and Szmigielski[4] have noted that in order to understand the effects of exposure to microwave and radiofrequency energy, one must have some knowledge of the mechanisms of radiant energy absorption and any direct interference with biophysical and biochemical phenomena in living systems. In this context they suggest:

(i) all detectable changes in function and structure above the molecular level, may be termed biological effects,
(ii) the intermediate effect at the site of primary interaction may induce further changes (secondary or indirect effects),
(iii) some time may elapse between the primary interaction and the detection of the biological effect,
(iv) measureable biological effects that remain within the range of normal compensation are not necessarily hazardous; some effects may improve the efficiency of certain physiological processes and are used for therapeutic purposes.
(v) biological effects that may be detrimental to the efficiency of a living system could be hazardous.

Tissues and organs of the human body are susceptible to effects from microwave or radiofrequency radiation exposure. Some reactions to these exposures may lead to measureable biological effects which remain within the range of normal physiological compensation of the body and thus lead to an effect which is not necessarily a hazard. Some reactions on the other hand may lead to effects which are outside the range of normal compensation of the body and which may be an actual or potential health hazard. Let us consider a few examples of effects which have been confirmed, so that adverse effects or health hazards can be evaluated further.

At a certain incident power density of radiofrequency radiation and under appropriate exposure conditions, it is possible to raise the rectal temperature (generally accepted as equivalent to the core temperature) of the human body by $1^{o}C$. Neglecting the effects of focal heating (hot spots), the thermoregulatory system of exposed persons would be able to cope with such a thermal load. A $1^{o}C$ temperature rise is well within the range of normal physiological compensation and the rectal temperature would return to normal following termination of the exposure. Should this be considered a hazard to health?

At much lower average power densities (as low as 0.1 mW/cm^2) of pulsed microwave radiation, exposed humans can perceive within the back of the head, a buzzing or clicking sound (microwave hearing) depending on the pulse repetition frequency and peak power density[5]. This hearing sensation could alter behavioral patterns but would not likely have any irreversible physical consequences. Where does one draw the line between biological effects and adverse health effects?

Let us give further consideration to the first example. Tell and Harlen[6] have completed an excellent review of the thermogenic biological effects expected in man from exposure to radiofrequency energy. In their review they considered man to be a thermal entity having a thermoregulatory mechanism to maintain a constant body temperature. Many homeostatic processes are involved in maintaining a constant body temperature by balancing internal heat generated from various metabolic functions and vigorous physical activity, and external thermal loads on the body from high ambient temperatures or absorbed microwave and radiofrequency energy. The thermal load from microwave and radiofrequency fields can be considered as one of many thermal stressors placed on man by the environment.

The ability of man to tolerate thermal stress depends on his environment and in particular such factors as air temperature, air movement, humidity level, duration of exposure to high temperatures and the level of work activity. Other factors that will influence man's tolerance to heat stress during work include type of clothing, age, weight and general physical condition. On the basis of a review of available data on the susceptibility of man to hot, thermally stressing environments, the National Institute for Occupational Safety and Health[7] issued their criteria which provided evidence that a 1°C rise in rectal temperature represented an upper limit for man's thermoregulatory mechanism to adapt to heat stress. In their review, Tell and Harlen[6] suggested that "An additional consideration, which may become most important under certain conditions of exposure, is the possibility of highly non-uniform deposition of energy within the body of man and subsequent non-uniform increases in localized tissue temperatures, the biological consequences of which may not be properly reflected by deep

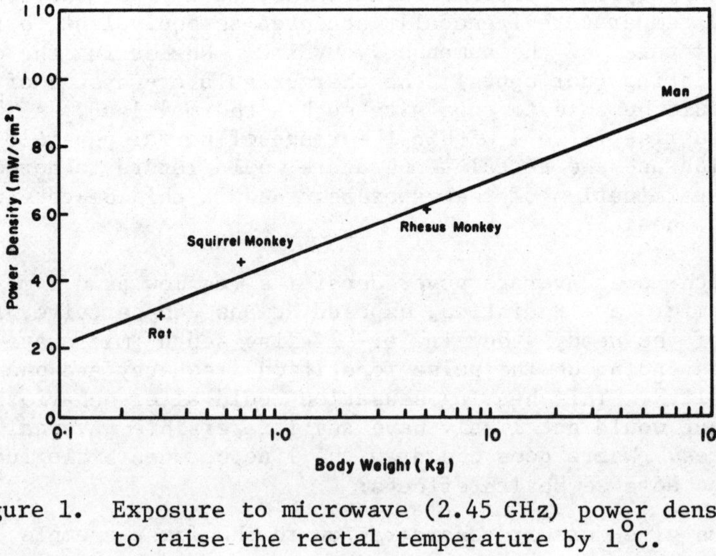

Figure 1. Exposure to microwave (2.45 GHz) power density to raise the rectal temperature by 1°C.

body average (rectal) temperature. With the proviso that for some conditions it may also be necessary to control local hot spots, it would seem reasonable to define intensity of radiofrequency irradiation as a function of frequencies that could potentially elevate man's rectal temperature by 1°C."

Using the data of de Lorge[8] on the increase in rectal temperature of rats, squirrel and rhesus monkeys exposed to microwaves, Tell and Harlen[6] made an extrapolation to determine the expected microwave power density exposure to give a rise in rectal of 1°C. These data are given in Figure 1 and show that exposure to a power density of about 92 mW/cm^2 of 2.45 GHz radiation would be expected to raise the rectal temperature of a 70 kg man by 1°C. However exposure of a resting 70 kg man to 30 mW/cm^2 of radiation in the whole body resonance region (approximately 79 MHz) could overload the thermoregulatory system and cause an uncontrolled excursion of the rectal temperature. Physical effort in addition to this exposure would reduce the duration before this overheating would occur[6].

Clothing will not screen out radiofrequency energy but will cause much of the heat generated by the absorbed radiation to be contained and reduce the ability of the body to dissipate the thermal load. Figure 2 gives the estimated[6] equilibrium rectal

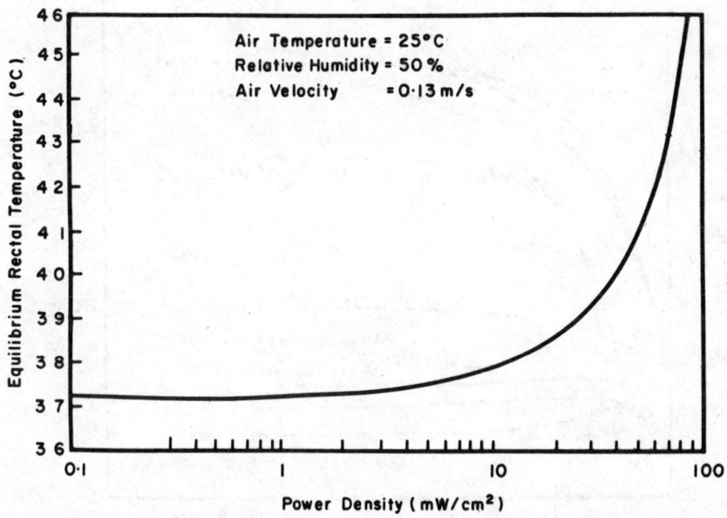

Figure 2. Estimated equilibrium rectal temperature of a resting man in a comfortable environment, dressed in standard miliatry uniform (fatigues) and exposed to varying power densities of 75 MHz radiofrequency radiation.

temperature of a resting man in a comfortable environment dressed in standard military uniform (fatigues) and exposed to varying power densities of 75 MHz electromagnetic radiation. It is apparent that at the resonant frequency, exposures to power densities above 10 mW/cm^2 can cause unacceptable increases in rectal temperature for a clothed, active person working in a hot environment.

Although man's rectal temperature may rise by 1°C when exposed to resonant frequency radiation, to estimate the total extent of potential thermal injury, one must determine what is happening at other points in the body. Using the modeling techniques by Emery et al[9], Guy et al[10] determined the temperature and sweating rates of various parts of man exposed to 79 MHz radiation at 10 mW/cm^2 (Figure 3). The hypothalamic temperature, which is approximately equivalent to the rectal temperature[6], rises by about 1°C. However, highly localized absorption of radiofrequency energy occurs in man's leg-core (thigh) such that the temperature rises to about 44°C in 3 h. This temperature could certainly result in irreversible tissue damage.

In addition to localized absorption of energy occurring within relatively large volumes such as the leg, similarly highly

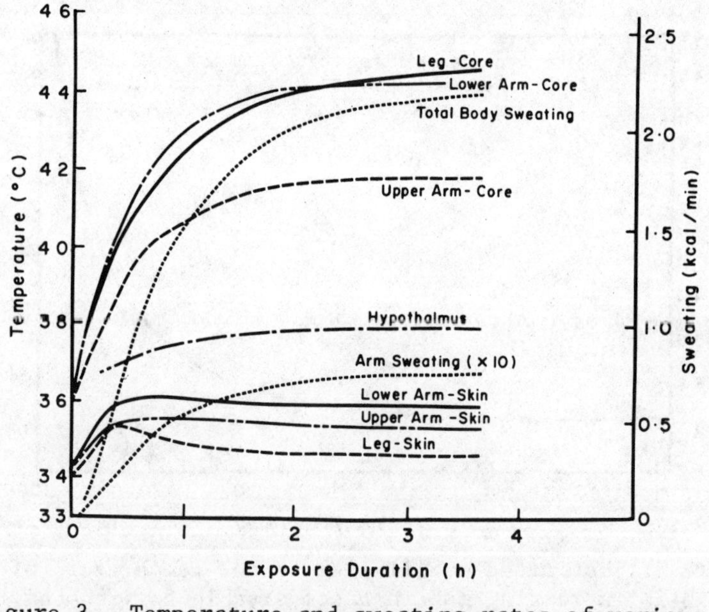

Figure 3. Temperature and sweating rates of various parts of man exposed whole body to 79 MHz radiofrequency radiation at an incident power density of 10 mW/cm^2.

localized absorption (hot spots) can occur in much smaller volumes such as the brain, even after allowing for heat conduction and heat convection due to blood flow. Depending on the size of the head and frequency of the incident radiation, regions of relatively intense absorption can occur, possibly at or near the centre of the brain, which probably has the lowest threshold for thermal damage. Damage to some of the sensors for the core temperature of the body, located in the hypothalamus deep within the brain, could be crucial to the body's thermoregulatory mechanism. Kritikos and Schwan[11] have demonstrated that exposure of a 10 cm diameter human head model to 1 GHz electromagnetic radiation of incident power density 10 mW/cm^2 (heat deposition rate 10 mW/g) can produce a hot spot in the central region having a 0.5 ^{o}C differential temperature rise over the surrounding tissues and blood. Smaller temperature rises would occur in larger models of man's head. Confirmation of this result was recently provided by Burr et al[12] using 1.2 and 2.5 GHz radiation, and by Burr and Krupp[13].

The main points from this discussion can be summarized as follows:

(i) Biological effects cannot be evaluated with respect to potential health hazard in isolation. Even for a biological effect as apparently straight-forward as an increase in temperature, the full implications must be studies under all possible conditions. Additional factors such as ambient environment, work activity, age, sex, weight and general physical condition of the person exposed as well as the effect of wearing clothing, must be all considered in the evaluation.

(ii) The frequency of the incident radiation is important as demonstrated in the example. Maximum energy absorption occurs at the body resonance frequency. At frequencies below body resonance, the rate of energy absorption falls as the square of the frequency. An indication of the absorption of electromagnetic radiation (10 - 100,000 MHz) in humans is given in Figure 4 (from Durney et al[14]). This figure shows the incident power density (mW/cm^2) of various frequencies of electromagnetic radiation needed to deliver a heat load of 3 W/kg in men, women and children.

Of particular importance with respect to absorption of microwave or radiofrequency radiation is the polarization (or orientation to the body) of the electric (E) and magnetic (H) fields. For example, at the resonant frequency and below, and for far-field exposures, the maximum absorption of energy occurs when the E-field is aligned with the long axis of a body. At frequencies above about 1 GHz the average SAR is greater for H-field polarization. For exposures in the near-field the E- and H-fields are no longer in phase producing a complex situation which still awaits proper evaluation.

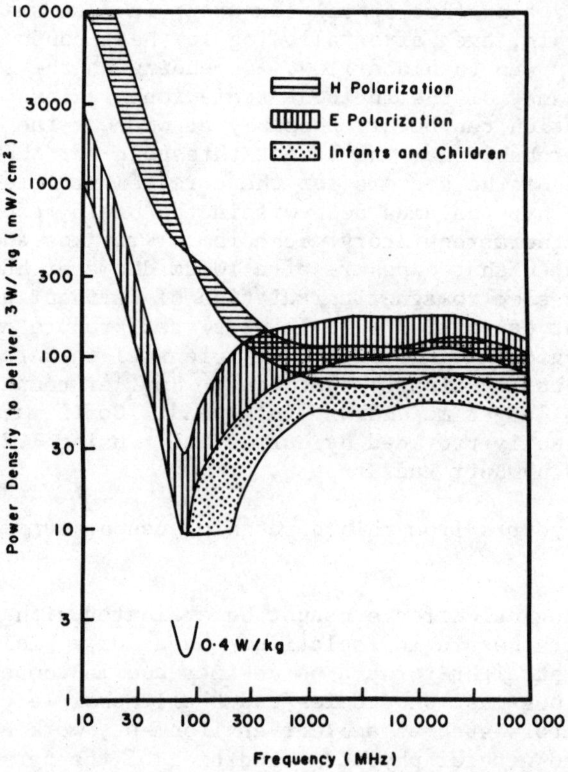

Figure 4. Incident power density as a function of frequency of electromagnetic radiation needed to deliver a heat load of 3 W/kg in men, women and children.

(iii) Distribution of energy deposition is of obvious importance. As a general guide it is apparent that a rectal temperature increase of 1°C above normal is within the body's normal range of physiological compensation. However, regardless of non-uniform deposition of energy possibly producing hot spots in the brain or other tissues, it is unlikely that most people would accept having their rectal temperatures increased in a manner over which they have little or no control.

Let us now consider the case of microwave hearing. Humans perceive an auditory sensation when the head is exposed to rectangular pulse-modulated microwave energy (200 - 3000 MHz) with peak incident power densities of the order of 300 mW/cm^2, average power densities as low as 0.1 mW/cm^2, and pulse widths varying from 1 to 100 μs. The auditory sensation is heard as a click, buzz or chirp depending on the pulse width and pulse repetition frequency, and is perceived as originating from within or near the back of the head[15]. The absorbed microwave energy produces a thermoelastic expansion of the brain tissue, causing an acoustic pressure wave which is detected by the hair cells of the organ of Corti (in the cochlea) via bone conduction. The deposition of energy needed to induce this auditory sensation is very small and has been estimated[16] to increase the temperature of the brain per pulse by less than 10^{-5} ^{o}C. The auditory sensation is loud enough to be clearly perceived humans in an ambient noise level of 65 dB (J. Lin - personal communication, 1981).

Could this microwave-induced auditory sensation pose a risk to the health of an individual? It is known that humans suffer a general stress reaction when exposed to high levels of sound or noise[17]. Lower noise levels can produce annoyance and elicit various behavioral responses in humans. It is suggested that perception of relatively loud acoustic pulses for prolonged periods of time could be particularly annoying and could induce an adverse health effect. It has been reported[15] that exposure of rats to 2880 MHz microwave pulses of width 2 - 3 μs and having a peak power density of 45 W/cm^2 and average power density of 10 mW/cm^2 (100 pps) can induce peak sound pressure levels inside the rat brain of about 120 dB. Human exposure to such peak sound pressure levels would likely induce much more than annoyance, and causes definite changes in normal behavior.

Microwave hearing has been studied for some 20 years and the phenomenon has been reasonably well characterized. It is an effect of pulsed microwave exposure and under certain conditions could pose a risk to health. Should consideration be given to formulating exposure standards to ensure that the general population is not exposed to microwave fields causing this auditory sensation?

Microwave hearing was used as an example for assessing biological effects in terms of health risk evaluation for the following reasons:

(i) the auditory sensation is induced at very low average power densities, and has been well substantiated scientifically,

(ii) it is a phenomenon that does not cause any apparent adverse physical reaction within the head but, depending on the exposure parameters, could cause varying degrees of annoyance to the exposed person,

(iii) the auditory effect will vary from a barely perceptible sound to a clearly distinguishable clicking, buzzing or squealing. At what stage does one suggest that the phenomenon becomes an annoyance and potentially elicit abnormal behavioral or stress reactions?

The opportunity for exposure to this microwave hearing phenomenon should be put in perspective. Under normal circumstances the general public is unlikely to experience this auditory sensation because such pulsed microwave beams generally come from certain radars. Thus radar operators or maintenance personnel are normally the only people likely to be subjected to this phenomenon.

Real or Imagined?

In the scientific literature there are many reports of behavioral or physiological effects produced in various biological organisms exposed to microwave or radiofrequency energy. Justesen[18] has conveniently categorized these effects into three groups:

1. Bona fide physiological reactions that give rise to changes in behavior following exposure of sensitive tissues to microwave fields,
2. Subjective or indeterminate physiological reactions, generally reversible, which include mild depression, headaches, nausea, dizziness and fatigue,
3. Imagined effects - afflictions provoked in the human psyche with microwave radiation as the supposed causative agent - effects not borne of physical forces in the usual sense of the word but nevertheless having consequences for human behavior.

Health agencies can make health risk assessments from the first category since they are normally the end-point of scientific research, performed under controlled conditions and hopefully reported as a reproducible effect. With sufficient data on an effect it can be studied and some evaluation made as to whether it constitutes a potential or actual health hazard.

The second two groups present a much greater problem. Subjective effects depend to a large extent on the individual (subject) concerned and the working environment. Unfortunately virtually all epidemiological or clinical studies reporting these effects as being due to exposure to microwave or radiofrequency radiation, did not use matched control groups to determine if their cause was due to other factors, such as a stressful environment. Reports of subjective effects are useful to regulatory agencies only if the studies are conducted in a truly scientific manner and the effects are shown to be statistically significant.

Imaginary effects are very real to some people. At the Radiation Protection Bureau we have received numerous calls from people claiming to be "monitored" or "observed" via microwaves by the Central Intelligence Agency (CIA) or Royal Canadian Mounted Police (RCMP). Such people have claimed to have slept behind the piano to avoid being monitored. Many of these people demand that microwave surveys be conducted around their homes. The latest device to endure the wrath of many operators is the much maligned video display terminal (VDT). These devices have been blamed for causing cataracts of the eye, miscarriages, skin irritation and a rash of other problems. Initially it was proposed that these complaints were due to the excessive X-ray emission from the VDT. Once people realized that X-ray production from VDTs was insignificant, the next obvious choice was microwaves. It would be fair to estimate that many hundreds of hours have been wasted by professionals pressured into surveying this class of device knowing them to be a non-existent radiation hazard.

Unfortunately many of these imaginary effects are given full play by the popular media. In some cases, news reporters lacking the scientific background and lusting for the big story, will present distortions and unsupportable speculations of effects. Too many of these stories are believed as gospel by an unknowing general public. A good example of this was cited by Justesen[18]. The statement that microwave ovens emit ionizing radiation appeared in such publications as Time (April 9, 1979) and U.S. News and World Report (April 16, 1979) following the incident at the Three Mile Island nuclear facility.

Although these "imaginary effects" produce adverse behavioral reactions they cannot be considered as health hazards by any self respecting health agency. The agency must spend time, however, attempting to disseminate factual information not only to the complaining public but to the purveyors of public information.

In-Vitro Versus In-Vivo

Let us give some consideration to the applicability of data from in-vitro experiments and how they can be used in the assessment of biological effects in-vivo. In-vitro experimentation allows one to determine the toxicity of an agent in increasingly complex steps. For example, the effects of microwave radiation on solutions of biological molecules might be used as a test system to study predominant mechanisms of action. Uncomplicated systems can be very useful for exploring and evaluating mechanisms and may serve as a useful basis for designing experiments at the cellular level - the next level of biological complexity. By restricting the complexity of the experimental system, there will be less chance of possible subtle effects being masked by gross or dominant effects.

There are certain limitations that must be recognized when assessing in-vitro results. One can only speculate that an effect or mechanism of interaction found in-vitro will occur in-vivo. Many have speculated that the responsible mechanism(s) and physical interactions will not pertain in-vivo, but such speculations have been wrong often enough that uncritical dismissal should be avoided. When in-vitro results are used to serve as a basis for the design of in-vivo studies, two important advantages are offered:

(i) such experimental designs which can circumvent perceived elements of inapplicability may disclose important biological phenomena of general applicability,
(ii) failure to obtain comparable results (in-vivo as in-vitro) may offer clues to, or confirmation of, biophysical phenomena relating to fundamental interactions of the physical agent with tissue.

One can conclude from the preceding that health agencies can place only limited value on in-vitro experiments and must await the results of similar experiments conducted in-vivo. The in-vitro results may indicate that a cautious or prudent approach should be adopted when setting standards. Once mechanisms of interaction are understood and found to occur in animals, the next step is to determine if it is possible to extrapolate the results to man.

Scaling From Animals

One can perform two types of extrapolation of results from animal experiments to those expected in man: physical and physiological scaling. Let us first consider physical scaling. Exposure to microwave or radiofrequency energy induces electric and magnetic fields within a biological system. At the frequencies of interest, animals and humans can be considered as lossy dielectrics - having finite conductivity through motion of charge in the form of free ions (conduction loss) and molecular rotation (dielectric loss). Both these processes result in energy being transfered from the field to the absorbing medium. The amount of energy absorbed varies with the frequency of the impinging radiation. Figure 5 shows the amount of energy absorbed (specific absorption rate (SAR)) as a function of frequency for man, mouse and monkey. The total amount of energy absorbed by an exposed animal will vary greatly depending on the animal size, its orientation to the field and frequency of the microwave and radiofrequency energy.

Durney et al[19] have a relationship for determining the equivalence of animal exposure to that expected for man under similar conditions. The equivalent human-exposure frequency (f_h) can be approximated using the following equation:

$$f_h = f_a \frac{l_a}{l_h}$$

where f_a = animal exposure frequency
l_a = length of animal

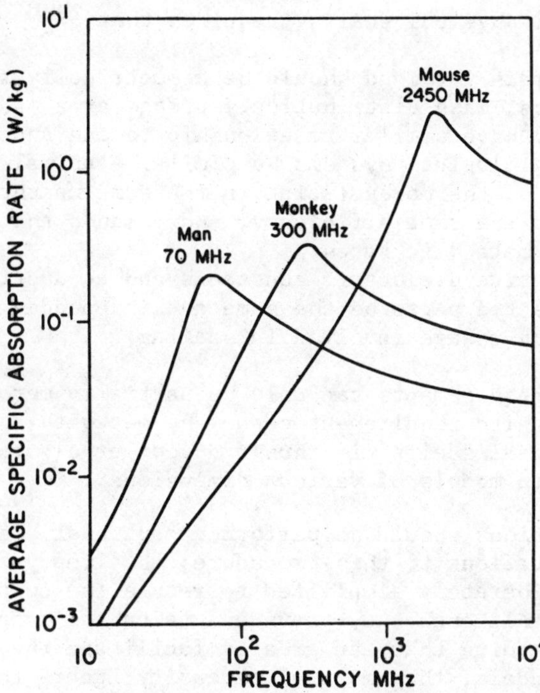

Figure 5. Average specific absorption rate as a function of frequency of electromagnetic radiation, for man, mouse and monkey.

l_h = length of human

f_h is then used to obtain the average SAR expected in man at this frequency by reading the SAR for the appropriate polarization from Figure 17 in Durney et al[14]. The equivalent human exposure or power density P_e (mW/cm^2) can then be determined using

$$P_e = \frac{SAR_a}{SAR_h}$$

where SAR_a = average SAR in exposed animal (W/kg)
SAR_h = average SAR in human per unit power density expected at the equivalent frequency (f_h) in W/kg/mW/cm^2.

This physical or frequency scaling can be used for extrapolating the results of experiments performed on different sizes of laboratory animals to those expected in man, or extrapolation from one species to another.

Successful physical scaling requires that:[20]

(i) the animals involved should be geometrically similar, so that mass, mass distribution, surface area and surface geometry have similar relationship to one another;
(ii) the physiological systems be similar - animals to be capable of thermoregulating in the same manner, or at least to the same efficiency, and demands that they have similar metabolic rates;
(iii) the relative dielectric constants and conductivities of the affected parts be the same and independent of the frequency change involved in scaling.

The first two requirements can only be partially met or taken into account. The third requirement cannot be met with any known animal species. Physical scaling is thus reduced largely to extrapolating data obtained in models of various dimensions.

Extrapolations should be performed cautiously as there are a number of limitations to this procedure, as already indicated. Models are deliberately simplified to reduce the complexity of the calculations. Although they provide a valuable insight and quantitative understanding that can greatly facilitate the analysis of more complex models, they must of necessity ignore the existence of limbs and the true geometry of the animal, which can lead to further distortions of the field. Most of the data have been obtained from models or phantoms having uniform properties. When consideration is given to the different properties of bone and muscle for example, the energy deposition might be expected to be much more uneven in live animals than the models predict.

There are other problems inherent in the use of whole body average SAR. Whole body average SAR is probably unsuitable for extrapolation of partial body and many near-field exposure situations. Further, SAR values are determined using the bulk electrical properties of the exposed medium and ignores local variations in electrical properties due to tissue inhomogeneities, and ignores possible effects from frequency - dependent resonances occurring, for example, at the subcellular or submolecular levels. Inherently SAR specifies a rate of delivery, not an amount of energy, implying the absence of cumulative effects, regardless of the exposure duration.

Physiological scaling can be performed on the basis of basal metabolic rates (BMR) for animals and man. In essence the scaling depends on relating the BMR to the effectiveness that a thermal load can be dissipated. This has already been discussed briefly in this text and has received extensive treatment by Tell and Harlen[6]. Temperature elevations occur in a body when the rate of energy absorbed from the incident fields exceed the energy dissipation rate and depends on such factors as the thermoregulatory mechanism, and the microwave or radiofrequency field characteristics and distributions within the body.

Both passive and active thermoregulatory mechanisms exist to dissipate a thermal load. Passive thermoregulatory mechanisms include heat radiation, evaporation cooling, conduction and convection. Fur-bearing animals and clothed humans lose heat by this mechanism predominantely via heat radiation and convection between the body and the immediate environment.

Active thermoregulatory mechanisms use internal circulating fluids (such as blood) to transfer heat to external parts of the body where passive heat convection and radiation are more effective. Some fur-bearing animals transfer internal heat via the blood to the lungs, dissipate the heat to inspired air by convection and expire it into the environment. Man uses the mechanism of cutaneous vasodilation to transfer internal heat via the blood to the skin where it can be radiated and convected away. Sweating from the human skin and the paws and nose of fur-bearing animals also provides a means of dissipating heat via evaporation of fluids.

Localized temperature rises or hot spots can occur if the rate of energy absorption is higher than the vascular heat transfer capacity of the local area (e.g. lens of eye, brain) or conversely if the rate of energy absorption is uniform throughout the region but the vascular system is such that pooling occurs (ie in the gut or the spleen), with a subsequent accummulation of heat in this pool.

It is apparent that the thermoregulatory mechanisms of animals and man are not the same. The efficiency of heat dissipation of fur-bearing animals is likely quite different to that of man under different environmental and exposure conditions. However it is a fact of life that most experiments must be performed on animals and one would like to have some method of scaling the observations in animals to predict the consequences of human exposure. At the present time, oversimplified as it may be, scaling on the basis of frequency is still the best available methods.

One can only make limited conclusions from such frequency scaling of biological effects. Further, such limited scaling could only have application to thermal effects. Apparent non-thermal effects such as the report of calcium ion efflux from isolated chick brain[21] would not appear to be able to be scaled.

Until about 5 years ago, virtually all reported biological effects were related to incident power density and not to absorbed energy, making it almost impossible to correlate or extrapolate data from animal experiments to those expected in man.

CONCLUSIONS

The question of whether a biological effect of exposure to microwave or radiofrequency radiation is a risk to health requires a very careful analysis. One would like to be able to obtain the necessary data on health effects directly from human experience, either through epidemiological studies or possibly from case reports that have been studied scientifically. Unfortunately this is not the case.

Reliance has to be placed on in-vitro experiments to elucidate fundamental interactions and phenomena, and obtain guidance with respect to experiments that should be performed in-vivo. Effects observed in-vitro do not necessarily mean that similar effects will occur in-vivo. This point cannot be over emphasized. The determination of adverse health effects cannot be made solely on the basis of effects found from in-vitro experiments. A prime example of such an effect that could potentially have widespread implications is the alteration of calcium efflux in brain tissue induced by modulated microwave fields. The best one could make of such a situation is to adopt a cautious approach to assessment in the hope that similar experiments conducted in-vivo will shed enough light to determine if a health hazard exists.

Health agencies rely heavily on the data from animal experiments. In this regard however, equal weight cannot be placed on all scientific publications. Unfortunately many conflicting reports occur in the scientific literature which further compound the problems of determining potential health hazards. Peer review of scientific reports to ensure that data were obtained from well performed and controlled experiments with good dosimetry, is of great value when making health assessments. Final assessments of biological effects being true health hazards can only be made from experiments confirmed in at least two independent laboratories.

What is perceived to constitute a risk to health in one country may not necessarily be considered a concern in another country - this obviously has to be taken into account in any health risk assessment.

In conclusion, I would like to give my own definition of what effects should be considered as health hazards. A biological effect is a health hazard if the effect either produces damage to tissue, albeit reparable, or causes changes to normal function that are outside the range of physiological compensation. Behavioral effects are generally a secondary reaction to the primary effect. Secondary reactions must be considered in this health risk assessment. As already discussed, adverse behavioral effects could be induced by being subjected to the microwave auditory sensations without knowledge or control of the circumstance.

The primary effect is an insignificant rise in temperature. Exposure standards should probably address this effect of pulsed radiation.

Acknowledgements

I would like to thank Dr. Jim Lin for helpful discussions on the microwave auditory effect. Many thanks to Dr. Maria Stuchly and Dr. Peter Waight for their reviews, Mr. David Lecuyer for preparation of the figures and Mrs. Judy Smith for typing this manuscript.

REFERENCES

1. S.M. Michaelson, Human exposure to non-ionizing radiant energy - potential hazards and safety standards, Proc. IEEE, 389-421, April (1972).
2. I. Matelsky, Non-ionizing radiations, in Industrial Hygiene Highlights, Vol. 1, ed. L.V. Cralley and G.D. Clayton, Industrial Hygiene Foundation of America, Pittsburg, Pa., pp. 140-179 (1968).
3. World Health Organization, Environmental Health Criteria for Radiofrequency and Microwaves, WHO, Geneva, Switzerland (1980).
4. P. Czerski and S. Szmigielski, Microwave bioeffects, current status and concepts, Proc. 5th European Microwave Congress, Hamburg (1975).
5. J.C. Lin, "Microwave auditory effects and applications", C.C. Thomas Pub., Springfield, Illinois, pp. 221 (1978).
6. R.A. Tell and F. Harlen, A review of selected biological effects and dosimetric data useful for development of radio-frequency safety standards for human exposure, J. Microwave Power, 14(4), 405-424 (1980).
7. "Criteria for a recommended standard: Occupational exposure to hot environments", U.S. Dept. of Health, Education and Welfare, National Institute for Occupational Safety and Health Technical Report, HSM 72-10269 (1972).
8. J. de Lorge, Disruption of behavior in mammals of three different sizes to microwaves: Extrapolation to larger mammals, In: Abstracts 1978 Symp. on Electromagnetic Fields in Biological Systems, Ottawa, Canada, June 27-30 (1978).
9. A.F. Emery, R.E. Short, A.W. Guy, K.K. Kraning and J.C. Lin, "The numerical thermal stimulation of the human body when absorbing non-ionizing microwave irradiation with emphasis on the effect of different sweat models", Symposium on Biological Effects of Electromagnetic Waves, Boulder, Colorado, October 20-23, 1975, In U.S. Dept. of Health, Education and Welfare Pub. (FDA) 77-8011, December (1976).

10. A.W. Guy, M.D. Webb, A.F. Emery and C.K. Chou, Determination of the average SAR and SAR patterns in man and simplified models of man and animals exposed to radiation fields from 50 - 2450 MHz and the thermal consequences. In abstracts: "Symposium on the Biological Effects of Electromagnetic Waves", Helsinki, Finland, August 1-8 (1978).
11. H.N. Kritikos and H.P. Schwan, Potential temperature rise induced by electromagnetic field in brain tissue, IEEE Trans. Biomed. Eng., BME-26(1), 29-33 (1979).
12. J.G. Burr, D.K. Cohoon, E.L. Bell and J.W. Penn, Thermal response model of a simulated cranial structure exposed to radiofrequency radiation, IEEE Trans. Biomed. Eng., BME-27(8), 452-459 (1980).
13. J.G. Burr and J.H. Krupp, Real-time measurement of RFR energy distribution in the Macaca Mulatta head, Bioelectromagnetics 1, 21-34 (1980).
14. C.H. Durney, C.C. Johnson, P.W. Barber, H. Massoudi, M.F. Iskander, J.L. Lords, D.K. Ryser, S.J. Allen and J.C. Mitchell, "Radiofrequency radiation dosimetry handbook" (second edition), Report SAM-TR-78-22, United States School of Aerospace Medicine, Brooks Air Force Base, Texas 78235 (1978).
15. J.C. Lin, The microwave auditory phenomenon, Proc. IEEE 68(1), 67-73 (1980).
16. A.W. Guy, C.K. Chou, J.C. Lin and D. Christensen, Microwave-induced acoustic effects in mammalian auditory systems and physical materials, Ann. N.Y. Acad. Sci., 247:194-218 (1975).
17. Health and Welfare Canada, "Noise hazard and control", Environmental Health Directorate Publication 79-EHD-29 (1979).
18. D.R. Justesen, Behavioral and physiological effects of microwave radiation, Bull. N.Y. Acad. Med., 55(11); 1058-1078, (1979).
19. C.H. Durney, M.F. Iskander, H. Massoudi, S.J. Allen and J.C. Mitchell, "Radiofrequency radiation dosimetry handbook" (third edition), Report SAM-TR-80-32, United States School of Aerospace Medicine, Brooks Air Force Base, Texas 78235, (1980).
20. S.M. Michaelson, "Microwave and radiofrequency radiation", World Health Organization, Regional Office for Europe, Copenhagen, Pub. No. ICP/CEP 803, pp. 98 (1977).
21. S.M. Barwin and W.R. Adey, Sensitivity of calcium binding in cerebral tissue to weak environmental electric fields oscillating at low frequency, Proc. Nat. Acad. Sci. (USA), 73:1999-2003, (1976).

DIELECTRIC PROPERTIES OF BIOLOGICAL TISSUES AND CELLS AT ELF-FREQUENCIES

H. P. Schwan

Max Planck Institut für Biophysik
Frankfurt a. Main, Germany

and

Department of Bioengineering D3*
University of Pennsylvania
Philadelphia, Pennsylvania 19104 USA

The dielectric properties of tissues and cell suspensions in the RF-and MW-range and mechanism responsible for such data have been summarized in our preceeding lecture[1]. Here we shall review low frequency data and what is known so far about possible mechanism involved.

Unfortunately not many data are available about dielectric properties of cell suspensions in the ELF range compared to the abundance of data in the RF- and MW-range. Reasons for this are the great experimental technical problems involved in the determination of the dielectric constant[2]. Electrode polarization is a major problem, causing large reactive deviations which have nothing to do with cellular dielectric properties and must be corrected for. Demands for exceedingly high resolution must be set in order to be able to detect the contribution of the dielectric constant to the total admittance observed. This problem is particularly severe for cell suspensions at low frequencies.

Let us assume a simple cellular model with a membrane surrounding the cell interior. This model does not yet incorporate more

---

* Permanent Address

complex structures and phenomena such as surface conductances and capacitances and their relaxational behavior caused by counterion movements and subcellular organelles connecting with the outer membrane. Then equations (4, 5) from the preceeding lecture[1] indicates that membrane capacity C_m and conductance G_m must change at low frequencies below the β-dispersion range if the dielectric constant and conductivity change, i. e. if α-relaxational effect exist. All other parameters of these equations are frequency in-

Table 1. Typical data are presented which characterize the α-dispersion of several biological systems. Characteristic frequencies f_c are given and apparent membrane capacitance changes $\Delta C = C_o - C_\infty$ with frequency as calculated from equation (5). These apparent membrane capacitance changes are not necessarily caused by the membrane since they integrate membrane responses with those in its immediate neighbourhood.

	ΔC	f_c
E. coli	> 10 μF/cm^2	3 KHz
Muscle	30	0.1
Ghosts	0.6	2.5
PPLO	0.1	100

dependant. We shall term these membrane changes in the α-range "apparent" since they are deduced from the stated model. Observed dielectric changes in the α-range can be expressed in terms of equivalent "apparent" membrane property changes, using equations (4, 5) of reference[1]. Examples are given in table 1. They demonstrate at first glance a confusing variety without any clear pattern. Possible mechanism responsible for these apparent membrane changes are discussed now.

low frequencies for typical membrane conductivities and capacitances[3]. But while this membrane model may have been acceptable in the Fifties, it is no longer so today. A simple double layer structure is not representative of the distribution of proteins through the membrane structure and membrane conductances cannot be individually assigned to the two layers as shown in Fig. 1. They occur instead at specific sites and are in parallel to the total membrane structure.

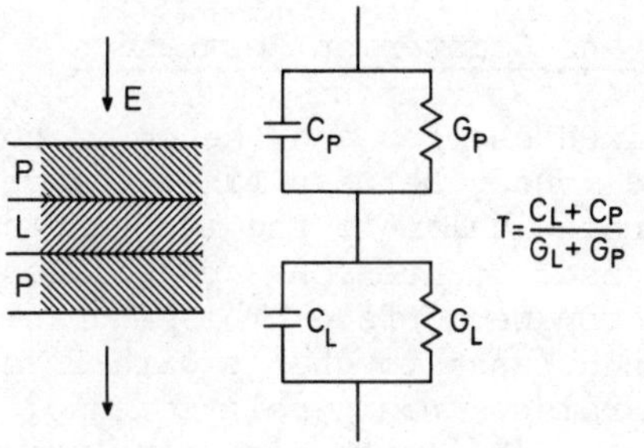

Figure 1. A membrane consisting of a lipid layer (L) covered by two protein layers (P) can be modelled by the network in the center. The two protein layers are combined into one network, assuming these two layers are identical. The network displays dispersion behavior with a time constant indicated in the equation.

MECHANISM

A Sandwich Type of Membrane Structure[3]

The membrane model assumes two layers of proteins and a lipid layer, figure 1. This model and its corresponding circuit indicated in Fig. 1 display an overall frequency dependence of its total capacitance and conductance characterized by a single time constant. Dispersion effects are anticipated to occur at

A "Polarization" Element in Series with Membrane

A boundary potential exists in the immediate neighborhood of the membrane which will be modulated by an alternating current. The modulation potential is proportional to the current density and thus defines an impedance element in series with the membrane. A double layer capacitive component of more than 10 μF/cm^2 can be estimated. This capacity, rather than the membrane capacitance, will determine the apparent capacitance of the total system at frequencies low enough to make the capacitive membrane susceptibility small compared to the membrane conductance. This happens at frequencies f so that $2\pi f < 1/T$ where T is the membrane time constant $T = R_m C_m$ (R_m, C_m membrane resistance and capacitance per 1 cm^2 area). Little attention has been directed so far to the role of cellular boundary potentials.

Surface Conductance and Counterion Relaxation

Cells possess fixed charges and, hence, a counterion atmosphere. Electrostatic forces between fixed charge and counterion prevent movement perpendicular to the membrane surface but not tangential to it. Hence, counterions are mobile in the direction tangential to the membrane surface. This mechanism causes the apparent surface conductance to change with frequency and, hence, as demanded by the Kramers-Kronig relationship, to contain an imaginary part. We were able with high resolution equipment to demonstrate that these changes are of the relaxational type[4, 5]. They can be well described by the Cole-Cole type relaxation equation

$$Y_s = Y_\infty + \frac{Y_o - Y_\infty}{1 + (j\omega T)^\alpha} \tag{1}$$

where Y_s is the surface admittance

$$Y_s = G_s + j\omega C_s \tag{2}$$

with G_s surface conductance and C_s surface capacitance and the subscripts o and ∞ indicating limit values for low and high frequencies compared to the characteristic frequency $f_c = 1/2\pi T$ and T the average time constant of the relaxation process. Confirming data with polysterene latex particles of various sizes, and fat particle emulsions had been collected[4, 5, 6]. Induced dipol moments caused by movement of counterions was proposed as responsible for this effect[5, 7]. A theory which explained the frequency dependent contribution to the surface conductance was developed[7]. The theory provided under circumstances not necessarily relevant to biological cells closed form solutions for the dielectric constant

$$\varepsilon_o = \varepsilon_\infty + \frac{e^2 \sigma R}{KT_o} \frac{9}{4} p \tag{3}$$

and the time constant

$$T = \frac{R}{2uKT} \quad , \tag{4}$$

with e elementary charge, σ charge density, R particle radius, K Boltzmann constant, T_o absolute temperature, p particle volume fraction, u ion mobility. It had to be assumed that the extent of the counterion atmosphere is small compared with the radius of the particle and that the effective dielectric constant of the particle makes only a negligible contribution to the total polarization. This latter assumption is unfortunately not correct for cells since the effective dielectric constants of biological cells are very high at low frequencies, reaching values of many thousands relative to free space. Thus, the theory is of limited usefulness for biological cells and needs to be extended. Counterion relaxation was suggested as possibly responsible for the high dielectric constants of muscle tissue and its α-dispersion at a time when a theoretical treatment of this effect was not yet available[5]. Later, Fatt confirmed the relaxation mechanism, but pointed out that the counterion hypothesis would require unusually high fixed charge densities[8].

Intracellular Organelles Connecting with Outer Membrane Surface

Access to a large membrane system such as the endoplasmic reticulum may be modeled as a resistor in series with the folded membrane surface. Model calculations demonstrate that the effect occurs at low frequencies. Falk and Fatt[8] suggested that the frequency dependent access to the tubular system is responsible for the very high dielectric constants of muscular tissue. The change from an apparent membrane capacitance of 1 $\mu F/cm^2$ to 30 $\mu F/cm^2$, ref. 3, 5, as the frequency changes from 1 KHz to 10 Hz would be explained by a total membrane system with a frequency independent value of 1 $\mu F/cm^2$ if the subcellular membrane area is 30 times larger than that of the outer membrane. Supporting evidence of this model was provided by Freygang et al.[9].

Membrane Relaxation Effects

It is readily shown from a linearization of the Hodgkin-Huxley equations that relaxation effects of the dielectric properties of the membranes can be expected at low frequencies. Such changes in membrane properties must proportionally reflect in low frequency dielectric properties since from equation 4, reference 1

$$\varepsilon_L = \varepsilon_\infty + \frac{9}{4}\,pRC_m \sim \frac{9}{4}\,pRC_m \qquad (5)$$

with ε_L dielectric constant at low frequencies, ε_∞ dielectric constant at very high frequencies, p volume fraction of cells, R cell radius, C_m membrane capacitance per unit area. Usually ε_∞ can be neglected and, hence, ε_L becomes proportional to C_m as indicated. The equation is based on spherical cellular shape, but the proportionality of ε_L and the apparent membrane capacitance C_m has general validity.

The perplexing variety of α-dispersion phenomena observed with biological cells was already indicated in Table 1. Erythrocytes apparently do not display an α-relaxation behavior at all[10], but red cell ghosts relax near 2.5 KHz[11] and the low frequency limit of the membrane capacitance is about 1.5 times larger than its high frequency value of about 0.9 $\mu F/cm^2$. The strongest α-dispersion effect observed so far is that of muscle tissue, with the dielectric constant increasing from 10^5 to 3.10^6 with a relaxation frequency of only 80 Hz[3, 5]. Other tissues with high water content display similar large increases[12]. Bacteria also display large increases[5], ranging from values ne 10^4 to values of about 10^5. But their low frequency behavior appears to be characterized by a rather broad spectrum of relaxation times. PPLO (Pleurapneumonia-like organisms) have a rather small α-dispersion occurring at a rather high relaxation of about 100 KHz[13]. Several vesicle systems have been investigated[14, 15], with one displaying α-dispersion and the other not. And, finally, the squid axon membrane has been reported to display dispersion near 2.5 KHz[16] by an amount similar to that of the erythrocyte ghost[11].

Table 2 indicates which phenomena have been explained in terms of some of the models outlined before. Carstensen and his coworkers[17] have done extensive work on bacteria and protoplasts, and extended the counterion theory[18] and applied it with due consideration of the large amount of fixed charges in the bacterial wall[19]. They have convincingly argued that the low frequency effects in bacteria are due to the counterion displacement mechanism. The same is true for the vesicle system investigated by Schwan et al.[14]. Electrophoretic measurements on these vesicles were conducted and a surface charge determined which explains the magnitude of the dispersion using equation (3), and the relaxation frequency fits that calculated from equation (4). The high relaxation frequency simply reflects the small size of the vesicles. The same calculation has been carried out for the PPLO, investigated by Schwan and Morowitz[13]. The characteristic frequency fits fairly well, but the magnitude could not be calculated since we did not know the surface charge.

Table 2. A summary of some α-dispersion studies and suggested dispersion mechanisms. For references, see text.

Bacteria	Carstensen et al.	Counterion
Vesicles	Schwan et al.	"
PPLO	"	" (?)
Muscle	Schwan	Counterion
"	"	Double Layer (?)
"	Fatt	Organelles
Eryth. Ghosts	Schwan & Carstensen	Counterion (?)
Sq. Axon	Takashima et al.	Membrane

Counterions had originally been suggested as possibly responsible for the α-dispersion of tissues[5] at a time when the counterion theory had not yet been formulated. But this explanation cannot be sustained since equation (3) would predict a magnitude much smaller than observed if typical charge densities are about one elementary charge per 10 Å squared area. This was pointed out by Fatt[20] who convincingly argued that a frequency dependent access to the tubular system is responsible[8, 20]. More recently it has been speculated that in many tissues a fuzzy "greater" membrane structure may contain filaments extending from the membrane and with high fixed charge densities[21]. This would demand a corresponding large counterion atmosphere. The counterion model developed by Einulf and Carstensen[18] may then be applicable. The relative contribution of counterions and the tubular system (and other organelles such as the reticulum) to the α-dispersion of muscle and other tissues remains unresolved.

In the case of erythrocyte ghosts the dispersion cannot be due to subcellular organelles connecting with the outer membrane since such organelles are not known to exist. The magnitude of the dispersion could be explained by a reasonable fixed charge density using equation (3). But the relaxation frequency calculated from equation (4) is much too low compared with the experimental value of 2.5 KHz.

While measuring the bulk dielectric properties of tissue and cell suspensions, fairly uniform fields are applied over cellular dimensions. This causes counterion displacement in the field direction and results in surface admittance disperion discussed above. Fields in a radial direction can be achieved with internal-external electrode pair arrangements. Such fields are less likely to move counterions in a radial direction since counterions interact with the fixed cellular charges by strong Coulombic forces. We decided, therefore, to employ radial fields and investigate the membrane of the giant squid axon in order to exclude counterion effects to contribute to membrane relaxation effects.

The relaxation observed with the squid axon membrane[16], was probably, at least in part, due to stray field effects. Later attempts to compensate for the stray field by variation in electrode length resulted in a reduction of the dispersion amplitude. Attempts to correct for the stray field were made by varying the length of the internal electrode and noting the differences between the results obtained with different lengths[22]. This technique should eliminate stray field contributions provided they do not change due to a changing diameter of the axon. A dispersion effect was observed, of smaller magnitude than originally stated. Fishman also obtained results which support the existence of the relaxation effect near 2.5 KHz[23]. More work is indicated to entirely resolve the problem of possible stray field contributions to relaxation effects in membranes.

We have not discussed the frequency dependencies which may result from an ion gating mechanism. We already stated that the Hodgkin-Huxley equations suggest such effects at the linear level. In recent years Fishman and his colleagues have studied the squid axon membrane at frequencies extending substantially below 1 KHz[23, 24 25]. Strong frequency dependencies are observed, which appear to correlate well with the predictions of the linearized Hodgkin-Huxley equations. De Felice and his colleagues have studied the squid axon membrane admittance as a function of frequency and clamped DC potential with small AC signals. They report sharp resonant-like admittance peaks for certain combinations of clamped DC potential and frequency[26], and second order admittances generating harmonics and suggesting nonlinear admittance components at AC potentials as small as 1 mV across the membrane[27, 28]. As stated in the introduction, this summary is entirely restricted to dielectric relaxation effects at the linear level.

In summary: So far no membrane system has been identified yet with certainty which displays dielectric relaxation behavior directly at frequencies above 1 KHz, except for some observations reported above. Counterion relaxation is possibly responsible in many cellular suspensions for the observed low frequency relaxation effects. But the amazingly high static dielectric constants of tissues may be caused primarily by subcellular organelles. Counterion contributions provide an alternate explanation only if very high charge densities outside a "greater" membrane are assumed. More work is needed to extend the theory of counterion relaxation so that it can be applied with more confidence to biological cells.

To what extent ion gating mechanisms contribute to dielectric relaxation mechanisms is presently under investigation.

PROPERTIES

As mentioned above good ELF-data on the dielectric properties of cellular suspensions are limited. This is to be regretted since cellular suspensions render themselves more easily to analysis than comparatively complex tissues. But also tissue data are limited as far as dielectric constants are concerned and are primarily those determined by Schwan and Kay[11]. However several conclusions can be readily drawn from available data:

1. Electrical properties at ELF are highly frequency dependent, just as RF- and MW-properties are.
2. Dielectric constants reach at frequencies below 100 Hz values which are extraordinarily high. They are so high that the imaginary component of tissue admittance values can not always be assumed to be small compared to the real one (i.e. conductivity).
3. The highly frequency dependant characteristics of tissues through the total frequency range from DC to many GHz suggests that mechanism of interactions of EM fields with biological matter must also be strongly frequency dependant.
4. Anisotropy of dielectric properties of tissues is suggested by their structure and supported by limited experimental evidence. This suggests that the direction of in situ fields which are induced in situ by external EM-sources may significantly influence interactions which take place at the cellular level.

ACKNOWLEDGMENT

Support by the Alexander von Humboldt-Stiftung, which provided a Senior U. S. Scientific Award is gratefully acknowledged.

REFERENCES

1. H. P. Schwan, Dielectric Properties of Biological Tissue and Cells at RF- and MW-Frequencies _in_: "Advances in biological Effects and Dosimetry of Low Energy Electromagnetic Fields," this volume (1981).
2. H. P. Schwan, Determination of Biological Impedances _in_: "Physical Techniques in Biological Research," Volume 6, W. L. Nastuk, Ed., Academic Press, New York (1963).
3. H. P. Schwan, Electrical properties of muscle tissue at low frequencies, _Zs. F. Naturforschung_ 9b:245 (1954).
4. H. P. Schwan, G. Schwarz, J. Maczuk and H. Pauly, On the low frequency dielectric dispersion of colloidal particles in electrolyte solution, _J. Phys. Chem._ 66:2626 (1962).

5. H. P. Schwan, Electrical Properties of Tissue and Cell Suspensions, *in*: "Advances in Biological and Medical Physics Vol. 5", J. H. Lawrence and C. A. Tobias, ed., Academic Press, New York (1957).
6. H. P. Schwan and J. Maczuk, Electrical relaxation phenomena of biological cells and colloidal particles at low frequencies, Proc. of the first National Biophysics Conference, p. 348 Yale University Press (1959).
7. G. Schwarz, A theory of low frequency dielectric dispersion of colloidal particles in electrolyte solution, *J. Phys. Chem.* 66:2636 (1962).
8. G. Falk and P. Fatt, Linear electrical properties of striated muscle fibers observed with intracellular electrodes, *Proc. Royal Soc. B* 160:69 (1964).
9. W. H. Freygang, Jr., S. I. Rapoport and L. D. Peachey, Some relations between changes in the linear electrical properties of striated muscle fibers and changes in ultrastructure, *J. Gen. Physiol.* 50:2437 (1967).
10. H. P. Schwan, T. P. Bothwell and F. J. Wiercinski, Electrical properties of beef erythrocyte suspensions at low frequencies, *Fed. Proc. Am. Soc. of Exp. Biol.* 13:15 1954).
11. H. P. Schwan and E. L. Carstensen, Dielectric properties of membrane of lysed erythrocythes, *Science* 125:985 (1957).
12. H. P. Schwan and C. F. Kay, Capacitive properties of living tissues, *Circulation Research* 5:439 (1957).
13. H. P. Schwan and H. J. Morowitz, Electrical properties of the membranes of the pleuropneumonia-like organism A 5969, *Biophys. J.* 2:395 (1962).
14. H. P. Schwan, S. Takashima, V. K. Miyamoto and W. Stoeckenius, Electrical properties of phospholipid vesicles, *Biophys. J.* 10:1102 (1970).
15. W. R. Redwood, S. Takashima, H. P. Schwan and T. E. Thompson, Dielectric studies on homogeneous phosphatidylcholine vesicles, *Biochim. Biophys. Acta* 255:577 1972).
16. S. Takashima and H. P. Schwan, Passive electrical properties of squid axon membrane, *J. Membr. Biol.* 17:51 (1974).
17. E. L. Carstensen, et al., Passive electrical properties of micro-organisms, I-IV *Biophys. J.* 5:289 (1965); 7:493 (1967); 8:536 (1968); and 9:634 (1969).
18. C. W. Einolf, Jr. and E. L. Carstensen, Low frequency dielectric dispersion in suspensions of ion-exchange resins, *J. Phys. Chem.* 75:1091 (1971).
19. C. W. Einolf, Jr. and E. L. Carstensen, Passive electrical properties of micro-organisms. V. Low frequency dielectric dispersion of bacteria, *Biophys. J.* 13:8 (1973).
20. P. Fatt, An analysis of the transverse electrical impedance of striated muscle, *Proc. Roy. Soc. B* 159:606 (1964).
21. W. R. Adey and S. M. Bawin, Brain interactions with weak

electric and magnetic fields, Neurosciences Res. Bull. 15, MIT Press, January (1977).

22. S. Takashima, Membrane capacity of squid axon during hyper- and depolarization, J. Membr. Biol. 27:21 (1976).
23. H. M. Fishman, Personal communication.
24. D. Poussart, L. E. Moore and H. M. Fishman, Ion movement and kinetics in squid axon. 1. Complex admittance, Ann. N. Y. Acad. Sci. 303:355 (1977).
25. H. M. Fishman, D. Poussart, L. E. Moore and E. Siebenga, K-conduction description for the low-frequency impedance and admittance of squid axon. J. Membr. Biol. 32:255 (1977).
26. L. J. De Felice, Personal communication.
27. L. J. De Felice, W. J. Adelman, Jr., D. E. Clapham and A. Mauro, Second order admittance in squid axon, Abstract, ASBC/Biophys. Soc. Mtg. (1980).
28. W. J. Adelman, Jr., Personal communication.

SOME FUNDAMENTAL ASPECTS OF BIOLOGICAL EFFECTS OF EXTREMELY LOW FREQUENCY (ELF)

W. Ross Adey

Veterans Administration Hospital, Loma Linda, CA 92357
and Departments of Physiology and Surgery, Loma Linda
University, School of Medicine, Loma Linda, CA 92350

INTRODUCTION

Environmental ELF fields in the spectrum below 100 Hz are an intrinsic aspect of the normal terrestrial environment. The entire gamut of terrestrial organisms from bacteria to man have evolved in this unceasing barrage of electromagnetic activity. Coupling of fields at these frequencies to tissues will be weak in comparison with radio or microwave fields having the same electric gradients in air, whether the tissues be in the near field of man-made devices, with direct capacitive coupling, or in the far field of propagating ELF disturbances, such as the Schumann resonances that encircle the earth as true Maxwellian radiation. Thus, the expected levels of induced components of environmental fields in the tissues of man exposed to a 10 kV/m power line field at 50 or 60 Hz would be in the range of 1.0 mV/cm. In assessing possible biological effects, the level of this induced gradient in extracellular fluid must be equated with the possibilities of direct modification of cell membrane potentials, where these membrane potentials are vastly greater, typically of the order of 10^5 V/cm. Since this clear disparity in gradients between the components of imposed fields and the membrane potential has been long known, it has been assumed that interactions were extremely unlikely.

Evidence that such interactions do indeed occur has suffered from inappropriate experiments, often with inadequate controls and lack of repeatability in the hands of others. Nevertheless, certain repeatable and otherwise credible observations have emerged. Some involve "extraordinary" sensitivities, based on special transductive systems. These include such structural devices as ferromagnetic particles in bacteria (Blakemore, 1975; Kalmijn and Blakemore, 1978) and the tissues of bees (Gould, Kirschvink and Deffeyes, 1978). Similarly, specialized sense organs in the skin of sharks and rays allow detection of oscillating low frequency fields, as weak as 10^{-8} V/cm (Kalmijn, 1971). In mammals, no such specialized receptor systems are known to exist, but equivalent sensitivities to environmental electric fields have been noted, based on modification of biological rhythms (Wever, 1968, 1975), intrinsic estimates of time intervals (Gavalas-Medici and Day-Magdaleno, 1976), and altered irritability of the central nervous system (Sagan, et al., 1981).

Low frequency pulsed magnetic fields, with typical peak values of less than 30 gauss accelerate union in ununited fractures, even though the induced tissue electric gradient in extracellular fluid is about six orders of magnitude less than the gradient of the membrane potential. These findings have lead to the application of similar magnetic field generators to other tissues under experimental conditions. These fields decrease sensitivity of osteoblast cultures to parathyroid and other peptide hormones. Similar fields sharply decrease insulin secretion in pancreatic islet cultures, and calcium binding and efflux are concurrently modified, as discussed below. Adjuvant effects of these fields on chemotherapy of mouse melanoma tumors *in vivo* has also been reported (Norton, Tansman, Pilla and Regelson, 1980). These endocrine and metabolic effects are highly nonlinear and exhibit all essential characteristics of cooperative processes.

By contrast with these effects of low level electric and magnetic fields, relatively little change has been reported in exposure of animals and man to extremely high electric field levels that occur in the immediate vicinity of high voltage power transmission lines. Many of these studies with appropriate controls are only now beginning and the data must be regarded as preliminary.

Biological Sensitivities To ELF Fields

In 1917 Parker and vanHeusen first reported sensitivity of fish to environmental electric fields. They noted that the blind-folded catfish is remarkably sensitive to metal rods in water in its vicinity. By contrast, a glass rod elicited no response. When long metal rods were introduced into the tank, the fish often swam away from it, but would approach and nibble at short segments of metal. They noted that this nibbling response could be elicited by a total current of approximately 1.0 μA between two electrodes about 2.0 cm apart. Avoidance reactions occurred with stronger currents.

Orientation, Navigation and Predation by Electrosensing in Marine Vertebrates

It became clear from these first observations that certain fish might utilize weak electric fields in their environment as important elements in their total sensory experience. From observations on weak electric fish (Gymnarchus) that emit continuous trains of pulses at rates between 300 and 1,000 Hz, Lissman (1958) proposed that these pulses are essential in locating environmental objects, and that weak electric fish have evolved from a preelectric fish lacking specialized electric organs but already sensitive to electric fields. Subsequent research has shown that catfish, sharks and rays, though lacking electric organs, detect tissue potentials arising in surrounding animals, including predators and prey, as well as fields arising within the animal's own body.

Studies of this electrosensitivity in fish have used weak DC and low frequency oscillating electric fields. Some studies have examined sensitivity to the earth's magnetic field in moving subjects; others have tested sensitivity to electric fields induced in moving sea water at field levels expected to occur through interaction of the moving fluid with the earth's magnetic field. Escape reactions occur in blindfolded sharks when a piece of steel wire comes within several centimeters of the body (Dijkgraaf, 1962). Escape reactions with local DC fields of 1-10 mV/cm. Square-wave 5.0 Hz fields elicited the same response and also caused eyelid contraction. Further studies by Kalmijn (1966, 1971) have strikingly demonstrated the extreme sensitivity of sharks and rays to these fields, and also suggest that the sensitivity is yet another of the "windowed" type of interaction. Square-wave fields at 5.0 Hz altered respiration of rays that had settled to the bottom of a tank where the gradient was only 0.1 μV/cm. The biological significance of this electrical sensitivity was tested in the shark by examining its feeding responses toward flatfish that form part of its natural diet. The shark approached randomly to within 10-15 cm of the flatfish as it lay buried in sand and then made well-aimed dives at the prey, uncovering it and eating it voraciously. The flatfish was then placed in an agar chamber in sand, and thus concealed visually, chemically and mechanically, but the animal's bioelectric field was unchanged. Both sharks and rays continued well-aimed frenzied attacks from the same distance as with unscreened prey. Odor leakage was excluded as a possible basis for the responses. Finally, a polyethylene film only 10 μm thick over the agar container eliminated all responses. It is therefore reasonable to conclude that this sensitivity arises by electric field detection.

The earth's magnetic field can provide an essential cue for rays trained to seek a food reward concealed in one of two identical buckets, symmetrically placed with respect to the earth's magnetic field (at 9.00 and 3.00 o'clock) against the walls of the tank (Kalmijn, 1978). When the tank was rotated 180 degrees with respect to the earth's magnetic field, the rays reversed their direction of circling to reach the food reinforcement. Calculated tissue electric gradients based on the rate of the animal's movement through the natural magnetic field were 0.5 μV/cm. These responses faded out with magnetic fields weaker than the natural levels and were not observed with imposed fields two orders of magnitude greater, suggesting an intensity "window." As discussed below, there is also an effective upper frequency limit of about 10 Hz.

ELF Field Effects on Human and Avian Circadian Rhythms

Human and avian circadian rhythms have been modified in an underground isolation unit shielded against natural electric and magnetic fields. Human circadian rhythms arise endogenously (Aschoff and Wever, 1962). Even without time cues in a constant environment, they deviate only slightly from 24 hours, with most autonomous human rhythms approximating 25 hours. Typically, oscillators governing different physiological and psychological variables are coupled and run synchronously (Wever, 1975) but may run asynchronously in "internal desynchronization." There rhythms also appear sensitive to 10 Hz, 2.5 V/m square-wave fields imposed in a shielded environment (Wever, 1968, 1974, 1977). Circadian periodicity was measured by sleep-wakefulness and rectal temperature periodicities. Dual identical chambers, one shielded and the other unshielded, allowed simultaneous testing of field-exposed and control subjects. For 57 subjects in the unshielded unit, the mean free-running period was 24.87±0.45 hours, with 4 subjects showing internal desynchronization; for 80 subjects in the shielded unit, the mean free-running period was 25.21±0.80 hours, with internal desynchronization in 28 subjects. All these differences were significant at P<0.01 or lower when considered separately Wever therefore hypothesized that the differences were due to natural EM fields present only in the unshielded unit. Subjects were then exposed to a 2.5 V/m, 10 Hz artificial field for one or two weeks, preceded and followed by control periods without fields. In 10 subjects, the period was shorter during field exposure than without it by an average of 1.3±0.7 hours (P<0.001). The shortening was greater for those subjects with the longest circadian cycles in the absence of the field. In some subjects, internal desynchronization occurred immediately after the field was switched off; in others it ceased immediately after the field was switched on. Shortened circadian rhythms were also seen in birds exposed to the same 10 Hz, 2.5 V/m square-wave fields (Wever, 1973).

Behavioral Effects of ELF Fields

The search for behavioral correlates of interactions between living organisms and environmental ELF fields presents serious experimental difficulties. The behaviors which may be modified by these interactions are generally subtle, and similarly amenable to modification by other weak environmental stimuli. Intercurrent conditions can therefore seriously influence the statistical validity of many reported reactions. Behavioral correlates have been sought with both natural and artificial ELF fields. Amongst the natural ELF oscillations are the Schumann (1957) resonances occurring in the background spectrum of natural ELF activity at frequencies between 8 and 32 Hz. They arise as a cavity resonance between the earth's surface and the concentric conducting shell of ionospheric particles at heights between 80 and 200 km (Keefe, Etzold and Polk, 1973; Polk, 1974). Reaction times in man have been reported as slowed at times of high natural activity between 3 and 6 Hz, with a converse effect at times of 10 Hz peaks (König, 1974). These natural oscillations have typical amplitudes of 1-2 V/m. Further studies from the same group with artificial fields at frequencies of 5-10 Hz and strengths of 0.3-5.0 V/m again showed trends consistent with effects of natural fields, but these trends were not amenable to statistical analysis. Other tests of human reaction times in ELF fields of 1-20 Hz have suggested that reaction time is inversely related to the field frequency (Hamer, 1968, 1969) but the statistical significance of these results has been questioned (Natl. Acad. Sci. USA, 1977). No changes in reaction time were seen in three squirrel monkeys tested for 1 hour daily before, during, and after exposure to a 45 Hz, 10 G magnetic field for 42 days (Grissett and deLorge, 1971).

These equivocal effects of ELF fields on reactions times suggested that this approach to psychophysiological effects might be unsuitable, and that "a broad range of very sensitive experiments are therefore required to evaluate properly the long-term effects of the ELF environment" (Grissett and deLorge, 1971). A more subtle and sensitive test involving subjective estimates of the passage of time by monkeys has been examined in two laboratories. Monkeys were required to estimate a time interval of 5.0 sec in the absence of behavioral cues. The results differed in the two laboratories, but the differences may relate seemingly minor differences in test procedures. In two separate studies, Gavalas-Medici and colleagues (Gavalas, Walter, Hamer and Adey, 1970; Gavalas-Medici and Day-Magdaleno, 1976) studied subjective time estimation in pigtail macaque monkeys to fields of 7, 45, 60 and 75 Hz at intensities of 1-100 V/m. At 7 Hz and 10 V/m, the mean time estimate was 5-10 percent shorter than in no-field conditions. There was an apparent threshold for the 7 Hz fields between 1 and 10 V/m. At 45 and 75 Hz, fields of 56 V/m produced smaller changes. At

100 V/m, no consistent effects were noted at any test frequency. Similar sensitivities were observed in monkeys with and without implanted cerebral electrodes. Measurements of total current (0.9 nA) induced in a phantom monkey head (Valentino, 1972) by a 10 Hz, 10 V/m field in this exposure chamber indicated expected extracellular electric gradients of 10^{-7} V/cm enhanced to 10^{-4} V/cm in the vicinity of the electrode tips.

In a similar study on rhesus monkeys exposed to weak (8.2-9.3 G) 15 and 45 Hz magnetic fields, deLorge (1973, 1974) interpreted the findings as equivocal. 3 of 4 subjects showed shorter interresponse times with the first series of exposures but not to the second. A test of the distributions was highly significant (Kalmogorov-Smirnov test, $P<0.001$). However, mean interresponse times were not altered by field exposure. Differing conclusions in these two studies that appear so similar may relate to details of the test procedures. Gavalas-Medici noted larger field/no field differences in interresponse times in the third and fourth hours of a 4-hour exposure. deLorge imposed an interresponse schedule 3 or 6 times in a 2-hour session, but for only 15 min for each task. If the findings of Gavalas-Medici validly indicate a gradual onset of altered subjective time estimation over several hours, there is a need for further studies of long-term exposure, particularly since investigator intervention was sometimes required in the later hours of the experiment to stimulate performance.

Behavioral Effects of 60 Hz Environmental Electric Fields on Laboratory Rats

Attempts to establish threshold levels for behavioral sensitivity to environmental ELF fields have lead to sharply differing results that appear related to the specific behavioral criterion under test. For this reason, there is much continuing research in which no final conclusions have yet been reached. Most of these studies are examining effects of fields at powerline frequencies. In simulating the environments around high voltage lines, it has been necessary to produce extremely high electric gradients in the range 50-100 kV/m. In turn, there are problems in assessing behavioral effects of such fields on test subjects with hairy skin, since these high field levels inevitably involve hair movement. For this reason, altered behavior seen in these fields requires consideration of at least two quite distinct mechanisms: those associated with peripheral sensory stimulation, including hair movement and those arising in direct interaction with internal organs and physiological systems.

Altered behavior has been reported with 60 Hz fields at levels below 10 kV/m, and thus not associated with significant hair movement. For example, during the first days of a 30-day field exposure, motor activity in male albino rats was considerably reduced by exposure to a vertical 1 kV/m 60 Hz field in the period after midnight. Normally, rats exhibit a major diurnal peak in their motor activity after midnight. This reduction was significant in comparison with animals exposed to 50 and 500 V/m fields and to control conditions. This decreased motor activity was not sustained beyond the first days of field exposure at 1 kV/m (Sagan, Adey, Sabbot and Bystrom, 1981).

In these same test subjects, the relative motor activity during the epoch from 0900 to 1000 hours was consistently but not significantly greater in the 1 kV/m period than in the 500 V/m and control conditions. The stimulus to this heightened activity related to the presence of animal handlers engaged in feeding procedures at this time.

These responses were interpreted as indicating a possible modification in circadian patterns of general motor activity associated with the start of exposure to a 1 kV/m field and a possibly enhanced sensitivity to external stimuli associated with the 1 kV/m condition.

Bird and Insect Orientation and Navigation in Environmental Electromagnetic Fields

Although there is good evidence that electromagnetic sensing in birds and insects offers a basis for biologically relevant activities, including navigation, uncertainties and controversies surrounding important aspects of these studies exemplify comparable problems in evaluation of related studies in mammals.

The earth's magnetic fields effects the orientation of the "waggle run" in the dance of honey bees (Lindauer and Martin, 1968, 1972). The gravitational field appears to be a symbol for the sun in this dance, so that the angle of the dance changes at approximately 15 degrees per hour relative to gravity as the bee compensates in time for the changing azimuth throughout the day. The most accurate runs occur at those times of day when the dance angle coincides with the magnetic vector. Errorless runs can be induced by artificial compensation of the magnetic field. Bees orient the sheets of comb within the hive to the geomagnetic field in the absence of other cues (Crane, 1974) and build bizarre combs in stronger or unusual fields (Martin and Lindauer, 1973). With fields changing as slowly as 1.5×10^{-6} G/min, bees are slowed in orienting responses to about 10 percent of normal rates and take about 30 min to adjust to a new field. Although a region of transversely oriented magnetic material has been reported on the front of the bees abdomen, appearing in the pupal state and

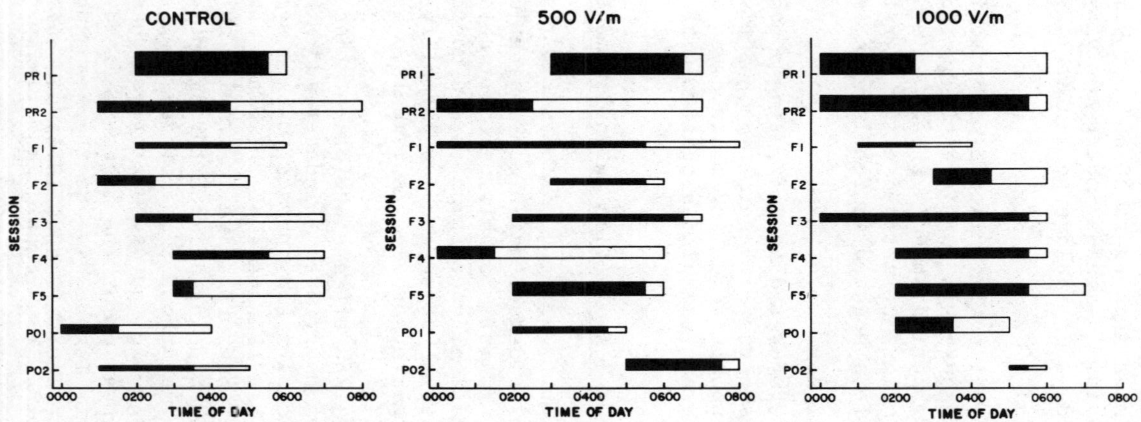

Fig. 1. The size, duration and time of occurrence of the late-night motor activity bout for selected sessions in rats exposed to 60 Hz fields for 30 days. Panel 1, control condition; Panel 2, 500 V/m field exposure. Each bar begins at the time the bout started and ends at the termination of activity. The area of each bar is proportional to the area between relative activity curve and the mean. The bars are divided to indicate the mode of the bout. (from Sagan *et al*., 1982)

persisting in adults (Gould, Kirschvink and Deffeyes, 1978), this period of adaptation argues against a role in simple reflex responses for either ferromagnetic particles within sensory cells or electric charge displacement by movement through the field. Termites (Becker, 1976) and beetles (Arendse and Vrins, 1976) are also sensitive to steady magnetic fields.

Evidence for insect sensitivities to electric fields is less substantial and the findings are somewhat contradictory. In 50 Hz high voltage fields (3-5 kV/m), bees have higher metabolic rates than controls, with higher food intake and activity and reduced life-span of worker bees (Altmann, 1959). Controls and data in these studies are difficult to evaluate, and the picture is further complicated by reported effects in plastic hives that are absent in wooden hives (Warnke, 1976).

There is now substantive evidence that birds may use a variety of cues in the course of a migratory flight, including landmark recognition, sun altitude, azimuth, a precise time sense, style patterns, the wind and weather, as well as the geomagnetic field. Many early studies of bird orientation to natural and artificial magnetic fields have been questioned on theoretical grounds, or for lack of statistical validation, or because of difficulties in reproducibility. A possible role for the geomagnetic field was first suggested by Middendorf in 1855, and since that time, experiments have tested models based on a comparison of field intensities, travel along a magnetic contour, and movement up or down a gradient (Keeton, 1977). Results have been conflicting, partly because of difficulties in designing experiments that are unequivocal in the evaluation of perception and response to signals that humans may not perceive (Adey, 1977). By contrast, there have been statistically significant results from experiments in which discrimination behavior in the magnetic environment was associated with unrestrained movement (Bookman, 1977). For example, pigeons were successfully trained in a flight tunnel 3 m long to discriminate between a simulated field of 0.5 G and the field reduced to 0.02 G at paired feeding stations at the termination of the tunnel. Discrimination was statistically significant in trials associated with "fluttering," defined as more than 3 sec of jumping, hovering or flight. "No-flutter" trials yielded random responses.

The extreme sensitivity to small differential changes in ambient magnetic field levels has been a striking aspect of these avian studies and a consistent finding among many of them. Minor fluctuations of 10^{-4} - 10^{-5} G associated with perturbations in solar particle fluxes are detected by homing pigeons (Keeton, Larkin, and Windsor, 1974). Orienting by the European robin becomes random after a certain change in the magnetic field strength by 0.1-0.2 G but may resume its directed character after adaptation over several days. Translated into expected levels of induced tissue gradients at flight velocities of tens of meters per second, these would probably not exceed 10^{-7} V/cm and might be several orders of magnitude lower for delta functions attributable to geomagnetic perturbations.

The Role of Specialized Receptors in Sensing ELF Environmental Fields

Specialized electroreceptive sensing organs have been found in some marine vertebrates, including sharks and rays. These systems have fascinating characteristics in relation to the animal as a whole, behaving as a volt meter without significant shunting of the imposed field. Their dynamic range is low, not more than 20-30 dB, so that range has been sacrificed in favor of sensitivity, a characteristic shared with the olfactory system (Adey, 1959). Two types of electroreceptors have been described, ampullary and tuberous. The ampullary receptors occur in both electric and nonelectric fish. Tuberous receptors are found exclusively in electric fish.

Ampullae of Lorenzini detect low fields originating externally, but they may also respond to certain nonelectric organ fields generated by the animals themselves. The ampullary electroreceptor opens on the skin surface by a minute pore connected to a subcutaneous jelly-filled canal with a terminal swelling, the ampulla proper. Sensing cells lie in the wall of this ampulla proper. Their outer surfaces face the lumen of the ampulla and thus appear to be connected to the external aqueous environment. Their inner surfaces synapse with afferent nerve fibers. Ampullary receptors are clustered along the snout region of the shark.

Tuberous receptors are sensitive only to high frequencies and seem to be specialized for detecting electric organ discharges (Scheich and Bullock, 1974). Discharges in this high-frequency receptor system are often synchronized with the electric organ discharge, with frequencies from 300 to 1000 Hz. There appeared to be thousands of receptor sites on the body. Each may oscillate at its own rate, not necessarily tuned to the electric organ frequency, although this is typical in organs with a higher frequency discharge (Bennett, 1971).

The ampullary canal has an extremely high wall resistance but a relatively low core resistance within the central canal and at the blind ampullary end. It therefore exhibits almost ideal cable properties at DC and for low-frequency electric oscillations. Typically, the wall resistance is around 6 $M\Omega/cm^2$, whereas core resistivity may be as low as 31 $\Omega.cm^{-1}$. The high wall capacity per unit length rapidly attenuates coupling of high-frequency oscillations in the length of the tube (Waltman, 1966). The low-pass frequency characteristic of the ampullary system gives it an effective upper frequency limit of about 10 Hz. Its sensitivity may be high for frequencies as low as 0.1 Hz, but it shows adaptation to DC fields. At frequencies between 0-10 Hz, the threshold for the first reaction of slight twitches in the body or appendages is about 1.0 μV/cm in fish with electrogenic organs and 10^4 V/cm in ordinary fish.

No such specialized electroreceptors are known to exist in the mammalian peripheral or central nervous systems, although intracellular ferromagnetic bodies have been described in the skull and muscles of pigeons (Presdi and Pettigrew, 1980). A region of transversely oriented magnetic material has been described on the front of the bee's abdomen, appearing in the pupal state and persisting in adults (Gould, Kirschvink and Deffeyes, 1978). The possible role of these inclusions in tissues of bees and pigeons in orienting to environmental magnetic fields is not yet known.

Microscopic examination of marine and freshwater muds collected from the Woods Hole area showed several forms of anaerobic and microaerophilic bacteria consistently swimming northward when separated from the sediments (Blakemore, 1975). Their direction of swimming was sensitive to introduction of a small bar magnet. Magnetosensitive bacteria include cocci, spirilla, and rods. Killed cells orient to the imposed field but do not swim. Some showed chains of crystals that stained with phosphotungstic acid, with typically two chains per cell. The crystals show a predominance of iron with significant amounts of magnesium phosphorus, sulphur and calcium.

Kalmijn and Blakemore (1978) reversed the north-seeking tendency by reversing the ambient magnetic field with Helmholtz coils. Strong, brief monophasic magnetic pulses reversed the internal permanent magnetic dipole, and the bacteria instantly turned around and from then on continued to swim in a southerly direction. The access of motility and the access of magnetization coincide. Their responsiveness fades out at magnetic levels below the natural fields and also disappears at levels about 100 times higher, strongly suggestive of a "window" phenomenon common to this and other bioeffects described here.

Cell and Tissue Biology of Interactions with ELF Fields

ELF electromagnetic fields influence important hormonal interactions with receptor cells *in vivo* and *in vitro*. Although these effects are now being studied in many laboratories, much of the work is in a preliminary phase and is the subject of continuing research. Representative experiments from our own and collaborating laboratories will be presented here, but they describe only limited aspects of a rapidly growing field. At the mechanismal level, there is strong evidence that calcium ions play a mediating role in many responses.

Freshly isolated chick and cat cerebral tissues exposed to sinusoidal electric fields at 1, 16, 32 or 75 Hz with electric gradients in air of 5, 10, 56 and 100 V/m exhibit a general trend toward a reduction in release of preincubated $^{45}Ca^{2+}$ (Bawin and Adey, 1976). Tissues were bathed in Ringer solution at 36°C. After 30 min of incubation with $^{45}Ca^{2+}$, each sample was immersed in the fresh solution and exposed to the field for 20 min. Efflux of $^{45}Ca^{2+}$ was then measured and compared with unexposed controls. Maximum decreases of 12-15% occurred at 6 and 16 Hz, with thresholds around 10 V/m for chick ($P < 0.01$) and 56 V/m for cat cortex ($P < 0.05$ at 6 Hz and $P < 0.01$ at 16 Hz), with estimated tissue gradients of the order of 0.1 μV/cm. Similar but nonsignificant trends occurred during other field exposures at 5 and 100 V/m. Thus the field effect on $^{45}Ca^{2+}$ was "windowed" in both frequency and amplitude domains. The curve of frequency dependence was a mirror image of that for the increased efflux induced by radio frequency fields modulated at the same low frequencies (see Fig. 1, Lectures 19 and 20).

Blackman, Benane and Kinney (1981) have examined effects of 16 Hz fields in the range 1 to 70 V/m (peak-to-peak incident field in air) on calcium efflux from chick brain tissue. This study used an exposure system in which appreciable current flowed in the plates establishing the electric field. Increased efflux (rather than the decrease noted by Bawin and Adey) occurred in these experiments, with evidence for multiple amplitude windows in this intensity range.

Stimulation of Bone and Bone Cells In Vitro by Low Frequency Pulsed Magnetic Fields

Clinical studies have demonstrated the usefulness of induced electromagnetic fields in stimulating feeling of chronically ununited fractures in man (Bassett, Pilla and Pawluk, 1977). Fields proven effective in clinical studies generate electrochemical gradients in the tissue fluid surrounding cells considerably weaker than levels required to depolarize cell membranes. These devices typically impose pulsed magnetic fields of about 20 Gauss. They induce current densities of about 1 μA/cm^2 and associated electric gradients of 1-10 mV/cm in extracellular fluids (Brighton *et al.*, 1981). Because of the high resistance of cell membranes, any transmembrane electrical components of imposed fields would be lower than the extracellular gradients by 2 to 3 orders of magnitude (Adey, 1981b), and thus would be as much as 5 orders of magnitude less than the typical excitatory threshold currents of 1 mA/cm^2 observed for axonal depolarization (Hodgkin and Huxley, 1952). Two types of generators developed by Bassett and Pilla and their colleagues at Columbia University have been approved for clinical therapy of nonunion in fractures. One generates a continuous train of pulses at around 72 Hz. Each pulse has a main deflection lasting 325 μsec, followed by a tail of opposite polarity lasting about 5 msec. The other produces recurrent bursts of 200 μsec pulses at a 4 kHz rate, with a burst duration of 5 msec and a burst repetition rate of 15 Hz.

These two generators have been tested on cultures of the osteoblast-like mouse bone cell line MMB-1 (Luben *et al.*, 1981). No significant differences were noted between effects of the two fields. Both fields significantly reduced the cellular production of cyclic adenosine monophosphate (cAMP) in response to parathyroid hormone (PTH) and osteoclast activating factor (OAF). Neither basal nor fluoride-activated levels of adenylate cyclase were altered in membranes from cells cultured in the fields. However, the same membrane preparation exhibited markedly inhibited responses to PTH. At the same time, the field blocked the inhibitory effects of PTH on synthesis of collagen by MMB-1 cells. However, there was no effect on the inhibition of collagen synthesis by 1,25-dihydroxyvitamin D3, which is believed to act primarily by a nuclear rather than a membrane-dependent mechanism. Responses in cultured fetal bone (mouse calvaria) were similar. We hypothesize that these field effects are mediated primarily at the plasma membrane of osteoblasts, either by interference with hormone-receptor interactions or by blocking of receptor-cyclase coupling within the membrane. These responses occurred with induced extracellular fields of 1 mV/cm or less, even though transmembrane potential gradients are typically 10^5 V/cm. The expected transmembrane current components of these extracellular fields would be on the order of 10^{-8} A/cm^2, five orders of magnitude less than the typical threshold for excitation based on a Hodgkin-Huxley model, implying the occurrence of a powerful amplification process in transduction of these exceedingly weak electrochemical triggers.

Response of Pancreatic Islet Cells to Low Frequency Pulsed Magnetic Fields in vitro

The pancreatic islets of Langerhans have been successfully isolated from the acinar tissue of the gland and thereafter transplanted to the liver in the therapy of human and animal diabetes mellitus (Jolley *et al.*,1982). Insulin secretion occurs from the β-cells of the islets, and the effects of low frequency pulsed magnetic fields on insulin secretion and on calcium uptake and efflux by the isolated islets in culture has been tested by Jolley *et al.* They used the Helmholtz Coil field generator described above, with recurrent bursts of 200 μsec pulses at a 4 kHz rate, with a burst duration of 4 msec and a burst repetition rate of 15 Hz. Insulin secretion was stimulated by 20 mM glucose solution.

During field exposure, insulin secretion was reduced by 35% as compared with control preparations ($P < 0.002$). Insulin secretion is a calcium-dependent process; calcium uptake by the islets was inhibited by 26% ($P < 0.004$) and calcium efflux fell by 27% ($P < 0.006$).

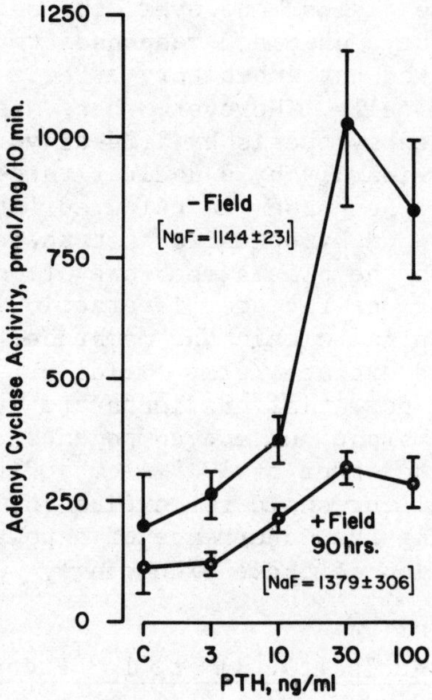

Fig. 2. Dose-response relationships for the effects of PTH on adenyl cyclase activity of bone cells in culture. MMB-1 cells were grown in the presence or absence of the 72 Hz pulsed magnetic field for 90 h without hormone treatment. The cells were then disrupted and a membrane preparation was isolated for adenyl cyclase assay. The membranes were treated for 10 min with indicated concentrations of parathyroid hormone (PTH) without field exposure, and production of cAMP determined (pmol cAMP formed per mg membrane protein per 10 min assay ± S.E.M.). (from Luben et al., 1981).

These data offer further support for models that emphasize the cell membrane as the site of primary interaction with an imposed electromagnetic field.

Models of cellular interactions with ELF Fields

The models of cellular interactions proposed for weak radio and microwave fields modulated at ELF (see Lectures 19 and 20) appear generally relevant to imposed ELF fields, since the experimental data have clearly established the requirement for ELF modulated, rather than unmodulated, RF fields in these responses, and thus implying that detection of the ELF envelope by a process of demodulation, presumably at cell membrane sites.

Classic models of membrane permeability changes during membrane excitation have been based on activation of ionic channels for the movement of Na^+ and K^+ ions, with an associated sharp rise in conductance (Hodgkin and Huxley, 1952). More recent theoretical studies have considered ionic behavior within the membrane in terms of an ionic plasma, and membrane behavior during excitation in terms of plasma oscillations (Vaccaro and Green, 1979; Triffet and Green, 1980; Lawrence and Adey, 1982).

Vaccaro and Green suggest that the sodium permeability hypothesis be replaced with one attributing the action potential to nonlinear plasma oscillations, and voltage clamp records to strongly damped oscillatory currents. In this model, the membrane phase is treated as a semielectrolyte with connected regions in which the ionic concentrations are not very different from those of the adjacent electrolytes. Mobilites of different ionic species in the membrane are identified with those measured in the steady state, and are not assumed to have large variations during excitation. The solution to the plasma model offered by Vaccaro and Green yields solutions in the millisecond range, consistent with the time course of the action potential and voltage clamp records. Polyvalent cations, such as Ca^{2+}, have a more pronounced damping effect on the electrolyte systems than monovalent cations. Plasma oscillations would allow transfer of ions at a much faster rate than could be achieved by ordinary conductance, an essential feature of the action potential. We have considered the possibility of entrainment of plasma oscillations by weak imposed fields (Lawrence and Adey, 1982). If we restrict attention to the region within the membrane in the Vaccaro, Triffet and Green model, the ionic fluctuations take on dispersive, rather than dissipative properties. The cold plasma equations used by Vaccaro and Green to show the existence of nonlinear waves as a special case may similarly be reduced to a single nonlinear equation with dispersive properties. We conclude that the action potential may be regarded as two critically damped Korteweg de Vries waves moving in opposite directions across the membrane.

SUMMARY

1) Biological sensitivities to ELF fields were reviewed. Much earlier research requires care in interpretation, due to lack of adequate controls and effects of intercurrent stimuli. 2) Orientation, navigation and predation in marine vertebrates (sharks and rays) involves electrosensing of gradients no larger than 10^{-7}V/cm for fields between 0 and 10 Hz. Human and avian cicadian rhythms appear sensitive to 10 Hz, 2.5 V/m square-wave fields. Subjective time estimation in monkeys suggests a threshold for 7 Hz fields between 1 and 10 V/m. From measurements of induced currents in phantom heads, expected extracellular gradients would be 10^{-7} V/cm. Specialized electroreceptive sensing organs have been found in sharks and rays, but are not known to exist in mammalian peripheral or central nervous systems. 3) Calcium binding and calcium-dependent cellular mechanisms are modified by weak ELF fields. Field effects on $^{45}Ca^{2+}$ efflux from isolated chick cerebral tissue is "windowed" in both frequency and amplitude in the spectrum from 6-20 Hz and at amplitudes in air between 10 and 100 V/m. Pulsed magnetic fields proven effective in therapy of ununited bone fractures generate electrochemical gradients considerably weaker than levels required to depolarize cell membranes. Induced current densities are about 1 $\mu A/cm^2$ and associated electric gradients of 1-10 mV/cm in extracellular fluids. Transmembrane gradients would be as much as 5 orders of magnitude less than typical excitatory threshold currents of 1.0 mA/cm^2. These fields reduced cellular production of cyclic adenosine monophosphate (cAMP) in response to the peptides parathyroid hormone (PTH) and osteoclast activating factor (OAF). The fields also blocked inhibitory effects of PTH on collagen synthesis, but excited no effect on the inhibition of collagen synthesis by 1,25-dihydroxyvitamin D3, which acts primarily by a nuclear, rather than a membrane-dependent mechanism. The same fields reduce insulin secretion and the binding and release of calcium in cultured pancreatic islets. 4) Models of mechanisms of bioeffects of ELF fields with ELF modulation (see Lectures 19 and 20). Observed effects are consistent with both dissipative (cooperative) and dispersive (soliton) processes at cell membranes. The sharp rise in cell membrane conductance associated with excitation has been modeled in terms of plasma oscillations, with sodium and calcium ions in a plasma state within the lipid bilayer. Plasma oscillations of this type would be susceptible to entrainment by imposed weak electromagnetic fields.

ACKNOWLEDGEMENTS

Studies from our laboratory described in these lectures were supported by the Office of Naval Research, the National Institute of Environmental Health Sciences, the Department of Energy, the Southern California Edison Company and the Bureau of Radiological

Health. It is a pleasure to acknowledge their patient help and guidance throughout the difficult initial phases of this research.

REFERENCES

Adey, W.R., 1959, The sense of smell, in: "Handbook of Physiology. Neurophysiology." Am. Physiol. Soc., Washington D.C. Sect.1, Vol. 1, ch. 21, pp. 535-549

Adey, W.R., 1977, The sensorium and the modulation of cerebral states: tonic environmental influences on limbic and related systems, Ann. NY Acad. Sci. 290:396-420

Adey, W.R., 1981a, Tissue interactions with nonionizing electromagnetic fields, Physiol. Rev. 61:435-514

Adey, W.R., 1981b, Ionic nonequilibrium phenomena in tissue interactions with electromagnetic fields, in: "Biological Effects of Nonionizing Radiation", K.H. Illinger, ed. Am. Chem. Soc. Symp. Ser., No 157. Am. Chem. Soc., Washington, D.C. pp. 271-297

Arendse, M.C., and Vrins, J.C.M., 1976, Magnetic orientation and its relation to photic orientation in Tenebrio Molitor L. (Coleoptera, Tenebrioniadae) Netherlands J. Zool. 25:407-437.

Aschoff, J., and Wever, R., 1962, Spontanperiodik des Menschen bei Ausschluss aller Zeitgeber. Naturwissenschaften 49:337-342

Bassett, C.A.L., Pawluk, R.J. and Pilla, A.A., 1974, Acceleration of fracture repair by electromagnetic fields, Ann. NY Acad. Sci. 238:242-249.

Bawin, S.M. and Adey, W.R., 1976, Sensitivity of calcium binding in cerebral tissue to weak environmental electric fields oscillating at low frequency. Proc. Natl. Acad. Sci. USA 73:1999-2003

Becker, G., 1976, Reaction of termites to weak alternating magnetic fields. Naturwissenschaften 63:201-202

Bennett, M.V.L., 1971, Electrolocation in fish, Ann. NY Acad. Sci. 188:242-269

Blackman, C.F., Bennane, S.G., and Kinney, L.S., 1981, Effects of ELF radiation on calcium ion efflux from brain tissue *in vitro*, Bioelectromagnetics Soc., 3rd Annual Conf. Washington, D.C. Abstracts, p. 47

Blakemore, R.P., 1975, Magnetotactic bacteria, Science 190:377-379

Bookman, M.A., 1977, The sensitivity of the homing pigeon, *Columbia livia*, to an earth strength magnetic field, Nature, London 267: 340-342

Brighton, C.T., Black, J., Friedenberg, Z.B., Esterhai, J.L., Day, L.J., and Connolly, J.F., 1981, A multicenter study of the treatment of nonunion with constant direct current. J. Bone Joint Surgery 63A:2-13

Crane, E., 1974, Directions in which bees build combs, Bee World 55:153-155

DeLorge, J., 1973, Operant behavior of rhesus monkeys in the presence of extremely low frequency-low intensity magnetic and electric fields. Experiment 2. Pensacola, FL Naval Aerospace Med. Lab. Publ. NAMRL - 1179. pp. 23

DeLorge, J., 1974, A psychological study of rhesus monkeys exposed to extremely low frequency-low intensity magnetic fields. Pensacola, FL Naval Aerospace Med. Lab. Publ. NAMRL - 1203

Dijkgraff, S., and Kalmijn, A.J., 1962, Verhaltensversuche zur Funktion der Lorenzinischen Ampullen. Naturwissenschaften 49:400

Gavalas, R.J., Walter, D.O., Hamer, J., and Adey, W.R., 1970, Effect of low-level, low-frequency electric fields on EEG and behavior in Macaca nemestrina, Brain Res. 18:491-501

Gavalas-Medici, R., and Day-Magdaleno, S., 1976, Extremely low frequency, weak electric fields affect schedule-controlled behavior of monkeys, Nature, London 261:256-258

Gould, J.L., Kirschvink, J.L., and Deffeyes, K.S., 1978, Bees have magnetic remanence. Science 201:1026-1028

Grissett, J.D., and deLorge, J., 1971, Central nervous system effects as measured by reaction time in squirrel monkeys exposed for short periods to extremely low-frequency fields. Pensacola, FL Naval Aeorspace Med. Res. Lab. Publ. NAMRL - 1137. pp 1-11

Hamer, J.R., 1968, Effects of low-level, low-frequency electric fields on human reaction time. Comm. Behav. Biol. 2(A):217-222

Hamer, J.R., 1969, Effects of low-level, low-frequency electric fields on human time judgement in: "Proc. 5th Internat. Biometeorologics Congress", Montreau, Switzerland. Trompe, S.W., and Weihe, W.H., eds. Springer, Berlin. p. 92

Hodgkin, A.L., and Huxley, A.F., 1952, A quantitative description of membrane current and its application to conduction and excitation in nerve J. Physiol., London 117:500-544.

Jolley, W.B., Hinshaw, D.B., Knierim-Hinshaw, K., and Hinshaw, D.B., 1982, Magnetic field effects on calcium efflux and insulin secretion in isolated rabbit islets of Langerhans, Bioelectromagnetics, in press.

Kalmijn, A.J., 1966, Electroperception in sharks and rays, Nature, London 212:1232-1233

Kalmijn, A.J., 1971, The electric sense of sharks and rays, J. Exper. Biol. 55:371-383

Kalmijn, A.J., 1979, Electromagnetic guidance systems in fishes, in: "Magnetic Field Effects on Biological Systems", Tenforde, T., ed. Plenum Press, New York

Kalmijn, A.J., and Blakemore, R.P., 1978, The magnetic behavior of mud bacteria, in: "Animal Migration, Navigation and Homing", Schmidt-König, K., and Keeton, W.T., eds. Springer, New York pp. 354-355

Keefe, W.T., Etzold, H., and Polk, C., 1973, Detection and processing of ELF (3-30 Hz) natural electromagnetic noise. Univ. Rhode Island, Kingston. US Air Force Report AFLRL-TR-73-0077

Keeton, W.T., 1977, Biological sensitivity to magnetic fields in orientational responses. Neurosci. Res. Program Bull. 15: 22-27

Keeton, W.T., Larkin, T.S., and Windsor, D.M., 1974, Normal fluctuation in the earth's magnetic field influence on pigeon orientation. J. Comp. Physiol. 95: 95-103

Lawrence, A.F., and Adey, W.R., 1982, Nonlinear wave mechanisms in interactions between excitable tissue and electromagnetic fields, Neurol. Res., in press.

Lindauer, M., and Martin, H., 1968, Die Schwereorientierung der Bienen unter dem Einfluss des Erdmagnet feldes. Z. Vgl. Physiol. 60: 219-243

Lindauer, M., and Martin, H., 1972, Magnetic effect on dancing bees in: "Animal Orientation and Navigation", Galler, S.R., Schmidt-König, K., Jacobs, G.J., and Belleville, R.E., eds. NASA Publ. SP-262. US Govt. Printing Office, Washington, D.C. pp. 559-567

Lissman, H.W., 1958, On the function and evolution of electric organs in fish. J. Exper. Biol. 35: 156-191

Luben, R.A., Chen, M., Rosen, D., Pilla, A.A., and Adey, W.R., 1981, Effects of therapeutic electromagnetically induced current on hormone responsiveness of bone cells in vitro, Proc. 157th Annual Meeting, Electrochem Soc., Bioelectrochemistry Symp., St. Louis, MO, 1980. Abstract 464, p. 75

Martin, H., and Lindauer, M., 1973, Orientierung in Erdmagnetfeld, Fortschr. Zool. 21:211-228

National Academy of Sciences, USA, 1977, "Biologic of Electric and Magnetic Fields Associated with Proposed Project Seafarer". Washington, D.C., p. 257

Norton, L., Tansman, L., Pilla, A.A., and Regelson, W., 1980, Electrochemical information transfer and the enhancement of in vivo anti-cancer chemotherapy, Proc. 157th Annual Meeting, Electrochem. Soc., Bioelectrochem. Symp., St. Louis, MO, 1980. Abstract 462, p. 75

Polk, C., 1974, Sources, propagation, amplitude and temproal variations of extremely low frequency (1-100 Hz) electromagnetic fields, in: "Biologic and Clinical Effects of Low Frequency Magnetic and Electric Fields", Llaurado, V., ed. Thomas, Springfield, Illinois

Presdi, D., and Pettigrew, J.D., 1980, Ferromagnetic coupling to muscle receptors as a basis for geomagnetic field sensitivity in animals, Nature, London 285: 99-101

Sagan, P.M., Adey, W.R., Sabbot, I.M., and Bystrom, B.G., 1982, Effects of 60 Hz environmental electric fields on laboratory rats, Bioelectromagnetics, in press.

Scheich, H., and Bullock, T.H., 1974, The detection of electric fields from electric organs, in: "Handbook of Sensory Physiology. Electroreceptors and Other Specialized Receptors in Lower Vertebrates", D. Albe-Fessard, ed. Springer, New York. Vol. 3, part 3, pp. 201-256

Schumann, W.O., 1957, Uber elektrische Eigen schwindungen des Hohlraumes Erd-Luft-Ionosphare, erregt durch Blitzenladungen, Zeits Angew. J. Phys. 9:373-378

Triffet, T., and Green, H.S., 1980, Information and energy flow in a simple nervous system, J. Theor. Biol. 86: 3-44

Vaccaro, S.R., and Green, H.S., 1979, Ionic processes in excitable membranes, J. Theor. Biol. 81: 771-802

Valentino, A.R., 1972, Evaluation of the E-field simulator at UCLA, Washington, D.C., Illinois Institute of Technology Research Institute, Tech. Memo

Waltman, B., 1966, Electrical properties and fine structure of the ampullary canals of Lorenzini Acta Physiol. Scand. 66, Suppl. 264: 1-60

Warnke, V., 1976, Effects of electric charges on honey bees. Bee World 57:50-56

Wever, R., 1968, Einfluss schwacher elektro-magnetischer Felder auf die circadiane Periodik des Menschen Naturwissenschaften 55: 29-33

Wever, R., 1973, Human circadian rhythms under the influence of weak electric fields and the different aspect of these studies. Internat. J. Biometeorol. 17: 227-232

Wever, R., 1974, ELF-effects on human circadian rhythms, in: "ELF and VLF Electromagnetic Field Effects", Persinger, M.A., ed. Plenum, New York. pp. 101-144

Wever, R., 1975, The circadian multioscillatory system of man. Internat. J. Chronobiol. 3: 19-55

Wever, R., 1977, Effects of low-level, low-frequency fields on human circadian rhythms. Neurosci. Res. Program Bull. 15: 39-45

POWER FREQUENCY ELECTRIC FIELDS: DOSIMETRY

John S.T. Looms

Central Electricity Research Laboratories
Leatherhead, Surrey
England

INTRODUCTION

The concept of "dose", when applied to the electric fields which are associated with high-voltage transmission apparatus, is artificial and potentially misleading.

In classical dosimetry of ionizing radiations "dose" is defined in terms of absorbed energy per unit mass of the subject's body. The unit of absorbed dose, the gray (Gy), is defined as one joule of absorbed energy per kilogram of body-mass. It is evident that many different processes may contribute to this absorbed energy, including interactions with photons and particles of widely different kinds. All, however, can produce ionization: ionization is known to be a cause of damage to living cells. Therefore dosimetry based on the assumption of a correlation between dose and risk of physiological consequences is a logical procedure, even though the relationship between dose and risk is still subject to research and argument (Mayneord and Wheatley, 1981).

So-called dosimetry of electric fields does not have a similarly rational foundation and analogies with classical procedures must be treated with caution. The only reason for attempting to quantify "exposure" of human beings to electric fields is to validate or disprove allegations that such exposure is harmful, either in direct physiological consequences or indirectly, e.g. in causing malfunction of heart-pacemakers. However, since human beings are able to perceive the existence of electric fields, in circumstances where currents, of milliampere order or above, are caused to flow in their bodies, they do not choose to remain in such regions. Dosimetry is thus only relevant when these induced currents are imperceptible. In intensities of field as low as these - which cover the overwhelming majority of practical cases - there is no evidence whatsoever of significant physiological effects (Gary, 1980).

Comparing the cases of ionizing radiation and of electric induction a priori we have, for radiation, several known processes whereby bombardment damages cells, these processes having incidental heating properties. In the case of induction the only effect, in practical field-intensities, is a flow of alternating current carried in the conductive tissue and blood. No mechanism is known whereby either these feeble currents, or the negligible and diffuse powers which they dissipate as heat, can have deleterious biological effects. The generation of perhaps a microwatt in a body having a natural metabolic output one hundred million times greater is not, in the case of induction, an indication of other insidious effects: not even a plausible theory about how such effects could occur has yet been proposed.

Much work has been put into the development of apparatus for estimating the "exposure" of human beings to power-frequency fields. This is reviewed below. The results must be treated with caution, for the reasons stated above.

Physical Principles

When a man enters a region of space, say under a transmission line, where the electric field intensity before his arrival was near-uniform and, say, 1 kV/m in value, he perturbs the field into a multiplicity of different values (Fig 1).

The intensities within his body are very low, of order mV/m (i.e. one hundred-thousandth of the original unperturbed value) because of his body's high electrical conductivity. Some of the external intensities are higher than the unperturbed value and some are lower: generally points and protrusions concentrate the field while concavities screen and disperse it.

At any point the induced displacement current-density and the external field intensity are related. At power-frequency of 50 Hz the relationship is

$$i(\mu A/m^2) = 2.78\ E_s\ (kV/m)$$

where i = current density and E_s = field intensity. Although high field intensity means high current density, both effects are local to protrusions. The man's finger-tip (Fig 1) is a high-point both for field intensity and current-density but the actual current which flows out of it is a very small fraction of the whole.

It is seen, therefore, that measurement of the current flowing from a small region of the body can be used to deduce the intensity of the field at that point and hence, provided calibration is feasible, to derive the intensity of the unperturbed field.

Hence a measurement of the product (current x time) at a given part of the body can be used to deduce a so-called "exposure-dose", here defined as (intensity of unperturbed field x time for which man is in this field).

The limitations to this procedure must be understood. The relationship between the local current, which is to be integrated, and the unperturbed field is not unique. The current varies with the man's stance, with the positions of his arms, legs and head, with the presence of local conductors which may concentrate the field or screen it. It also varies with the man's height, so that calibration relates only to one combination of man + detecting instrument.

More fundamentally, if an attempt is to be made to relate physiological effects to exposure, since any such effects must be

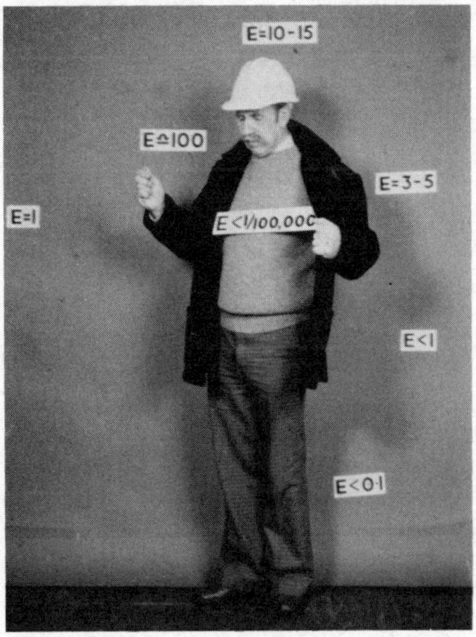

Fig 1 Field-intensities on surface of man standing in region where unperturbed field was unity, E = 1. (E<1/100,000) represents intensity <u>inside</u> body.

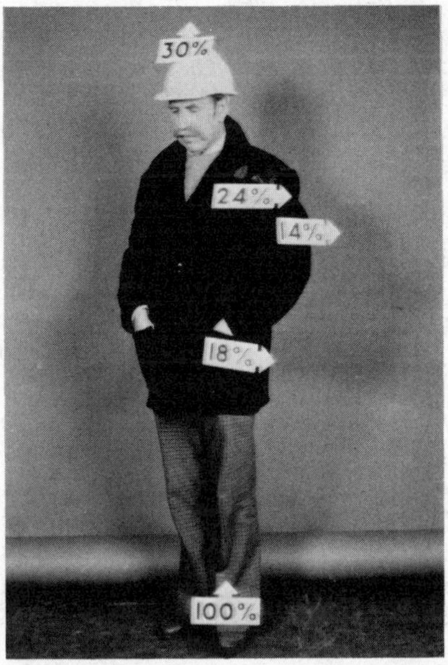

Fig 2 Distribution of induced current in man standing on flat ground.

current-related, it clearly must matter where the body-currents flow as well as how large they are. If we are interested in possible effects, say, on the man's brain we should not measure the quantity of charge which flows across his chest. The distribution of current in a standing man (Fig 2) shows that only about 30% of the induced flow is through his head: the relatively large flow from large areas of low field-intensity (thorax, arms, legs) is also noteworthy.

Basic Methods

A thorough analysis of the currents induced in human bodies in attitudes relevant to work on high-voltage transmission apparatus, including measurement and calculation of distribution and dose, is given by Deno (Deno, 1977). He shows how the flow of induced current varies with the stance of the man and position on his body. He also introduces the principle of deducing the product (current x time) from an electrolytic storage cell.

The cell is mounted on the man's body, at a determined place, and the combination of man + detector is calibrated by immersion in a known electric field. The electrolytic cell is of a type which can be "read out" by reversing it with suitable ancillary apparatus. In this way a quantity of induced charge is determined from the time required to reverse the cell at a known current rate, and this quantity of charge is related to the known time spent at a location where the unperturbed field, before the introduction of the man + detector, was known.

Different calibrating factors are determined depending on the position of the detector on the man's body and on his height. The best location is the top of the head, associated with the protective helmet, but in practice an arm band is generally found to be convenient.

Because of the existence of thresholds, it is seen, as pointed out by Bridges, (Bridges, 1979) that a less-misleading indication of exposure is obtained by timing the duration in fields of different intensity than by a single integration. Bridges suggests a THEF meter (Time Histogram Electric Field) which, for example, could measure the time spent in 0 to 2.5, 2.5 to 5, 5 to 10, 10 to 15, and above 15 kV m^{-1} intensities.

Modern Applications

Two detectors are illustrated, (Figs 3,4) respectively a single level and THEF design. Their small size and convenient portability, made possible by the development of solid state electronics, are noteworthy.

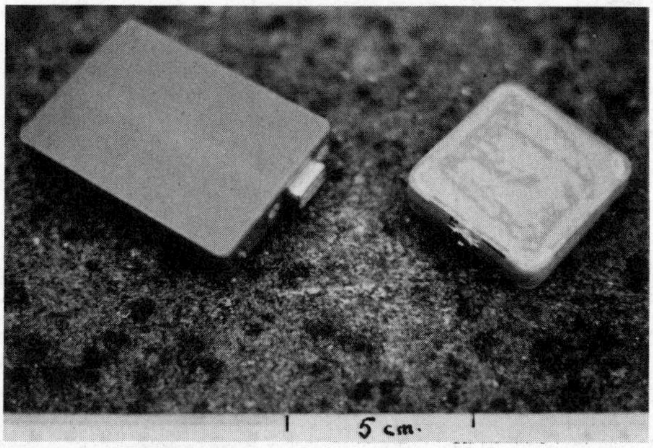

Fig 3,4 Detectors
Four-level THEF "All-intensity"

In the THEF the switching of the induced current into the appropriate levels is accomplished wholly by means of solid state devices without moving parts (Fig 5).

A means of fixing the detector to the man's body is provided by the conducting band (Fig 6). The underside of this band makes electrical contact both with the man and with one electrode of the detector; the second electrode, the "live" one, receives the electric flux from the inducing source, overhead line, substation component, etc.

Because the basic circuitry must include a rectifier, to convert the alternating induced current into direct currents suitable for operating the electrolytic cell, precautions must be taken to avoid false registration arising from the detection of other fields than power frequency, for example, radio broadcasts. Filtration is therefore usually provided.

The detectors used in U.K. (Figs 3,4) are small and light in weight. These are essential design-features: linesmen and sub-station attendants are liable to refuse to wear instruments which are bulky or heavy. If these are worn they may well alter the normal working-pattern, because of their inconvenience.

Discussion

Measurements of "exposure" to electric fields by the methods described here so far have been on a limited scale. As far as can be seen the integrated (intensity x time) which is measured is much less than the simple product (maximum local intensity x working time) as deduced from the calculated or measured field intensity and known exposure-duration. When results are analyzed the following matters must be borne in mind.

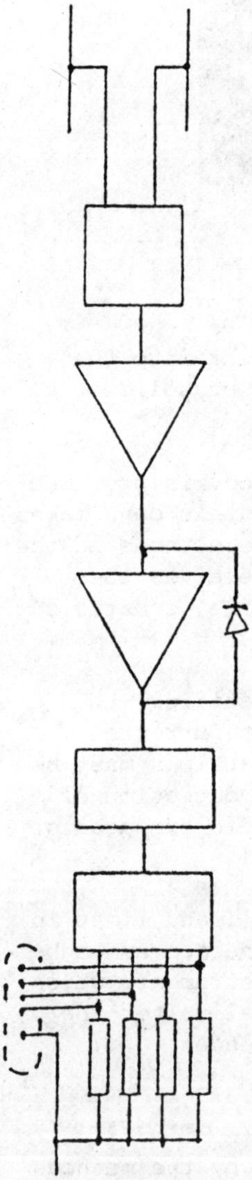

Fig 5 TIME HISTOGRAM ELECTRIC FIELD METER
Four-level design by A.E.T. Nye

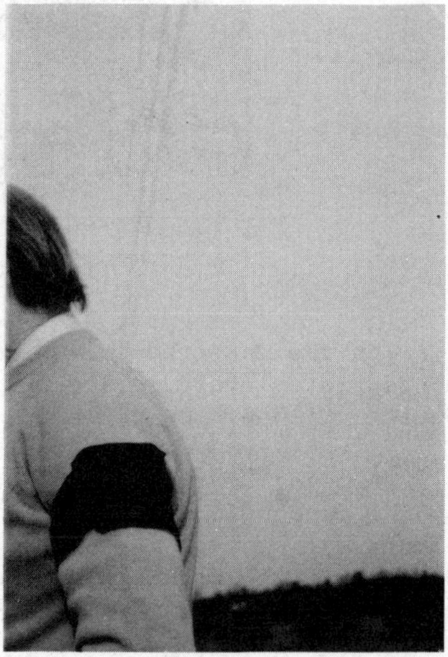

Fig 6 Detector mounted in pocket on armband. Man stands on level ground under live test-line for calibration of detector. Unperturbed intensity can be accurately fixed from conductor-bundle geometry, height above ground, applied voltage. Residence-time then gives calibrating "exposure".

In everyday life, in an industrial environment especially, alternating currents circulate within the human body because of leakage from appliances, as a result of interactions with magnetic fields and by capacitive coupling from such sources as electric blankets. Some of these currents are comparable with those induced by transmission apparatus but none would be indicated by a dosimeter of the described type.

Expert opinion is opposed to the very basis of dosimetry in the realm of electric fields.

"I found no evidence to support the dosimetry concept either from a physical or biological viewpoint, ... Thresholds render meaningless the dose concept. ..... A 100 mA, three-second shock is regarded as a likely fibrillation threshold for human adults. On the other hand, a 1 mA body current for 300 seconds (the same 300 mA x second dose) is clearly not hazardous." (Bridges, 1977.)

Comparing the thermal input to a man's body by induction from, say, a high voltage line with normal backgrounds, like solar radiation, the former is seen to be quite negligible. If a man spent a complete <u>year</u>, night and day, at a distance of 25m from a typical 400 kV line, he would absorb the same thermal dose as from 10 <u>seconds</u>' exposure of his face to full sunlight! (Gary, 1980.)

It is therefore hardly surprising that intermittent residence by linesmen and substation-attendants in comparable field-intensities, giving even smaller thermal doses, does not give a rise to physiological symptoms.

CONCLUSIONS

1. The concept of dosimetry as applied to power-frequency electric fields is artificial and requires some caution in its application.

2. The derived quantity, (unperturbed electric field intensity x time of exposure to induction), is likely to be ambiguous because of the existence of thresholds. Large currents for short time are known not to be equivalent to small ones for long times.

3. Satisfactory apparatus has been developed for both "all-intensity" and THEF registration (THEF = Time Histogram Electric Field).

4. The quantity of induced charge flow in an exposed human being is likely to be much less than that calculated from maximum local intensity of field and time spent in region of field.

5. In energy terms the absorbed dose in all practical cases will be negligible in comparison with both metabolic output and background inputs, e.g. from sunlight.

ACKNOWLEDGEMENTS

This work was done at the Central Electricity Research Laboratories and is published by permission of the Central Electricity Generating Board. The author is indebted to his colleagues Mr. G.C. Stringfellow, Mr. A.E.T. Nye and Mr. R.H. Minors, by whom the experimental work, the instrument development and much of the analysis were done.

REFERENCES

Bridges, J.E., Discussion on Paper F77-258-7, IEEE, 1977.

Deno, D.W., "Currents Induced in the Human Body", Paper F77-258-7, IEEE, 1977.

Gary, C., "Electric and Magnetic Fields Produced by Transmission Lines: Description of Phenomena and Practical Guide to Calculation" CIGRE 36 WG 01, 1980.

Mayneord, W.V. and Wheatley, B.M., "Nuclear power: putting the risks into perspective", CEGB Research No. 11, January 1981.

ANALYSIS OF EXPERIMENTAL AND EPIDEMIOLOGICAL DATA FROM EXPOSURE TO MICROWAVE/RADIOFREQUENCY (MW/RF) ENERGIES

Sol M. Michaelson

Department of Radiation Biology and Biophysics
University of Rochester
School of Medicine and Dentistry
Rochester, New York 14642

INTRODUCTION

Much of the research on biological effects of microwave/radiofrequency (MW/RF) energies has been done with small rodents having coefficients of heat absorption, field concentration effects, body surface areas and thermoregulatory mechanisms significantly different from man. Even closely related species can differ widely in their responses. The literature is replete with "anomalous" reactions. Thus, results of exposure of common laboratory animals cannot be readily extrapolated to man unless a comparative biology approach and some form of "scaling" among different animal species, and from animal to man, is used in an appropriate manner to obtain quantitatively valid extrapolation relationships from the observed data.

Even by using approaches where absorbed energy patterns in test animals closely approximate those that may exist in man under certain exposure conditions, the intrinsic physical and physiological dissimilarities between species further confounds the problem of extrapolating between animals and humans. In addition to the obvious external geometric differences, physiologic differences are important for MW/RF exposures. Body size and orientation are critical in such studies.

Principles of Animal Experimentation

Biological experiments using human subjects, have either been few in number or inapplicable to the specific biological parameter one desires to study. It is often important, therefore, to use data obtained from experiments using other biological organisms, such as small animals, to predict the human response to a specific stimulus. There are general principles which allow the results of experiments on one organism (an animal) to be extrapolated to predict biological responses in organisms different from those tested (i.e. a human).

In making such extrapolations we must be particularly mindful of the limitations and pitfalls in the use of animal experimentation data. Many factors must be considered in the design of experiments using organisms other than man as a test subject. These include the species, strain, sex, age of the animal, the methods of caring for the test animals, the animals' feeding patterns, the roles of seasonal and circadian rhythms, temperature and humidity.

The reliability of laboratory studies using experimental animal models depend on the following considerations: (1) the selection of the animal model with consideration of its cognitive limits, (2) scaling factors associated with the nature of the field in the laboratory investigation of the biological processes using animal models, and (3) the method by which the extrapolation of data gathered using the animal models relates to human studies.

The cognitive value of the animal model increases sharply in relation to the physiologic and biochemical similarities of the experimental animal to man. Regrettably, criteria for assessing similarity are not always available or apparent. Concomitantly, with physiologic and biochemical similarities, the investigator must recognize (1) the biological parameters of systems reacting on exposure to the selected stimulus, (2) the quantitative indices of response in relation to the energy-intensity-time effect relations, and (3) the characteristics of the physiology and biochemistry involved.

In any review of biological experiments one has to be aware of the critical importance of how experiments are designed and executed and how results are interpreted. Even in experiments that appear to be impeccably planned, it is easy to come to incorrect conclusions. There are a number of cases where a claimed electromagnetic field effect was actually due to some interacting variable in the experiments. It is also possible that no effect is found but the design of the experiment is such that probably none could have been found even if it did exist.

Some of the criteria used for assessing the results of research on MW/RF biological effects are:

1) The techniques used should be such that possible effects of intervening factors i.e. changes in ambient temperature, noise, vibration and chemicals in the environment such as air, bedding, etc., are avoided.

2) The sensitivity of the experiment should be adequate to ensure a reasonable probability that an effect would be detected if indeed any exists.

3) The experiment and observational techniques, methods and conditions should be objective. Wherever there is a possibility of investigator bias special safeguards such as double blind techniques, blind scoring or codes should be employed.

4) All data analyses should be objective and subjected to acceptable analytical methods with no relevant data deleted from consideration.

5) If an effect is claimed, the results should demonstrate it at an acceptable level of statistical significance by application of appropriate tests.

6) A given experiment, should be internally consistent with respect to the effect of interest.

7) Finally, the results should be quantifiable and susceptible to confirmation by other investigators.

Analysis of Scientific Literature

In an analysis of scientific literature to determine the probability of a biological response from exposure to a physical agent, we must consider the consistency of experimental results claimed, both the nature of the response and the biological system involved, the ability to replicate the results of studies with consistency and whether the results claimed and observations reported can be explained by previously accepted biological principles or must be explained only upon the basis of new, untested hypotheses.

Experiments with small animals, such as mice and rats, which are undertaken to evaluate the potential effects of a stressor, such as an electromagnetic field, must be carefully designed and performed. The observations may be the result of another, unrelated stressor inadvertently introduced into the experimental design rather than the stressor intended to be studied. The fact that a living organism responds to many stimuli is a part of the process of living; such responses are examples of biological "effects". Since biological organisms do have adaptive, compensatory ability and tolerance to change, these "effects" may be well within the capability of the organism to maintain a normal equilibrium or condition of homeostasis. If, on the other hand, an effect should compromise the individual's ability to function properly or overcomes the recovery capability of the individual, then the "effect" may be considered a "hazard". In any discussion of the potential for biological "effects" from exposure to electromagnetic energies we must first determine whether any "effect" can be demonstrated; and then determine whether such an observed "effect" is "hazardous".

The reason for discussing this distinction is to note that while many biological "effects" have been claimed as a result of exposure to electromagnetic fields, it is highly questionable whether such effects, even if substantiated, can be considered to be hazardous simply because we do not understand to the absolute degree the mechanism by which they are caused.

If a specified electromagnetic environment should produce a characterizable biological reaction, the effect must be evaluated as to its potential hazard to humans. Since initial experiments are usually performed on animal models, this necessitates an extrapolation from the experimental animal to man.

To rationally review the literature and assess the implications of the reported results of exposure to microwaves, it is essential to consider fundamental principles and concepts related to biomedical research in the laboratory and extrapolation to man.

Experimental animal models are extensively used for the study of physical factors in the environment to assure human health and safety. The best we can do experimentally is to create an arbitrary set of conditions which we consider to be as relevant as possible for the purpose of the study. Many factors such as methods of animal care, the role of seasonal and circadian rhythms, temperature, and humidity, etc., as well as psychosocial interactions must be considered in experimental design and analysis of results. Reliability of laboratory studies depends on the following:

1) selection of the animal model with consideration of its cognitive limits,

2) methods applied for investigation of biological processes in animals,

3) extrapolation of data from animals to man.

Obviously, direct extrapolation from animal experiments to man cannot be performed *a priori*. This is due not only to their physiologic differences but also the physical dimensions and shape.

Among the problems in studying biologic effects are the selection of the most appropriate animal species and extrapolation to man. Animals are quite often selected only on the basis of convenience, economy, or familiarity and without regard to their suitability for the problem under study. One should not extrapolate to larger animals or man, results obtained in small laboratory animals, without consideration of size distributions as well as metabolic and physiologic differences. Meticulous care must be exerted in defining experimental conditions. These are shown in Tables I and II.

TABLE I. FACTORS THAT AFFECT MICROWAVE/RADIOFREQUENCY ABSORPTION

I. PHYSICAL PARAMETERS OF THE EM SOURCE:

1. FREQUENCY
2. POLARIZATION
3. MODULATION (AM, FM, PULSE, CW)
4. POWER DENSITY
5. FIELD PATTERN (NEAR, INTERMEDIATE, OR FAR FIELD: UNIFORMITY)
6. MEASURING TECHNIQUE
7. CALIBRATION TECHNIQUE
8. POWER
9. TRANSMITTING AND RADIATING EQUIPMENT
10. CHAMBER MATERIAL AND DIMENSIONS

II. BIOLOGICAL PARAMETERS:

1. TISSUE DIELECTRIC PROPERTIES
2. SIZE; GEOMETRY
3. RELATION TO POLARIZATIONS
4. SPATIAL RELATIONS OF ANIMALS

III. ARTIFACTS:

1. GROUND OR CONDUCTOR PLATE
2. CONTAINER (MATERIAL, SIZE)
3. METAL IMPLANTS
4. METAL OR NON-METALLIC OBJECTS IN THE FIELD
5. SHIELDING MATERIALS

Extrapolation from Animals to Man

In order to extrapolate observatons in animals to predict results that might be obtained during human exposures, some method of scaling must be employed. The best method available at present, albeit fraught with oversimplifications, is frequency scaling. This approach assumes the use of shorter wavelengths (higher frequencies) for smaller animals and longer wavelengths (lower frequencies) for larger animals. Approximating the bodies of all animals and man as prolate spheroids, an attempt has been made to ascertain what (lower) frequency must illuminate the larger animal if the total absorbed dose rate (at the same plane wave exposure field intensity) is to be the same as that obtained at a higher frequency for a smaller animal.[1]

Where absorbed energy patterns in a test animal are used to approximate the pattern that may exist in man under certain exposure conditions, the intrinsic physical and physiological

TABLE II. FACTORS THAT INFLUENCE BIOLOGICAL RESPONSES TO THE SAME SPECIFIC ABSORPTION RATE

I. SUBJECT VARIABLES:	
1. SPECIES: SEX; AGE; WEIGHT	4. INTERVENTIONS (ANESTHETICS; DRUGS; ELECTRODES; LESIONS)
2. SENSITIVITY	
3. NUMBER OF SUBJECTS	5. ANIMAL HUSBANDRY
II. ENVIRONMENTAL VARIABLES:	
1. TEMPERATURE; HUMIDITY; AIR FLOW	3. TIME OF DAY OF EXPOSURE AND SAMPLING
2. LIGHTING	4. NOISE; ODOR
III. CONCOMITANT VARIABLES:	
1. GENETIC PREDISPOSITION	3. FUNCTIONAL AND METABOLIC DISORDERS
2. BASE-LINE OF THE RESPONSE	
IV. EXPERIMENTAL VARIABLES:	
1. ACCLIMATION PROCEDURES	5. SAMPLING TECHNIQUE
2. DURATION OF EXPOSURE	6. TIME BETWEEN EXPOSURE AND SAMPLING
3. NUMBER AND SCHEDULE OF EXPOSURES	7. RESTRAINT DEVICES
4. MODE OF EXPOSURE (PARTIAL- OR WHOLE BODY	8. INVESTIGATOR--ANIMAL INTERACTION

dissimilarities between species further confounds the problem of extrapolating between animals and to the human. In addition to the obvious external geometric differences, the differences in internal vascular anatomy and mechanisms of heat dissipation in fur-bearing animals compared to man, allows only limited conclusions from such frequency scaling.

The need for proper dosimetry in experimental procedures and the importance of realistic scaling factors required for extrapolation of data obtained with small laboratory animals to man are clearly required. Detailed discussions that serve as bases for scaling have been presented by several authors.[1-4]

Responses induced by exposure to MW/RF energies depend on the amount of energy absorbed which is a function of the wave-length and on the geometry, orientation, and electrical properties of the object(s) being irradiated.[1] Maximum absorption, (maximum SAR), during whole-body irradiation of small animals apparently occurs at frequencies between approximately 0.5 and 3 GHz, and for man, at around 60-100 MHz with a peak at about 80 MHz. At frequencies below 30 MHz, absorption drops off rapidly and is also much less at frequencies above 500 MHz.

MW/RF energy absorption which is dependent on polarization, frequency, and the immediate physical environment is rapidly converted to thermal energy. This thermal energy is then rapidly redistributed by conduction, convection (e.g. blood flow) within and, to a lesser extent, radiation from the biological target. The tissue heat capacity and heat transfer processes influence the dose and dose distribution within the body.

An effort is being made to standardize dosimetric measures of MW/RF exposure by employing a quantity called - the Specific Absorption Rate (SAR). The unit-mass, time-averaged rate of MW/RF energy absorption is specified in SI units of watts per kilogram ($W\ kg^{-1}$).[5] The SAR depends on a finite period of exposure to yield the amount of energy absorbed by a given mass of material, which is termed specific absorption (SA), i.e., Joules per kilogram = J/kg. Thus, the <u>specific absorption</u> rate is the time rate at which radiofrequency electromagnetic energy is imparted to a component or mass of a biological body. The SAR is applicable to any tissue or organ of interest or, is expressed as a whole-body average.

Durney *et al.*[1] have made calculations of the Specific Absorbed Rate (SAR) as a function of frequency for different sizes of laboratory animals and of man. This concept is useful in allowing limited extrapolation from one species to another but it should be used cautiously in view of its limitations. Except for spherical models the bodies studied have had uniform properties. Because of the different properties of various tissues energy deposition may be much more uneven in animals than the models predict.

Whole-body absorption rates approach maximal values when the long axis of a body is parallel to the E-field vector and is four tenths the wavelength of the incident field. At 2450 MHz, (λ = 12.5 cm) for example, Standard Man (long axis 175 cm) will absorb about half of the incident energy. If the human whole-body SAR is divided by the BMR for man, a ratio is obtained that provides a measure of the thermal load incurrred due to a known incident power density.[6] Table III illustrates the variation of this ratio with frequency at two incident power densities. In the region of human whole-body resonance (60-80 MHZ), this ratio reaches a maximum value (about 0.16 for an incident far-field power density of 1 mW/cm^2). The ratio drops off rapidly on either side of this peak, and at 10 MHz and below, the ratio would be less than 0.001.[7]

At frequencies that result in maximal absorption, which defines whole-body resonance, the electrical cross section of an exposed body increases in area. This increase occurs at a frequency near 70 MHz for Standard Man and results, as shown in Table IV in an approximate seven-fold increase in absorption relative to that in a 2450-MHz field.

TABLE III. RATIO OF SPECIFIC ABSORPTION RATE TO BASAL METABOLIC RATE FOR AN AVERAGE MAN EXPOSED TO FAR-FIELD INCIDENT POWER DENSITIES OF 1 mW/sq cm AND 5 mW/sq cm*

Frequency (MHz)	AV. SAR/BMR (%) 1 mW/sq cm	5 mW/sq cm
10	0.13	0.65
20	0.60	3.00
50	5.80	29.00
60	10.00	50.00
80	16.00	80.00
100	12.00	60.00
200	5.20	26.00
500	3.70	18.50
1,000	2.90	14.50
2,000	2.50	12.50
5,000	2.50	12.50
10,000	2.50	12.50
20,000	2.50	12.50

*based on Stuchly[6]

Human Exposures

There have been a few epidemiologic studies of MW/RF exposure but these have generally beeen limited in scope.[8,9] Persons exposed while assigned to the military services or occupationally exposed in industrial settings have been the principal groups studied. A few other populations living or working near generating sources or exposed to medical diathermy have been or are being investigated.[8-11] Information about health status has come from medical records, questionnaires, physical and laboratory examination, and vital statistics. Sources of exposure data include personnel records, questionnaires, environmental measurements, equipment emission measurements, and (assumed adherence to) established exposure limits. Although there have been advances in measurement, microwave dosimetry still presents formidable problems for meaningful assessment in most epidemiologic studies.[8,9]

An early study on U.S. Navy personnel during World War II did not reveal any conditions that could be ascribed to radar exposure.[12] Ten years later a four-year surveillance of a relatively large group of radar workers in the U.S. did not demonstrate any significant clinical or pathophysiologic differences between the exposed and control groups.[13,14] On the other hand, surveys of East European workers revealed functional changes in the nervous and cardiovascular systems.[15-17]

In an extensive 12-year survey Czerski and associates, examined persons occupationally exposed to microwaves for various periods of time, for the incidence of functional disturbances and disorders considered as contra-indications for occupational exposure to microwaves according to the criteria employed in Poland.[18-23] The population was involved in identical work conditions except for the exposure levels, which constituted two subgroups. Workers in the first subgroup (507 individuals) were exposed to varying power densities between 0.2 and 6 mW/cm^2; in the second subgroup power densities were below 0.2 mW/cm^2. No dependence of incidence of disorders, such as organic lesions of the nervous system, changes in translucency of the ocular lens, primary disorders of the blood system, neoplastic diseases or endocrine disorders on exposure level, duration, or work history could be demonstrated. The incidence of functional disturbances ("neurasthenic syndrome", gastrointestinal tract disturbances, cardiovascular disturbances with abnormal ECG) was found not to be related to the level or duration of occupational exposure. There were no instances of irreversible damage or disturbances caused by exposure to microwave energy.[18]

The Medical Follow-up Agency of the National Academy of Sciences of the United States studied mortality and morbidity among 40,000 personnel of the United States Navy. Graduates of technical schools for training in the use of radar and maintenance of equipment were compared with graduates of technical schools not involved with microwave energy. There was no indication of any adverse affect due to exposure to microwaves.[24] This study was preceded by a survey to investigate physiological and physical effects among U.S. Navy crewman who could be exposed to 0.1 - 1 mW/cm^2 aboard an aircraft carrier.[25] No significant differences were found, with respect to task performance, psychological tests, or biological effects. Blood study findings were within the normal range.

Table IV. Specific Absorption Rate (SAR) for Animals and Man
(W/kg for 1 mW/cm^2 incident PD)

SPECIES	MAX. ABSORPTION (MHz)	FREQUENCY (MHz) 20-30	70	300	1000	2450	3000	10,000
MOUSE	2000	8×10^{-4}	0.008	0.06	0.4	1.00	0.965	0.322
		(0.05)	(0.04)	(1.50)	(13)	(36)	(36.60)	(12.40)
RAT	600	1.8×10^{-3}	0.0125	0.3	0.6	0.23	0.26	0.25
		(0.12)	(0.06)	(7.50)	(20)	(8)	(9.60)	(9.60)
RABBIT	320	0.015	0.050	0.80	0.250	0.15	0.08	0.07
		(1.00)	(0.22)	(20)	(8.30)	(5.40)	(2.96)	(2.69)
RHESUS	300	1.7×10^{-3}	0.0125	0.195	0.10	0.07	0.065	0.060
		(0.01)	(0.06)	(5.00)	(3.33)	(2.50)	(2.41)	(2.30)
DOG	200	1.5×10^{-3}	0.010	0.100	0.050	0.040	0.037	0.030
		(0.10)	(0.04)	(2.50)	(1.67)	(1.40)	(1.40)	(1.15)
HUMAN (1 YR)	150	0.004	0.040	0.15	0.065	0.055	0.050	.042
MAN (AVG)	70	0.015	0.225	0.04	0.03	0.028	0.027	0.026

*(   )SAR relative to average man

A study of 4,388 employees and 8,283 dependents of the U.S. Embassy in Moscow, some of whom had possibly been exposed to levels of microwave intensities of 5-15 $\mu W/cm^2$ for variable periods of time (9-18 hours/day) up to 8 months revealed no differences in health status as indicated by their mortality experience and a variety of morbidity measures.[26,27] Exhaustive comparative analyses were made of all symptoms, conditions, diseases and causes of death among employees and dependent groups of adults and children. No differences in health status by any measure could be attributed to microwave exposure.[9]

This study was preceded by a cytogenetic evaluation for possible mutagenesis performed on 250 samples from 71 State Department employees and family members before, during, and after exposure to microwaves at the Moscow Embassy.[27] No genetic or other adverse biologic effect among employees and dependents attributable to microwave exposure could be established.

A study was also conducted to determine the blood lymphocyte counts of adult employees and dependents of the American Embassy in Moscow.[27] Approximately 350 adults who were Embassy employees during the study period were examined; approximately 1,000 foreign service personnel in the United States served as a comparison group. The higher average lymphocyte count found in the Moscow population did not correlate in time or space with microwave irradiation in the Embassy and was believed to be of microbial origin.

Ocular effects

Several cases of cataract attributed to microwave exposure have been reported in the literature, but substantiation has not been established. There is no clinical or experimental evidence that ocular lens damage allegedly due to microwave exposure is morphologically different from lens abnormalities from other causes, including the aging process.

Numerous surveys of ocular effects of MW/RF energies in man have been made, especially in the United States.[8,9] Most investigations have involved armed services personnel and civilian workers at military bases and in industrial settings. The principal subject of interest has been the significance of minor lens changes in the cataractogenic process and cataracts (opacities impairing vision).

Lenticular defects too minor to affect visual acuity have been studied as possible early markers of microwave exposure or precursors of cataracts. The studies have been mainly prevalence surveys although the time periods are often variable or not specified; reexamination data rarely permit estimates of incidence.[8,9] Some generalizations, however, can be made about observations of lens changes in microwave workers and comparison groups.

1. Lens imperfections occur normally and increase markedly with age among employed males studied. There is evidence that lens changes increase with age even during childhood.[28] By about age 50, lens defects have been reported in most comparison subjects, based on data from various studies.

2. Although a few suggestive differences have been reported,[28-30] there is no clear indication that minor lens defects are a marker for microwave exposure in terms of type or frequency of changes, exposure factors or occupation.[8,9] The reported earlier appearance of lens defects in microwave workers than in comparison groups cannot be adequately assessed because there is considerable variation in the type, number and size of defects recorded, in the scoring methods used by different observers, and in the numbers examined.[8,9]

3. Clinically significant lens changes, which would permit selection of individuals to be followed have not been identified.[31]

4. There is no evidence from ophthalmologic surveys to date that minor lens opacities are precursors of clinical cataracts.[8,9]

Although there has been much interest in the cataractogenic effect of MW/RF energies, only a minimal effort has been made to investigate cataracts as such, as distinct from their precursors.[8,9] A case-control epidemiologic study of World War II and Korean War veterans was negative for cataract.[32]

Neither definitions nor methods of detection of cataract are standardized.[8,9] The common meaning of cataract, a lens opacity that interferes with visual acuity, is open to many interpretations as to degree and nature of the opacity and loss of visual acuity. Specific disorders, physical agents and injuries are known to cause cataracts but many cataracts are loosely called "senile" when they occur after middle age. Alleged "microwave cataracts" are not distinguishable from other cataracts, in the opinion of most ophthalmologists.[8,9]

The most prominent characteristic of cataracts is their age distribution. Although estimates of frequency are not comparable because of differences in population groups surveyed, as well as nonuniform methods of detection and definition, all point to low frequencies until about the fifth decade of life, when sharp increases occur. Although not comparable with general population figures, recorded mean annual incidence rates are extremely low, of the order of 2 per 100,000.[8,9] In a preliminary national estimate by age of the total prevalence of cataracts in the civilian noninstitutionalized population 1-74 years of age in the United States, one or more cataracts was found in 9 percent of the population.[33] For the various age groups under 45, frequency of the condition increased gradually from 0.4 percent in those 1-5 years of age to 4 percent in the 35-44 year age group. The marked increase that occurs after age 45 reaches a maximum in the oldest group examined: of those 65-74 years of age, more than half had cataracts. Cataract data for personnel on active duty in the armed services (who are mainly healthy, relatively young males) are available as incidence rates which show similar age dependence up to about age 55.[34]

Nervous System and Cardiovascular Effects

Clinical and laboratory studies of workers in the U.S.S.R. and other Eastern European countries employed in the operation, testing, maintenance, and manufacture of microwave-generating equipment have described central nervous and cardiovascular reactions to MW/RF exposure.[16,17,35] According to some reports exposures have been mainly low-level (microwatts up to a few milliwats per cm^2) and long-term.

With few exceptions[23], functional disturbances of the central nervous system have been described as a typical kind of radiowave sickness, the neurasthenic or asthenic syndrome. The symptoms and signs include headache, fatigability, irritability, loss of appetite, sleepiness, sweating, thyroid gland enlargement, difficulties in concentration or memory, depression and emotional instability. This clinical syndrome is generally reversible if exposure is discontinued.[8,9]

Another frequently described manifestation is a set of labile functional cardiovascular changes including bradycardia (or occasional tachycardia), arterial hypertension (or hypotension) and changes in cardiac conduction. This form of neurocirculatory asthenia is also attributed to nervous system influence. More serious but less frequent neurologic or neuropsychiatric disturbances have occasionally been described as a diencephalic syndrome.[8,9] The identification and assessment of these poorly defined, nonspecific complaints, symptom-complexes and illnesses is extremely difficult.[36,37]

Growth and Development

A case-control study of Down's syndrome in relation to exposure to ionizing radiation yielded an unexpected finding regarding paternal exposure to radar.[38] Apparently, fathers of children with mongolism gave more frequent histories of occupational exposure to radar during military service than did fathers of unaffected children, a difference that was of borderline statistical significance. Exposure during military service occurred prior to the birth of the affected child. After publication of the first report in 1965, expansion of the study group, follow-up of all fathers to obtain more detailed information about radar exposure, and search of available military personnel records were undertaken. The suggestive excess of radar exposure of fathers of Down's syndrome cases was not confirmed on further study.[39]

A report of congenital anomalies at a U.S. Army base[40] suggested that during the 3-year period 1968-1971 the adjoining communities in which the base was located, had a reported number of clubfoot cases among white babies that greatly exceeded the expected number (based on birth certificate notifications for the State). A more detailed investigation revealed that in the 6-county area surrounding the base, there was, during the same time period, a considerably higher rate of anomalies (diagnosed within 24 hours after birth) among births to military personnel than in the State as a whole. This base was a training facility for fixed-wing and helicopter aircraft, situated within 35 miles of dozens of radar stations. Analysis revealed that there apparently were errors in malformation data on birth certificates and probable over-reporting from the Army base. Thus convincing evidence was lacking that radar exposure was related to congenital malformations.[41] The higher malformation rate across a group of counties of the State was presumably environmentally induced but no specific agent was suggested.[8,9]

A few human data are available from studies in which radiofrequency heating of the pelvic region was used in the treatment of gonorrhea, pelvic inflammatory disease, endometriosis, carcinoma of the uterus, or pelvic peritonitis. In one report[42] the pelvic temperature in women was raised to 115°F. Although the author was concerned about possible harmful effects, he did not allude to specific complications. Rubin and Erdman[43] reported case histories of four women treated with microwave diathermy (2450-MHz, 100 W output) for chronic pelvic inflammatory disease who were or became pregnant during the course of the therapy. Three women delivered normal infants; the fourth, who received eight treatments during the first 59 days of pregnancy, aborted on day 67 but delivered a normal baby following a subsequent pregnancy during which she again received microwave therapy. The authors concluded that microwaves did not interfere with ovulation, conception, and pregnancy.

The use of microwave heating to relieve the pain of uterine contractions during labor, has been reported by Daels.[44,45] The analgesic effect was found helpful in 2,000 selected patients without obstetric pathology, and the babies were born healthy with good circulation. No evidence of injury had been manifested in a 1-year folow-up of the children. There was no evidence of mental retardation. Four cases of chromosome anomalies in controls and two cases in the irradiated group were noted. It is important to note that the human fetus at partuition is almost fully developed. Thus gross structural defects at this late stage of development would not be expected.

There are reported case studies of increases in congenital abnormalities in women working in RF fields in Eastern Europe[46] but there are no uniquivocal reports of microwave-induced teratologies in the human being.

Cancer

Microwave-induced cancer has not been reported experimentally or suspected in medical surveillance examinations of microwave workers or military personnel.[8,9] Two recently completed cohort epidemiologic studies[24,26] have looked into the question systematically. Neither has revealed an excess of any form of cancer to date that can be interpreted as microwave-related.[8,9]

Eastern European Reports

Nervous system perturbations and behavioral reactions of exposure of man to microwave energy have been reported mostly in Eastern European literature which describes subjective complaints consisting of fatigability, headache, sleepiness, irritability, loss of appetite and memory difficulties.[46-49] Psychic changes that include unstable mood, hypochondriasis and anxiety have been reported. Most of the subjective symptoms are reversible, and pathological damage to neural structures is insignificant.[50] Several reviewers[51-57] have noted the difficulties in establishing the presence of, and quantifying the frequency and severity of "subjective" complaints. Individuals suffering from a variety of chronic diseases may exhibit the same dysfunctions of the central nervous and cardiovascular systems as those reported to be a result of exposure to microwaves;[57] thus, it is extremely difficult, if not impossible, to rule out other factors in attempting to relate microwave exposure to clinical conditions.

Critique of Epidemiologic Studies

An important concept of disease causation is that, in general, disease is not caused by a single factor or agent, but rather is influenced by multiple, interactive factors including the subject and his environment. Health effects or manifestations of disease have a spectrum of intensity ranging all the way from the barely discernible and rapidly reversible symptomatic disorders, through an increasing gradient of severity to the point of irreversibility, and finally, to disease states of such gravity as to ultimately cause death. For electromagnetic fields, in common with most other agents, biological or physical, the trivial end of this severity scale includes detectable physiological effects, which are well within the range of physiological adaptation and do not constitute disease in any meaningful sense.

The validity of application of the epidemiologic method to the study of the health impact of an agent is largely determined by the ascertainability and definition of an effect. Perhaps the main limitation of epidemiologic studies of MW/RF esposure is the lack of recognized pathophysiologic manifestations at realistic levels of exposure as indicators for measuring the effects of the fields on man.

Eastern European reports describe such symptoms as listlessness, excitability, headache, drowsiness, fatigue and cardiovascular deficits in persons occupationally exposed to electromagnetic fields. These symptoms are also caused by many other occupational factors, so it is not possible to define a cause-effect relationship. Many other factors in the industrial setting or home environment as well as psychosocial interactions can cause similar symptoms. In addition to smolking and obesity, genetic factors and emotional stress, psychological personality factors that determine an individual's reactivity to environmental conditions are proven risk factors in the development of cardiac ischemia.[57] Thus, these factors are important in assessing the effects of environmental insults.

Reports of effects in man must be put in perspective. Epidemiologic and incidence studies suffer from inadequate design and examination as well as lack of data on actual power levels and duration of microwave exposure. It is essential that evaluation be made of the multiple environmental factors which may interact among themselves and with personal characteristics of the individual. There is always the danger that real factors may be overlooked leading to false association with factors of initial interest.

Analysis of occupational exposure to MW/RF energies is fraught with many difficulties. Of utmost importance is assessment of the relationship between exposure levels and the health status of the examined groups of workers. The problem of adequate control groups is controversial and hinges mostly on what one considers "adequate". Quantitation of occupational exposure is extremely difficult. This is particularly true when personnel move around in the course of their duties and are exposed to non-stationary fields, i.e., moving beams or antennas, as well as to near- and far-fields at random. The possible role of other environmental factors and of socioeconomic conditions must be taken into account. As often happens in such studies, it is difficult to demonstrate a causal relationship between a disease and the influence of environmental factors, at least in individual cases.[19]

Recommendations

Because of the difficulties in extrapolating from animal experiments to man, epidemiologic studies, including appropriate clinical and laboratory examinations are essential to improve our understanding of possible health hazards from exposure to MW/RF energies. As noted by Silverman,[8,9] it is difficult to identify exposed populations, select suitable controls and obtain exposure data. Some study groups already characterized can be improved by the acquisition of additional exposure data, some groups should be followed for longer periods of time, and some should be investigated for additional endpoints.

A careful search should be made for exposed groups not yet investigated or considered for study. In epidemiologic studies, as in experimental or clinical work, there is rarely a single study, positive or negative that can be accepted as definitive. Replication and validation are needed at all exposure levels.

The reports from Eastern Europe of a wide variety of functional changes and possible nervous system effects have yet to be confirmed. In appropriate epidemiologic studies, medical reports should be augmented to include assessment of emotional and psychologic status.

Although there is no direct evidence that microwaves are carcinogenic, more intensive and extended morbidity monitoring to identify malignancies would be appropriate.[8,9]

ACKNOWLEDGEMENT

This paper is based on work performed under Contract No. DE-AC02-76EV03490 with the U.S. Department of Energy at the University of Rochester Department of Radiation Biology and Biophysics and has been assigned Reprot No. UR-3490-1967.

REFERENCES

1. C. H. Durney, C. C. Johnson, P. W. Barber, H. Massoudi, M. F. Iskander, J. L. Lords, D. K. Ryser, S. J. Allen and J. C. Mitchell, Radiofrequency Radiation Dosimetry Handbook (2nd Edition), USAF Report SAM-TR-78-22, Brooks Air Force Base, TX (1978).
2. A. W. Guy, J. C. Lin and C. K. Chou, Electrophysiological effects of electromagnetic fields on animals, in: "Fundamental and Applied Aspects of Non-ionizing Radiation," S. M. Michaelson, M. W. Miller, R. Magin, and E. L. Carstensen, eds., Plenum Press, New York (1975).
3. O. P. Gandhi, State of knowledge for electromagnetic absorbed dose in man and animals, Proc. IEEE 68:24 (1980).
4. H. Massoudi, "Long Wavelength Analysis of Electromagnetic Power Absorption by Prolate Spheroidal and Ellipsoidal Models of Man." Salt Lake City: University of Utah, Ph.D. Thesis, 217p. (1976).
5. National Council on Radiation Protection and Measurements: Radiofrequency Electromagnetic Fields. NCRP Report No. 67, Washington, DC (1981).
6. M. A. Stuchly, Health Aspects of Radiofrequency and Microwave Radiation Exposure, Part 2. Dept. Nat. Health and Welfare, Ottawa, 107p. (1978).
7. C. C. Johnson, C. H. Durney, P. W. Barber, H. Massoudi, S. J. Allen and J. C. Mitchell, "Radiofrequency Radiation Dosimetry Handbook," SAM-TR-76-35. Brooks AFB, AFSC, AMD, SAM, 125p. (1976).
8. C. Silverman, Epidemiologic approach to the study of microwave effects, Bull. N.Y. Acad. Med. 55:1166 (1979).
9. C. Silverman, Epidemiologic studies of microwave effects, Proc. IEEE 68:78 (1980).
10. BRH, Bureau of Radiological Health, "Annual Report of the Division of Biological Effects," Fiscal Year 1979, HHS Publication (FDA) 81-8152, p. 34, Rockville, MD (1980).
11. P. S. Ruggera, "Measurements of Emission Levels During Microwave and Shortwave Diathermy Treatments, Bureau of Radiological Health, HHS Publication (FDA) 80-8119 (1980).
12. L. Daily, A clinical study of the results of exposure of laboratory personnel to radar and high frequency radio, U.S. Nav. Med. Bull. 41:1052 (1943).
13. C. I. Barron and A. A. Baraff, Medical considerations of exposure to microwaves (radar), JAMA 168:1194 (1958).
14. C. I. Barron, A. A. Love and A. A. Baraff, Physical evaluation of personnel exposed to microwave emanations, J. Aviat. Med. 26:442 (1955).
15. Z. V. Gordon, "Biological Effect of Microwaves in Occupational Hygiene," Izd. Med., Leningrad (TT 70-50087, NASA TT F-633, 1970) 164p. (1966).

16. Z. V. Gordon, Occupational health aspects of radiofrequency electromagnetic radiation, in: "Ergonomics and Physical Environmental Factors." Occupational Safety and Health Series, No. 21, Geneva, International Labour Office, p. 159 (1970).
17. M. N. Sadchikova, Clinical manifestations of reactions to microwave irradiation in various occupational groups, in: "Biological Effects and Health Hazards of Microwave Radiation," P. Czerski et al., eds., Warsaw, Polish Medical Publishers, p. 261 (1974).
18. P. Czerski and M. Piotrowski, Proposals for specifications of allowable levels of microwave radiation, Medycyna Lotnicza (Polish) 39:127 (1972).
19. P. Czerski and M. Siekierzynski, Analysis of occupational exposure to microwave radiation, in: Fundamental and Applied Aspects of Non-Ionizing Radiations, S. M. Michaelson, M. W. Miller, R. Magin and E. L. Carstensen, eds., Plenum Press, New York p. 367 (1975).
20. P. Czerski, M. Siekierzynski and A. Gidynski, Health surveillance of personnel occupationally exposed to microwaves. I. Theoretical considerations and practical aspects, Aerospace Med. 45:1137 (1974).
21. M. Siekierzynski, A study of the health status of microwave workers, in: "Biologic Effects and Health Hazards of Microwave Radiation," P. Czerski et al., eds., Polish Medical Publishers, Warsaw, p. 273 (1974).
22. M. Siekierzynski, P. Czerski, H. Milczarek, A. Gidynski, C. Czarnecki, E. Dziuk and W. Jedrzejczak, Health surveillance of personnel occupationally exposed to microwaves. II. Functional disturbances, Aerospace Med. 45:1143 (1974).
23. M. Siekierzynski, C. Czarnecki, E. Dziuk, et al., Microwave radiation and other harmful factors of working environment in radiolocation: method of determination of microwave effects, J. Microwave Power 11:144 (1976).
24. C. D. Robinette, C. Silverman and S. Jablon, Effects upon health of occupational exposure to microwave radiation (radar) 1950-1974, Am. J. Epidemiol. 112:39 (1980).
25. U.S. Senate, "Radiation Health and Safety", Hearings before the Committee on Commerce, Science, and Transportation, 95 Congress, First Session on Oversight of Radiation Health and Safety, June 16, 17, 27, 28 and 29, 1977, Serial No. 95-49, pp. 284, 1195, 1196 (1977).
26. A. M. Lilienfeld, J. Tonascia, S. Tonascia, C. H. Libauer, G. M. Cathen, J. A. Markowitz and S. Weida, "Foreign Service Health Status Study: Evaluation of Health Status of Foreign Service and other Employees from Selected Eastern European Posts, Final Report," July 31, 1978 Contract No. 6025-619073 Dept. of Epidemiol. Johns Hopkins Univ. Baltimore, NTIS PB-288, 1963 (1978).

27. U.S. Senate, Committee on Commerce, Science, and Transportation. Committee Print, "Microwave Irradiation of the U.S. Embassy in Moscow," April, 1979, (43-949) U.S. Government Printing Office, Washington, DC (1979).
28. S. Zydecki, Assessment of lens translucency in juveniles, microwave workers and age-matched groups, in: "Biological Effects and Health Hazards of Microwave Radiation," P. Czerski, K. Ostrowski, C. Silverman, et al., eds., Polish Medical Publishers, Warsaw, 306p. (1974).
29. S. F. Cleary and B. S. Pasternack, Lenticular changes in microwave workers, a statistical study, Arch. Environ. Health 12:23 (1966).
30. K. Majewska, Study of effects of microwaves on visual organs, Klin. Oczna (Polish) 38:323 (1968).
31. M. M. Zaret, S. F. Cleary, B. Pasternack, M. Eisenbud and H. Schmidt, "A Study of Lenticular Imperfections in the Eyes of a Sample of Microwave Workers and a Control Population," Final contract report for Rome Air Development Center, RADC-TDR-6310125, March 15 (1963).
32. S. F. Cleary, B. S. Pasternack and G. W. Beebe, Cataract incidence in radar workers, Arch. Environ. Health 11:179-182 (1965).
33. U.S. Department of Health, Education and Welfare, National Center for Health Statistics, Division of Health Examination Statistics, Medical Statistics Branch, March 2 (1977).
34. L. T. Oland, Observations on microwave hazards to USAF personnel, J. Occup. Med. 14:544 (1972).
35. S. Baranski and P. Czerski, "Biological Effects of Microwaves, "Dowden, Hutchinson and Ross, Inc., Stroudsburg, PA (1976).
36. C. Silverman, "The Epidemiology of Depression," Baltimore, Johns Hopkins Press (1968).
37. C. Silverman, Nervous and behavioral effects of microwave radiation in humans, Am. J. Epidemiol. 97:219 (1973).
38. A. T. Sigler, A. M. Lilienfeld, B. H. Cohen, et al., Radiation exposure in parents of children with mongolism (Down's Syndrome), Bull, Johns Hopkins Hosp. 117:374 (1965).
39. B. H. Cohen, A. M. Lilienfeld, and S. Kramer, et al., Parental factors in Down's Syndrome-results of the second Baltimore Case-Control study, in: "Population Cytogenetics, Studies in Humans, E.B. Hook and I.H. Porter, eds., Academic Press, New York, 301p. (1977).
40. P. B. Peacock, J.W. Simpson, C. A. Alford, et al., Congenital anomalies in Alabama. J. Med. Assoc. State Ala., July, pp. 42-50 (1971).
41. J. A. Burdeshaw and S. Schaffer, "Factors Associated with the Incidence of Congenital Anomalies: A Localized Investigation", Environmental Protection Agency, Final Report, Contract No. 68-02-0791, March 31 (1976).

42. S. Gellhorn, Diathermy in gynecology, _J. Am. Med. Assoc._ 90:1005 (1928).
43. A. Rubin and W.J. Erdman, Microwave exposure of the human female pelvis during early pregnancy and prior to conception. _Am. J. Phys. Med._ 38:219 (1959).
44. J. Daels, Microwave heating of the uterine wall during parturition, _Obstet. Gynecol._ 42:76 (1973).
45. J. Daels, Microwave heating of the uterine wall during parturition, _J. Microwave Power_ 11:166 (1976).
46. K. Marha, J. Musil and H. Tuha, "Electromagnetic Fields and the Life Environment," State Health Publishing House, Prague, 1968 San Francisco Press (1971).
47. I. R. Petrov, ed., "Influence of Microwave Radiation on the Organism of Man and Animals," Lenigrad, Meditsina Press (NAS TT F-708) (1970).
48. A. S. Presman, "Electromagnetic Fields and Life," Izd-vo Nauka, Moscow (Transl. Plenum Press, New York, 1970) (1968).
49. Z. V. Gordon, The problem of the biological action of UHF, _Tr. Gig. i. Prof. AMN SSR_, No. 1:5 (1960).
50. T. N. Orlova, Clinical aspects of mental disorders following protracted human exposure to super-high frequency electromagnetic waves, _in_: "Cerebral Mechanisms of Mental Illness," Kazan', 16p. (1971).
51. S. M. Michaelson, Human exposure to non-ionizing radiant energy - potential hazards and safety standards, _Proc. IEEE_ 60:389 (1972).
52. S. M. Michaelson, Effects of exposure to microwaves: Problems and perspectives, _Environ. Health Perspect._ 8:133 (1974).
53. S. M. Michaelson, Radiofrequency and microwave energies, magnetic and electric fields, Chapt. 1, Vol. II, Book 2, _in_: "The Foundations of Space Biology and Medicine", M. Calvin and O.G. Gazenko, eds., NASA, Washington, DC, 409p. (1975).
54. S. M. Michaelson and C. H. Dodge, Soviet views on the biologic effects of microwaves: An analysis, _Health Physics_ 21:108 (1971).
55. C. H. Dodge and Z. R. Glaser, Trends in non-ionizing radiation bioeffects research and related occupational health aspects, _J. Microwave Power_ 12:319 (1977).
56. R. M. Albrecht and E. Landau, Microwave radiation, An epidemiologic assessment, _Reviews on Environmental Health_ 3:44 (1979).
57. A. K. Guskova and Y. H. Kochanova, Some aspects of etiological diagnostics of occupational diseases as related to the effects of microwave radiation, _Gig. Truda i. Prof. Zabol._ 3:14 (1975).

DEVELOPMENT OF STANDARDS - ASSESSMENT OF HEALTH HAZARDS AND OTHER FACTORS

Michael H. Repacholi

Radiation Protection Bureau
Health and Welfare Canada
Ottawa, Ontario K1A 0L2

INTRODUCTION

Applications of microwave and radiofrequency energy are increasing in number and diversity in industry, medicine, commerce, research, communications and the home. Although these applications provide significant benefits to mankind, they may also constitute hazards to the individual through uncontrolled and excessive emissions of radiant energy. It has been substantiated that at sufficiently high levels, exposure to microwave and radiofrequency fields can produce not only biological effects but pose a definite risk to health. Thus there is a need to set limits on the amount of exposure which individuals can receive without sustaining any injury.

In most biological interactions with physical agents, there is a certain range of exposure levels between which no apparent or observable effects are produced and at which effects are clearly detectable. Although an effect is detected, it is not necessarily one that is irreparable or even a sign that a threshold of damage has been reached. In any assessment of reported biological effects, a clear distinction must be made between those effects which do not result in either immediate or latent functional impairment and those that result in some injury through impairment of normal activity either temporarily or permanently. Unfortunately however, there is not a clearly defined relationship between the radiofrequency or microwave exposure level and patho-physiological effect. This makes the problem of drafting standards much more complex. There are many variables to consider, as was outlined by Repacholi[1], and in most cases it is extremely difficult or impossible to obtain the information needed to draw valid conclusions regarding the dose-effect relationship. Ideally one would like to base standards on firm human data. However since insufficient data are available, extrapolations from well-designed, adequately-performed and properly analysed animal experiments are necessary.

In developing standards one should bear in mind that a potential hazard to health is created either as a result of direct exposure to the human body or by interactions with certain devices which themselves are susceptible to electromagnetic radiation and cause health hazards (e.g. interference with cardiac pacemakers, electromedical devices, unintended triggering of electronically activated detonators, ignition of flammable materials). A review of potential electromagnetic devices was recently given by Reis[2].

In this presentation is a discussion of standards, their applicability and usefulness, and various concepts on which they should be based. The development of exposure standards is of primary importance. These are described with respect to the population at risk, selection of the scientific data base, approaches one could take in determining maximum exposure limits, and other factors which should be considered. Detailed requirements which must be a part of any exposure standard to make it internally consistent and cause as little confusion as possible in the minds of persons who must determine compliance with such a standard, are also discussed. Finally the susceptibility of a regulatory agency to external influences is touched upon.

STANDARDS

A standard is a general term, incorporating both regulations and guidelines, and is defined for this presentation to be a set of specifications or rules laid down to promote the safety of an individual or group of people. A regulation is promulgated under a legal statute and is referred to as a mandatory standard. A guideline generally has no legal force and is issued for guidance only - a voluntary standard. Standards can specify maximum exposure limits and other safety rules for personal exposure, or provide details on the performance, construction, design or functioning of a device.

Standards should only be developed if there is a real need for them. Either persons can be exposed to sufficient amounts of radiation to cause adverse health effects or devices can emit or leak sufficient radiation that injury can result from their use. The potential severity and the frequency of the hazard should influence whether the standard is made into a guideline or a regulation.

Prior to the development of standards for devices or personnel exposure one generally has to give some consideration to the following:[3]

1. Does microwave or radiofrequency energy really present a problem to humans? Are there confirmed biological effects from exposing human beings or other mammalian species? Do these confirmed effects constitute a health hazard?
2. What sources of microwave and radiofrequency radiation could be potentially hazardous, how rapidly are they proliferating, and how can they be controlled?
3. Will the existence and implementation of regulations or guidelines alleviate the problem?
4. In developing standards, what is the acceptable risk to health of exposure to microwave and radiofrequency fields considering the benefits that can accrue from its use?
5. What would be the economic impact of such controls on device manufacturers, retailers and users?
6. What national and/or international standards exist, their scientific basis, and associated philosophy of acceptable risk?

Thus, before proceeding with the development of standards on microwave and radiofrequency energy, one must review thoroughly the available scientific literature on biological effects, study the various sources of this radiant energy, and evaluate the current national and international standards on the subject. This analysis will generally provide answers to the above questions with varying degrees of satisfaction. It is then up to the individual regulatory agencies or standards setting organizations to determine if there is a need for standards, and if so, whether compulsory regulations or voluntary guidelines should be developed.

Development and implementation of regulations to limit the exposure to microwave and radiofrequency energy can provide beneficial effects to the health of exposed persons and industry in the following ways:

1. The existence of regulations serves as a signal to industry and the general public that there is a concern about exposure to this radiant energy and that they should become aware of the potential hazards.
2. Regulations provide goals to be achieved at the planning stages by manufacturers of devices and by organizations involved in the installation and construction of microwave or radiofrequency radiation facilities.
3. Devices or facilities producing leakage fields of microwave or radiofrequency energy in excess of the levels permitted by the regulations should be identified and appropriate remedial action taken.
4. Regulations form the basis for safe working practices to ensure that employees are not exposed to excessive levels

of radiation.

Safe-use guidelines may have a number of advantages over regulations:

1. they can be introduced more rapidly than regulations,
2. modifications to the guidelines can normally be made quickly if necessary,
3. they can be made with more flexibility to adjust to changes in technology, and
4. they are not restricted in their scope by legal statute or act.

On the other hand safe-use guidelines have limitations:

1. they are voluntary and thus need not be followed,
2. they are less useful to manufacturers, since regulations provide detailed requirements on design, construction or functioning, and
3. regulations, being mandatory, protect good manufacturers from 'fly by night' operations.

Types of Standards

To protect the general population and persons occupationally exposed to microwave or radiofrequency fields, two types of standards are generally promulgated:

1. Exposure standards are basic standards of personnel protection which do not apply to particular devices or equipment but generally refer to maximum levels to which whole or partial body exposure is permitted from any number of radiation emitting devices. This type of standard normally incorporates safety factors and provides the basic guide for limiting personnel exposure.
2. Emissions standards are protective standards designed to limit the health risks from exposure to excessive leakage radiation emitted from products or devices. Normally these standards set maximum emissions of leakage radiation from a device at a specified distance. Detailed specifications on the design, construction, functioning and performance of the device are usually given to ensure that the maximum exposure or leakage levels are not exceeded. An example is the Canadian regulation on microwave ovens, where the power density is not permitted to exceed 1 mW/cm^2 at a distance of 5 cm from any external surface of the oven while a water load of 275 ml is placed inside the oven cavity. Requirements for safety interlocks, labelling and quality control are also included.

Exposure standards differ from emission standards in that

they are determined from biological effects data and consideration of many other factors, and would normally represent an exposure level, below which, no biological effects have been detected. Maximum levels of emission or leakage radiation for a particular device would then be derived and set below that provided for in an exposure standard, since personnel could conceivably be exposed to radiation from more than one source at a time, or because the device is used in an "uncontrolled" environment by "uneducated" operators.

Standards development should preferably be preceded by publication of a criteria document which summarizes the experimental data on exposure of various biological systems to microwave or radiofrequency energy, the known mechanisms of interactions of this energy with biological tissue, a health risk assessment of the scientific data and an analysis of the various national and international standards. The criteria document then forms an important scientific basis for regulations, from which the maximum exposure levels incorporated into standards can be justified. There are many standards today which have been developed without such a rationale or criteria document, and it is thus difficult to interpret their basis.

Development of Exposure Standards

1. Population at risk. There are a number of factors which must be considered prior to the promulgation of exposure standards. One must initially define the population the exposure standard is intended to protect. In this regard a distinction must be made between persons occupationally exposed and the general public. Occupational health exposure standards are aimed at protecting healthy adults exposed under controlled conditions, who are aware of the occupational risk and who are likely to be subjected to medical surveillance.

Exposure standards for the general public must be based on broader considerations, including health status, special sensitivities, possible effects on the course of various diseases, as well as limitations in adaptation to environmental conditions and responses to any kind of stress in old age[4]. In essence the general public comprises a spectrum of health status - from the physically healthy to the sick, obese, aged and stress sensitive individuals. In addition, exposure standards for the general public must be set at a level considered acceptable for exposures of 24 h per day. Occupational exposure standards can be set for exposure durations of 8 h per day.

2. Selection of biological effects data base. Of all the factors involved in the development of exposure standards, probably the most important is the selection of biological effects

data on which the standards are to be based. In this respect it is extremely important to select data that has been:

(i) scientifically derived through adequately controlled and properly performed studies, using reliable dosimetry, and reporting correctly interpreted data,

(ii) reproduced by independent laboratories, to the point that the evidence is irrefutable,

(iii) published in a peer reviewed journal,

(iv) studied to the extent that sufficient information becomes available so that a reasonable assessment of health risk can be made.

One of the major factors for the extreme variations in exposure standards in various countries around the World has been the significance placed on certain data and the exclusion of other data when making a health risk assessment. In some cases, undue weight may be placed on biological effects data that, although they have not received adequate study, appear to have health risk implications. This is not to say that a health agency should not take note of effects that have potential for concern. For example, the effect that has created a lot of interest is the alteration of calcium efflux in chick brain tissue following exposure to modulated microwave fields[5]. Although this effect has been confirmed and studied in a very scientific manner, it is impossible from the information gathered to date to make any rational assessment of potential health risk in humans. All that a health agency can do in this situation is monitor the progress of scientific experimentation.

3. Methods to determine the maximum exposure levels. There are a number of approaches that can be taken to determine exposure limits. On the basis of a health risk assessment of the scientific data, a threshold exposure level may be derived. This is judged as being the lowest exposure level, below which no adverse health effects have been found. Since there will be a certain amount of imprecision in determining this threshold, primarily because of an incomplete knowledge of the biological effects, a range of uncertainty will exist. The degree of uncertainty will then be directly proportional to the value of a safety factor that should then be incorporated to arrive at the final maximum exposure limit.

This approach requires a good understanding of the interaction mechanisms involved and indeed supposes that a true threshold exists. It also assumes that cumulative effects do not occur. Evidence for cumulative damage would suggest that small amounts of damage may be occurring from low level exposure and that an accumulation of this damage is necessary before it becomes detectable. Further, there is a dependence on information from extensive research, including long-term follow-up studies. Without such studies, it is possible that illnesses or effects which manifest themselves after a long latency period, would be excluded from consideration.

Another way of determining exposure limits is to adopt a phenomenological approach. From the scientific data base a threshold exposure level is determined below which no biological effect is observed. This method alleviates the necessity of making a health risk assessment of the biological effects data and assumes an incomplete knowledge of the interaction mechanisms. There is always the problem that such an approach will result in an unduly conservative standard which could not only restrict technological advances but would be unacceptable in terms of the loss of benefits accruing from technology for protection against questionable risks.

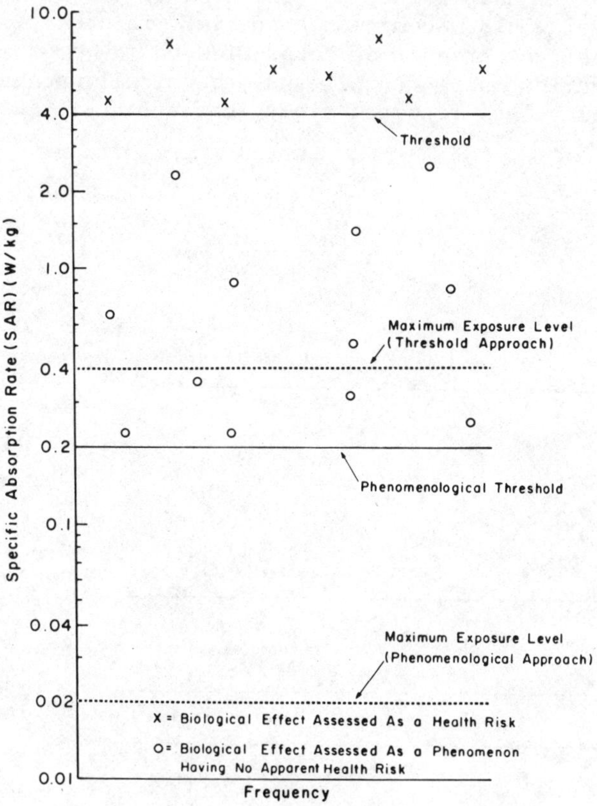

Figure 1. Determination of maximum exposure levels using the threshold and phenomenological approaches.

A third approach to defining exposure limits is to adopt the ALARA principle. The ALARA principle (as low as readily achievable) is used extensively for radiation protection in the ionizing radiation field and has as its basis the assumption that any exposure to radiation should be avoided since it might involve some degree of risk. The International Commission on Radiological Protection[6] incorporates this philosophy as its primary recommendation for ionizing radiation safety. However if there is a well established threshold exposure level for an effect, then the ALARA principle would not apply. This principle is applicable if a well quantitated dose-response relationship does not exist. The conservative philosophy reflected in the ALARA principle may be useful as an interim measure until such a relationship for microwave and radiofrequency exposure to man has been well quantitated[6].

To actually define the exposure limits using the ALARA principle still involves a study of the biological effects data. One would arrive at a limit that is below the level of reported biological effects (and well below the level of potential adverse health effects) to the extent that the cost of protection for an even lower level would become unreasonable. In other words the limit is reached as a result of compromise on the economic cost. The limit is as low as is readily and economically achievable and yet below the level of reported biological effects.

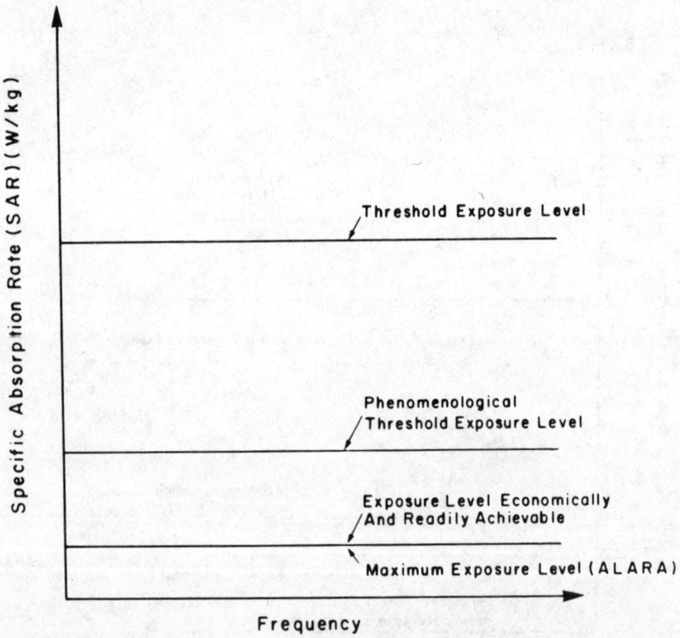

Figure 2. Determination of maximum exposure levels using the ALARA Principle.

Exposure standards in most countries will tend to be developed with more than one of the above approaches. Although a complete knowledge of biological effects from exposure to microwave and radiofrequency radiations may never by fully gained, enough information is available on which standards can be formulated. The precision with which the standards are determined is then a reflection on how extensive one feels that the knowledge of biological effects and interaction mechanisms is.

4. Environmental and health status factors. Prior to promulgation of any standard, an assessment of the effects that these levels will have on persons working or living under all environmental conditions must be made. In making this assessment, one should assume that the maximum allowable levels of exposure will exist in the environment or the workplace. All too often standards have been set under the premise that such levels would never be reached in practice. This attitude is irresponsible and does not properly address the problem of setting standards on the basis of the scientific evidence.

If general public exposure standards are to be set at given levels, account must be taken of the effect these levels will have under various temperature, wind velocities and humidity. In practice the level of exposure, if based on thermal considerations alone, should be safe for older, obese people undergoing work or recreation that requires a reasonable level of metabolic activity, in an environment of high temperature, high humidity, low air movement, and wearing appropriate clothing. In addition, if the scientific data base suggests it, consideration should be given to the normal spectrum of sensitivities to heat stress that would exist in any population, to the possibility that certain drugs may produce adverse reactions in patients exposed to a microwave or radiofrequency environment, and to people who are diseased or sick to the extent that they may be particularly sensitive to additional stress. These considerations will generally require that certain safety factors be incorporated. The same safety factors may not be needed in occupational exposure standards, since one is normally dealing with a healthy population working under controlled environmental conditions.

5. Actual exposure conditions. Exposure standards must incorporate sufficient safety factors to account for actual exposure situations that can occur in practice, such as higher exposure levels caused by reflections of microwave and radiofrequency energy. In the vicinity of flat and corner reflectors, for specific positions of the reflectors, the ratio of the rate of energy absorption to the basal metabolic rate can be as large as 70 (at resonance)[7] for an incident plane wave at a power density of 10 mW/cm^2. This figure should be kept in perspective however since such enhancement is critically dependent on the position,

shape and dimensions of the reflector, and in practice only limited possibilities exist for such exposure conditions. Nevertheless some account for these possibilities must be made.

6. Exposure standard requirements. To ensure that an exposure standard has all the elements necessary to be complete, the following must be addressed:

(i) frequency - since the absorption of electromagnetic radiation is frequency dependent, one would expect that the same maximum limit on incident power density would not be applicable over the whole frequency range. Here the absorption of energy in man as indicated in a determination of SAR as a function of frequency, could be an initial guide,

(ii) exposure level - the level of exposure can be practically expressed in terms of power density, however to provide guidance for exposures occurring in the near-field, both the electric and magnetic field strengths should also be given. Situations where exposures can occur to fields of different frequencies must be accounted for in the standard,

(iii) exposure duration - the time of exposure to various power densities should be quite precise. In many standards a power density level is set for continuous exposure for 8 or 24 h per day, but higher levels of exposure are generally permitted for short periods of time. In this respect, the time over which the exposure level is averaged is very important - whether it be over a 1 min or 1 h time period to average the effect of intermittent exposures, higher levels for shorter periods of time, or for pulsed beams. The exact means of averaging exposures must be clearly indicated so that no confusion arises in the minds of persons responsible for compliance,

(iv) pulsed beams represent a problem for standards setting organizations because inadequate information is available to determine whether a pulsed beam with a high peak power density but low average power density, incurs similar biological effects to a continuous wave beam with the same average power density. To date no real account has been taken of pulsed beams, except to indicate that the average power density of these beams should not exceed the maximum exposure level. The same solution is generally applied to the case of exposure to stationary and rotating antennas or alternatively some arbitrary factor may be applied to the cw power density to account for the lower average power density one would receive from a rotating antenna,

(v) whole-body and partial-body exposure - exposure levels are generally determined for whole-body exposure. Unfortunately very little work has been conducted on the effects of microwave or radiofrequency on individual parts of the body. Certainly at this time there is insufficient information to make any separate assessment of health risks from partial-body exposure. In some standards however, high exposure levels are allowed to the extremities (arms and legs). In any exposure standard however, the concern of partial-body exposures should be addressed, even if the standard merely allows the same levels of exposure for both whole- or partial-body exposure.

7. Complexity of a standard. How precise can an exposure standard be made? If one takes the stance that the permitted exposure will be set at a level below which no significant biological effects have been reported, one could in essence be quite conservative and adopt a single value over the whole frequency range. There are many standards that have adopted this approach. Sufficient information is now available that should allow standards to be based to a greater extent on the amount of energy deposited in the body. Since energy absorption is frequency dependent, one should expect some dependence of the maximum exposure level on frequency.

If the exposure standard was to be based purely on heat stress considerations, it would be tempting to define the permitted exposure limits by using the curve[8] (Figure 3) of the power density required to deliver a heat load as a function of the frequency of the incident electromagnetic radiation. In effect this seems to be the approach taken by the latest U.S. ANSI[9] and ACGIH[10] Committees (Figure 4). Both the ANSI and ACGIH Committees found that the reported biological effects were related to the amount of energy absorbed by the living system studied, and so had a good rationale for curve fitting around Figure 3. A standard having such a precise reliance on the frequency of the incident radiation may be too complex. The scientific basis is understandable but its practical application with regard to determining compliance can be a nightmare. This is especially true in situations when exposure levels are near the maximum recommended and result from multiple sources emitting fields with different frequencies. The Canadian standard (Figure 4) contains basically the same degree of protection as the ANSI and ACGIH proposals - but is more practical for compliance purposes.

The more complex and precise a standard is set, the greater confidence one has placed in the accuracy and comprehensiveness of knowledge of the biological effects data and on the depth of understanding of interaction mechanisms on which the standard is based. I believe the state of knowledge is sufficient to make

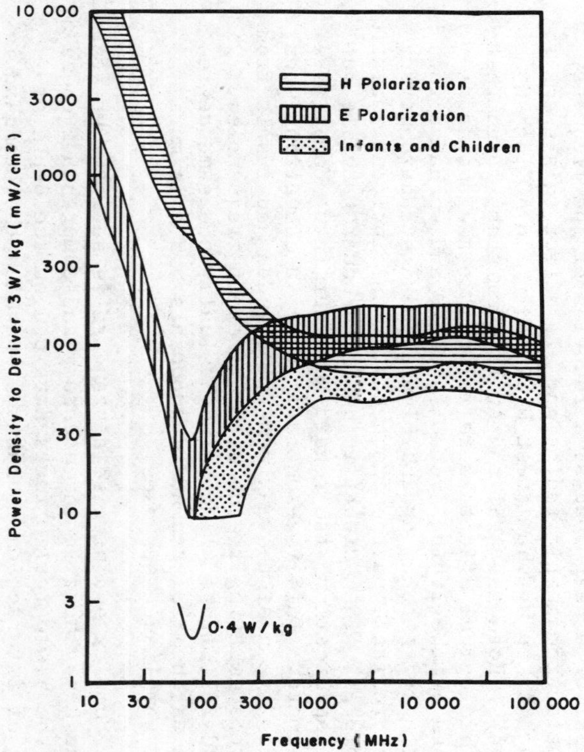

Figure 3. The incident power density as a function of frequency to deliver a heat load of 3 W/kg in men, women and children.

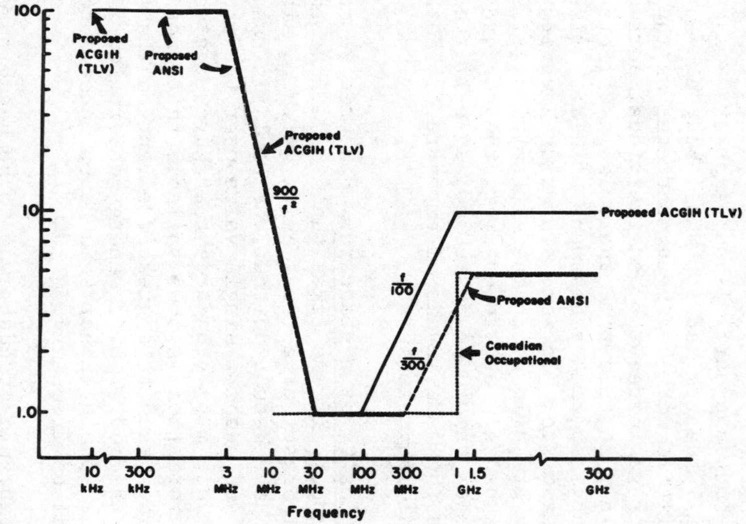

Figure 4. Complexity of standards - a comparison of the Canadian occupational exposure standard with that proposed by ANSI and ACGIH.

generalized assumptions only and this should be reflected in a stepped as opposed to a ramped dependence on frequency.

8. Influence of other standards and public pressure. Many governments and especially regulatory agencies are being pressured by a concerned general public to adopt safety standards for microwave and radiofrequency exposure. Part of this concern stems from an active but uninformed press, as well as popular publications (e.g. The Zapping of America by Paul Brodeur) which tend to distort the scientific facts. Another component of this pressure to develop conservative exposure standards comes from the fact that many scientists or "pseudo-authoritative" experts are seen by the general public as being in a never-ending debate over the interpretation or misinterpretation of biological effects data. Until the scientific community can put its own act together, one cannot expect an uneducated general public to reduce its level of concern.

Real influence on standards-setting regulatory agencies is exerted by preceding standards. In particular one notes that virtually all Eastern European countries have tended to adopt, what is regarded in the West, as very conservative exposure standards. By contrast many Western countries have adopted exposure standards similar to those developed in the United States. Pressure is now being placed on many Western countries to adopt somewhat more conservative standards which fall somewhat between those in Eastern Europe and those in the United States. The biological effects data and a better developed understanding of the deposition of microwave and radiofrequency energy in the body, have tended to support a move to this compromise position.

Conclusions

The development of standards is not something that can be taken lightly - these standards have a very direct impact not only on our quality of life but an economic impact - through higher cost consumer products and potential restriction of technological advances. Although the final decision to promulgate a standard is normally at the political level, all possible consequences must be explored.

There are many factors that go into the development of an exposure standard - these are itemized below.

1. Determining the population to be protected,
2. Selection of a good scientific biological effects data base,
3. Making a health risk assessment of the bioeffects,
4. Assessing the effects of exposure limits for various environmental conditions and health status,
5. Accounting for microwave and radiofrequency exposure conditions

that occur in practice,

6. Ensuring that the exposure standard is internally consistent and addresses all possible characteristics of the radiation as well as requirements of partial body and intermittent exposures.

Once the basic exposure standard has been developed, emission standards for various radiation emitting devices can be derived. Incorporation of safety factors into any standard is a result of:

(i) the degree of conservatism to be adopted,
(ii) pressure from outside influences, and
(iii) the degree of complexity.

The role of a regulatory agency is not easy. A clear course must be set between the often opposing demands of a concerned public on the one hand and the economic concerns of manufacturers on the other. It is only by basing standards on unimpeachable scientific evidence that these two demands can often be satisfied.

Acknowledgements

I would like to thank Dr. Maria Stuchly and Dr. Peter Waight for their reviews and Mrs. Judy Smith for typing the manuscript.

REFERENCES

1. M.H. Repacholi, Differentiation between biological effects and health hazards: Scaling from animals, Presented at the 4th course: Advances in biological effects and dosimetry of low-energy electromagnetic fields. Erice, Sicily, March 28-April 8, 1981.
2. R. Reis, Potential interference with medical electronic devices, Bull. N.Y. Acad. Med. 55(11): 1216-1221 (1979).
3. M.H. Repacholi, Proposed exposure limits for microwave and radiofrequency radiations in Canada, J. Microwave Power 13(2): 199-211 (1978).
4. World Health Organization, Environmental Health Criteria for Radiofrequency and Microwaves, WHO Geneva, Switzerland (1980).
5. S.M. Barwin and W.R. Adey, Sensitivity of calcium binding in cerebral tissue to weak environmental electric fields oscillating at low frequency, Proc. Nat. Acad. Sci. (USA), 73:1999-2003 (1976).
6. International Commission on Radiological Protection, Implications of Commission recommendations that doses be kept as low as readily achievable, ICRP Publication, No. 22, Pergamon Press, Oxford (1973).
7. O.P. Gandhi, E.L. Hunt and J.A. D'Andrea, Electromagnetic power deposition in man and animals with and without ground and reflector effects, Radio Science, 12-65: 39-47 (1977).

8. R.A. Tell and F. Harlen, A Review of selected biological effects and dosimetric data useful for development of radiofrequency safety standards for human exposure, J. Microwave Power 14(4):405-424 (1979).
9. American National Standards Institute (ANSI) Committee C95.4, "Safety level with respect to human exposure to radiofrequency electromagnetic fields (300 kHz - 100 GHz)", Eighth Draft, 24 March (1980).
10. American Conference of Governmental and Industrial Hygienists (ACGIH) Committee on Physical Agents. Proposed Radiofrequency Radiation Threshold Limit Value. Meeting, Rockville, Maryland, March 12-13, (1981).

ASSESSMENT OF HEALTH HAZARD AND STANDARD PROMULGATION IN CHINA

Chiang Huai

Microwave Institute
Chekiang Medical College
Hangchow, China

In general, radiofrequency and microwave radiation at sufficient levels of intensity and duration of exposure could cause harmful effects on a living organism, but the bioeffects and their mechanism are not yet well known. There are many uncertainties and differences of opinions, so that the safe exposure limits proposed in various countries differ from each other greatly, and there are two different types of safe exposure standards to consider depending on the population to be protected. There is an occupational standard which is used to protect persons working in the RF or MW environment, and an environmental standard to protect the general public. The safe exposure level of the latter is often as low as one tenth of the former, because the general population includes children, pregnant women, and individuals with various diseases. Both of these exposure standards differ from the emission or performance standards which restrict the emission of radiation from devices, such as the emission standards for microwave ovens in the United States and Canada. An exposure standard refers to the maximum permissible exposure level to the body, which must be based mainly on realistic assessment of health hazard, and which is to be discussed here.

Setting of the standards is not a simple task. It is necessary to establish a quantitative relationship between power densities of incident radiation and all biological effects for human beings. Quantification of the biological response to microwaves is a complex problem because of the wide range of the frequency spectrum. There are a large number of physical and biological variables and complex interrelationships among these variables. Most of the scientific data has been obtained from experiments on small animals or simpler organisms, and extrapolating laboratory results to man is not a clearly defined process. Additionally, there is a large amount of uncorroborated and controversial evidence of various biological effects. In these cases, the assessment of health hazard for "Standard" promulgation should rely mainly on the health status of personnel professionally exposed to RF and MW, although the information available in this field is limited. In various radiation conditions of human exposure, since it is impossible to make quantitation precisely and distinction between various radiation conditions strictly, the results of experiments with animals on bioeffects of RF and MW should be supplemented to the human exposure data.

Assessment of Health Status of RF and MW Workers

Some cases of acute reaction to microwave overexposure have been encountered [1]. The syndrome seems to consist mainly of subjective complaints of headaches, nausea, vertigo, and sleeplessness. Objectively, hypertonia, changes in cardiac rhythm, and a skin rash may be encountered. EEG examination may show a decrease in amplitude of alpha waves. In all cases the symptoms were transient and disappeared completely after a few days of sedation and rest. In one case, noted by the present author, the patient was extremely excited, highly unsteady in body temperature and heart rate, and evidenced reversible impairment of visual acuity and ventricular block. The symptoms lasted several weeks, even months. In general, the power density of microwave exposure causing acute reaction must be above at least 30 mW/cm^2. There is no doubt that the maximum permissible exposure level should be far below that level.

In setting a standard, one of the most important considerations has to be chronic exposure. As the assessment of the relationship between exposure levels and the health status of personnel professionally exposed to RF and MW is difficult, large groups must be observed in order to obtain epidemiological data with statistical significance. Many contributions in this field have been made by Soviet authors. Papers have also been published by authors from Czechoslovakia, Poland, USA, Sweden and so forth. In recent years, some investigations have been carried out in China. A large part of these findings concerning health hazard will be discussed here jointly.

The first topic is quantitation of human exposure. In view of the lack of personal dosimeters, the quantitation of exposure during work is extremely difficult, particularly where the personnel move around in the course of their duties and are exposed to moving beams or antenna of radars. Additionally, it is impossible to evaluate the exposure over a period of several years. So on the basis of analysis of working conditions, authors usually roughly divide the personnel examined into two or three groups named high, (middle), and low power density groups. In fact, the exposure levels generally range from some tens to several hundred uW/cm^2 for professional microwave workers. One or two hundred uW/cm^2 as the demarcation line between high and low power densities has been adopted by some researchers. Only in a few working places do the microwave exposure levels exceed 1 mW/cm^2 or 10 mW/cm^2.

The principal part of the clinical findings from observed microwave workers is similar in different countries. Symptoms of functional disturbance in the central and vegetative nervous systems are the main manifestation. These will be described in the following with the results of investigations in China being compared with those in other countries. The investigation [2] on which the "Chinese Tentative Standard" is mainly based was conducted in 11 factories and institutes. The microwave workers observed had worked with microwave equipment (most of them were PW in cm range) more than one year, and a large part of them had 5 - 15 years of working experience. Everyone in the study had been in an ordinary work setting for the last three months. There were 841 workers given clinical observation, with 471 persons observed as a control group, their sex and age distribution similar to that of the microwave workers. The microwave workers were divided into two groups in terms of power density exposed. The first group, 306 workers, was exposed to a higher power density of >200 uW/cm^2 and the second group of 535 workers, to a lower <200 uW/cm^2. There was no significant difference in ages and working experience of these two groups ($p<0.05$).

1. Effects on the Nervous System

The results confirm the previous findings of Soviet authors on the occurrence of subjective complaints (Table 1). Another finding in the microwave workers was the partial loss of hair. The most pronounced symptoms were headache, fatigue, disturbance of sleep (insomnia or somnolence) and decrease in memory. The persons who complained of any of the three symptoms mentioned above were defined as "neurasthenia" and the incidence of neurasthenia is shown in Table 2. It is indicated that there were significant differences between any two groups.

A part of the observed persons (106 in all) were examined for EEG. The microwave workers' EEG revealed an increase in theta and delta waves, but there were no significant differences in statistics.

Similar complaints and incidences of neurasthenia symptoms were observed in RF workers in China, and the places where they worked were at the field strengths of several hundred V/m.

TABLE 1 Complaints of Microwave Workers (%)

Authors	No. of workers	Headache	Fatigue	Sleep disturbances		Memory decrease	Irritability	Hyperhidrosis	Abnormal menstruation
				Sleepless	Sleepiness				
Present authors (1979)	841	41-44.8	38-40.5	25.5-26	11-11.1	46.4-50	14.4-19	12.1-18	14.6-20
Sadcikova (1974)	1180	41-45	47-57		11-14	10-22	28-38	32-58	
Ramzen-Evaokinov (1970)	155	44	29	35			36	25	
Tjagin (1966)	573	33.5	46.2	25.3			9.6	25.5	
Uspenskaja (1963)	100	37	31	29			9	7	
CONTROL									
Present Authors	471	27.6	14.4	18.3	4.3	17.2	9.6	6.6	6.6
Sadcikova	200	12	7		2	1	6	12	
Ramzen-Evdokinov	50	7	8	3				4	
Tjagin	184	10.8	5.9	8.7				2.7	
Uspenskaja	100	15	22	2				4	

TABLE 2: Incidence of Neurasthenia Symptoms

Group	Incidence (%)	Groups for X^2	p
1	32	among all	<0.001
2	24.1	high to lower	<0.02
3	11	lower to control	<0.001

2. Effects on the Cardiovascular System

The microwave workers who complained chiefly of palpitation and pains around the cardiac region were in the high power density microwave radiation group; the incidences were much higher than for the control group ($p<0.001$). The incidences of hypotonia (≤ 100 mm Hg) were higher in the microwave groups (high and lower density group in 25.5% and 22.6% respectively) than in the control group (15.3%). Reviewing the reports [3,4,5] published by Soviet authors, we could find that the incidence of hypotonia in RF and MW workers mostly is 20-40%, and in the most recent ten years, the incidence of hypertonia is higher than hypotonia. It has been suggested that hypertonia increases with working age, and occurs in advanced stages of the disease. Glotova observed the dynamic alteration of blood pressure of microwave workers. She divided the observed persons into three groups according to their initial pressure. They all were near thirty years of age.

TABLE 3: Dynamic Alteration of BP in MW Workers

Group No.	Observed Time	Total	BP (mm Hg) 90-95	100	105-135	140-145	150-160
1	initial	17	8	9	0	0	0
	after 3-6 years		3	6	2	3	3
2	initial	17	0	0	17	0	0
	after 3-6 years		0	0	5	6	6
3	initial	9	0	0	0	8	1
	after 3-6 years		0	0	0	1	8

The microwave exposure effects on ECG showed changes in cardiac rate, minor downward displacement of the S-T segment, lowering of T deflection, and slight deviations from normal in excitability and conduction of cardiac-electric activity (Table 4).

TABLE 4: Changes in ECG (Incidence %)

Group No.	Deep Bradycardia 50/min	Tachycardia 100/min	ST-T lower male	ST-T lower female	P 0.1s	QRS 0.1s	High potential at left ventricle (male)
1	1.63	6.54	11.8	34.29	6.86	10.78	11.92
2	3.93	3.36	11.2	14.61	7.85	11.59	12.89
3	0.42	4.25	5.6	18.07	3.18	4.03	8.95

In order to observe the microwave exposure effects on vascular functional state, rheoencepalogram, rheogram of finger hemodynamics and oculi fundus were examined. There were no significant findings in the results.

The data mentioned above show that microwave action was characterized by autonomic vascular symptoms of a vagotonic character, expressed especially in hypotonia and bradycardia. Sadchikova and many Soviet authors [4,5,6] state that the asthenic syndrome in the initial stages included mainly a complex of asthenic symptoms dominated by autonomic vascular changes with a vagotonic tendency. In the advanced stages of the disease, the astheno-autonomic syndrome with vascular dysfunction of the hypertonic type was most frequent. At a certain stage of development of autonomic vascular disturbances, the hypothalamic syndrome (autonomic vascular form) appeared and was characterized by sudden crises, predominantly of a sympathico-adrenal character. In our investigations, the autonomic vascular symptoms of most persons maintained a vagotonic character, while they were observed over a period of five years. Nothing of such severity as to be described as hypothalamic syndrome was found. It seems that the nature and sensitivity of cardiovascular reactions to prolonged exposure depend, to a large extent, on the individual characteristics. Further study on clinical manifestations and its mechanism could be valuable, as some doctors in our country are now interested in using microwave in treatment for hypertension.

The hypotonia and bradycardia were also observed in RF workers in China, but the incidence was not so high as that in microwave workers.

3. Effects on peripheral blood

No characteristic changes in peripheral blood picture were found, only a slight leukopenia and thrombocytopenia occurring in the first group as compared to the others ($p<0.001$).

Table 5 Incidence of Leukopenia and Thrombocytopenia

Group No.	Leukocyte (%) $<5{,}000/mm^3$	Leukocyte (%) $>9{,}000/mm^3$	Thrombocyte (%) $<100{,}000$
1	29.41	1.96	26.79
2	18.69	8.6	14.02
3	21.23	7.2	17.2

Diversified WBC responses are found in many reports. In general, slight or moderate leukopenia may be found in microwave workers working at high power densities. In a number of cases leukocytosis was encountered in the initial period of professional exposure. Absolute lymphocytosis may also be found in microwave workers.

4. Effects on eye

Several epidemiological surveys of lenticular effects of microwave workers have been performed. None of the surveys reported a statistically significant increase in the number of cataracts in personnel occupationally exposed to microwave radiation. The surveys were mostly concerned with minor lenticular defects. Some of the surveys indicated a statistically significant increase in lenticular defects in microwave workers. Zydecki [7] examined 3,000 persons divided equally into three groups. Group A comprised two subgroups. A_1 contained 542 individuals exposed directly to microwave radiation at power density of about 0.1 mW/cm^2 up to 6 mW/cm^2. Group A_2 comprised 458 individuals exposed to MW at about 0.01 mW/cm^2. Group B comprised 1,000 age-matched individuals not exposed to microwave, while Group C was made up of children and juveniles aged 5 to 17 years. The examination of the lens was made using a slit lamp after dilatation of the pupil. Lens translucency was assessed using a 5-grade scale:

1° No lens changes
2° Numerous small, multishaped opacities, which may be counted
3° Numerous small, multishaped opacities, which are difficult to count
4° As above, but with a tendency to increase in number or size on successive examinations
5° Any change impairing visual acuity

Statistically significant differences in the frequency of various grades of lens translucency exist between Group A and Groups B and C. Moreover the comparison between A_1 and A_2 also demonstrates significant differences (Table 6). The author indicated that long-term overexposure to low doses of microwaves may tend to accelerate the normal aging process of the lens.

Table 6 Percentage incidence in various lens translucency grades

Lens Tranclucency Grade	Group A A_1	A_2	A_1+A_2	Group B	Group C
1	13.0	31.3	21.7	29.7	68.8
2	62.0	52.6	57.7	50.3	26.9
3	19.7	12.2	16.2	16.6	3.6
4	4.8	3.5	4.1	2.6	0.3
5	0.5	-	0.3	0.8	0.4

In our investigation, the lenticular transparency was examined in 227 microwave workers and 117 age-matched persons as control. No significant differences in incidence of lens opacities were found. The incidence of lens vacuole in the first group was higher than that in the control group ($p<0.025$). A few cases of cataracts or retina hemorrhage points were found in the microwave workers.

Table 7 Incidences of lens changes (%)

Group No.	Lens opacity	Lens vacuole
1	71.21	24.24
2	76.4	15.53
3	79.4	10.26

Tengroth and Aurell [8] reported an increased number of retinal lesions in 68 workers in a Swedish factory where microwave equipment was tested. The retinal lesions were characterized by their resemblance to chorioretinal scars after inflammatory reactions. No data on the intensity of the radiation were provided, but the authors considered that the maximum permissible exposure of 10 mW/cm^2 is too high. The problem should be further investigated.

5. Reproduction and Genetic Effects

Microwave radiation can induce sterility in humans when the incident power density is high enough. In recent years, microwave has been used for birth control in some hospitals in our country. In some workers occupationally exposed to RF or MW, the spermatogenesis or menstrual pattern was altered, and even impotence occurred. But the total number of cases are too few to conclude a cause/effect relationship.

RF and MW radiation are teratogenic to experimental animals exposed at specific times during gestation, but there is no evidence of such in humans. The use of microwave heating as diathermy to relieve the pain of uterine contractions during labor was reported from Belgium. It was said that the babies were born healthy. Nevertheless, extreme caution must be exercised. A few cases of multiple inborn defects in the offspring of women irradiated immediately before or during the early stages of pregnancy with shortwave diathermy have been reported by Coccorza Erdman et al.

Siglor et al suggest that mongolism occurs more frequently among the offspring of fathers professionally exposed to microwaves. However, an intensive follow-up study failed to confirm the association. In general, there seems to be no hazard under ordinary professional exposure conditions.

In the United States, a study [9] of American Embassy personnel in Moscow was reported. The purpose of the study was to compare the morbidity and mortality experience of U.S. Government employees at the Moscow Embassy during the period 1953 to 1976 with the experience of employees who had served in other selected, nonirradiated Eastern European embassies during the same period. The study population consisted of 1827 employees at the Moscow Embassy and over 3000 of their dependents and 2561 employees at the eight comparison posts and 5000 of their dependents. Comparative analyses were made of all symptoms, conditions, diseases, and causes of death according to the abstract of the medical records, response to the Health History Questionnaire, diseases reported on the Questionnaire, and acquisition of death certificates. No differential health risks associated with presumed exposure to microwave radiation were demonstrated. The maximum exposure levels measured at or near the windows of the upper central building ranged from 1 uW/cm^2 to 15 uW/cm^2. Another study [9] was reported of a three year investigation that was aimed at the determination of health risks from microwave radiation of U.S. Naval persons. A population of approximately 40,000 (half constituted the exposed group, and half the control group) were examined for mortality, morbidity, reproductive performance and health of children. The data did not show any differences between the two groups. It did not assign the exposure doses to any individuals in this study. Some of the observed persons were exposed to microwave in excess of the 10 mW/cm^2 limit. Accidental exposure was at estimated levels exceeding 100 mW/cm^2. Radiomen and radar operators were generally exposed to levels well below 1 mW/cm^2.

It may be summarized that there are great differences in the methods, contents and results of investigations for evaluating the health hazard of microwave radiation between different countries, causing great controversy. Additionally, the health hazard in microwave usually is not so serious and so certain as that in any other disease. Numerous questions concerning the clinical course and pathogenesis of certain lesions caused by RF and MW radiation have not been clearly elucidated up till now, and the symptoms usually are reversible, but the existence of health hazardous effects of RF and MW can not be denied. An investigation [6] of the patients suffering from microwave sickness reported by Sadechikova illustrates this. It showed that, despite repeated therapeutic courses and temporary withdrawal from work with microwave sources, upon returning to previous work conditions symptoms increased in severity, particularly among patients with advanced stages of the disease. In such patients autonomic vascular disturbances dominated, crises of cerebral and coronary insufficiency progressed and development of ischaemic heart disease and hypertension was observed. Cessation of work involving irradiation frequently resulted in stabilization of the initial stage of illness (Table 8).

Table 8 Clinical course of microwave radiation during and after exposure

Clinical syndromes	Period of observation	No. of cases	Clinical course		
			Recovery	Stabilization	Progression
Asthenic	A	25	-	13	11
	B	5	3	2	-
Astheno-autonomic with vascular dysfunction	A	47	-	-	47
	B	16	-	15	1
Hypothalamic (autonomic vascular form)	A	2	-	-	2
	B	6	-	5	1
Total		100	3	35	62

A: under MW exposure B: after cessation of exposure

This implies that those syndromes are not easy to recover, and it is important to lower exposure level and improve work conditions for protection from hazardous radiation.

Radiation conditions related to health hazard and standard promulgation in China

In order to set a reasonable safety standard of RF and MW radiation, conditions related to health hazard should be reviewed. Several exposure standards [10,11,12,13,14] in different countries are reported.

1. Radiation intensity

It might be considered that according to epidemiological data from exposure to microwave energy, long-term exposure at several mW/cm^2 may induce alteration not only in nervous and cardiovascular systems, but in the normal aging process of the lens and peripheral blood picture. The function of the nervous and cardiovascular systems might be influenced at about one or two hundred uW/cm^2. Considering that the lower power density group (<200 uW/cm^2) in our investigation mentioned above had more alteration in blood pressure and ECG, we selected 238 persons who had been exposed to microwave power density less that 50 uW/cm^2 and their age- and sex-matched individuals as control. There were still significant differences in the incidence of neurasthenia symptoms. However, there was no difference in objective indexes between the two groups in statistics. Although some reports stated that the microwave exposure group at a few hundredths of a mW/cm^2 had similar functional changes in the nervous and cardiovascular systems, it seems that there is no correlation between the exposure intensity and the changes. Gordon and other authors indicated that in low level exposure groups similar effects were observed, but symptoms were less evident and easily reversed. This impression is strengthened by the fact that after reducing the exposure levels, no further cases with pronounced dysfunction syndrome were noted.

In order to search for the threshold level of microwave bioeffects on animals, acute and chronic experiments were conducted.

Acute effects of microwave radiation on blood pressure, respiration, rectal temperature, subcutaneous temperature and ECG were observed [15]. In this experiment using rabbits, the whole body was radiated on its abdominal side with 2450 MHz continual microwave for 1 hr. There were five groups with 68 rabbits in all divided into 80 mW/cm^2, 40 mW/cm^2, 20 mW/cm^2, 10 mW/cm^2 and control. The microwave radiation induced a drop in blood pressure, acceleration of respiration, and elevation of subcutaneous and rectal temperature (Table 9).

Table 9 Variation on acute experiment

Investigated items	80 mW/cm^2	40 mW/cm^2	20 mW/cm^2	10 mW/cm^2	Control
Blood pressure drop mean (mm Hg)	25	18	22	-	-
Respiratory rate increase mean (per min.)	109	55	-	-	-
Subcutaneous tem. pure rise mean (°C)	5	3.1	1.6	-	-
Rectal tem. pure rise mean (°C)	2	1.3	0.3	-	-

- no significant changes

The chronic experiment was conducted with 16 rabbits and 40 rats. The rabbits were divided into four groups at random from which three groups were irradiated with three levels (10, 1, and 0.1 mW/cm^2) and one served as control. The rats were divided into four groups, from which three groups were irradiated with the other three levels (5 mW/cm^2, 0.2 mW/cm^2 and 0.01 mW/cm^2) and one was control. The exposed groups were irradiated six hours daily for four and a half months. A certain power density of microwave (300 mW/cm^2) induced EEG frequency slowing and amplitude increasing. The most pronounced changes of ECG were bradycardia, tachycardia and R wave widening. Leukocyte and leukocytic alkali phosphatase increased in the first half a month and then there were no changes. Blood presure fluctuated. Mistakes at Y-labyrinth test appeared to tend to increase. The relationship between these variations and power densities is shown in Table 10.

Table 10 Relation between the variance of observed indexes and power densities

Items	10 mW/cm^2	5 mW/cm^2	1 mW/cm^2	0.2 mW/cm^2	0.1 mW/cm^2	0.01 mW/cm^2	control
EEG							
amplitude	++	/	-	/	-	/	-
frequency	++	/	++	/	-	/	-
ECG							
heart rate	/	++	/	-	/	-	-
R widen	/	++	/	++	/	-	-
Leukocyte	/	++	/	-	/	-	-
L A P	/	+	/	-	/	-	-
Blood pressure waved	++	/	-	/	/	-	-
Rectal tem.	-	-	-	-	-	-	-
Body weight	/	+	/	-	/	-	-

++ represents the variance with significant difference
\+ represents the variance only with a tendency change
/ represents no animal exposed at this power density level
\- shows no significant changes

The experimental data are preliminary and limited. A large number of experiments have been carried out in other countries.

The threshold of biological effects, which differs from health hazards, is extremely low. The average heart rate decreased during the pulsed microwave energy affected on frog hearts under certain conditions at only 0.003 mW/cm^2 average power density presented (Frey). The threshold of auditory responses for cats, the threshold of avoidance by rats of pulse modulated microwave, and the threshold of incidence efflux of calcium ions from the isolated chick or rat cerebral tissue (with frequency "window" modulated in amplitude) are far below or near 0.1 mW/cm^2. The threshold of hazardous effects in acute experiment is rather high and usually depends, to a great extent, on overheating.

The most important experiments, on which to base a set of safety standards, are long-term low level exposures. Dumenskij [16] reported an investigation performed at 10, 2.4, 1.9, 0.06, 0.01, and 0.006 uW/cm^2 for wavelength 6 m and 20, 10, 5 and 1 uW/cm^2 for 12 cm wavelength. The animals (rats and rabbits) were irradiated 8-12 hr. daily for 120 days. The experiment showed that in the conditioned reflex activity, the latent period was longer, reflex reactions to positive stimuli weakened, and the number of these missing increased. In this investigation these changes in the central nervous system were supplemented and confirmed by EEG, and biochemical studies including cholinesterase activity and sulphydryl (SH) groups in the blood. Changes in blood composition and morphologic structure of the tissues and organs of the animals were also observed. The author pointed out that prolonged action of electromagnetic energy of low intensities in the UHF and SHF ranges resulted in appreciable changes. The biologically active intensities of electromagnetic fields were 10-0.06 and 20-5 uW/cm^2 for UHF and SHF ranges respectively. Such low thresholds of hazardous effects of RF or MW radiation have not been supported by other reports. In some studies observed on the same systems and functions, negative results were obtained with even much higher power densities. However, a number of chronic experiments on bioeffects of RF and MW showing lower thresholds have been made by other Soviet authors.

In the United States, D'Andrea [17] reported a chronic experiment of exposure to 2450 MHz microwave. Long-Evans male rats were exposed 8 hr. a day for 16 weeks to microwaves at an average power density of 5 mW/cm^2. The dose rate was 1.23 mW/g. After exposure, it revealed a significant depression of behavioral activity. There were no effects on body mass, mass of adrenals, and levels of 17-ketosteroids in urine. Another long term experiment recently was presented by Guy and McRee [18,19]. Four rabbits were exposed to 2450 MHz microwave for 6 months. Daily duration of exposure was 23 hr. and continued across 180 consecutive days. The power density at the body axis of the animals was 7 mW/cm^2 and at the head location was 10 mW/cm^2. The average whole body SAR was 1.5 W/Kg. Eosinophil percentage, albumin and calcium levels were significantly lower in exposed than in control rabbits. Thirty days after termination of exposure, no change in hematological parameters was observed, but a significant decrease in albumin/total globulin ratio was measured in the exposed animals. Lymphocytes from exposure animals showed a significant suppression in responsiveness to pokeweed mitogen. That microwave radiation may suppress immunological competence was reported by other studies. It seems that the power density of several mW/cm^2 may be critical to the effects observed on the immune system.

If we review the animal and human data on biological effects of MW and RF radiation, we find that there are considerable differences and controversy in this field. That the safety standard must be able to protect the health of the workers without obstructing the microwave techniques in extensive application. In accordance with our investigation and experiments, and referring to the experience of other countries, the power density at average 50 uW/cm^2 in the working place for a duration of six hours daily has been proposed as the tentative microwave occupational exposure standard in our country. If it is eight hours exposure a day, it must be less than 40 uW/cm^2. 300 uW/cm^2 is the limited dose for a whole working day. However, it is not permissible to be over 5 mW/cm^2. This tentative exposure standard has been adopted in local areas in our country for two years. It will be further perfected and decided by the end of this year.

2. Radiation frequency.

Because of the different reflection, propagation and absorption for different frequencies of electromagnetic field, the specific absorption rate must be different in a biological target from the same incident power density. Additionally, some special effects may occur at a certain frequency range. It is necessary to set separate standards for some frequency ranges.

Ermolajev and Subbota [20] suggested a formula to express the relation between the frequencies and electric field strengths, in which the equivalent bioeffects could be observed.

$$E_1 = E_2 \cdot \sqrt{\frac{f_2}{f_1}}$$

E_1 electric field strength in V/m for f_1 (MHz)
E_2 electric field strength in V/m for f_2 (MHz)

The formula was derived from the following data (Table 11).

Table 11 Relation between frequencies and electric field strengths (V/m)

Bioeffects	Species	3 MHz	14 MHz	22 MHz	69.7 MHz	150 MHz	300 MHz
Functional alteration	rabbit	500 (615)	250 (285)	200 (220)	150 (125)	100-150 (90)	60 (60)
Death	mice	10000		3000			1000
	rat		5000		2000		

The properties of electromagnetic energy absorption and distribution under various frequency ranges were studied and manifested by many scientists (Schwan, Guy, Gandhi et al). In humans, maximum whole body SAR occurs in the frequency range of 60-100 MHz, with a peak at approximately 70 MHz. Human absorption at frequencies below 30 MHz and above 500 MHz is much less than that at the resonant frequency. Partial body resonant absorption occurs at 150 MHz for the arm and at 350 MHz for the head. In general, small animals absorb MW energy maximally at frequencies near or above 500 MHz. In view of this, the formula mentioned above is not fit for humans. It seems that the minimum intensity of maximum permissible exposure level should be at the frequency range of 30-300 MHz which is adopted in Canada's new standard. A new proposed exposure standard in America which is based on the whole body SAR equal to 0.4 W/kg is also the strictest at the resonant frequency range.

The lower limit of frequency regulated in the exposure standard is 10 MHz in some countries. The frequency range of electromagnetic field now widely used in industry of our country is from 0.25 MHz to 40 MHz and microwave. It seems that the frequency lowest limit of exposure standard should be at least at 0.2 MHz in RF range. Some cases of workers who suffered from typical neurasthenia resulting from RF radiation were found by the present author. A worker was exposed to 250 KHz near zone field at the electromagnetic field strength of about 400 V/m and 20 A/m over 5 years. Systolic blood pressure of this patient was highly unsteady with a 60 mm Hg fluctuation or so within a day. Bradycardia (ECG), slight leukopenia, emission and sterility occurred. Decrease in activity of sperms was found by laboratory examination. Slight abnormality in EEG appeared with more θ waves. After transient withdrawal from work with RF sources, the neurasthenia symptoms were observably relieved. After cessation of exposure to RF radiation over one year, the neurasthenia symptoms disappeared and disfunction of the cardiovascular system tended to recover. Similar, less extensive symptoms also occurred in a few other persons working at the same radiation condition. Another case is a woman who lived near a radio broadcast antenna with working frequency at 800 KHz. Keratoconjunctivitis resulting from lack of tear occurred while the patient was living there, and alleviated after she left there for several weeks. This phenomenon happened several times. The electric field strength in her bedroom was about 20 V/m. Perhaps the patient was extremely sensitive to such an RF electromagnetic field. Perhaps disfunction of the endocrine system resulting from RF radiation was the main cause in reducing secretion of tears. Epidemiological data on RF radiation in China and some other countries also demonstrated that sufficiently intense RF radiation including the frequencies from 0.1 MHz to 10 MHz also can produce harmful effects. Several decades V/m will be adopted as the maximum permissible electric field strength for RF range in China.

3. Other radiation conditions

Several factors other than intensity, dose, and frequency range may also influence the harmful effects of RF and MW radiation. Pulsed and continual microwave may be different for their bioeffects. In Czechoslovakia, the exposure standards for them are different. In the new exposure standard of Canada, the maximum permissible level was differentiated between whole-body exposure and exposure of extremities. A distinction between continuous (stationary field) and intermittent (nonstationary field) exposure was made in Poland and then accepted by the Soviet Union in their microwave safety exposure standards. The ambient temperature and the presence of X-ray radiation are also considered in the USSR occupational exposure standard. All those factors should be investigated and studied further.

Finally it should be pointed out that the safety exposure standard will continue to be perfected with increasing knowledge.

REFERENCES

1. S. Baranski and P. Czerski, "Biological Effects of Microwave", DHR Inc., Stroudsbury (1976).
2. Chiang Huai and Yee Ko-ching, "A study of microwave safety standard", J. Zhejiang Medical University, 8:57 (Chinese) (1979).
3. M.H. Sadchikova, K.V. Nikonova, E.A. Denisova, G.V. Snegova, E.N. Lvovskaya and V.A. Soldatova, "Arterial pressure under the effect of low-intensity microwave and high temperature", Gig Tr Prof Zabol, 2:17 (Russian) (1977).
4. V.P. Medvedev, "The cardio-vascular system of man under the effect of super-high frequency electromagnetic fields", 1:18 (Russian) (1977).

5. K.V. Glotova and M.N. Sadchikova, "Characteristics of the development and clinical course of changes in the cardiovascular system under chronic exposure to ultrahigh frequency electromagnetic field", Gig Tr Prof Zabol, 7:24 (Russian) (1970).
6. M.N. Sadchikova, "Clinical manifestations of reactions to microwave irradiation in various occupational groups", in: Biological Effects and Health Hazard of Microwave Radiation, P. Czerski, Ch. Silverman, K. Ostrowski, M.L. Shore and B. Waldeskog, ed., Polish Medical Publishers, Warsaw (1974).
7. S. Zydecki, "Assessment of lens translucency in juveniles, microwave workers and age-matched groups", in [6].
8. B. Tengroth and E. Aurell, "Retinal changes in microwave workers", in [6].
9. C. Silverman, "Epidemiologic studies of microwave effects", Proceedings of the IEEE, 68:78 (1980).
10. R.F. Cleveland and J.K. Kielman, "Biological effects of radiofrequency and microwave radiation and their relevance to occupational safety and health standards in the United States, Presented at the 1979 Microwave Power Symposium, Monaco (1979).
11. National Telecommunications and Information Administration, "Fifth Report on Program for Control Pollution of the Environment: The Assessment of Biological Hazards of Nonionizing Electromagnetic Radiation", U.S. Department of Commerce (1979).
12. N.H. Steneck, H.J. Cook, A.J. Vomder and G.L. Kane, "The origins of U.S. safety standards for microwave radiation", Science, 208:1230 (1980).
13. M.H. Repacholi, "Proposed exposure limits for microwave and radiofrequency radiation in Canada", J. Microwave Power, 13:199 (1978).
14. Environmental Health Directorate Health Protection Branch (Canada), "Safety Code-6: Recommended Safety Procedures for the Installation and Use of Radiofrequency and Microwave Devices in the Frequency Range 10 MHz - 300 GHz", published by authority of the Minister of National Health and Welfare (1979).
15. Yee Ko-ching and Chiang Huai, "Experimental research on acute biological effects of microwave exposure", Acta Physiol Sinica, 32:10 (Chinese) (1980).
16. J.D. Dumenskij and M.G. Sandala, "The biological action and hygienic significance of electromagnetic fields of superhigh and ultrahigh frequencies in densely populated areas, in [6].
17. J.A. D'Andrea, O.P. Gandhi, J.L. Lords, C.H. Durney, C.C. Johnson and L. Astle, "Physiological and behavioral effects of chronic exposure to 2450 MHz microwaves, J. Microwave Power, 14:351 (1979).

18. A.W. Guy, P.O. Kramar, C.A. Harris and C.K. Chou, "Long-term 2450 MHz CW microwave irradiation of rabbits: methodology and evaluation of ocular and physiologic effects", _J. Microwave Power_, 15:37 (1980).
19. D.I. McRee, R. Faith, E.E. McConnell and A.W. Guy, "Long-term irradiation: evaluation of hematological and immunological effects", _J. Microwave Power_, 15:45 (1980).
20. E.A. Ermolajev, A.G. Subbota and B.A. Tchuchlovia, "Effects of HF and UHF electromagnetic radiation on organism and the principle of their normalization", _Voen Med Zh_, 4:65 (Russian) (1980).
21. O.P. Gandhi, "Dosimetry - the absorption properties of man and experimental animals", _Bull NY Acad Med_, 55:999 (1979).

MICROWAVE/RADIOFREQUENCY PROTECTION GUIDE AND STANDARDS

Sol M. Michaelson

Department of Radiation Biology and Biophysics
University of Rochester
School of Medicine and Dentistry
Rochester, New York 14642

Exposure Standards - The first standards for controlling exposure to MW/RF were introduced in the 1950's, in the USA and the USSR. The maximum permissible exposure levels proposed then have remained substantially unchanged, i.e., for continuous exposure these are respectively 10 mW/cm^2 and 10 $\mu W/cm^2$. Most countries that developed national standards based them on either the US[1] or the Soviet[2] values. Subsequently, however, some countries have proposed standards intermediate between these extremes.

In the U.S. the American National Standards Institute (ANSI), a voluntary body with members from government, industry, various associations and the academic community develops consensus standards (guides) in various areas. ANSI issued a nonionizing radiation safety standard in 1966 with maximum permissible exposures of 10 mW/cm^2, as averaged over any 6 minute period, for frequencies from 10 MHz to 100 GHz. This standard was reviewed and reissued with minor modifications in 1975. New recommendations [1], based on frequency dependence and specific absorption rates (SAR) state: For human exposure to electromagnetic energy of radiofrequencies from 300 kHz to 100 GHz, the radiofrequency protection guides, in terms of equivalent plane wave free space power density, and in terms of the mean squared electric ($\underline{E}^2$) and magnetic ($\underline{H}^2$) field strengths as a function of frequency, are:

Table I

(1) Frequency (MHz)	(2) Power Density (mW/cm^2)	(3) E^2 (V^2/m^2)	(4) H^2 (A^2/m^2)
0.3 - 3	100	400,000	2.5
3 - 30	$900/f^2$	4,000 ($900/f^2$)	0.25 ($900/f^2$)
30 - 300	1.0	4,000	0.025
300 - 1500	f/300	4,000 (f/300)	0.025 (f/300)
1500 - 100,000	5	20,000	0.125

Note: f is the frequency, in megahertz (MHz)

These standards do not apply to practitioners of the Healing Arts. For near field exposure, the only applicable radiofrequency protection guides are the mean squared electric and magnetic field strengths given in columns 3 and 4. For convenience, these guides may be expressed in equivalent plane wave power density (column 2).

For both pulsed and non-pulsed fields, the power density, the mean squares of the field strengths, and the values of SAR or input power as applicable, are averaged over any 0.1 hour period and should not exceed the values given in Table I. For situations involving exposure of the whole body, the radiofrequency protection guide is believed to result in energy deposition averaged over the entire body for any 0.1 hour period of about 144 joules per kilogram (J/kg) or less. This is equivalent to a specific absorption rate (SAR) of about 0.40 watts per kilogram (W/kg) or less, spatially and temporally averaged over the entire body mass. This recommendation will no doubt be adopted with only minor modifications if any.

The ANSI Standard applies to the total population. In other words, the Standard applies to non-occupational as well as occupational exposures.

In the United Kingdom the 10 mW/cm^2 standard is followed. The maximum permissible occupational levels (MPL'S), adopted in Canada are shown in Table II. The MPL's apply for the frequency range of 10 MHz to 300 GHz; no distinction is made between CW and pulsed waveforms.

The State Committee on Standards of the Council of Ministers of the USSR has promulgated "Occupational Safety Standards for Electromagnetic Fields of Radiofrequency (GOST 12.1.006-76)," effective January 1, 1977. It specifies the maximum permissible magnitudes of electric and magnetic field strengths and power

Table II

	Frequency	Limits			Comments*
Canada		power density	rms E strength	rms H strength	Safety Code - 6 (1979)
Occupat.	10 MHz - 1 GHz	1 mW/cm^2	60 V/m	0.16 A/m	averaged over 1 h period
		25 mW/cm^2	300 V/m	0.8 A/m	averaged over 1 m period
	1 GHz - 300 GHz	5 mW/cm^2	140 V/m	0.36 A/m	averaged over 1 h period
		25 mW/cm^2	300 V/m	0.8 A/m	averaged over 1 m period
	*additional provisions for exposures shorter than 1 h and exposure of extremities				
General public	10 MHz - 300 GHz	1 mW/cm^2	60 V/m	0.16 A/m	averaged over 1 m period

densities in the workplace. It does not apply to personnel of the Ministry of Defense. Maximum permissible RF fields in the workplace must not, during the course of the workday, exceed the levels noted in Table III.

Table III

Frequency Range	P (mW/cm^2)	E (V/m)	H (A/m)
60 kHz-1.5 MHz			5
1.5 MHz-3.0 MHz		50	
3.0 MHz-30 MHz		20	
30 MHz-50 MHz		10	0.3
50 MHz-300 MHz		5	
	0.01	(entire workday)	
300 MHz-300 GHz	0.10	(2 hr. period during workday)	
	1.00	(20 min. period during workday)	

This standard also applies in environments with ambient temperatures above 28°C and/or in the presence of X-ray radiation, except, under these conditions, the maximum during a 20 minute period is restricted to 0.1 mW/cm^2.

In 1972 and 1977, the Polish Council of Ministers and the Minister of Health and Social Welfare promulgated a change in the Polish Standard.[3-6] For the general population the values of 10 and 100 microwatts/cm^2 were adopted for continuous and intermittent exposures respectively. These values were taken as the upper limits of a safe zone, in which occupation is unrestricted. Three other zones are also defined, based on power density. For stationary (continuous) fields, these are defined as follows:

1. <u>safe zone</u> - the mean power density cannot exceed 10 $\mu W/cm^2$, human exposure is unrestricted;
2. <u>intermediate zone</u> - minimal value 10 $\mu W/cm^2$ upper limit 200 $\mu W/cm^2$ occupational exposure is allowed during a whole working day (normally 8 hours, but in principle can be extended to 10 hours);
3. <u>hazardous zone</u> - minimal value 200 $\mu W/cm^2$, upper limit 10 mW/cm^2 occupational exposure time per 24 hours is determined by the formula:

$$t = 32/p^2$$

where t = exposure time in hrs
p = mean power density in W/m^2;

4. <u>dangerous zone</u> - mean power density in excess of 100 W/m^2 (10 mW/cm^2), human exposure is forbidden.

For exposures to non-stationary fields, i.e., intermittent exposure the following values were adopted:

1. <u>safe zone</u> - mean power density does not exceed 1 W/m^2 (100 $\mu W/cm^2$);
2. <u>intermediate zone</u> - minimal value 1 W/m^2 (100 $\mu W/cm^2$), <u>upper limit</u> 10 W/m^2 (1 mW/cm^2).
3. <u>hazardous zone</u> - the exposure time is determined by the formula:

$$t = 800/p^2$$

where the symbols t and p designate the same values as above. The minimum value is 10 W/m^2; upper limit is 100 W/m^2.;
4. <u>dangerous zone</u> - mean power density in excess of 100 W/m^2 (10 mW/cm^2), human exposure is forbidden.

The Swedish National Board for Industrial Safety, promulgated a nonionizing radiofrequency standard (Worker Protection Authority Instruction No. 111) effective January 1, 1977.[7] This regulation applies to all work which may involve exposure to radiofrequencies between 10 MHz and 300 GHz. The instruction specifically excludes applications involving the treatment of patients. Maximum permissible exposures (as averaged over a six minute period) are:

Frequency Range	Power Density
10 MHz - 300 MHz	5 mW/cm^2
300 MHz - 300 GHz	1 mW/cm^2

According to WHO (World Health Organization) and the IRPA (International Radiation Protection Association), the exposure range of 0.1 to 1 milliwatt per centimeter square has a high enough safety factor to permit continuous exposure over the whole frequency range[8]. Environmental exposure should be based on the ALARA principle - as low as reasonably achievable - with social and economic benefits considered.

<u>Product Emission Standard</u>. The "Radiation Control for Health and Safety Act of 1968" (PL 90-602), administered by HEW/FDA (BRH)*, provides authority for controlling radiation from electronic devices. According to the BRH microwave oven standard, effective October, 1971: Ovens may not emit (leak) more than 1 mW/cm^2 at time of manufacture and 5 mW/cm^2 subsequently, for the life of the product--measured at a distance of 5 cm and under conditions specified in the standard.

The Canadian standard[9,10] restricts the maximum leakage to 1 mW/cm^2 at 5 cm from the oven (consumer, commercial and industrial). In contrast the U.S. standard[11] specifies a maximum emission level at 5 cm of 1 mW/cm^2 before purchase and

*U.S. Department of Health, Education and Welfare/Food and Drug Administration, (Bureau of Radiological Health)

5 mW/cm^2 thereafter which is consistent with standards for the general population in the USSR and Poland.[12] The standard applies to domestic and commercial ovens, but not to industrial equipment. A similar standard has been adopted in Japan and most of Western Europe.[13] Computation of human exposure during typical operation of a microwave oven leaking up to 1 mW/cm^2 at a distance of 5 cm indicate that actual exposure of the body is 5-20 $\mu W/cm^2$. An emission level of 10 $\mu W/cm^2$ at a distance of 50 cm from the oven's surface has been adopted in the USSR.

A review of international standards reveals numerous differences. In all cases, however, the recommended permissible exposures provide safety for individuals in the workplace as well as for the general public. Protection guides for microwave/radiofrequency energies, as for standards in general, are a reflection not only of scientific knowledge but also encompass philosophic and socio-political considerations.

ACKNOWLEDGEMENT

This paper is based on work performed under Contract No. DE-AC02-76EV03490 with The U.S. Department of Energy at the University of Rochester Department of Radiation Biology and Biophysics and has been assigned Report No. UR-3490-2090.

REFERENCES

1. ANSI. Safety Level of Electromagnetic Radiation with Respect to Personnel, American National Standards Institute, New York: C95.1-1966, C95.1-1974. Safety Levels with Respect to Human Exposure to Radiofrequency Electromagnetic Fields (300 kHz to 100 GHz) C95.1-1981.
2. USSR. Temporary Sanitary Rules for Working with Centimeter Waves. Ministry of Health Protection of the USSR, 1958.
3. Czerski P, Piotrowski M. Proposals for specifications of allowable levels of microwave radiation, Medycyna Lotnicza (Polish) 1972;39:127-139.
4. Rozporzadzenie Rady Ministrow z dnia 25.02 1972 w sprawie bezpieczenstwa i hygieny pracy przy stosowaniu urzadzen wytwarzajacych pole elektromagnetcyzne w zakresie mikrofalowym. Dziennik Ustaw PRL No. 21 II, 1972, pp. 153.
5. Zarzadzenie Ministra Zdrowia i Opieki Spolecznej z dnia. 9.08.1972 w sprawie okreslenia pol elektromagnetycznych w zakresie mikrofalowym oraz dopuszczalnego czasu pracy w strefie zagrozenia. Dziennik Urzedowy mzios, Nr 17, poz 78, 20.09.1972.

6. Rozporzadzenie Ministrow Pracy Placy i Spraw Socjalnych oraz zdrowia i Opieki Spolecznej w sprawie berpieczenstwa i higieny pracy przy stosowaniu urzadzen wytwarzajacych pola elektromagnetyczne w zakresie 0.1 MHz de 300 MHz. Dzienni k Ustaw PRL Nr 8 z dn 17.03, 1977 poz. 8.
7. Royal Swedish Academy of Engineering Sciences. Biological Effects of Electromagnetic Fields, (ISBN91.7082.123.2) Stockholm, 1976;160p.
8. World Health Organization (1981) Environmental Health Criteria 16 Radiofrequency and Microwaves 134 p., WHO, Geneva.
9. Repacholi MH. Proposed exposure limits for microwave and radiofrequency radiations in Canada. J Microwave Power 1978;13:199-277.
10. DHEW Canada. Radiation emitting devices regulations. SOR/74-601 23 October 1974. Part III Microwave Ovens Canada Gazette Part V, 1974;108:2822-2825.
11. USDHEW. Regulations for Administration and Enforcement of the Radiation Control of Health and Safety Act of 1968 paragraph 1030.10 Microwave Ovens DHEW Publ. No. (FDA) 75-8003 pp. 36-37, July, 1974.
12. Baranski S, Czerski P. Biological Effects of Microwaves. Stroudsburg, PA: Dowden, Hutchinson and Ross, 1976, 234 p.
13. IEC. Internat. Electrotechnical Commission. Particular Requirements for Microwave Cooking Appliances. IEC 335-25 pt 2, 1976.

LECTURERS

ADEY W.R.
J.L. Pettis Memorial Veterans' Hospital
11201 Benton Street
Loma Linda, Ca. 92357 USA

BERTEAUD A.J.
C.N.R.S.
2, Rue Henry Dunant
94320 Thiais, France

GRANDOLFO M.
Istituto Superiore di Sanità
Viale Regina Elena, 299
00161 Rome, Italy

GRANT E.H.
Queen Elizabeth College
Campden Hill Road
London W8 7AH, U.K.

GRUNDLER W.
Ges. fuer Strahlen und Umweltforschung
Ingolstaedter Landstrasse 1
8042 Neuherberg, FRG

GUY A.W.
Bioelectromagnetics Research Lab.
University of Washington
Seattle, Wa. 98195 USA

HARLEN F.
National Radiation Protection Board
Harwell, Didcot
Oxfordshire OX110RQ, U.K.

Huai CHIANG
Microwave Institute
Chekiang Medical College
Hangchow, China

KAISER F.
Institut fuer Theoretische Physik
Pfaffenwaldring 57/v
7000 Stuttgart-80, FRG

KEILMANN F.
Max Planck Institut
Heisenbergstrasse 1
P.O. 800665
7000 Stuttgart-80, FRG

LOOMS J.S.T.
Central Electricity Gen. Board
Kelvin Avenue
Leatherhead, Surrey, U.K.

MICHAELSON S.M.
University of Rochester
Medical Center
601 Elmwood Avenue
Rochester, N.Y. 114641 USA

REPACHOLI M.H.
Environmental Health Centre
Tunney's Pasture
Ottawa, Canada

RINDI A.
I.N.F.N. National Laboratory
Via Enrico Fermi
00044 Frascati, Italy

ROBERTS N.
University of Rochester
Medical Center
601 Elmwood Avenue
Rochester, N.Y. 14641 USA

SCHWAN H.P.
Max Planck Institut fuer Biophysik
Kennedyallee 70
6000 Frankfurt a.M. 70, FRG

SERVANTIE B.
Hôpital d'Instruction des Armées
Sainte-Anne
83800 Toulon Naval, France

STUCHLY M.
Environmental Health Centre
Tunney's Pasture
Ottawa, Canada

TELL R.
U.S. Environmental Protection Agency
P.O. Box 18416
Las Vegas, Nv. 89104 USA

TENGROTH B.M.
Karolinska Instituet
Ogonkliniken Karol. Sjukhuset
104 01 Stockholm, Sweden

YEE K.C.
Microwave Institute
Chekiang Medical College
Hangchow, China

PARTICIPANTS

BARKER A.T.
Department of Medical Physics
Royal Hallamshire Hospital
Sheffield, U.K.

BERGSMA J.
I.R.I. - Interuniversitair Reactor Instituut
Mekelweg 15
2629 JB Delft, The Netherlands

BIAZZI VALMARIN L.
Istitute Radiologia e Terapia fisica
Università degli Studi
27100 Pavia, Italy

BINI M.
I.R.O.E. - C.N.R.
Via Panciatichi, 64
50127 Florence, Italy

BOSNJAKOVIC B.F.M.
Ministerie van Volksgezondheid en Millieuhygiene
Koopmansstraat 1
2288 Rijswijk, The Netherlands

BOZZETTI M.
Instituto Elettrotecnico
Fac. Ingegneria
Via Re David, 200
70125 Bari, Italy

CAPEL-BOUTE C.
Université Libre de Bruxelles
Avenue F.D.Roosevelt, 50
1050 Brussels, Belgium

CASPERS F.
Ruhr-Universitaet Bochum
Universitaetsstrasse 150, IC 6
D 4630 Bochum-Querenburg, FRG

CASTELLANI F.
Istituto di Impianti Nucleari
Via Diotisalvi, 2
56100 Pisa, Italy

CHIABRERA A.
Istituto di Elettrotecnica
Facoltà di Ingegneria
Università degli Studi
16145 Genoa, Italy

CIAMPA R.
CAMEN
56010 S.Piero a Grado, Italy

CONTE L.
Ospedale di Circolo
Viale L.Borri, 57
21100 Varese, Italy

CULLEN P.
Fac.of Science
School of Optometry
University of Waterloo
Waterloo, Ontario, Canada

D'INZEO G.
Istituto di Elettronica
Facoltà di Ingegneria
Via Eudossiana, 2
00100 Rome, Italy

DARDALHON M.
Institut Curie
Sec.de Biologie
26, Rue d'Ulm
Paris V, France

DI POFI M.
C.N.E.N.
Viale Regina Margherita, 125
00198 Rome, Italy

DRAGO G.
C.N.R. - Lab. Circuiti Elettronici
Via all'Opera Pia, 11
16145 Genoa, Italy

FREIJ J.C.
Rijks Geneeskundige Dienst
Postbus 20012
2500 EA's-Gravenhage, The Netherlands

FURIA L.
Istituto Elettrotecnico
Facoltà di Ingegneria
Via Claudio, 21
80125 Naples, Italy

GOMEZ VELA D.
Facultad de Medicina
Policlinicos
Cadiz, Spain

GRANT J.P.
Department of Physics
University of Surrey
Guildford, Surrey GU2 5XH, U.K.

HAMNERIUS Y.
Research Laboratory of Electronics
Chalmers Univ.of Technology
41296 Goteborg, Sweden

HANSSON H.A.
Inst. of Neurobiology
Univ.of Goteborg
Box 33031
400 33 Goteborg, Sweden

IGNESTI A.
I.R.O.E. - C.N.R.
Via Panciatichi, 64
50127 Florence, Italy

KREMER F.
Max Planck Institut
Heisenbergstrasse 1
P.O.800665
7000 Stuttgart 80, FRG

LAOGUN A.A.
Physics Department
University of Benin
Benin City, Nigeria

LOMAGLIO F.
Selenia S.p.A.
Via Tiburtina, km 12,4
00100 Rome, Italy

MANNO M.
Istituto di Medicina del Lavoro
Via Facciolati, 71
35100 Padua, Italy

MARIUTTI G.
Istituto Superiore di Sanità
Viale Regina Elena, 299
00161 Rome, Italy

McAVOY G.
Dpt.of Physics
University of Calgary
2500 University Drive N.W.
Calgary, Alberta, Canada

MONET-DESCOMBEY C.
Centre d'Orsay
Batiment 200
91405 Orsay Cedex, France

MONTELEONE G.
Istituto Superiore di Sanità
Viale Regina Elena, 299
00161 Rome, Italy

MORE' C.
Org.Moleculaire et Macromoleculaire
2, rue Henry Dunant
94320 Thiais, France

PAULY H.
Inst.fuer Radiologie
Univ.Erlangen-Nuernberg
Krankenhausstrasse 12
8520 Erlangen, FRG

RESCH W.
Inst.fuer Medizinische Physik
Univ.Wien
Waeringerstrasse 13
1090 Wien, Austria

RIDELLA S.
C.N.R.
Laboratorio Circuiti Elettronici
Via all'Opera Pia, 11
16145 Genoa, Italy

RIGHI E.
I.N.F.N. - National Laboratory
Via Enrico Fermi
00044 Frascati, Rome

RINALDI P.
Studio Tecnitest
Via Volturno, 1
00053 Civitavecchia, Italy

STURM J.
Ministry of Social Affairs
P.O.Box 69
Voorburg, The Netherlands

TERRANA T.
Clinica del Lavoro
Università degli Studi
Via S.Barnaba, 8
20122 Milan, Italy

TUYN J.W.N.
CERN
Rue de Merin
1211 Geneva, Switzerland

VUKCEVIC M.
Rad.Prot.Dept.
Inst.of Nuclear Sciences
P.O.Box 522
11001 Belgrade, Yugoslavia

YERUSHALMI A.
Radiation Unit Wolfson Bldg.
The Weizmann Inst.of Science
Rehovot, Israel

INDEX